Andreoli

Comprehensive Cardiac Care

Andreoli's

Comprehensive Cardiac Care

Edited by

Marguerite R. Kinney, RN, DNSc, FAAN
Professor and Associate Director of Nursing
Center for Nursing Research
School of Nursing
University of Alabama at Birmingham
Birmingham, Alabama

Donna R. Packa, RN, DSN
Professor of Nursing and
Associate Dean for Academic Affairs
University of Mississippi School of Nursing
University of Mississippi Medical Center
Jackson, Mississippi

EIGHTH EDITION
with 333 illustrations

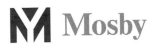 Mosby

A *Harcourt Health Sciences Company*
St. Louis   Philadelphia   London   Sydney   Toronto

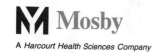

A Harcourt Health Sciences Company

Editors: Tim Griswold, Barry Bowlus
Developmental Editors: Jolynn Gower, Brian Morovitz
Project Manager: Carol Weis
Senior Production Editor: Pat Joiner
Designer: Sheilah Barrett
Manufacturing Manager: David R. Graybill

EIGHTH EDITION

Copyright © 1996 by Mosby Inc.

Previous editions copyrighted 1968, 1971, 1975, 1979, 1983, 1987, 1991

Printed in the United States of America

Mosby Inc.
11830 Westline Industrial Drive, St. Louis, Missouri 63146

ISBN 0-8016-7887-0

00 01 02 03 / 9 8 7 6 5 4

Contributors

Erin L. Abramczyk, RN, MSN, CCRN
Cardiovascular Case Manager
Capital Health System
Harrisburg, Pennsylvania

Linda Baas, PhD, RN, CCRN
Assistant Professor
College of Nursing and Health
University of Cincinnati
Cincinnati, Ohio

Lynne T. Braun, PhD, RN
Teacher-Practitioner/Associate Professor
Department of Medical Nursing
Rush University
Chicago, Illinois

Mary-Michael Brown, RN, MS, CCRN
Clinical Nurse Specialist
Intermediate Care Unit
Mercy Hospital and Healthcare
San Diego, California

William J. Combs, MSEE
Senior Staff Scientist
Medtronic, Inc.
Minneapolis, Minnesota

Barbara A. Erickson, PhD, RN, CCRN
Clinical Nurse Specialist/Case Manager
Case Western Reserve System
Youngstown, Ohio

Dorothy K. Gauthier, PhD, RN
Associate Professor of Nursing
University of Alabama School of Nursing
University of Alabama at Birmingham
Birmingham, Alabama

Doris F. Glick, RN, PhD
Assistant Professor
School of Nursing
University of Virginia
Charlottesville, Virginia

Nancy Houston Miller, RN, BSN
Associate Director
Stanford Cardiac Rehabilitation Program
Stanford University School of Medicine
Palo Alto, California

Flerida Imperial-Perez, RN, MN
Clinical Nurse Specialist
Cardiothoracic ICU
UCLA Medical Center
Los Angeles, California

Sharon Lobert, RN, PhD
Associate Professor
University of Mississippi Medical Center
Jackson, Mississippi

Marcia Pencak Murphy, MS, RN
Practitioner-Teacher
Rush Presbyterian St. Luke's Medical Center
Chicago, Illinois

Darlene A. Rourke, RN, MSN
Clinical Nurse Specialist
Cardiothoracic Surgery
UCLA Medical Center
Los Angeles, California

Ruth Stanley, PharmD
Coordinator, Clinical Pharmacy Services
Department of Pharmacy
Baptist Medical Center-Montclair
Birmingham, Alabama

Nancy Stephenson, BSN
Manager, Physician Relations
Medtronic, Inc.
Minneapolis, Minnesota

Stephen "Pete" Stribling, RN, MSN, CCRN
Cardiovascular Clinical Nurse Specialist
Service Line Manager/Cardiology
The Heart Center at Baptist
Mississippi Baptist Medical Center
Jackson, Mississippi

Elizabeth Van Beek Carlson, DNSc, RN
Teacher-Practitioner/Associate Professor
Department of Medical Nursing
Rush University
Chicago, Illinois

Connie White-Williams, RN, MSN
Senior Cardiac Transplant Coordinator
Department of Critical Care Nursing
University of Alabama at Birmingham
Birmingham, Alabama

Preface

In 1968, when Kathleen G. Andreoli, Virginia K. Hunn, Douglas P. Zipes, and Andrew G. Wallace prepared the first edition of *Comprehensive Cardiac Care,* the cardiovascular landscape was very different from today. Coronary care units, begun just a few years earlier in Pennsylvania and in Kansas, were springing up in hospitals across the United States. Between 50% and 60% of patients with acute myocardial infarction were dying before they reached a hospital, and the inhospital mortality rate was about 15%, down from the 30% seen in the pre-CCU era. This decline was attributed to the early detection and treatment of dysrhythmias. Although rehabilitation was acknowledged as an important component of care, patients were placed on complete bed rest, perhaps for weeks, and exercise prescriptions were rarely explicit. Heart failure remained a significant clinical problem, and the centerpieces of treatment were morphine sulfate, intermittent positive pressure breathing, tourniquets to retard venous return, and a few drugs such as digitalis, diuretics, and aminophylline.

Much has been learned in the past 27 years about heart disease and its treatment. Today, about 20% of people experiencing myocardial infarction die before reaching the hospital, and the mortality rate has declined steadily. We have witnessed amazing developments in patient care with new generations of drugs and sophisticated technologies, and advances continue at a rapid pace.

We are indebted to the four original editors for their vision in recognizing a need for a text that would guide clinicians in their care of patients with heart disease and for the leadership of Dr. Andreoli in subsequent editions that reflected the important advances being made in the field. This eighth edition marks the first time that Drs. Andreoli and Zipes have not actively participated in the effort. You will notice that beginning with this edition the text has been renamed *Andreoli's Comprehensive Cardiac Care* to honor Dr. Andreoli. In this way we acknowledge with much gratitude her contributions to the care of patients with cardiovascular disease and herald the placing of her name in the title of this text.

We wish to express our appreciation to the individuals who have contributed in many ways to the preparation of this edition. We thank contributors to the previous edition, on whose work we have built: Martha Branyon, RN, EdD; Mary Sue Craft Baldwin, RN, MSN; Cathie E. Guzzetta, RN, PhD; Janine M. Neely, RN, MSN; Joann M. Pillion, RN, MSN; Patricia C. Seifert, RN, MSN; and Laurel J. Sutherland, RN, MSN.

We are especially indebted to the authors of the present edition whose dedication to the task resulted in the timely receipt of outstanding manuscripts. Their willingness to share their knowledge and expertise is appreciated more than we can adequately express. The author of Chapter 15, Dr. Doris F. Glick, wishes to acknowledge the contribution and capable assistance of Karen Thompson, RN, MSN, in preparing the revision of this chapter.

Jolynn Gower and Pat Joiner at Mosby deserve our heartfelt thanks for the many ways in which they contributed to this text and made our work a pleasant experience. We also want to thank Ann Wilcox for her assistance in the preparation of this text. Finally, we again thank our readers who transfer the words on these pages into skilled and artful patient care, which is, of course, the ultimate purpose of this text.

Marguerite R. Kinney
Donna R. Packa

Contents

1 Anatomy and Physiology of the Heart, 1
Dorothy K. Gauthier

Anatomy of the Heart, 1
Blood Flow, 2
Pulmonary Circulation, 5
Coronary Circulation, 5
Excitation of the Heart, 6
Regulation of Cardiac Function, 7
  Control of cardiac output, 8

2 Cardiovascular Assessment, 10
Sharon Lobert

Interview, 10
  Establishing a nurse-patient relationship, 10
  Guiding the interview, 10
  Communication, 14
Health History, 14
  Current health problems, 14
  Previous illness, hospitalization, surgeries, and
    problems, 14
  Current medications, 14
  Risk factors, 15
  Family history, 15
  Perception or knowledge of illness and
    expectations, 15
  Spiritual concerns, 16
  Social and economic history, 16
  Health-seeking behaviors, 16
  Nutrition, 19
Physical Examination, 20
  Peripheral circulation, 22
  Cardiac assessment, 29
  Oxygenation, 37
  Abdomen, 38
  Neurologic functioning, 39
  Physical integrity, 39
  Physical regulation, 40
Formulating Nursing Diagnoses, 41

3 Patient Assessment: Diagnostic Studies, 42
Stephen "Pete" Stribling

Serum Enzyme Levels in Acute Myocardial
  Infarction, 42
Stress Testing, 43
Radionuclide Imaging, 45
  Myocardial perfusion imaging, 45
  MI imaging, 45
  Radionuclide angiocardiography, 46
Other Cardiac Imaging Techniques, 46
Ambulatory ECG, 47

Echocardiography, 48
  Techniques, 49
  Applications, 49
  Doppler echocardiography, 52
Bedside Right-Sided Heart Catheterization Using a
  Flow-Directed, Balloon-Tipped PA Catheter, 53
Cardiac Catheterization and Cardiac Angiography, 55
Cardiac Electrophysiologic Studies, 56
Endomyocardial Biopsy, 56

4 Introduction to Electrocardiography, 58
Barbara A. Erickson

Basic Considerations, 58
  Standardization, 58
  Deflections, 58
Electrophysiologic Principles, 59
Waves and Complexes, 60
  P wave, 60
  QRS complex, 61
  ST segment, 64
  T wave, 64
  QT interval, 65
  U wave, 65
ECG Leads, 66
  Standard limb leads, 66
  Augmented leads, 66
  Precordial leads, 67
Vector Approach to ECG, 68
  Sequence of electric events in the heart, 69
  Mean cardiac vector, 70
  Mean QRS axis, 71
  Clinical significance of axis, 72
  Electric heart positions and electric axis, 73
Causes of Axis Deviation, 74
  Determination of the horizontal plane projection
    of the mean QRS vector, 74
Left Ventricular Enlargement, 74
Left Atrial Enlargement, 76
Right Ventricular Enlargement, 77
Right Atrial Enlargement, 79
Myocardial Infarction, 79
  Q wave, 79
  Vector abnormalities, 79
  Localization of infarction, 81
  Evolution of a myocardial infarction, 82

5 Dysrhythmias, 86
Barbara A. Erickson

Normal Cardiac Cycle, 86
Determination of Heart Rate, 86

Electrophysiologic Principles, 89
Dysrhythmia Analysis, 91
Therapy of Dysrhythmias, 92
  General therapeutic concepts, 92
  Electrophysiologic and hemodynamic consequences, 92
  Normal sinus rhythm, 93
  Sinus tachycardia, 93
  Sinus bradycardia, 99
  Sinus dysrhythmia, 100
  Sinus arrest, 102
  Sinus exit block, 102
  Wandering pacemaker, 104
  Premature atrial complexes, 104
  AV nodal reentry, 108
  Preexcitation syndrome, 113
  Atrial flutter, 121
  Atrial fibrillation, 125
  Atrial tachycardia with and without AV block, 127
  Premature AV junctional complexes, 129
  AV junctional rhythms, 129
  Nonparoxysmal AV junctional tachycardia, 129
  Ventricular escape beats, 133
  Premature ventricular complexes, 134
  Ventricular tachycardia, 138
  Torsades de pointes, 143
  Long QT syndrome, 144
  Accelerated idioventricular rhythm, 144
  Ventricular flutter and ventricular fibrillation, 145
  Atrioventricular block, 148
  Bundle branch block, 154
  Parasystole, 160
AV Dissociation, 161
Supraventricular Dysrhythmia with Abnormal QRS
  Complexes, 162
  Identification of atrial activity, 164
  Analysis of QRS contours and intervals, 165
  Esophageal pill electrode, 165
Electrolyte Disturbances, 166
  Potassium, 166
  Sodium, 166
  Calcium, 166
Invasive Electrophysiologic Studies, 166
  Artifacts, 170
Dysrhythmia Test Section, 171

6 Artificial Cardiac Pacemakers and Implantable Cardioverter Defibrillators, 220
Nancy Stephenson
William J. Combs

Artificial Cardiac Pacemakers, 220
  Indications, 220
  Modalities, 221
  Pacemaker programmability, 229
  Power sources, 229
  Electrode systems (leads), 230
  Follow-up, 234
  Troubleshooting, 235
  Equipment, 235
  Conclusions, 240

Implantable Cardioverter Defibrillators, 240
  Indications, 241
  Modalities, 242
  Programmability, 243
  Power sources, 246
  Electrode systems (leads), 246
  Waveform and current pathways, 248
  Follow-up, 249
  Troubleshooting, 250
  Equipment, 250
Nursing Care of Patients with Permanent Cardiac
  Pacemakers and ICDs, 250
Summary, 252

7 Coronary Artery Disease, 256
Elizabeth Van Beek Carlson
Lynne T. Braun
Marcia Pencak Murphy

Incidence, Prevalence, Morbidity, and Mortality, 256
  Pathogenesis, 256
  Natural history and prognosis, 257
Risk Factors, 258
  Age, Gender, and Race, 258
  Hypertension, 258
  Hypercholesterolemia, 260
  Smoking, 262
  Physical inactivity, 264
  Glucose intolerance, 265
  Personality factors, 266
  Stress, 266
  Obesity, 267
  Caffeine and alcohol intake, 267
  Other risk factors, 267
  Summary, 268
Prevention in the Community, 268
  Home, 268
  School, 268
  Worksite, 268
  Community, 268
National Priorities, 271
Research Needs in Health Promotion, 271

8 Care of the Cardiac Patient, 276
Linda Baas

Priorities in Admission to the CCU, 277
  Immediate monitoring of cardiac rate and rhythm, 277
  Establishment of intravenous access, 277
  Relief of pain and anxiety, 277
  Supplemental oxygen, 279
  Decrease in myocardial oxygen consumption, 279
  Completion of database, 279
Equipment, 281
  Monitoring system, 281
  Electrodes, 283
  Interference with monitoring, 284
  Electric hazards, 284

Complications of Coronary Artery Disease, 286
  Angina pectoris, 286
  AMI, 287
  Heart failure, 296
  Left venticular failure, 297
  Right venticular failure, 298
  Cardiogenic shock, 300
  Care of the patient and PA equipment, 304
  Additional approaches to hemodynamic
   monitoring, 305
  Dysrhythmias, 310
  Defibrillation and cardioversion, 311
  Circulatory arrest, 315
  Sudden cardiac death, 322
Psychologic Adjustment to Coronary Heart
  Disease, 331
  Prehospital phase, 331
  Hospital phase, 331
  Posthospital phase, 332
Care Issues, 334
  Sociocultural considerations, 334
  Daily care, 335
  Transfer from CCU, 337
  Priorities during intermediate care, 338
  Preparation for discharge, 338

9 Valvular Heart Disease, 342
Erin L. Abramczyk
Mary-Michael Brown

Structure and Function of Valves, 342
Murmurs of Valvular Heart Disease, 343
Aortic Valve Disease, 343
  Aortic stenosis, 343
  Aortic regurgitation, 348
Mitral Valve Disease, 349
  Mitral stenosis, 349
  Mitral regurgitation, 351
  Mitral valve prolapse, 353
Tricuspid Valve Disease, 354
  Tricuspid stenosis, 354
  Tricuspid regurgitation, 355
Pulmonary Valve Disease, 355
  Pulmonary stenosis, 356
  Pulmonary regurgitation, 357
Summary, 358

10 Surgical Management of Heart Disease, 359
Flerida Imperial-Perez
Darlene A. Rourke

Myocardial Revascularization, 359
Preoperative Considerations, 360
Intraoperative Events, 360
  CPB, 360
  Cardioplegia, 362
  Surgical procedure, 362
Postoperative Management, 363
  Admission to the unit, 363
  Cardiovascular subsystem, 363

  Pulmonary subsystem, 368
  Renal subsystem, 370
  Neurologic subsystem, 370
  Pain, 372
Other Considerations, 372
  Infection, 372
  Nutrition, 372

11 Cardiomyopathy, 376
Connie White-Williams

Classification, 376
Dilated Cardiomyopathy, 376
  Pathophysiology, 376
  Pathology, 379
  Clinical presentation, 379
  Diagnostic tests, 379
  Medical and surgical interventions, 380
Hypertrophic Cardiomyopathy, 381
  Pathophysiology, 381
  Clinical presentation, 382
  Diagnostic tests, 382
  Medical and surgical interventions, 383
Restrictive Cardiomyopathy, 383
  Pathophysiology, 383
  Clinical presentation, 383
  Diagnostic tests, 384
  Medical and surgical interventions, 384
Conclusion, 384

12 Cardiac Transplantation, 387
Connie White-Williams

Recipient Selection, 387
  Referral and cardiac transplant evaluation, 389
  Listing for transplantation and waiting for a donor
   organ, 389
Donor Selection and Operative Procedure, 390
Postoperative Care and Long-Term Follow-Up, 391
  Immediate postoperative concerns, 391
  Immunosuppression, 392
  Complications, 395
  Long-term follow-up, 397
Conclusion, 397

**13 Cardiac Rehabilitation: Management of the Patient
After Myocardial Infarction, 402**
Nancy Houston Miller

Rehabilitation Periods, 403
  In-hospital rehabilitation, 403
  Outpatient recovery period, 406
Exercise Benefits and Training, 406
  Exercise prescription, 407
  Supervised vs. unsupervised exercise, 408
Modification of Lifestyle, 408
  Managing coronary risk factors, 408
Other Rehabilitation Issues, 411
  Sexual activity, 411
  Return to work, 411
Summary, 412

14 Cardiovascular Drugs, 415
Ruth Stanley

Clinical Pharmacokinetics, 415
Clinical Pharmacology, 416
    Subclassification of α-adrenergic receptors, 416
    Subclassification of β-adrenergic receptors, 416
Inotropes, 417
    Digitalis glycosides, 417
    Dopamine, 419
    Dobutamine, 421
    Phosphodiesterase inhibitors, 422
Sympathomimetics, 423
    Epinephrine, 423
    Norepinephrine, 424
    Isoproterenol, 425
    Phenylephrine, 426
α-Adrenergic Blockers, 426
Central α Agonists, 427
Ganglionic Agents, 429
β Blockers, 429
Vasodilators, 432
    Nitrates, 432
    Nitroprusside sodium, 433
    Direct arteriolar vasodilators, 434
    Doxazosin, prazosin, and terazosin, 435
Diuretics, 436
ACE Inhibitors, 438
Calcium Channel Blockers, 439
Thrombolytic Agents, 443
Heparin, 445
Warfarin, 447
Antiplatelet Agents, 452
Antidysrhythmics, 453
    Disopyramide, 453
    Procainamide, 455
    Quinidine, 456
    Lidocaine, 456
    Mexiletine, 457
    Tocainide, 457
    Flecainide, 458
    Propafenone, 458
    Sotalol, 459
    Amiodarone, 459
    Bretylium, 460
Antilipemic Agents, 460
    Bile acid–binding resins, 460
    Niacin, 462
    Fibric acid derivatives, 462
    Probucol, 463
    3-Hydroxy-3-methylglutaryl coenzyme A reductase
        inhibitors, 463

Miscellaneous Agents, 464
    Atropine, 464
    Edrophonium, 464
    Sodium bicarbonate, 465
    Potassium, 465
    Magnesium, 465
    Adenosine, 468

15 Home Care of Patients with Cardiac Disease, 470
Doris F. Glick

Perspective on Home Care, 470
    Development of home care, 470
    Scope of home health services, 471
    Costs and benefits of home care, 471
Continuity of Care, 472
    Case management, 472
    Discharge planning: collaboration among agencies, 473
    Home health care team: collaboration among
        disciplines, 474
    Community resources, 474
Assessment for Home Care, 475
    Family, 475
    Patient, 477
Plan of Care, 478
    Documentation of the treatment plan, 478
    Diet, 478
    Medications, 482
    Pain management, 482
    Activity and rest, 482
    Sexual activity, 484
    Psychosocial considerations, 484
Home Care for Patients with Technically Complex
    Needs, 485
    Pacemakers, 485
    Home ECG, 486
    Supplemental oxygen, 486
    Intravenous therapy, 487
    Implantable cardioverter defibrillators, 489
    Ventricular assist devices, 490
Dying at Home, 491
Research Needs, 491

Andreoli's

Comprehensive Cardiac Care

CHAPTER 1

Anatomy and Physiology of the Heart

Dorothy K. Gauthier

This chapter contains a review of the anatomy and physiology of the heart and related aspects of the systemic and pulmonary circulations. It is intended to be a brief overview of the various topics and to serve as a starting point for further study.

ANATOMY OF THE HEART

Cardiac muscle cells are characterized by their branched appearance and the presence of *intercalated discs* (areas where adjacent cells meet end-to-end, with partial fusion of their cell membranes). These structures form low-resistance bridges that allow electrical impulses to pass from cell to cell. The anatomic arrangement of cells gives cardiac tissue a syncytial appearance (Fig. 1-1, *A*); that is, it resembles a network of cells with no separation between the individual cells. The heart contains an atrial syncytium (the muscle of the two upper chambers) and a ventricular syncytium (the muscle of the two lower chambers) that are separated by fibrous tissue.

Each cardiac muscle cell or fiber contains *myofibrils* (the contractile elements) and mitochondria (the energy-producing units) (Fig. 1-1, *B*). Viewed with a microscope, myofibrils exhibit alternating light and dark bands because of the orderly arrangement and overlap of two protein filaments, the thin *actin* and the thick *myosin*. When the muscle is excited, projections on the myosin filaments interact with adjacent actin filaments to form cross-bridges. These cross-bridges use energy released from adenosine triphosphate (ATP) to bend, sliding the actin filaments over the myosin and causing the myofibrils and the entire muscle fiber to shorten.

The muscle fiber also contains two systems of tubules and two regulatory proteins. *T tubules,* or *transverse tubules,* which are extensions of the cell membrane, conduct the impulse to the interior of the cell. *L tubules,* or *longitudinal tubules,* also referred to as the *sarcoplasmic reticulum,* store calcium (see Fig. 1-1, *B*). The regulatory proteins troponin and tropomyosin normally form a complex with the actin filament to prevent it from forming cross-bridges with myosin. In this state, the muscle is relaxed.

Excitation of the muscle fiber is initiated by passage of an electric impulse over the cell membrane (sarcolemma) and T tubule membranes to the interior of the cell. Passage of the impulse over these membranes permits calcium ions to enter the sarcoplasm from outside the cell through the sarcolemma and T tubule membrane and from the nearby sarcoplasmic reticulum. Calcium ions bind to troponin, causing an alteration in the position of tropomyosin. This permits the interaction of actin and myosin, and the muscle fiber shortens.[1] Because each muscle fiber membrane is connected to its immediate neighbors by the low-resistance intercalated discs, the excitatory impulse can spread to all cells in the atrial or ventricular syncytium.

When the electrical stimulation is ended, calcium ions are transported back into the sarcoplasmic reticulum and the extracellular fluid, lowering the calcium concentration in the sarcoplasm. At the lower calcium level, the regulatory proteins can again interfere with the interaction of actin and myosin; therefore these filaments return to their original position, and the muscle relaxes.

Located between the atria and ventricles is the fibrous skeleton of the heart, which consists of four fibrous rings, or annuli (arranged as shown in Fig. 1-2), and the tissue that connects them. Each annulus is the supporting structure for one of the four valves of the heart and the connecting site for muscular networks that form the heart's four chambers. This fibrous skeleton is nonconductive and insulates the atrial syncytium from the ventricular syncytium. Specialized conduction pathways responsible for initiating an impulse and conducting it through the fibrous skeleton from the atria to the ventricles and within the walls of the chambers are discussed later in the chapter.

The wall of the heart can be divided into three layers. The inner *endocardium* is composed of endothelial cells supported by fibrous tissue. The endothelial layer is continuous with the endothelial lining of the blood vessels. The middle *myocardium* is primarily cardiac muscle. The

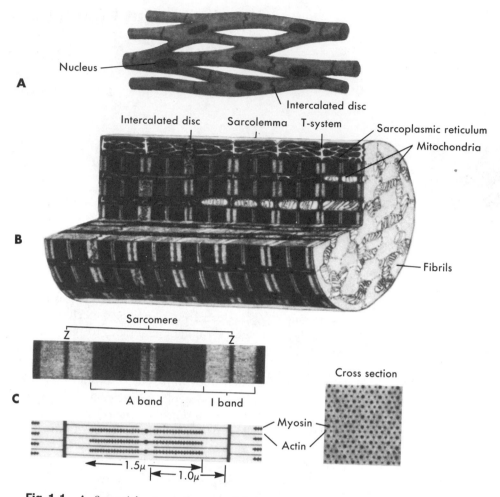

Fig. 1-1 **A,** Syncytial nature of myocardial tissue, with intercalated discs between cells. **B,** Cardiac muscle fiber. *Fibrils,* myofibrils. **C,** Arrangement of the protein filaments actin and myosin to produce dark (A) and light (I) bands. The protein filaments of the myofibril form subunits (sarcomeres) bounded on either end by a dark Z line. The arrangement of filaments is shown in microscopic, schematic, and cross-sectional views.   (From Sonnenblick EH: *Myocardial ultrastructure in the normal and failing heart.* In Braunwald E, editor: *The myocardium: failure and infarction.* New York, 1974, HP Publishing. Illustration by Seward Hung.)

outer *epicardium* contains fibrous connective tissue and mesothelial cells. The heart is surrounded by the *pericardium,* a double layer of fibrous tissue and mesothelial cells. The inner layer of the pericardium forms the epicardium. Accumulation of blood or other fluid in the space between the two layers of the pericardium can lead to compression of the heart (cardiac tamponade) and compromise the heart's ability to fill with blood.

BLOOD FLOW

The heart is a double pump that is divided anatomically into right and left sides. It receives blood from the venous (return) system and propels it into the arterial (delivery) system (Fig. 1-3). The right atrium receives deoxygenated venous blood from the superior vena cava, which drains the upper half of the body; the inferior vena cava, which drains the lower half of the body; and the coronary sinus (not shown), which contains blood that has nourished the heart itself. Blood flows from the right atrium through the *tricuspid valve* into the right ventricle. During contraction, the ventricle ejects blood through the *pulmonary valve* into the pulmonary artery (pulmonary trunk), which branches and conducts the blood to the lungs for oxygenation. Oxygenated blood returning from the lungs enters the left atrium through four pulmonary veins (only two are shown in Fig. 1-3). It passes from the left atrium through the *mitral valve* to the left ventricle. Contraction of the left ventricle causes ejection of blood through the *aortic valve* into the aorta, which distributes the blood to the peripheral circulation.

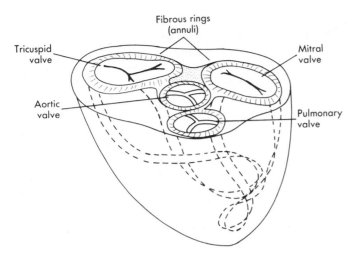

Fig. 1-2 Fibrous skeleton of the heart, including the fibrous rings that support the four heart valves.

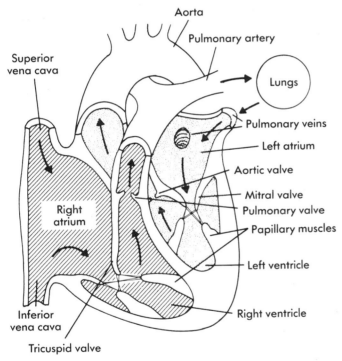

Fig. 1-3 Internal anatomy of the heart.   (Modified from Guyton AC: *Textbook of medical physiology,* ed 8, Philadelphia, 1991, Saunders.)

The leaflets of the tricuspid and mitral valves (the atrioventricular [AV] valves) are attached by fibrous bands, the chordae tendineae, to the papillary muscles, which are anchored in the ventricular walls (see Fig. 1-3). Contraction of the papillary muscles during ventricular contraction ensures tight closure of the valves and prevents their leaflets from everting into their respective atria because of the increased pressure of blood in the ventricles.

The pumping action of the heart can be divided into a period of ventricular relaxation and expansion *(diastole)* and a period of ventricular contraction *(systole).* During diastole, the mitral and tricuspid valves are open, and the aortic and pulmonary valves are closed. Blood flows freely into the atria and ventricles, filling the ventricles to about 75% of their ultimate *end-diastolic volume* (EDV).[2] Toward the end of diastole, the atria contract and propel the remaining blood into the ventricles. At the beginning of systole, ventricular contraction occurs, increasing the pressure within the ventricles and closing the AV valves. With both sets of valves closed, the pressure in each ventricle increases rapidly until it forces the pulmonary and aortic valves open and ejects blood into the pulmonary artery and aorta.

With each ventricular contraction, 70 to 80 ml of blood are ejected. This *stroke volume* represents 60% to 75% of the total volume of blood in the ventricle at the end of diastole, producing an *ejection fraction* of 0.60 to 0.75.[1] *Cardiac output* (the total volume of blood pumped per minute from either ventricle) is the product of stroke volume and heart rate and is approximately 5.6 L/min for a normal adult in the supine position.[3] *Cardiac index* is calculated by dividing the cardiac output by the square meters of body surface area. Use of this value takes into consideration the fact that stroke volume and cardiac output depend in part on the size of the person. The normal cardiac index ranges from 2.8 to 4.2 L/min/m².[1]

The major physiologic roles of the circulatory system are the delivery of oxygen and other essential nutrients to tissues of the body and the removal of carbon dioxide and other products of cellular metabolism. Many of the substances carried to and from the tissues are dissolved in plasma, and their transport depends on the volume of flow. However, almost all of the oxygen is transported by hemoglobin in red blood cells, making red blood cell and hemoglobin concentrations, as well as blood flow, important for the transport of this nutrient. Carbon dioxide is carried on hemoglobin and in the plasma.

As blood from the right side of the heart passes through the pulmonary capillaries, oxygen from air in the pulmonary alveoli enters the blood and attaches to the hemoglobin in red blood cells. Carbon dioxide diffuses from blood into the alveolar air. As blood from the left side of the heart passes through systemic capillaries, red blood cells surrender a portion of their oxygen (the exact amount depending on the needs of the tissue at the time), and the blood picks up carbon dioxide to be transported away. The rate of metabolism in a specific tissue affects not only the ability of blood passing through this tissue to exchange gases but also the diameter of blood vessels in the tissue, thereby regulating blood flow. The local rate of metabolism is probably the most important determinant in the distribution of cardiac output. During exercise, for example, blood flow increases in areas involved in the activity (such as specific skeletal muscle groups and the heart) and decreases in areas of little metabolic activity (such as the kidneys, stomach, and intestines). Blood flow to the brain remains the same at rest or during exercise.

SYSTEMIC CIRCULATION

The systemic circulation is composed of the arteries, arterioles, capillaries, venules, and veins. Blood flows through the system because of the downward pressure gradient along these conduits from the aorta to the superior and inferior venae cavae, which lead into the right atrium (Fig. 1-4). When blood is pumped from the left ventricle into the aorta, a relatively high pressure is created, and the aorta becomes distended. During ventricular diastole, the elastic aorta recoils, providing additional pressure to pump blood into the systemic circulation. Blood pressure in the aorta gradually falls as blood flows into peripheral vessels. Pressure in the aorta and large arteries normally fluctuates between 120 mm Hg (the *systolic pressure*) and 80 mm Hg (the *diastolic pressure*). The difference between systolic and diastolic pressures, the *pulse pressure*, can be noted in arteries and arterioles. The *mean arterial pressure* is the arterial pressure averaged during one cardiac cycle (systole and diastole); it can be accurately estimated as the diastolic pressure plus a third of the pulse pressure.

The major arteries branch to form smaller ones, which eventually give rise to arterioles. Arterioles have muscular walls that can dilate or constrict, controlling blood flow into capillary beds. The relatively high vascular resistance of arterioles causes a drop in blood pressure to less than 35 mm Hg as the blood enters the capillaries (see Fig. 1-4). Vasodilatation or vasoconstriction in systemic arterioles is controlled in part by *local conditions*. Arterioles respond to a decrease in oxygen or an increase in carbon dioxide or certain other waste products in the fluid around them by dilating to increase blood flow. Because of this local control of blood vessel size, a tissue that needs extra oxygen can receive increased blood flow. Arterioles in some tissues also respond to changes in pressure. A local increase in blood pressure causes the arterioles to constrict to protect the smaller vessels in the tissue from increased pressure. If pressure in arterioles suddenly decreases, the arterioles dilate to ensure that the tissue receives sufficient blood flow for nutrition. This local regulatory mechanism (sometimes called *autoregulation*) is believed to be important in maintaining a relatively constant blood flow in the cerebral circulation despite fluctuations in mean arterial pressure.

Once blood is in the capillary bed, its velocity of flow is at its slowest. This allows sufficient time for the exchange

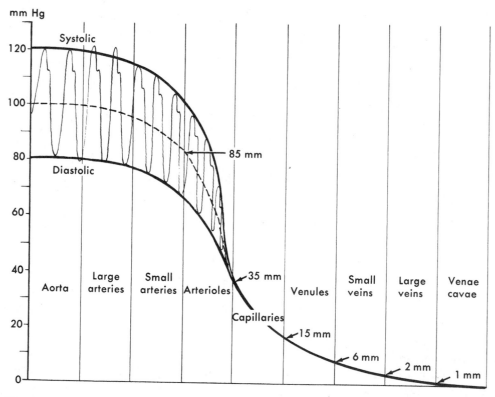

Fig. 1-4 Blood pressures in the vessels of the systemic circulation. The dotted line is an approximation of the mean pressure in arteries and arterioles. A more precise value for the mean pressure would be as follows: Diastolic pressure + ⅓ (Systolic pressure − Diastolic pressure). (From Thibodeau GA: *Structure and function of the body*, ed 9, St Louis, 1992, Mosby.)

of nutrients and wastes between the blood and the fluid that bathes the cells (interstitial fluid). Capillary walls are very thin and have a large total surface area, permitting rapid exchange. Capillaries are unique because they can produce intermittent blood flow. At any given time, some of the capillaries in a tissue are open and others are closed by constriction of a band of muscle at the capillary's proximal end (the precapillary sphincter) or by constriction of the vessel from which the capillary arises.[2] The length of time that a capillary is open or closed depends on the nutrient needs of the tissue.

Blood flows from the capillaries into venules, which converge to form veins. At this level of the systemic circuit, pressure is low (see Fig. 1-4). Venous walls are thin and compliant, yet muscular and contractile, which allows the veins to easily accommodate a greater or lesser volume of blood. Thus veins can adjust the total volume of blood in the circulatory system to the amount of blood available to fill it and thus contribute to the regulation of blood pressure.

Constriction of blood vessels is subject to *central* (or *systemic*) *control* as well as control by the local conditions previously described. One systemic factor affecting the diameters of blood vessels (especially arterioles and veins) is the *sympathetic nervous system*. Increased sympathetic stimulation usually causes constriction, whereas decreased sympathetic stimulation results in vasodilatation. In addition to this nervous regulation of the circulation, blood vessels respond to *vasoactive chemicals* that may be present in the blood. Vasoconstrictor chemicals include norepinephrine, epinephrine, antidiuretic hormone (vasopressin), angiotensin II, and certain prostaglandins. Vasodilators include histamine, bradykinin, and certain prostaglandins.[2]

PULMONARY CIRCULATION

Like the systemic circulation, the pulmonary circulation is a continuous circuit. Blood is pumped by the right ventricle into pulmonary arteries, which branch into arterioles and capillaries, where oxygen and carbon dioxide are exchanged. The pulmonary capillaries converge into venules and veins, which return oxygenated blood to the left atrium.

Gas exchange between the blood in pulmonary capillaries and the alveolar air takes place through the *pulmonary membrane,* or respiratory membrane. The pulmonary membrane consists of a thin layer of fluid that lines the alveolar wall, the alveolar wall itself, a thin layer of interstitial fluid, and the wall of the pulmonary capillary. Despite its complex nature, this membrane is only 0.6 micrometers thick. It has a total area (for both lungs) of approximately 50 to 100 m² to further facilitate gas exchange.[2] When the body is at rest, blood flows through a pulmonary capillary in about 1 second, but with increased activity and increased cardiac output, this time can be shortened to less than ½ second. However, the exchange of oxygen and carbon dioxide occurs so fast that even this shortened time is adequate to permit the normal exchange of blood gases.

An important feature of the pulmonary circulation is the ability of certain pulmonary vessels to adjust their diameters in response to local conditions. This allows the vessels to regulate the distribution of blood flow in the lungs. Local control of blood vessels in the pulmonary circulation is converse to that in the systemic circulation. Because gas exchange between blood and air is the major reason for blood flow in the pulmonary circulation, vessels in areas of the lung that do not have an adequate oxygen supply (because of bronchiolar obstruction, for example) constrict to shunt the blood to a more well-ventilated part of the lung.

Pulmonary blood vessels, which have thin walls and are easily stretched, offer little resistance to blood flow, so blood can flow through the lungs with a smaller pressure gradient than is needed in the systemic circulation. Mean pressure in the pulmonary artery is approximately 15 mm Hg,[4] compared with that of approximately 100 mm Hg in the aorta. Because the pulmonary and systemic circulations occur in series, the volume of blood flowing through the lungs per unit of time equals that flowing through the systemic circulation in the same amount of time. The lungs must be prepared to accept as much as a fivefold increase in blood flow during strenuous exercise without causing undue strain to the right ventricle and without developing a significant increase in blood pressure in the pulmonary vessels, which might cause pulmonary edema. The ability of the pulmonary vessels to stretch to accommodate extra blood flow prevents an excessive increase in pressure in this situation.

CORONARY CIRCULATION

The function of the coronary artery system is maintenance of an adequate blood supply to the myocardium. The two major coronary arteries, the left and right, arise from the aorta immediately above the cusps of the aortic valve. Shortly after its origin, the *left coronary artery* (sometimes called *left main coronary artery*) divides into two branches (Fig. 1-5), the *anterior descending branch* and the *circumflex branch*. The anterior descending branch passes down the groove between the two ventricles on the anterior surface of the heart. From it arise diagonal branches, which supply the left ventricular wall, and septal perforating branches, which supply the anterior portion of the interventricular septum and the anterior papillary muscle of the left ventricle. The anterior descending branch usually supplies the entire apical portion of the interventricular septum before turning upward at the apex (lower tip) of the heart. The circumflex branch of the left coronary artery passes under the left atrial appendage (one of the earlike flaps found on each atrium). It then passes posteriorly in the groove between the left atrium and left ventricle. It gives off several small and one or two large marginal branches that supply the lateral aspects of the left ventricle.

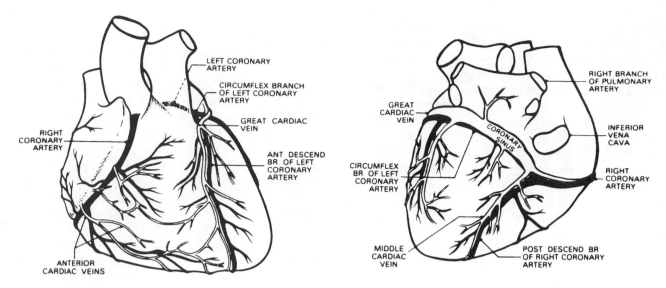

Fig. 1-5 Coronary arteries supplying the anterior aspect of the heart *(left)* and the inferior aspect of the heart *(right)*. Major veins that drain the respective aspects of the heart are also shown. (From Smith JJ, Kampine JP: *Circulatory physiology: the essentials,* ed 3, Baltimore, 1988, Williams & Wilkins.)

The *right coronary artery* passes in the right AV groove, giving off several branches to the right ventricle and a large posterior descending branch, which descends in the posterior interventricular groove and supplies the inferior aspect of the septum and the posterior left ventricular papillary muscle. The right coronary artery gives off important branches that supply the sinoatrial (SA or sinus) node in 55% of human hearts and the AV node in 90%. In the remainder of human hearts, the SA and AV nodes are nourished by branches of the circumflex artery.[5]

Coronary blood flow at rest averages about 250 ml/min, which represents 4% to 5% of the total cardiac output.[4] Blood flow is controlled primarily by the local rate of metabolism, responding especially to myocardial oxygen demand. With normal activity, 65% to 70% of the arterial oxygen content is extracted by the myocardium, the highest rate of extraction of any tissue during normal activity and one that cannot be significantly improved. Thus the heart can improve its oxygen uptake only by increasing coronary blood flow. With strenuous activity, coronary blood flow can increase threefold to fivefold to ensure an adequate oxygen supply to the myocardium.[3]

Impairment of coronary circulation by atherosclerosis constitutes the most frequent cause of heart disease. The atherosclerotic process causes a decrease in the luminal diameters of the coronary vessels, which decreases blood flow to the myocardium. Symptoms of coronary artery disease are not usually manifested, however, until blood flow to an area of the heart is compromised by at least 60%.[6]

EXCITATION OF THE HEART

The normal cardiac impulse arises in specialized pacemaker cells of the *SA node,* which is located about 1 mm beneath the right atrial epicardium at its junction with the superior vena cava (Fig. 1-6). A spontaneous change in membrane potential in these cells (Fig. 1-7) initiates a wave of excitation (an impulse) that passes over the atrial myocardium. Spread of the impulse is facilitated by *internodal pathways,* which conduct the impulse faster than ordinary atrial muscle can (see Fig. 1-6). Bachmann's bundle (a branch of the anterior internodal tract) conducts the impulse to the left atrium, and the anterior, middle, and posterior internodal tracts conduct the impulse toward the *AV node.* As the impulse spreads over the atrial syncytium, the atria depolarize, producing the P wave on the electrocardiogram (ECG) (see Fig. 1-7). Depolarization results in atrial contraction, which propels extra blood into the ventricles.

Conduction slows markedly when the impulse reaches the AV node (see Fig. 1-6), which is specialized for slow conduction. This accounts for the long PR interval on the ECG and allows sufficient time for blood to flow from the atria into the ventricles before ventricular contraction. After the impulse emerges from the AV node, it enters the rapidly conducting tissue of the *AV bundle* (bundle of His) and the right and left bundle branches. The bundle branches supply the endocardium of their respective ventricles with a profusely branching terminal network of *Purkinje fibers.* The rapid spread of the impulse throughout these structures allows almost simultaneous depolarization

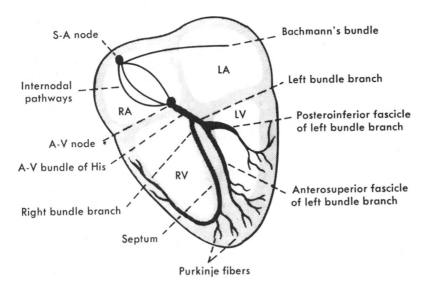

Fig. 1-6 Transmission of the cardiac impulse from the SA node over the atrial myocardium, Bachmann's bundle, internodal pathways; through the AV node and bundle of His; and down the left and right bundle branches to the Purkinje fibers, which distribute the impulse to all parts of the ventricle.

of the entire muscle mass of both ventricles, which is necessary for efficient contraction and pumping action. Ventricular depolarization produces the QRS complex on the ECG (see Fig. 1-7) and the mechanical contraction of the ventricles that propels blood forward into the pulmonary artery and aorta. The return to a resting electric state (repolarization) of the ventricles is recorded on the ECG as the T wave and results in ventricular relaxation. Repolarization of the atria cannot be noted on the ECG because it is masked by depolarization of the ventricles, which occurs at the same time and involves greater tissue mass.

REGULATION OF CARDIAC FUNCTION

Cardiac function is regulated by an intrinsic mechanism (the response of the heart to the amount of blood to be pumped) and by nervous reflexes involving the autonomic nervous system. *Intrinsic regulation* of the heart is based on the principle that if cardiac muscle is stretched *before* it contracts, it contracts with greater force. The consequences of this property on cardiac muscle performance are set forth by Starling's law, which states that, within limits, the greater the EDV, the greater the force of contraction and the resulting stroke volume. For example, if extra blood returns to the heart every minute from the systemic and pulmonary circulations (increased venous return), as happens during exercise, the ventricles are stretched and contract with greater force, pumping out the extra volume of blood. Thus a healthy heart is able to adjust its force of contraction to handle changes in the amount of blood it receives from the systemic and pulmonary circulations.

The other major regulator of cardiac function is the *autonomic nervous system*, which alters the rate of impulse generation by the SA node, the speed of impulse conduction, and the strength of cardiac contraction. It regulates the heart through sympathetic and parasympathetic nerve fibers (Fig. 1-8). The sympathetic fibers supply all areas of the atria and ventricles. Parasympathetic fibers conducted to the heart via the vagus nerves innervate primarily the SA and AV nodes, and the atrial muscle mass. At their synapses with cardiac tissue, sympathetic neurons secrete the neurotransmitter norepinephrine, whereas parasympathetic neurons secrete acetylcholine. These neurotransmitters bind to specific receptors on cardiac cells and exert their effects on the heart.

Sympathetic effects on the heart include increased heart rate, increased conduction speed through the AV node (which shortens the PR interval), and increased force of contraction. Vagal (parasympathetic) stimulation produces decreased heart rate, decreased conduction rate through the AV node (with a longer PR interval), and decreased force of atrial contraction. There is some evidence that parasympathetic fibers invest the ventricles and that they decrease the vigor of ventricular contraction.[3] When sympathetic neurons to the heart are activated, their effect is reinforced by the hormones epinephrine and norepinephrine, which are secreted by the adrenal medulla and reach the heart via the bloodstream.

Sympathetic and parasympathetic control of the heart occurs by reflexes coordinated at the medulla of the brain. Groups of neurons in the medulla that affect heart activity

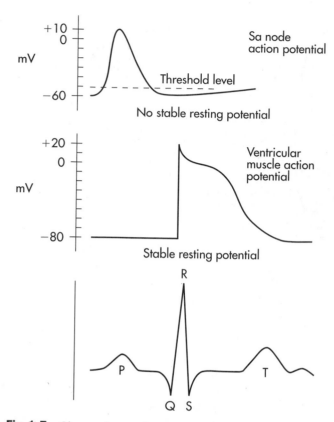

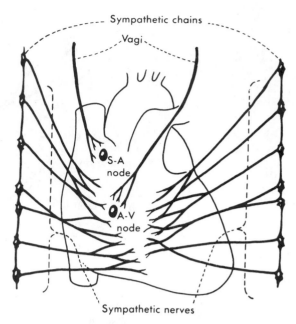

Fig. 1-8 Connections of parasympathetic nerves (vagi) and sympathetic nerves with the heart. (From Guyton AC: *Textbook of medical physiology,* ed 8, Philadelphia, 1991, Saunders.)

Fig. 1-7 Changes in membrane potential of SA node cells and ventricular muscle cells when they become excited. The pattern of changes is called an *action potential.* During the depolarization phase of the action potential, the membrane potential becomes more positive. During the repolarization phase, the membrane potential returns to its resting state. The gradual change in membrane potential during the resting state in SA node cells causes them to depolarize spontaneously, whereas atrial and ventricular muscle cells will not depolarize unless they are stimulated by an impulse transmitted from adjacent cells. A typical electrocardiographic (ECG) tracing is shown at the bottom of the figure, using the same time scale on the horizontal axis as was used for the action potentials.

can be referred to as a *cardioacceleratory area* and a *cardioinhibitory area,* and the group that affects blood vessels is referred to as a *vasomotor area.* These three areas are referred to collectively as the *cardiovascular center.* The cardiovascular center can be stimulated by impulses from various nervous receptors. These include pressoreceptors (baroreceptors) located in the walls of the arch of the aorta and the carotid sinuses in the internal carotid arteries. These pressoreceptors alter their rate of impulse generation in response to changes in blood pressure. They transmit impulses to the cardiovascular center via the vagus and glossopharyngeal nerves. A sudden elevation of blood pressure within the aorta or the carotid artery increases impulse transmission to the cardioinhibitory area, producing changes in sympathetic and parasympathetic output to decrease the heart rate and

force of contraction. Sympathetic stimulation to blood vessels also is altered, lowering vascular resistance and blood pressure. The opposite reactions occur if the pressoreceptors detect a decrease in blood pressure.

The cardiovascular center also responds to changes in the chemical composition of the blood (a decrease in oxygen or an increase in carbon dioxide or hydrogen concentrations) and to changes in blood volume. These changes are detected by specific nervous system receptors in various areas of the body. The cardiovascular center then adjusts sympathetic and parasympathetic output to regulate the heart and blood vessels as needed to bring more oxygen to the tissues and to carry away accumulating waste products.

In addition to the nervous reflexes mentioned, heart activity is affected by higher centers in the brain that can stimulate sympathetic or parasympathetic neurons. This is evident when a change in heart activity and blood vessel tone occurs in response to fear, pain, or intense emotion. In these cases, cardiac and vascular changes are probably initiated by the cerebral cortex and hypothalamus.[2]

Control of Cardiac Output

The adequacy of cardiac function is reflected by cardiac output, which is the total volume of blood pumped per minute and which can be calculated using the following equation:

$$\text{Cardiac output} = \text{Heart rate} \times \text{Stroke volume}$$

Factors that influence cardiac output are those that influence its two components. *Heart rate* is determined by the autonomic nervous system. Stroke volume has three major determinants: preload, afterload, and contractility of the heart.

Preload can be thought of as the amount of stress (tension) on the ventricular muscle fibers just *before* they contract. This is related to the EDV.[2] As previously discussed in relation to intrinsic regulation of the heart, an increase in EDV (preload) increases stroke volume and cardiac output. A decrease in EDV has the opposite effect.

Afterload is the force that the ventricles must overcome *during* contraction (that is, while they are ejecting blood). The major component of afterload is blood pressure in the aorta. Two additional contributors to afterload are the resistance offered by the size of the aortic valve opening (which is an important consideration for persons with aortic stenosis) and the resistance in peripheral vessels. Anything that increases afterload increases the work of the heart and decreases stroke volume and cardiac output.

Myocardial *contractility* (inotropy) can be thought of as a change in cardiac performance that cannot be attributed to a change in muscle fiber length (preload), afterload, or heart rate.[7] This property of cardiac muscle is increased by sympathetic stimulation or inotropic drugs and is decreased by a decrease in the "health" of cardiac muscle cells (for example, as in heart failure). An increase in contractility produces increased stroke volume and cardiac output, whereas a decrease in contractility has the opposite effect.

By making adjustments in the heart rate, preload, afterload, and contractility, the nervous and endocrine systems regulate cardiac output to ensure the adequate nutrition of tissues. Medical interventions used to change or stabilize cardiac output are also directed at altering these same parameters.

REFERENCES

1. Schlant RC, Sonnenblick EH: *Normal physiology of the cardiovascular system.* In Hurst JW and others: *The heart, arteries and veins,* ed 7, New York, 1990, McGraw-Hill.
2. Guyton AC: *Textbook of medical physiology,* ed 8, Philadelphia, 1991, Saunders.
3. Little RC, Little WC: *Physiology of the heart and circulation,* ed 4, St. Louis, 1989, Mosby.
4. Smith JJ, Kampine JP: *Circulatory physiology: the essentials,* ed 3, Baltimore, 1990, Williams & Wilkins.
5. Conover MB: *Understanding electrocardiography: arrhythmias and the 12-lead ECG,* ed 6, St. Louis, 1992, Mosby.
6. Bullock BL, Rosendahl PP: *Pathophysiology: adaptations and alterations in function,* ed 3, Philadelphia, 1992, Lippincott.
7. Cohn PF: *Clinical cardiovascular physiology,* Philadelphia, 1985, Saunders.

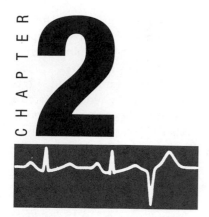

Cardiovascular Assessment

Sharon Lobert

People who have cardiovascular disease enter the health care system at varying stages of disease progression. Thus for identification of patient problems and determination of objectives of care, a thorough patient assessment is needed. This chapter describes the first step in the nursing process—the assessment phase—emphasizing assessment from a holistic and nursing point of view. The discussion includes a review of principles of communication, including interview techniques, and summarizes the important parts of the database (history and physical examination) for cardiovascular patients.

INTERVIEW

Interviewing and communicating skills are essential for performing a thorough assessment. Interviewing is a goal-directed method of communication. Its purpose is to elicit pertinent information about the patient so that problems or health-related issues can be identified. The accuracy and completeness of the data gathered during assessment depends on the nurse's ability to communicate effectively and elicit pertinent information. By showing concern and sensitivity to patients, the nurse can help establish meaningful nurse-patient relationships.

Thus the key to achieving a comprehensive and holistic assessment is to be wholly involved with patients during interviews. This means that the nurse needs to be relaxed and focused.[1] Astute and sensitive nurses function at their highest level when open to subtle cues, environmental exchanges, and intuitive feelings that can have an impact on the data collected and the conclusions formulated during patient assessment.

The timing of the interview may vary. Data should be collected within a time period that reflects the gravity of the patient's condition. If patients are critically ill or easily fatigued, priority sections can be completed first, and other sections can be completed later (usually within 24 hours) (Fig. 2-1).

Establishing a Nurse-Patient Relationship

To facilitate data collection, the nurse should remember the following guidelines for establishing an effective nurse-patient relationship:

1. Provide as much privacy as possible for the assessment.
2. Introduce yourself.
3. Call patients by their preferred names.
4. Tell patients the purpose of the assessment.
5. Sit at eye level, establish eye contact, and lean toward patients.
6. Probe and listen for concerns and beliefs about patients' conditions and health problems.
7. Show caring and concern for patients as human beings.
8. Be nonjudgmental in your responses.
9. Use language that is appropriate for the patients' educational, cultural, and psychosocial backgrounds.
10. Observe nonverbal behavior such as facial grimacing or wringing of hands.

In addition to establishing a good nurse-patient relationship, the nurse should be familiar with alternatives in guiding an interview and responding to patients. Nurses often use only one or two alternatives.

Guiding the interview

The use of the following techniques can help structure the interview and facilitate a more complete and accurate data collection.

1. Use open-ended questions and statements: "Tell me about your chest pain."
2. Clarify words, phrases, or statements: "What do you mean by 'a little bit'?"
3. Summarize data during and after the interview to ensure accuracy.
4. Reflect words, phrases, statements, and feelings: "You've been having trouble sleeping?"

MISSISSIPPI BAPTIST MEDICAL CENTER

NURSING ADMISSION
HISTORY & ASSESSMENT

---

*Vital Signs:

T _____ P _____ R _____ B/P _____

Weight _____ Height _____
(circle)   recent gain or loss

I. ADMISSION DATA

  A. **TO BE COMPLETED AT TIME OF ADMISSION** (may be done by NA)

    *Date _____ **Time** _____

    How Admitted (circle)

    Ambulatory   Stretcher   Wheelchair   Arms

  B. **TO BE COMPLETED AT TIME OF ADMISSION BY EXTERN, LPN, OR RN:**

    *Reason for admission (include summary of pt.'s statement regarding present problem-symptoms, duration treatment):

    _____

    _____

    *Date last admitted to MBMC _____ Reason for last admission _____

    Other Health Problems:

      Past Medical: High B/P   Diabetes   Respiratory   Cardiac   Heart Murmur   Rheumatic Fever

        Seizures   Thyroid   Glaucoma   Ulcer   GI   GU   Arthritis   Other _____

    Previous Surgery or Injury _____

*Special Requests:

(No Smoking, Visitors, Phone Calls, Etc.) _____

*Prosthesis: (circle if app.)

Glasses   Contact Lens   Hearing Aid   Dentures: upper or lower

Partial Plate: upper or lower   Denture cup given to patient: YES or NO

W/C or other personal item (identify) _____

SECTION A — Completed By: _____

*ALLERGIES None Known ☐	**REACTION**					***PRESENT MEDS**			
(food, medication, environment)	Rash	Hives	Dyspnea	N/V	Other	Drug Name	Dose	Freq.	Time of Last Dose
1.									
2.									
3.									
4.									
5.									

Did patient bring meds with them?   Yes _____ No _____
If yes, disposition of meds:
  Sent home with family   Treated as valuable

Diet _____ **Appetite** (circle)   GOOD   FAIR
    Number of meals/day _____
Sleep/Rest: Pattern _____ Problems _____

Social Habits: (circle)
Smokes (how much?) _____ Alcohol (how much?) _____
*Valuables: Watch _____ Billfold _____ Rings _____
Disposition (check approp.): _____ with pt.
Receipt # _____ Approp. slip to pt./family _____

Discharge Plans: See Discharge Planning Assessment Form

*Information supplied by _____

Signature and Title of Person Admission

_____

*Identification Band on: Yes _____ No _____
*Allergy Armband on: Yes _____ No _____

CCTV Instructions   Yes _____ No _____
*Presence of (circle any applicable):
 Tubes—indicate patency and character of drainage in Nurses Notes
 Catheter(s) _____ NG _____ Other _____
*Supportive Measures (circle if app.)
 Oxygen _____ Cast: (where) _____
 IV: location _____ IV: solution _____
 Amount in IV: _____
      Money _____ Other _____ None _____
 sent home with _____ to Business Office _____
      Put on Chart _____

SECTION B — Completed By: _____

ORIENTATION TO UNIT:
Introduction (if app.):   _____ Primary Nurse
                 _____ Assoc. Nurse
Environment: _____ Bed Control & Rails   _____ Meal Routine
             _____ Phone   _____ Thermostat
             _____ Hospital Booklet   _____ Nurse Call
             _____ Bedside Unit   _____ Unit Routine
             _____ Overbed Table
             (Will Roll — Do Not Use for Support)

Physician notified of admission: _____ **signature** _____ **Date/Time**

*If patient has been admitted within the last 30 days for the same reason as this admission, complete these items. Up-date any other items that have been changed.

Fig. 2-1   Example of a health history data collection form, first page.   (Courtesy Mississippi Baptist Medical Center, Jackson, Miss.)   *Continued.*

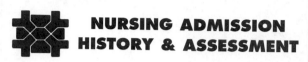

MISSISSIPPI BAPTIST MEDICAL CENTER

NURSING ADMISSION HISTORY & ASSESSMENT

I. NURSING OBJECTIVE ASSESSMENT: (To be completed within 8 hours by RN)

General Appearance _____

Language Barrier   YES   NO   Describe _____

REVIEW OF SYSTEMS: (circle those appropriate to patient)
HEENT: (WNL or impaired)

Sight _____	Speech _____	Hoarseness _____
Hearing _____	Sinus _____	Freq. Sore Throat _____

Comments: _____

MOUTH:
Mucous Membranes

Moist _____	Teeth Missing _____
Pink _____	Tongue Color: _____
Teeth Loose _____	Gums: Swollen _____
	Bleeding _____

Comments: _____

RESPIRATORY SYSTEM:

Regular Rate _____	SOB _____
Unlabored _____	Rales _____
Cough _____	Congested _____
Quiet _____	Breath Sounds:
Hemoptysis _____	Left _____
	Right _____

Comments: _____ Char. of Sputum _____

CARDIOVASCULAR:

Apical Pulse: Regular _____	Irregular _____	
Quality: Strong _____	Weak _____	Murmur _____

Chest Pain _____
Palpitations _____
Edema _____
Orthopnea _____
Peripheral Pulses: (if pertinent)
(Rate Using Scale):

Carotid	L _____	R _____	0 - Absent
Brachial	L _____	R _____	+1 - Diminished
Radial	L _____	R _____	+2 - Normal
Femoral	L _____	R _____	+4 - Bounding
Popliteal	L _____	R _____	
Post Tibial	L _____	R _____	
Dorsalis Pedis	L _____	R _____	

Nailbeds: Pink _____	Cyanotic _____	Clubbing _____
Extremities: Warm _____	Cool _____	

Claudication _____
Comments: _____

G.I.:

Heartburn _____	Bowel Sounds _____
Abdominal Pain _____	Bloody Stools _____
Difficulty Swallowing _____	Jaundice _____
Flatulence _____	Hemorrhoids _____
Nausea _____	Abd. Tenderness _____
Vomiting _____	Abd. Distention _____
	Ostomy _____ Type _____

Comments: _____

BOWEL HABITS:
Frequency _____ Last BM _____
Color _____
Consistency _____
Problem with: Diarrhea _____   Constipation _____
If so, treatment _____
Comments: _____

GENITOURINARY SYSTEM: Urinary:

Normal Female _____	Voiding Freely _____	Hematuria _____
Normal Male _____	Distention _____	Burning _____
Rash _____	Urgency _____	Ostomy _____
Redness _____	Frequency _____	History of Urinary
Excoriation _____	Hesitancy _____	Problems _____
Discharge _____	Incontinence _____	Nocturia _____
Swelling _____		Dysuria _____

Comments: _____

WOMEN:

LMP _____	
Breast Mass _____	
Vag. Itching _____	
Menses Irregularity _____	

Comments: _____

MEN:

Penile Discharge _____	
Lesions _____	
Testicular Pain/Swelling _____	
Prostate Trouble _____	

MUSCULOSKELETAL SYSTEM: (Yes or No)

Deformity _____		Ambulatory _____
Swelling _____		Braces _____
Cramps _____		Walker _____
Pain _____		Cast _____
Stiffness _____		Amputation _____

Comments: _____

NEUROLOGICAL SYSTEM: (Yes or No)
Level of Consciousness:

Alert _____	Lethargic _____
Unresponsive _____	

Mental Status:

Oriented _____	PERRLA _____	Extremities:
Confused _____	Epistaxis _____	Weakness of _____
Combative _____	Headache _____	Paralysis of _____
Cooperative _____	Seizure Activity _____	Numbness of _____
Calm _____	Moves all	
Anxious _____	Extremities _____	Gait: Steady _____
Irritable _____	Grip R _____ L _____	Unsteady _____

Comments: _____

EMOTIONAL:

SKIN: (May use figure)
Appearance of skin: (color)

Pale _____	Diaphoretic _____	Lesions _____
Cyanotic _____	Dry _____	Decubitus _____
Jaundice _____	Hot _____	Skin Turgor:
Flushed _____	Cool _____	Elastic _____
Mottled _____	Rash _____	Loose _____
Other _____	Hives _____	Tight _____

INDICATE AREAS ON FIGURES:
1. Burn   2. Rash   3. Scar   4. Bruises   5. Ulcers   6. Dryness
7. Other _____

RN/GN SIGNATURE _____ **DATE** _____ **TIME** _____

Fig. 2-1, cont'd   Example of a health history data collection form, second page.

MISSISSIPPI BAPTIST MEDICAL CENTER

DISCHARGE
PLANNING ASSESSMENT

DATE STARTED:

A. **DATA COLLECTION** (RN, GN, LPN, GPN, PCP, NT):

ADMISSION STATUS

MENTAL & EMOTIONAL: ___ ALERT ___ MENTAL DEFICITS ___ CONFUSED ___ ANXIETY ___ ANGER
___ DEPRESSED ___ BEREAVEMENT ___ DENIAL ___ OTHER _____
___ COPING ADEQUATELY: NO SIGNIFICANT MENTAL/EMOTIONAL PROBLEMS REQUIRING INTERVENTION
PRE-ADMISSION STATUS: ___ INDEPENDENT ___ SUPERVISED ___ ASSISTED ___ HOME HEALTH ___ NURSING HOME
PT. INTERVIEW (INTERVIEW FAMILY/SO IF PT. UNABLE TO ANSWER):
IS PATIENT ABLE TO MAKE OWN DECISIONS? ___ YES ___ NO ___ MINOR PT. ABLE TO READ/WRITE? ___ YES ___ NO
IF NO, DO YOU HAVE A GUARDIAN? ___ NO ___ YES, NAME_____
INDICATE YOUR CAPABILITY IN CARING FOR YOURSELF: ___ EXCELLENT ___ GOOD ___ FAIR ___ POOR
CONTINENT: BOWELS: ___ YES ___ NO BLADDER: ___ YES ___ NO
OCCUPATION _____ PERSON AVAILABLE TO HELP AFTER DISCHARGE_____
DAYTIME PHONE NO. _____

DISCHARGE SERVICE DEPARTMENTS

CHECK ALL SERVICES UTILIZED AT HOME. REVIEW AND UPDATE PRN — INCLUDE DATE IDENTIFIED:

SOCIAL SERVICES

LIMITATIONS: ___ BLIND ___ DEAF; DEAF/FOREIGN INTERPRETER NEEDED ___ YES ___ NO
HOME ENVIRONMENT: ___ NO HEAT ___ NO ELECTRICITY ___ STAIRS ___ NO RUNNING WATER
HOME SERVICES: ___ TRANSPORTATION ___ EQUIPMENT ___ DAY CARE ___ SITTER
___ HOME DELIVERED MEALS ___ HOME HEALTH ___ LIFELINE
ADL CAPACITY: ___ ASSISTANCE NEEDED ___ COMPLETELY IMPAIRED
HOME EQUIPMENT: ___ BED ___ W/C ___ WALKER ___ CANE ___ HOYER LIFT ___ OXYGEN ___ APNEA MONITOR
___ IV THERAPY ___ T-TUBE ___ VENOUS ACCESS DEVICE OTHER _____
DO YOU FEEL FINANCIAL RESOURCES ARE INADEQUATE? ___ YES ___ NO

D/C NEEDS FOR: ___ YES ___ NO ACTIVITIES DAILY LIVING (Bathing, Eating, Feeding, Toileting, Taking Medicine, Shopping, Dressing)
(Circle needs, if applicable) ___ YES ___ NO EQUIPMENT (Bed, W/C, Walker, Cane, Hoyer Lift, Oxygen, Apnea Monitor, IV Therapy, T-Tube,
Venous Access Device, Other _____)
___ YES ___ NO HOME HEALTH ___ YES ___ NO NURSING HOME

RESPIRATORY CARE SERVICES

PRE-ADMISSION: ___ NONE ___ TRACH CARE ___ SUCTIONING ___ NCPAP ___ BREATHING EQUIPMENT
HOME SERVICES: ___ VENTILATOR ___ AEROSOL TX. ___ POSTURAL DRAINAGE ___ O₂ THERAPY

POST-DISCHARGE ___ NONE ___ TRACH CARE ___ SUCTIONING ___ NCPAP ___ BREATHING EQUIPMENT
SERVICES: ___ VENTILATOR ___ AEROSOL TX. ___ POSTURAL DRAINAGE ___ O₂ THERAPY

PHYSICAL THERAPY
___ NONE INDICATED
___ EVALUATION/INSTRUCTION FOR ASSISTIVE DEVICE (i.e. WALKER, CANE, ETC.)
___ EVALUATION/INSTRUCTION FOR GAIT TRAINING
___ OTHER _____

SPEECH THERAPY
___ NONE
___ EVALUATION/INSTRUCTION FOR SPEECH/LANGUAGE/SWALLOWING DISORDER

FOOD/NUTRITION SERVICES
___ NONE INDICATED
___ EVALUATION/INSTRUCTION(S) NEEDED RE: _____ DIET

NURSING SPECIALTIES
___ NONE INDICATED . . . . PREVIOUSLY SEEN (INFORMATIONAL)
___ DIABETIC CLINICAL NURSE SPECIALIST. Y N
___ ENTEROSTOMAL THERAPY . . . . Y N
___ MATERNAL/NEWBORN EDUCATORS. Y N
___ MENTAL HEALTH CLINICAL NURSE . . . . Y N
___ CV THERAPY. . . . . Y N
___ OTHER _____

SIGNATURE OF PERSON COMPLETING "A"

B. **COMPLETED BY RN/GN:** DISCHARGE PLANNING CONSULTS NEEDED *(CONTACT SERVICES IDENTIFIED ABOVE:)* (PLEASE ✔)

CONSULTS

	DATE	PERSON NOTIFIED	STICKER ON CHART	NURSE'S SIGNATURE
___ SOCIAL SERVICES				
___ RESPIRATORY CARE SERVICES				
___ PHYSICAL THERAPY				
___ SPEECH THERAPY				
___ DIETARY				
___ NURSING SPECIALTY				
___ OTHER				

SIGNATURE OF RN

Fig. 2-1, cont'd Example of a health history data collection form, third page.

5. Use silence to organize your thoughts and allow patients time to answer questions.
6. Use supportive statements and gestures: "That must have been difficult—tell me more." (Nod head yes.)
7. Focus the interview on the current topic: "Let's talk some more about your chest pain."

Communication

Gathering of data about the patient history depends on the ability of the patient to communicate. Thus it may be necessary to initially obtain information from the family members or significant other or to validate the data with them.

Reading, writing, and understanding English

Begin the assessment by evaluating the patient's ability to understand, speak, read, and write English. Is there a physiologic or psychologic reason for any difficulty (for example, reduced circulation to the brain, stroke, brain tumor, oral anatomic defect, severe anxiety, psychosis, lack of stimuli)?

Other languages

Identify the primary language spoken in the home and other languages spoken. If the patient's primary language is not English and communication is difficult, an interpreter is recommended.

Intubation or speech impairment

Evaluate whether the patient has any barriers in communicating. Document whether the patient is unable to speak and determine the cause. If the patient is intubated or has had a tracheostomy, for example, why was it done and how long ago? Inability to speak may be related to other causes, such as severe shortness of breath, facial paralysis, facial laceration or burns, or a mandibular fracture. Assess whether the patient is able to modulate speech, find words, name words, identify objects, and speak in sentences.[2,3]

Alternative forms of communication

When assessing the communication pattern, also recognize whether the patient can use alternative forms of communication such as sign language, a sign board, writing, a typewriter, or a computer.[3]

HEALTH HISTORY

The health history begins with an assessment of patient knowledge about current and past health status, medications, and risk factors. Data regarding knowledge and perception of illness (for example, misconceptions, readiness to learn, orientation and memory, and coping and decision-making skills) are collected. Assessment of spiritual concerns is also important because spirituality may affect perception of illness. A thorough social and economic history and identification of health-seeking behaviors should

be included. The current level of comfort, including physical, psychologic, and emotional aspects, is determined. Activity and rest, nutrition, and elimination patterns are assessed. Discharge planning (see Fig. 2-1) also begins with this interview.

Current Health Problems

Asking "What brought you to the hospital?" is generally most effective in determining information about current health problems. Attempt to elicit information about the signs, symptoms, and problems in the order that they occurred. Determine when, where, and under what circumstances each sign or symptom occurred. Also determine the location, quality, quantity, and duration of the sign or symptom and any aggravating, alleviating, or associated factors. It is also important to identify the absence of certain signs and symptoms often associated with the problem (for example, absence of weight gain or dyspnea in patients suspected of having decreased cardiac output). In seriously ill patients, priority is given to information that appears most relevant to the immediate situation.

Previous Illness, Hospitalizations, Surgeries, and Problems

The history of previous health problems is collected in the review of systems (see Fig. 2-1). Information regarding previous illnesses, hospitalizations, and surgeries is identified. In this part of the assessment the nurse should briefly do the following:

1. Identify any history of heart problems, including cardiac enlargement, heart failure, murmurs, myocardial infarction, dysrhythmias, and heart infections.
2. Determine any history of peripheral vascular disease or intermittent claudication (for example, calf cramping and fatigue that occurs when walking or exercising and is relieved by rest).
3. Inquire about a history of lung disease such as tuberculosis, asthma, lung infections, or bronchitis.
4. Identify any history of liver disease, such as liver enlargement or hepatitis; kidney disease such as infections or stones; cerebrovascular problems such as dizziness, fainting, strokes, or high blood pressure; rheumatic fever; thyroid problems; gallbladder problems; gastrointestinal problems; or genitourinary problems.
5. Also determine whether the patient has a history of drug abuse, including what kind of drug, how long it lasted, how long ago it occurred, and how it was treated.

Current Medications

Identify medications that the patient is taking. Determine the name of the medication, dosage, frequency, length of time that it has been taken, and any side effects. Also determine whether the patients is taking over-the-counter medications such as aspirin, acetaminophen, ibuprofen, laxatives, sleeping pills, cold medications, or diet pills. It may be useful to ask the patient to pick a typical day and describe all medications (physician- and self-prescribed) taken from morning until bedtime. A medication history is particularly necessary with the older patient, who may see more than one health care provider and consume drugs that have synergistic or mutually inhibitory effects.[4]

Risk Factors

Determine whether patients have coronary artery risk factors and assess their perception and level of understanding of each.[4,5] Query patients about hypertension, hyperlipidemia, smoking, obesity, diabetes mellitus, sedentary lifestyles, high levels of psychophysiologic stress, alcohol abuse, and for women, the use of oral contraceptives, cessation of menses, or the beginning of menopause.

Family History

The family background may also contribute important information to the assessment. Identify the age, gender, and health status of living family members, including parents, siblings, children, and spouses or significant others. Determine the age, gender, and cause of death for each deceased family member. In addition, certain familial diseases that grandparents, parents, and close relatives may have had are pertinent to the assessment. Determine any family history of cancer, other heart diseases, peripheral vascular disease, cerebrovascular disease, hypertension, stroke, respiratory disease, diabetes mellitus, nervous or mental conditions, kidney disease, arthritic conditions, hematologic abnormalities, rheumatic fever, sickle cell anemia, or thyroid disease.

Perception or Knowledge of Illness and Expectations

It is important to determine what the patient knows and perceives about the illness, tests, or surgery. Query patients about their biggest health problem at the moment. Ask them to discuss the problem and the cause. Likewise, evaluate what patients know and understand about the tests, procedures, or surgery they are about to undergo. Patients can have diverse expectations about their hospitalizations and therapies. Determine how patients expect their health problems to be treated and what they think the results of this treatment will be.

Misconceptions

Throughout the assessment, evaluate any misconceptions or lack of understanding regarding the hospitalization, illness, tests, surgery, or therapy. Assess the areas of risk factors, perception and knowledge of the current situation, and expectations of therapy. Evaluate the answers given by patients and family members. Determine whether the information is correct, whether patients and family members have a good understanding of the information, and whether the understanding is realistic for the situation.

Readiness to learn

In the critical care unit, patients may request information that relates only to the immediate situation. Assess the kinds of questions being asked and evaluate the kind of information being requested. For example, are patients asking questions about the therapy, treatments, illness, or prognosis? Are they acknowledging or denying that a health problem exists?[4] When assessing readiness to learn, it is important to determine educational level so that teaching content and material can be appropriately selected. Evaluate also whether there are any barriers to learning such as pain, environmental distractions, or other physical, emotional, or psychologic conditions that have an impact on learning.

Orientation and memory

Evaluate whether the patient is alert, lethargic, comatose, and oriented to person, place, and time. Assess also whether behavior and communication are appropriate for the situation or whether the patient is confused. Determine if the patient's memory is intact. Assess *recent memory* by asking the day, month, and year or the patient's address, and assess *remote memory* by asking if the patient recalls the holidays celebrated in the previous month or in another month.

Coping
Patient's ability to cope

Evaluate *individual coping* behaviors.[6] Question patients as to whether they satisfactorily solve problems, who helps them to solve problems, and if it is easy or hard for them to accept help. Also ask patients how they deal with major problems. For example, do they become depressed, anxious, or nervous; eat food, drink alcohol or take drugs; ask someone for help; call the family; or try to solve the problem alone? Inquire about activities used to reduce stress, such as listening to music, exercising, or using relaxation techniques. Verify these perceptions by asking the family members whether patients ask others for help.

Evaluate *defensive coping behaviors.* Assess whether patients are denying obvious problems or weaknesses. Observe whether patients blame others for health or functioning. Do they rationalize failures or project a falsely positive self-evaluation?

Family's ability to cope and give support

When evaluating for *disabling family coping,* observe whether family members or significant others are neglectful of the patient regarding basic needs, attention, or treatment.[6] Do they deny the patient's health problem and its extent and severity? Do they demonstrate rejection, intolerance, or abandonment? Evaluate whether family members or significant others make decisions or demonstrate behavior detrimental to the patient's psychophysiologic, social, or economic well-being.

To assess for *compromised family coping,* determine whether the patient expresses concerns regarding the family members' responses to the illness. Discover inadequate knowledge of the patient's illness, treatment, or recovery that interferes with the family member's ability to support and assist the patient.

Acceptance and adjustment to illness

Evaluate the degree of *denial.* Patients who are denying frequently fail to recognize the importance and danger of symptoms, minimize symptoms, or displace the source of symptoms to other organs; for example, chest pain may be dismissed as gastrointestinal gas. These patients also tend to delay seeking health care when symptoms appear and often dismiss distressing events even when they are dangerous to their health.[6]

Investigate the level of *adjustment* to the illness. Does the patient accept changes in health status brought about by the illness? Observe whether the patient demonstrates an unwillingness to become involved in problem solving or goal planning. Does the patient exhibit a prolonged period of shock, disbelief, or anger regarding the current health status?[6] Evaluate for movement toward independence.

Judgment: decision-making ability
Patients' perspectives

To evaluate *decision-making abilities,* query patients about whether they usually make good decisions. Investigate the circumstances under which they have difficulty making a decision or whether they find it difficult to decide what to do. If patients are faced with decisions regarding treatment, observe whether they verbalize uncertainty regarding the possible choices, vacillate between the possible alternatives, or demonstrate unusual delay in making decisions.[6]

Others' perspectives

To validate patients' perspectives, ask family members about the soundness of the patients' decisions and whether the patients are usually able to make timely decisions.

Spiritual Concerns

Data are collected to identify religious preferences and to evaluate whether the patient practices the religion, how often church or synagogue is attended, and how important religion is in the patient's life.[6] Determine whether the patient would like to talk to a religious representative and whether any specific religious items are important to have while in the hospital. Also appraise whether the religious beliefs and practices might affect treatment. For example, are any treatments forbidden by the religion?

Social and Economic History
Culture

Identify patients' cultural background or heritage. Patients may have strong ties to the customs and practices of their country. Identify special customs that might be important. Determine how the culture defines the role of the family in illness. Ask patients whether any medical treatments are unacceptable because of cultural beliefs.[6,7]

Role
Marital status, age, and health of significant other and children

Begin the assessment by determining the patient's marital status. Determine the ages and health of significant others. Inquire about children, their ages, and whether they are living in the home.

Role in the home

Focus the line of questioning to determine the patient's role in the home. For example, determine whether the patient is responsible for running the household, making the major decisions in the home, and providing discipline for the children. Discover whether the illness might affect the ability to complete tasks expected at home, and inquire about feelings about such changes.

Financial support

Financial concerns frequently precipitated by illness also are assessed. Identify whether the patient is the major breadwinner in the family and whether the patient believes that there is money available to meet expenses or that financial assistance is needed.

Occupation

The patient's occupation is identified. Note specifically the hours worked per week, the amount of physical or mental energy involved, and the amount of stress perceived. Evaluate whether the patient likes the job, verbalizes major concerns or problems, or believes that this current illness will affect the ability to return to work.

Sexual relationships

The patient's sexual role is appraised. Illness can have an impact on the ability to perform sexual activity and interest in the activity. Identify reports of difficulties, limitations, or changes in sexual behaviors, interests, or activities.[6] Assess the risk for human immunodeficiency virus (HIV) infection (that is, whether the patient has received blood transfusions; has a history of homosexuality, prostitution, or intravenous drug abuse; admits to multiple sexual partners or to sexual contact with a person who is HIV positive).

Socialization
Quality of relationships with others

Ask patients how they relate to others, if they are comfortable in most social situations, and whether they feel a sense of belonging, caring, and interest when they are with family members or friends. Determine whether the patient prefers to be alone most of the time or if the patient feels isolated or rejected by family members and friends.[5] If it is important, corroborate the patient's perceptions with family members or significant others. Observe how the patient interacts with and relates to family members, friends, and staff members to validate the patient's perceptions.

Health-Seeking Behaviors

Evaluate the patient's health-seeking behaviors. Explore whether the patient is interested in finding ways to alter personal health habits or the environment to move toward a higher level of wellness. Does the patient express a need to change unhealthy habits such as smoking or overeating, and is the patient familiar with programs or resources that can be used for health promotion? Determine whether the patient accepts responsibility for meeting basic health needs. Inquire if the patient routinely has physical and dental checkups. Evaluate whether the patient demonstrates an understanding of basic health practices such as the need for prophylactic antibiotics before and after invasive procedures if the patient has a heart murmur. Does the patient express an interest in improving health behaviors? Does the patient indicate a need for special equipment or personal resources? Identify whether the patient has health insurance or is in need of any financial assistance.[5,6,8]

Assess the patient's past and current adherence to the nursing and medical regimen, since this could affect the plan of care and course of recovery. Ask patients whether they have had difficulty remembering to take their medication, following their diet, or adhering to a prescribed exercise program. Also ask patients what problems they have had in doing these tasks and why they believe such problems occurred.[6]

Determine the patient's motivation and willingness to adhere to the newly prescribed health care regimen. Ask patients whether they will have difficulty following the new diet, exercise program, prescribed activities, and treatments or taking medications. Observe whether patients express an interest in following the health care regimen and whether they foresee any problems. Ask the patient if there is anything that is particularly unpleasant or difficult regarding the health care instructions.[5,6] Also evaluate whether the patient has the motivation to comply.

Ask family members if they believe that the patient will adhere to the health care regimen. Determine whether the family members understand the regimen and will support the patient in adherence.

Comfort
Pain or discomfort

Ask the patient about any *pain* or *discomfort*. Determine if the pain or discomfort is acute or chronic, when it began, whether it was sudden or gradual, and if the patient has ever had it before.[4] Assess how long the pain lasts; where it is located; whether it is intermittent, continuous, dull, sharp, mild, or severe. Identify whether the pain travels or radiates to other parts of the body and whether there are associated, aggravating, or alleviating factors. Explore whether the patient has experienced *palpitations* with premature beats or other cardiac rhythm disturbances or whether the patient has experienced the subjective sensation of dyspnea or shortness of breath.

Objective manifestations

Assess the patient for objective psychophysiologic manifestations of pain or discomfort. Observe for guarding or protective behaviors such as self-focusing (for example, altered time perception, withdrawal from social contact, impaired thought processes), moaning, crying, restlessness, and grimacing. Evaluate alterations in muscle tone or autonomic nervous system response to pain such as diaphoresis or blood pressure, pulse, respiratory rate, and pupillary changes. With chronic pain, observe for fear of reinjury, physical and social withdrawal, anorexia, and weight or sleep pattern changes.

Stress
Recent stressful life events

Discover if patients have had recent stressful life events such as family, financial, or work-related problems or if anything has been particularly upsetting lately. Determine whether they have had any feelings of anxiety, fear, or grieving.[5,6]

Verbalization of the feeling, source of stress, and its physical manifestations

When assessing for *anxiety*, recognize if patients are experiencing threats to self-concept, threats of death, or threats or changes in health status, socioeconomic status, role functioning, environment, or interactional patterns. Evaluate verbal complaints of increased tension, apprehension, uncertainty, inadequacy, or shakiness. Ask patients whether they feel jittery, distressed, rattled, overexcited, or scared. To assess for *fear,* explore feelings of dread related to an identifiable source that can be validated. Also observe for physical manifestations of anxiety and fear, such as elevated heart rate and blood pressure; darting eye movements; startle reflex to normal sounds; nonpurposeful activity such as picking at the sheets, hair, or fingernails; or constant leg motion.[3,6]

To assess for *grieving,* query patients about personal or anticipated losses. Are patients denying the losses or having difficulty expressing them? Determine whether patients are having difficulty concentrating, eating, sleeping, or performing normal daily activities.[6]

Emotional integrity
Perception of self and situation

Body image and self-esteem can be dramatically altered because of the effects of illness. To assess *self-esteem,* ask patients to describe themselves, how they feel about themselves, and whether they are comfortable about the way they look, feel, and function. Evaluate the effects of illness or surgery on self-esteem. Ask patients to describe what the illness or surgery means to them and their families.

Observe for self-negating talk, shame, or guilt. Determine whether patients feel that they are unable to deal with events, project blame on to others, or rationalize positive and exaggerate negative feedback about themselves. Distinguish whether negative verbalization about the self is of a *chronic* nature or is *situational* in response to the illness.

Description of body structure and functioning

To assess for *body-image* disturbance, assess the patient for verbal or nonverbal expressions of an actual or perceived change in body structure or functioning.[5] For example, if there is a missing body part, does the patient refuse to look in a mirror? Refuse to look at a body part? Hide or overexpose a body part? Ignore, neglect, or traumatize a body part?[2] Refuse to discuss the illness, injury, or surgery? Have negative feelings about the body or a preoccupation with a change or loss of a body part?[5] Observe whether the patient demonstrates responsibility for self-care or demonstrates self-neglect.

Hopelessness

Illness may produce feelings of hopelessness and powerlessness. It is important to diagnose such problems because of their potentially profound effects on illness and recovery. To assess for *hopelessness,* ask patients to describe possible solutions to the problem, their feelings about the future, and their plans. Observe for negative feelings, passivity, decreased verbalization, flat affect, a lack of initiative, decreased appetite or response to stimuli, increased sleep, lack of involvement in care, and sighing or verbal clues such as "I can't."[6]

Powerlessness

To evaluate powerlessness, observe for verbalization that indicates a perceived loss of control. Ask the patient to describe what can be done to change, improve, or help the situation or problem. Does the patient verbalize perceived physical deterioration despite total adherence to the health care regimen? Determine whether the patient perceives a loss of control regarding self-care and the outcomes of medical and nursing care. Verify whether the patient chooses not to participate in decision making even when opportunities are provided or whether dissatisfaction or frustration is expressed because of an inability to perform previous tasks or activities.[3,6]

Activity and rest

Issues related to self-care capabilities, usual activities, and rest patterns are assessed to provide a baseline for nursing care. A summary of an activity-sleep history is given in the box. In the nursing admission history, habits related to activity and rest are assessed for planning care for the hospital and for discharge.

Self-care
Ability to perform self-care

Evaluate patients' ability to perform *self-care.* Determine whether patients are able to feed themselves, adequately swallow fluids and solids, bathe themselves, wash their hair, brush their teeth, dress themselves, maintain satisfactory appearances, and use toilets or commodes. Discharge planning needs regarding self-care deficits are identified during this section of the assessment. The following suggested

---

ACTIVITY-SLEEP HISTORY

Activity

Usual time of arising
Activities during a typical day
    In-home activities and outside activities
    Occupation and number of hours worked/shift
Equipment/prosthesis needed for activity/walking
    (cane, walker, wheelchair, braces, artificial limbs)
Environmental factors influencing mobility
    Physical surroundings (home, neighborhood)
    Financial resources
Motivation to be active
    Effort made to be active
    Enjoyment of activity
Leisure activities
    Time spent daily (frequency/regularity)
    Type of activity (sedentary vs. active)
    Exercise patterns (type, frequency, duration, regularity)
Special abilities (creative, athletic)
Past history of activity/exercise; recent change
Attitudes about exercise and motivation to exercise
Current exercise/fitness goals

Sleep

Usual bedtime and relationship of activity to bedtime
Sleep environment
    Light and noise tolerance
    Temperature preference
    Equipment needed (pillows, blankets)
    Type of bed (size, firmness, position)
    Sleep alone or in a room or bed with others
Bedtime rituals/routines/aids to sleep (for example,
    reading, drinking, bathing, eating, watching TV, smoking)
Medications/drugs taken (over-the-counter [OTC],
    prescription, street, alcohol, stimulants, depressants)
Arousals during sleep (number and reason)
Difficulty falling or staying asleep
Naps (number, length, time of day)
Changes in usual patterns
Difficulties caused by changes in patterns
Client's perception of adequacy/quality

From Bellack JP, Edlund BJ: *Nursing assessment and diagnosis,* ed 2, Boston, 1992, Jones & Bartlett.

codes can be used to define the level of functional ability. These codes are also used to classify the nursing diagnoses listed under self-care deficits (for example, feeding, impaired swallowing, bathing/hygiene, dressing/grooming, and toileting deficits), as well as the diagnosis of impaired physical mobility.

Suggested codes for functional level classification[6]

0 = Is completely independent
1 = Requires use of equipment or device
2 = Requires help from another person for assistance, supervision, or teaching
3 = Requires help from another person and equipment or device
4 = Is dependent and does not participate in activity

Home maintenance management

The size and arrangement of the home may impose obstacles for the patient. Explore any difficulty entering the home because of entrance steps and determine whether the kitchen, bedroom, and bathroom are accessible. Will steps make movement inside the home difficult? Inquire about any safety needs such as a safety rail in the bath and repair of frayed electrical cords or torn carpets. Ask about the patient's activities on a typical day—including meal preparation, shopping, cleaning, child care, bill paying, and household chores—and determine whether the illness might interfere with such activities.

Activity

Limitation of movement

Ask the patient about any limitations in movement (physical mobility), including the ability to get in and out of a chair and bed. Determine whether the patient has observed a decrease in muscle size, tone, strength, or control. Observe the patient for limitations of movement such as a reluctance to move, limited range of motion, or impaired coordination; and identify whether the patient has perceptual, cognitive, neuromuscular, or musculoskeletal impairments. To classify the patient's functional level, use the functional code previously outlined.

Limitation in activities

Ask whether the patient has noticed pain or discomfort when performing activities (activity intolerance). Has the patient observed decreased strength or endurance? Are there activities that can no longer be performed? Observe the patient's psychophysiologic response to activity and identify symptoms associated with or precipitated by such activity.

Verbal reports of fatigue

Fatigue can have an enormous impact on the moving pattern. Fatigue, a subjective feeling, is common in older patients and can be associated with cardiac complications, particularly congestive heart failure. Ask patients if they have felt constantly tired, weak, or exhausted. Determine whether they verbalize a lack of energy, irritability, listlessness, or an inability to concentrate or maintain usual routines that might validate the diagnosis of fatigue.

Exercise habits

Determine whether the patient is involved in an exercise program; ask about the type of program, the number of times per week the exercise is performed, and the duration of each exercise session. Because illness can interfere with normal exercise patterns, inquire about the importance of the exercise to the patient's psychophysiologic well-being. For example, a marathon runner who has suddenly developed angina during exercise may be devastated if the daily exercise routine is curtailed. Query the patient also about the amount of exercise involved with job, outside activities, sports, and household or yard work.

Leisure activities

Ask patients what they do in their leisure time (for example, participating in sports, reading, listening to music, or playing cards). Inquire about hobbies. Explore complaints of boredom and evaluate whether the environment, condition, or treatments prohibit involvement in diversional activities. Is it possible for patients to engage in usual hobbies or activities while in the hospital?

Social activities

Discover whether the patient is involved in social activities such as church groups, clubs, or organizations. Determine the extent of the involvement and the importance of the activities to the patient.

Rest

Sleep and rest pattern

When assessing sleep and rest pattern, inquire about patients' usual bedtime, number of hours slept per night, and rest periods routinely set aside for naps, relaxation, or meditation. Ask about the use of sleep aids such as alcohol, tranquilizers, hypnotics, warm showers, music, or food. Explore whether patients have trouble falling asleep, remaining asleep, or returning to sleep once awakened or have recurring nightmares. Ask patients if they usually feel rested after sleeping. If they verbalize difficulty sleeping, inquire about changes in behavior such as irritability, restlessness, lethargy, or listlessness and observe for signs of sleep pattern disturbances such as mild, fleeting nystagmus; a light hand tremor; ptosis of the eyelids; expressionless faces; dark circles under the eyes; frequent yawning; or changes in posture.

Nutrition

Eating patterns

Nutritional status can have a profound impact on illness and recovery. The box gives a summary of important data related to nutritional status. Collect data to determine the number of meals patients eat each day. Ask patients to de-

---

NUTRITIONAL HISTORY

Client Profile

Age, sex, and race

Client/Family Data

Number and ages of people living in household
Race, ethnic, and cultural background
Religious affiliations that affect food
Education level
Financial status (money available for food)
"Gatekeeper" of food (who purchases, prepares, and serves food)
Participating in nutrition planning and food preparation and consumption
Motivation to eat balanced meals
Family composition
Recent changes in family

Environmental Data

Place of residence—urban, suburban, rural, geography, climate, and other factors affecting food availability
Occupation (place and work schedule, availability of food, snacks, changes in nutrient needs related to occupational environment and activities)
Hobbies and leisure activities (that may influence nutrient needs or actual food intake)
Home and neighborhood facilities for purchase, storage, preparation, and serving of foods

Health History

Present height, usual weight, and current weight
Recent changes in weight or health
Recent attempts in changing nutrient intake
Health habits affecting nutrient intake, such as alcohol and medications (prescription and over-the-counter)
Usual bowel habits
Use of laxatives
Past and present exercise patterns
Health problems, physical handicaps, or surgery

Dietary History

Usual intake of foods and fluids with types and amounts
Food preferences and aversions
Number, frequency, and time of meals and snacks
Appetite changes
Lifestyle habits affecting dietary intake
Vitamin, mineral, and nutrition supplements used
Changes in dietary intake
Use of dentures
Chewing and swallowing problems
Food allergies and symptoms
Problem foods that cause gas, diarrhea, or indigestion

From Bellack JP, Edlund BJ: *Nursing assessment and diagnosis,* ed 2, Boston, 1992, Jones & Bartlett.

---

scribe what they eat or drink in a typical day. Investigate dietary needs or restrictions such as low-sodium, low-fat, low-calorie, low-sugar, or low-protein diets. Find out if most of the meals are eaten at home or in restaurants. Identify types of foods that patients prefer. Explore whether there are foods that patients do not tolerate and whether there are food allergies. Determine the number of caffeinated beverages (including caffeinated coffee, teas, or soft drinks) that are consumed each day and identify the amount of chocolate intake per day.

Appetite changes

Query patients about changes in appetite such as eating or drinking more or less. Do they have an explanation for this change in eating pattern? Have they experienced nausea or vomiting?

Current nutritional therapy

Identify whether the patient is currently receiving nothing by mouth; nasogastric suctioning; tube feedings, including the type, amount, and frequency; or total parenteral nutrition (TPN), including the type, additives, and rate.

Elimination
Usual bowel habits

Investigate patients' usual bowel habits and whether they use laxatives, enemas, suppositories, bran, or fruits to regulate bowel movements.

Alterations in bowel habits

Do patients complain of difficulty with constipation, hemorrhoids, bowel cramping, diarrhea, or bowel incontinence? Do they have pain or bleeding with defecation? Do they have colostomies or ileostomies? Why and for how long?[2]

Usual urinary patterns

How many times per day does the patient urinate? Determine whether the patient limits fluid during the day or night or whether excessive amounts of fluid are consumed.

Alterations in urinary patterns

Investigate complaints of incontinence or retention of urine. Ask the patient to describe any frequency, burning, pain, dribbling, urgency, hematuria, nocturia, oliguria, or polyuria. Determine whether the patient has a urostomy or is receiving dialysis (type, frequency, and cause).

PHYSICAL EXAMINATION

The review of systems and the physical examination are often performed simultaneously. However, parts of the physical examination important for cardiovascular patients are summarized separately in this section. Special emphasis is given to cardiovascular and oxygenation assessment. Assessments of the abdomen, neurologic functioning, physical integrity, and physical regulation are also discussed. Fig. 2-2 is an example of a flow sheet used to record this data.

NURSING OBSERVATIONS

	SHIFT/TIME		2300-0700 /		0700-1500 /		1500-2300 /	
NEURO	ALERT/ORIENTED × 4							
	CALM/COOPERATIVE							
	PERRLA 2-5 mm							
MUSCULO-SKELETAL	MOVING ALL EXTREMITIES							
	STRENGTH EQUAL BILAT.							
	EXTREMITIES WARM/PINK							
INTEGUMENTARY	SKIN WARM/DRY							
	COLOR PINK/NORMAL							
	MUCUS MEMBRANES PINK/MOIST							
	SKIN TURGOR NORMAL							
	SKIN INTEGRITY INTACT							
RESPIRATORY	RESP. EVEN/UNLABORED							
	RESP. RATE							
	LUNGS: RUL							
	RLL							
	RML							
	LUL							
	LLL							
	COUGH/SPUTUM							
	O2 - TYPE/FLOW							
CARDIOVASCULAR	HEART TONES AUDIBLE							
	RHYTHM							
	CAROTID PULSE R/L							
	RADIAL PULSE R/L							
	FEMORAL PULSE R/L							
	POPLITEAL PULSE R/L							
	P.T. PULSE R/L							
	D.P. PULSE R/L							
	JVD < 3cm. @ 45°							
	CAPILLARY REFILL < / = 3 Sec.							
	PERIPHERAL EDEMA							
GI	ABDOMEN SOFT/NON-TENDER							
	BS + × 4							
	BOWEL MOVEMENT							
	CONSTIPATION/DIARRHEA							
GU	VOIDS WITHOUT DIFFICULTY							
	URINE CLEAR/YELLOW							
	CATHETER/TYPE							

Fig. 2-2 Example of a flow sheet for physical examination data. (Courtesy Mississippi Baptist Medical Center, Jackson, Miss.)

Peripheral Circulation
Arterial pulses

Determine the patient's pulse rate and evaluate each set of peripheral pulses. If the presence of a pulse is questionable, Doppler ultrasonography can be used to determine its audible quality, symmetry, and the presence of bruits.[9,10]

The arterial pulse is a propagated wave of arterial pressure resulting from left ventricular contraction. The pulse wave begins with the opening of the aortic valve and the ejection of blood from the left ventricle (Fig. 2-3). The pressure in the aorta rises sharply, since blood enters the vessel more rapidly than it runs off to the peripheral vessels. An *anacrotic notch* may appear during the sharp rise in the central arterial pressure curve. After peak pressure has been reached, aortic pressure decreases, ventricular ejection slows, and blood continues to flow to peripheral vessels. As the ventricles relax, there is a brief reversal of flow (from the central arteries back toward the ventricle), and the aortic valve closes. This produces the *dicrotic notch* on the peripheral pressure pulse tracing. After this, aortic pressure increases slightly and then decreases as diastole continues, and blood flows to the periphery. In the graphic recording of aortic pressure in Fig. 2-3 the peak of the pulse wave represents systolic pressure, and the lowest point on the wave represents diastolic pressure.

The pulse wave changes in shape as it travels to the periphery. The height, or amplitude, of the wave (the systolic reading) increases as it moves from the aortic root to the peripheral arteries, with a slight decrease in the diastolic pressure. The ascending part of the wave becomes steeper, and the peak becomes sharper.

The examination covers the carotid, brachial, radial, femoral, popliteal, dorsalis pedis, and posterior tibial pulses. These pulses can best be evaluated with the patient in a reclining position and the trunk of the body elevated about 30 degrees.

The pulse is examined for *rate and rhythm, equality of corresponding pulses, contour,* and *amplitude.* The pulses should be palpated on both sides and simultaneously at the brachial and femoral arteries. To obtain information about *rate and rhythm,* the pulse should be palpated for 30 seconds if there is a regular rhythm and for 1 to 2 minutes if there is an irregular rhythm. If an irregularity exists, the apical and radial pulses should be checked for deficits (see section on apical rate and rhythm).

The *character of the arterial wall,* which normally feels soft and pliable, is noted by palpation. With significant atherosclerotic disease the vessel may be resistant to compression and feel like a rope.

The pulse *contour* is assessed by extending the patient's arm and palpating the radial or brachial pulse or the carotid pulse in the neck. The artery should be compressed lightly with a finger while the examiner ascertains the contour of the pulse wave.[11] Variations in the contour of the arterial pulse are depicted in Fig. 2-4.

The *normal arterial pulse* (Fig. 2-4, *A*) has a pulse pressure of 30 to 40 mm Hg; the systolic pressure is measured by the peaks of the waves, and the diastolic pressure is measured by the troughs. The examiner can feel a sharp upstroke and a more gradual downstroke (the dicrotic notch of the descending slope of the wave is too weak to be palpable). The contour of the normal pulse is smooth and rounded.

With *large bounding pulses* (Fig. 2-4, *B*), the pulse pressure is increased, and a rapid upstroke, a brief peak, and a fast downstroke are felt. This type of pulse wave is encountered most often with exercise, anxiety, fear, hyperthyroidism, anemia, aortic regurgitation, and hypertension. It is also found as a result of generalized arteriosclerosis and rigidity of the arterial system in older people.

Small, weak pulses (Fig. 2-4, *C*) are characterized by diminished pulse pressure and a pulse contour felt as a slow, gradual upstroke; a delayed systolic peak; and a prolonged downstroke. This pulse is found in severe cases of left ventricular failure as a result of decreased stroke volume and in moderate or severe cases of aortic stenosis as a result of slow ejection of blood through the narrowed orifice.

Pulsus alternans (Fig. 2-4, *D*) refers to a pulse pattern in which the heart beats with a *regular* rhythm, but the pulses alternate in size and intensity.

The *bigeminal pulse* (Fig. 2-4, *E*) is usually produced by a premature ventricular extrasystole that occurs regularly after a normally conducted beat. The stroke volume of the premature beat is less than that of the normal beat, since contraction occurs before complete ventricular filling. The rhythm is *irregular,* since the time between the normal beat and the premature beat is shorter than the time between the pairs. The irregularity may be consistent. Simultaneous arterial palpation and cardiac auscultation assist in diagnosing this cardiac irregularity.

The *amplitude* of pulses is categorized into levels using the following code and compared bilaterally:

$$
\begin{array}{ll}
0 & = \text{Not palpable} \\
+1 & = \text{Faintly palpable} \\
+2 & = \text{Palpable} \\
+3 & = \text{Bounding}
\end{array}
$$

In patients with significant vascular disease it is useful to draw the following small stick figure and label the amplitude of pulses accordingly:

Pulsus paradoxus (Fig. 2-4, *F*) refers to the phenomenon in which the pulse diminishes perceptibly in amplitude during normal inspiration.[12] Although the differences in pulse volume can be palpated, they can be more precisely

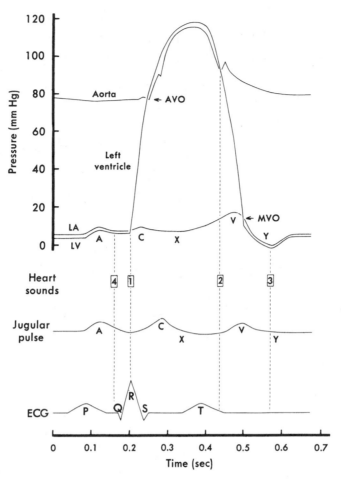

Fig. 2-3   Simultaneous ECG pressures obtained from the left atrium, left ventricle, aorta, and jugular pulse during one cardiac cycle. For simplification, right-sided heart pressures have been omitted. Normal right atrial pressure closely parallels that of the left atrium, and right ventricular and pulmonary artery pressures time closely with their corresponding left-sided heart counterparts, being reduced only in magnitude. The normal mitral and aortic valve closure precedes tricuspid and pulmonic closure, respectively, whereas valve opening reverses this order. The jugular venous pulse lags behind the right atrial pressure. During one cardiac cycle, the electrical events *(ECG)* initiate and therefore precede the mechanical *(pressure)* events, and the latter precede the auscultatory events *(heart sounds)* they produce. Shortly after the P wave, the atria contract to produce the a wave reflected in the jugular venous pulse because of backflow of blood into the vena cava; a fourth heart sound may succeed contraction. The QRS complex initiates ventricular systole, followed shortly by left ventricular contraction and the rapid buildup of left ventricular *(LV)* pressure. Almost immediately LV pressure exceeds left atrial *(LA)* pressure to close the mitral valve and produce the first heart sound. When LV pressure exceeds aortic pressure, the aortic valve opens *(AVO),* and when aortic pressure is again greater than LV pressure, the aortic valve closes to produce the second heart sound and terminate ventricular ejection. The decreasing LV pressure drops below LA pressure to open the mitral valve *(MVO),* and a period of rapid ventricular filling commences. During this time, a third heart sound may be heard. In addition to the a wave, the jugular venous pressure changes are reflected in the c wave produced by the closure of the tricuspid valve, the x slope produced by displacement of the bases of the ventricles during systole and subsequent atrial filling, the v wave produced by increasing pressure in the atria during filling, and the y slope produced by opening of the tricuspid valve.   (Modified from Hurst JW and others: *The heart: arteries and veins,* ed 8, New York, 1994, McGraw-Hill.)

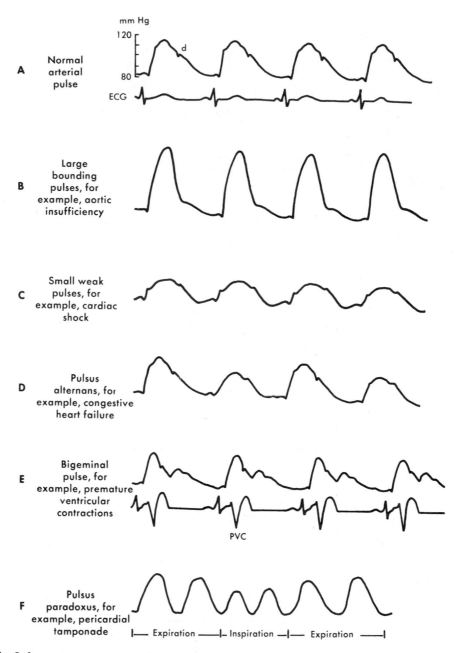

Fig. 2-4 Variations in contour of the arterial pulse with correlated electrocardiograms (ECGs). See text for description. *PVC*, Premature ventricular contraction.

demonstrated with sphygmomanometry. Under normal conditions of rest the systolic blood pressure ordinarily decreases by 3 to 10 mm Hg. The procedure for detecting pulsus paradoxus is as follows:

1. Have the patient breathe *normally.*
2. Pump up the sphygmomanometer and then lower the pressure until the first heart sound (systolic) (S_1) is heard.
3. Observe the patient's respirations. The systolic sound may disappear during normal inspiration.

4. Slowly deflate the cuff until all systolic sounds are heard, regardless of phase in the respiratory cycle.

The change (in millimeters of mercury) from the point at which systolic sounds were first heard to the point where they are heard during the entire respiratory cycle represents the millimeters of paradox observed. A paradox greater than 10 mm Hg is usually abnormal.

To be significant, a paradoxical pulse must occur during the normal cardiac rhythm and with respirations of normal rhythm and depth. In short, it is an exaggeration of a normal response during respiration. Pulsus paradoxus is found in cases of pericardial tamponade, adhesive pericarditis, severe lung disease, advanced heart failure, and other conditions.

Auscultation of arteries

Arteries are normally silent when auscultated with the stethoscope. Occlusive arterial disease such as arteriosclerosis interferes with normal blood flow through the artery, resulting in a blowing sound called a *bruit.* Auscultation of the carotid arteries should be done with the patient holding the breath so that the bruits can be distinguished from the sounds of respiration. Often these abnormal arterial vibrations can be felt as *thrills.* Auscultation is also done over the abdominal aorta and femoral arteries to detect bruits.

Arterial blood pressure

Determine the patient's systolic and diastolic blood pressure. The arterial blood pressure is an overall reflection of ventricular function.

Normal blood pressure in the aorta and large arteries such as the brachial artery varies between 100 and 140 mm Hg systolic and 60 and 90 mm Hg diastolic. Pressure in the smaller arteries is somewhat less, and in the arterioles, where the blood enters the capillaries, it is about 35 mm Hg. The difference between systolic and diastolic pressures is called the *pulse pressure;* it represents the range of pressure in the arteries. In contrast, the *mean arterial pressure* is the average pressure in the aorta and its major branches during the cardiac cycle.[13]

Wide variations of normal blood pressure exist, and the value may fall outside the normal range in healthy adults. The normal range also varies with age, gender, and race. A pressure reading of 100/60 mm Hg may be normal for one person but hypotensive for another. Blood pressure trends, rather than absolute numbers, must be analyzed and treated in light of the patient's clinical situation.

Arterial blood pressure can be measured indirectly or directly. *Indirect blood pressure monitoring* can be achieved manually or by automated devices. The most convenient and noninvasive method of measuring *manual indirect blood pressure* is auscultatory monitoring using a stethoscope and a sphygmomanometer. For routine indirect blood pressure monitoring the patient may sit or recline. In some cases, blood pressure may change with body position, and in this situation the pressure should be recorded with the patient lying, sitting, and standing. Severe decreases in pressure from lying to sitting or standing indicate postural hypotension. If this type of decrease occurs, the nurse assesses the patient for the cause; possible causes are dehydration, hemorrhage, medications, neurologic impairment, or prolonged bedrest associated with decreased muscle tone. Blood pressure is checked in both arms, and any differences are noted. Normally, there may be a 5 to 10 mm Hg difference between the two arms.

The collapsed cuff is affixed snugly to the patient's arm, with the distal margin of the cuff at least 2.5 cm above the antecubital fossa. The cuff width should be 40% of the circumference of the arm, and the length of the bladder should more than encircle the arm (that is, 1½ times around the arm).[14] With the arm resting on a table or bed at heart level, the brachial artery is palpated. Pressure in the cuff is rapidly increased to about 30 mm Hg above the point at which the palpable pulse disappears. As the cuff is deflated, observations may be made by palpation or auscultation. For *palpation,* the point at which the pulse can be felt is recorded as the palpable systolic pressure.

The *auscultatory method* is usually preferred to palpation. With this method, turbulence, vibrations, and sound occur (Korotkoff sounds) as indicators of blood pressure. The stethoscope is placed over the brachial artery while the cuff is slowly deflated (2 to 3 mm Hg per heartbeat). As intermittent blood flow returns, sounds become audible. The *systolic pressure* is the point at which at least two consecutive beats can be heard. As the cuff is further deflated, the sounds become louder for a brief period, then become muffled, and finally disappear. The *diastolic pressure* is the point at which the sounds disappear, although there is conflict as to whether the point of muffling is a more accurate indicator of the diastolic pressure.[14] If the diastolic sound continues until 0 mm Hg, as can occur with aortic regurgitation, the systolic, muffled, and zero values should all be recorded (for example, 120/70/0 mm Hg).

Although the sounds may disappear at a certain reading on the sphygmomanometer, one must continue listening to the zero pressure to detect a possible *auscultatory gap.* In this situation the nurse may first detect systolic sounds at a high level, only to have the sounds suddenly disappear and then reappear at a lower level. The silent period is called the *auscultatory gap* and is usually 20 to 40 mm Hg in length (Fig. 2-5). If the gap is not recognized, incorrect systolic and diastolic pressures may be recorded.

Another primary method of measuring indirect blood pressure is the use of *automated blood pressure monitors.* Several devices are available. For example, one type uses a double air bladder cuff that is applied in the same manner as a conventional cuff. The bladder senses the arterial wall oscillations and records the systolic, mean, and diastolic pressures.

The *Doppler method* of recording systolic blood pressure is similar to the auscultatory method. The Doppler technique is commonly used during low-flow, hypotensive states to augment Korotkoff sounds when they cannot be heard by auscultation. As the blood pressure cuff is slowly deflated, the Doppler device is applied with conduction gel over the brachial artery. The device uses amplified reflected ultrasound to audibly identify the systolic pressure.

Arterial line

Direct blood pressure monitoring is accomplished by inserting a catheter or needle into an artery and attaching

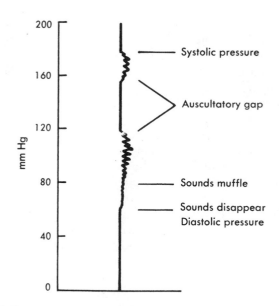

Fig. 2-5 Detection of an auscultatory gap in blood pressure measurement. The systolic sounds are first heard at 180 mm Hg. They disappear at 160 mm Hg and reappear at 120 mm Hg; the silent interval is the auscultatory gap. Korotkoff sounds muffle at 80 mm Hg and disappear at 60 mm Hg. The blood pressure is recorded as 180/80/60 with auscultatory gap.

the catheter to plastic tubing filled with heparinized saline solution. The tubing is connected to a transducer, which converts the mechanical energy that the blood exerts on the recording membrane into electrical voltage or current that can be calibrated in millimeters of mercury. The electrical signal is then transmitted to an electronic recorder and an oscilloscope, which continually record and display the pressure waves (see Fig. 2-4, *A*).

In some situations, major discrepancies exist between direct and indirect blood pressure measurements. Such inconsistencies suggest that when a high degree of accuracy is required, direct monitoring should be used. Thus in patients whose Korotkoff sounds might be diminished or absent, making auscultatory techniques unreliable, direct arterial measurements should be used. This method is used for patients who are in shock, who have high peripheral vascular resistance, and who are hypothermic, obese, or edematous. Direct blood pressure monitoring is also indicated when titrating intravenous drugs, especially those used for hypertension or hypotension. An arterial catheter is also beneficial in providing continuous pressure monitoring without disturbing the patient, and it allows for frequent arterial sampling to determine blood gas levels and pH in patients on ventilators or with cardiogenic shock or respiratory insufficiency.[14]

Venous pulse

Assess the venous pulse by examining the neck veins to gather information about right-sided heart functioning. For this clinical evaluation, the examiner must study the waveform of the venous pulsations, correlate them with the cardiac rhythm, and determine the venous pressure.

The examination begins with observation of the external and internal jugular veins. For accurate evaluation of the venous waveform the *right internal jugular vein* is usually selected. If the venous pressure is relatively normal, the patient can assume a comfortable recumbent position with the head and trunk elevated to about a 30-degree angle without flexing the neck. If the venous pressure is greatly elevated, the pulses can be examined better with the patient in a completely upright position so that the pulsations appear at the jugular level.

The patient's head should be gently rotated away from the examiner. A light shining tangentially across the area being examined may help detect a slightly distended vein. A series of undulant waves more clearly seen than felt characterize the venous pulse, a graphic recording of which is shown in Fig. 2-6.

a Wave. The a wave is produced by right atrial contraction and the retrograde transmission of the pressure pulse to the jugular veins. It occurs at the time of the fourth heart sound (S_4), preceding S_1. The a wave can be easily identified by placing the index finger on the carotid pulse opposite the side being inspected. Because of the compliance of the great veins and the low pressures in the right side of the heart, the a wave will be seen to start just slightly before the carotid pulse is palpated. The a wave is absent during atrial fibrillation. Giant a waves reflect an elevated right atrial pressure and may be seen in pulmonary hypertension and pulmonic and tricuspid stenosis.

c Wave. The c wave begins shortly after S_1 and may result from the pressure generated by the bulging tricuspid valve during right ventricular systole. The c wave is often difficult to visualize by inspecting the neck veins.

v Wave. Continued atrial filling during ventricular systole produces the v wave, which peaks just after the second heart sound (S_2), when the tricuspid valve opens. Tricuspid insufficiency causes a very large v wave.

x Descent. The x descent is the downslope of the a and c waves; it results from right atrial diastole plus the effects of the tricuspid valve being pulled downward during ventricular systole.

y Descent. The y descent represents the fall in the right atrial pressure from the peak of the v wave after tricuspid valve opening; it occurs during rapid atrial emptying in early diastole.

Venous pressure

Information about the right side of the heart also can be obtained by determining the venous pressure. *Venous pressure* refers to the pressure exerted within the venous system by the blood. It is highest in the venules of the extremities and lowest at the point where the vena cava enters the heart. Venous blood flow is continuous rather than pulsatory. In the arm, venous pressure ranges from 5 to 14 cm

H_2O, and in the inferior vena cava, it ranges from 6 to 8 cm H_2O.

The external and internal jugular veins are inspected to estimate venous pressure, right atrial pressure, and right ventricular function. The internal jugular veins are preferred for observation because the external jugular veins are smaller and do not adequately transmit pressure changes.[4] When the *internal jugular vein* is evaluated, the patient's trunk is elevated to an optimum angle to observe the venous pulse. The highest point of visible pulsation is determined, and the vertical distance between this level and the level of the angle of Louis is recorded. The angle of elevation is also recorded (Fig. 2-7). The *angle of Louis,* or sternal angle, is located at the junction of the sternum with the second rib; it lies approximately 5 cm above the right atrium for all positions between supine and 90 degrees upright. Pressures of more than 5 cm above the angle of Louis are considered to be elevated.

The sternal angle is used as a bedside reference point for the sake of convenience. The ideal reference level for venous pressure measurement is the midpoint of the right atrium. This level is established by running an imaginary anteroposterior line from the fourth interspace halfway to the back. A horizontal plane through this point is the zero level for the venous pressure measurement. The vertical distance from this plane to the head of the blood column, or the meniscus, approximates the venous pressure (Fig. 2-8). Elevations of pressure above 10 cm H_2O measured from the right atrial midpoint are considered abnormal.

Central venous pressure

Direct measurement of central venous pressure (CVP) is indicated if there is doubt about the venous pressure value estimated by using the indirect method and when precise measurements are needed to monitor critically ill patients. The CVP indicates right atrial pressure, which primarily reflects alterations in right ventricular pressure and only secondarily reflects changes in pulmonary venous pressure or the pressures in the left side of the heart. The CVP provides valuable information about blood volume, right ventricular function, and central venous return.

The CVP is obtained by cannulating a vein and threading the catheter into the vena cava. The pressure can be measured in centimeters of water by a water manometer or in millimeters of mercury by a pressure transducer. The normal CVP ranges from 4 to 15 cm H_2O or 3 to 11 mm

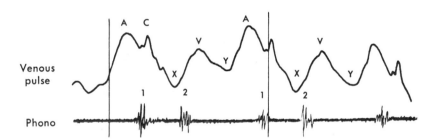

Fig. 2-6 Relationship of the jugular venous pulse to right atrial activity. (See the text and Fig. 2-3 for a description of waveforms.) The phonocardiogram *(phono)* recording indicates the first and second heart sounds.

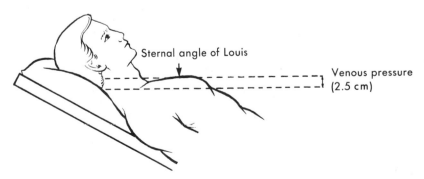

Fig. 2-7 Angle of Louis, or sternal angle, as a reference point for measuring venous pressure. The height of the distended fluid column in the internal jugular vein is less than 3 cm above the sternal angle.

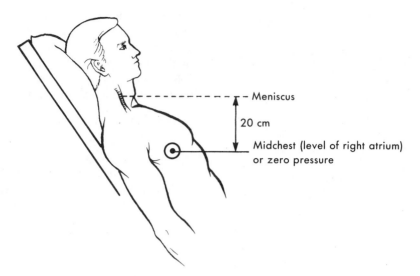

Fig. 2-8   Estimation of venous pressure is accomplished by elevating the head until the meniscus is visualized. Venous pressure is measured as the vertical distance between the meniscus and midchest, or right atrial level, in this case 20 cm and elevated above normal.

Hg.[4] Centimeters of water can be converted to millimeters of mercury by dividing the former by 1.36 because 1 mm Hg = 1.36 cm H_2O. Elevated CVPs may indicate right ventricular failure, pulmonary disease such as pulmonary hypertension or embolism, or cardiac tamponade. A low CVP may indicate hypovolemia or peripheral blood pooling, as in septic shock. Serial measurements must be interpreted according to the patient's clinical situation and correlated with other physical findings.

Skin temperature and color

Evaluate the patient's skin temperature to determine whether it is normal, warm, hot, cool, clammy, or moist. Also evaluate skin color. Does the patient exhibit pink, pale, or red coloring? Is there pallor, jaundice, mottling, increased pigmentation, or blanching?

Cyanosis. Determine whether the patient is cyanotic. *Cyanosis* is a bluish discoloration of the extremities and lips caused by poor circulation. It is brought on by cold temperatures or a severe dysfunction such as pulmonary disease or shock. Examine the color of the earlobes, nose, lips, nail beds, and mucous membranes. *Central cyanosis* occurs with low arterial oxygen saturation associated with congenital right-to-left shunts or pulmonary diseases such as pneumonia. It is observed in the mucous membranes such as the conjunctiva and the inside of the lips and cheeks. With *peripheral cyanosis* the arterial oxygenation saturation may be normal, but the oxygen within the peripheral vascular bed is inadequate. This may occur with heart failure and shock.[15]

Capillary refill. Describe whether the patient's capillary refill is normal. Capillary refill is assessed by pressing the nail bed, earlobe, or forehead so that it blanches; re-leasing the pressure; and observing whether the skin color returns to normal within 2 seconds.[15]

Clubbing. Determine whether the patient exhibits clubbing of the nail beds.[4] With clubbing, the proximal nail beds are convex and rise above the flat plane of the finger. The skin proximal to the nail bed feels spongy, and in some cases, the fingernails pulsate and flush. Clubbing is associated with certain pulmonary and cardiac diseases[11,12] (Fig. 2-9).

Edema

Determine whether the patient has edema. Edema occurs when fluid pressure in the interstitium increases. Peripheral edema accompanies right-sided heart failure. Fluid tends to accumulate in the dependent areas of the body, including the hands, ankles, and feet in the ambulatory patient and the sacral area of the patient on bedrest. Edema is assessed by firmly indenting the skin with the fingertips. When the patient on bedrest is examined, it is important to press over the sacrum, buttocks, and posterior thighs. The degree of pitting is quantified and described by the following scale[9]:

> 0 = None present
> +1 = Trace—disappears rapidly
> +2 = Moderate—disappears in 10 to 15 seconds
> +3 = Deep—disappears in 1 to 2 minutes
> +4 = Very deep—present after 5 minutes

Sudden weight gain may be a sign of edema. Pulmonary edema occurs with left-sided heart failure. Assessment of pulmonary edema is discussed in the section on oxygenation.

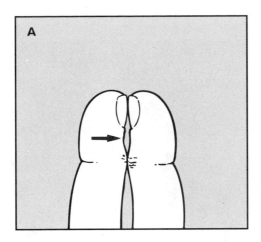
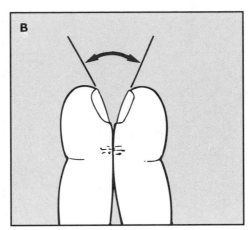

Fig. 2-9 Early clubbing is sometimes evidenced by a nail-to-nail bed angle of more than 180 degrees. **A,** Patient with normal nails. *Arrow,* Normal space. **B,** Patient with clubbing. *Arrow,* Abnormal space and angle.   (From Seidel H and others: *Mosby's guide to physical examination,* ed 3, St Louis, 1995, Mosby.)

Cardiac Assessment
Point of maximum impulse

Cardiac assessment is begun by inspection and palpation of the precordium. The anterior part of the chest is inspected with the patient in a supine position and the trunk elevated to about 30 degrees.

The approach should be made from the patient's right side. Certain landmarks on the anterior chest wall are useful as points of reference in describing the location of the heart. The heart rests on the diaphragm and is located beneath and to the left of the sternum. The base of the heart is situated approximately at the level of the third rib; the apex of the heart lies approximately at the level of the fifth rib in the midclavicular line (Fig. 2-10). The anterior surface of the chest closest to the heart and aorta is called the *precordium.* The precordium is inspected for abnormal pulsations. Tangential lighting helps in the effort to detect these pulsations. Any visible impulse medial to the apex and in the third, fourth, or fifth intercostal space generally originates in the right ventricle and is usually abnormal. The point of maximal impulse (PMI) is normally visible between the fourth and sixth intercostal spaces just medial to the left midclavicular line. However, it is also normal not to see this impulse. In pronounced right ventricular enlargement, the lower sternum can be observed to heave with each heartbeat. It is important to determine when the movements occur by correlating them with heart sounds or carotid artery pulsations.

After inspection, palpation of the precordium is performed to confirm the findings of inspection and to locate other impulses or thrills. The palmar bases of the fingers are used because this area is most sensitive to vibrations. First, areas where pulsations are visible are palpated, and then specific areas of the precordium systematically are felt (Fig.

2-11). The PMI is palpated at the left midclavicular line in the fifth intercostal space. Palpation of other precordial areas and abnormal findings are described in the box.

Pacemaker

Observe for an internal or external pacemaker. If an internal pacemaker is present, record the type and how it is functioning. If an external pacemaker is present, record the type, settings, and how it is functioning.

Apical rate and rhythm

Determine the patient's apical heart rate. Evaluate whether the rhythm is regular or irregular. If irregular, is it regularly irregular or irregularly irregular? If the rhythm is irregular, determine whether a peripheral pulse deficit is present. An *apical-radial deficit* indicates that the apical heart rate (counted by auscultation) exceeds the radial pulse rate (counted by palpation). A deficit means that not every cardiac systole is forceful enough to produce a palpable radial pulse. This may occur with premature extrasystoles or atrial tachydysrhythmias such as atrial fibrillation.

Heart sounds and murmurs

Auscultate the heart to identify the normal first (S_1) and second (S_2) heart sounds and to determine whether there is a third (S_3) or fourth (S_4) heart sound or whether there are ejection sounds, midsystolic clicks, opening snaps, or heart murmurs.

Selection and use of the appropriate stethoscope can influence the reliability of the findings. The stethoscope should have properly fitting earpieces and should be equipped with a diaphragm and a bell. The diaphragm is used to evaluate high-pitched sounds, such as S_1 and S_2, and it is pressed firmly against the skin. The bell is used to

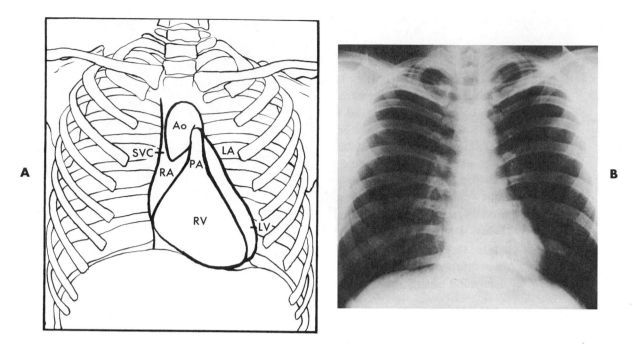

Fig. 2-10 **A,** Schematic illustration of the parts of the heart, whose outlines can be detected in **B.** *Ao,* Aorta; *SVC,* superior vena cava; *RA,* right atrium; *PA,* pulmonary artery; *LA,* left atrium; *RV,* right ventricle; *LV,* left ventricle. **B,** Frontal projection x-ray film of the normal cardiac silhouette.

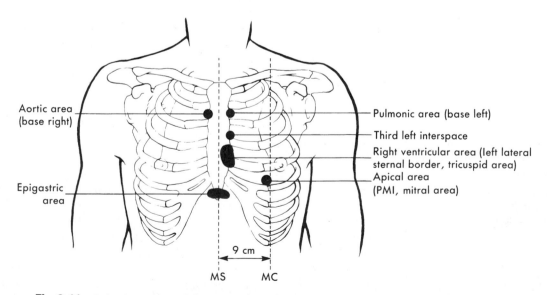

Fig. 2-11 Palpation areas on the precordium for detecting normal and abnormal cardiac pulsations. See text for description. *MS,* Midsternum; *MC,* midclavicular.

PALPATING PRECORDIAL AREAS

Aortic Area

The second interspace to the right of the sternum is felt for a pulsation, thrill, or vibration of aortic valve closure. A vibratory thrill is associated with aortic stenosis. Thrills at the base can best be palpated with the patient sitting and leaning forward.

Pulmonic Area

The second and third left interspaces are evaluated for abnormalities in the pulmonary artery or valve. A forceful pulsation of the pulmonary artery may be felt in mitral stenosis and primary pulmonary hypertension. A palpable sustained pulse and a thrill are associated with pulmonary stenosis.

Right Ventricular Area

The lower left sternal border, incorporating the third, fourth, and fifth intercostal spaces, is palpated. Abnormal pulsations here are most commonly found in conditions associated with right ventricular enlargement. When the sternum can be felt to move anteriorly during systole, this movement is termed *a substernal heave or lift.*

Apical Area

The *PMI* is evaluated for its location, diameter, amplitude, and duration. In normal adults the PMI is located at or within the left midclavicular line in the fifth intercostal space (Fig. 2-11). The impulse is normally less than 2 cm in diameter and often is smaller. It is felt as a light tap, beginning approximately at the time of S_1 and it is sustained during the first third and half of systole.

Epigastric Area

The upper central region of the abdomen can have visible or palpable pulsations in some normal individuals. Abnormally large pulsations of the aorta may be produced by an aneurysm of the abdominal aorta or by aortic valvular regurgitation. In right ventricular hypertrophy, right ventricular pulsations may also be detected in this area.

---

detect low-pitched sounds, such as S_3 and S_4, and it is placed lightly on the skin, with just enough pressure to seal the edge of the bell. The environment and the patient's position also are important during auscultation. The room should be quiet, with the patient resting comfortably on a bed or table that will easily accommodate lying flat, turning to the side, or sitting.

Auscultation of the heart requires selective listening for each component of the cardiac cycle as the nurse inches the stethoscope over the five main topographic areas for cardiac auscultation (Fig. 2-12). Note that these auscultatory areas do correspond not to the anatomic locations of the valves but rather to the sites at which the particular valve sounds are best heard. Accordingly, one listens with the stethoscope over the following areas:

1. *Aortic area* at the base of the heart in the second right intercostal space close to the sternum
2. *Pulmonic area* at the second left intercostal space close to the sternum

3. *Third left intercostal space,* where murmurs of aortic and pulmonic origin may be heard
4. *Tricuspid area* at the lower left sternal border
5. *Mitral area* at the apex of the heart in the fifth left intercostal space just medial to the midclavicular line

Auscultation is conducted in a systematic fashion. By beginning at the aortic area, one can determine the heart rate and the cardiac cycle time by identifying S_1 and S_2. This serves as a frame of reference as the examiner moves to other auscultatory areas of the precordium. At each site the procedure is as follows:

1. Listen to S_1, noting its intensity and splitting.
2. Listen to S_2, noting its intensity and splitting.
3. Note extra sounds in systole, identifying their timing, intensity, and pitch.
4. Note extra sounds in diastole, identifying their timing, intensity, and pitch.
5. Listen for systolic and diastolic murmurs, noting their timing, intensity, quality, pitch, location, and radiation.
6. Listen for extracardiac sounds such as a pericardial friction rub.

If an abnormal sound is detected, the surrounding area is carefully explored to evaluate the radiation of the sound. The patient's position should be changed for better evaluation of abnormal sounds. For example, an aortic murmur may be heard best by having the patient sit, lean forward, exhale, and hold the breath. Changes with respiration or during Valsalva maneuver may be important.

Changes in the intensity of heart sounds may be clinically significant. S_1 at the mitral area (apex) may become softer at the aortic area (base). Similarly, S_2 loses intensity as the stethoscope is moved toward the apex. The diagrams in Fig. 2-13 indicate the intensity and splitting of the S_1 and S_2, their relationship to S_3 and S_4, and the areas where these sounds can best be auscultated.

First heart sound

S_1 is associated with the closure of the mitral and tricuspid valves. It is synchronous with the apical impulse and corresponds to the onset of ventricular systole (Fig. 2-14). It is louder, longer, and lower pitched than S_2 at the apex (Fig. 2-13, *A*). As the ventricles begin to contract and pressure rises within, the tricuspid and mitral valves close. Valvular sounds of the left side slightly precede those of the right and are of higher intensity; the mitral valve closes before the tricuspid valve. *Splitting* of S_1 may therefore be heard, particularly in the tricuspid area (Fig. 2-13, *B*). When the PR interval is prolonged, the intensity of S_1 is decreased, and when the PR interval shortens, S_1 is increased.

As the pressure within the ventricles continues to rise and exceeds the pressure within the pulmonary artery and aorta, the pulmonic and aortic valves open. Opening of these valves is usually inaudible. If opening of the aortic valve is heard, this is called an *aortic ejection sound* or *click.* The same is true for the pulmonic valve. *Early systolic ejec-*

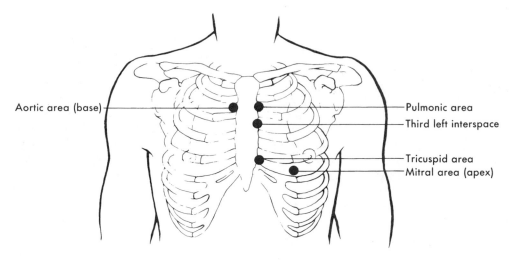

Fig. 2-12 Topographic areas on the precordium for cardiac auscultation. Auscultatory areas do correspond not to the anatomic locations of the valves but to the sites at which the particular valves are heard best. See text for description.

tion clicks occur shortly after S_1, as depicted in Fig. 2-14. Aortic ejection clicks are associated with aortic stenosis, dilatation of the aorta, and hypertension and are heard at the base and apex.

Second heart sound

S_2 is associated with closure of the aortic and pulmonic valves. With completion of ventricular contraction, pressure within the ventricles and great vessels decreases. The ventricular pressure decreases more rapidly than the pressures within the aorta and pulmonary arteries, causing the aortic and pulmonic valves to close. This is followed by the start of ventricular diastole. At the aortic area, or base, S_2 is almost always louder than S_1 (Fig. 2-13, *C*).

The aortic component is widely transmitted to the neck and over the precordium. It is, as a rule, entirely responsible for S_2 at the apex. The pulmonary component is softer than the aortic and is normally heard only at and around the second left interspace (pulmonic area). Splitting of S_2 is therefore usually heard best in this region.

Again, events of the left side of the heart occur before those on the right, and aortic valve closure slightly precedes that of the pulmonic valve. Transient *splitting* of S_2 may be demonstrated in most normal people during inspiration. Closure of the aortic and pulmonary valves during expiration is synchronous because right and left ventricular systoles are approximately equal in duration. With inspiration, venous blood rushes into the thorax from the large systemic venous reservoirs. This action increases venous return and prolongs right ventricular systole by temporarily increasing right ventricular stroke volume, which delays pulmonary valve closure. At the same time, venous return to the left heart diminishes because of the increased pulmonary capacity during inspiration, which decreases left ventricular stroke volume and shortens left ventricular systole. Thus the aortic valve tends to close earlier. These two factors combine to produce transient *physiologic splitting* of S_2 (Fig. 2-13, *D*).

As the pressure in the ventricles decreases below the pressure in the atria, the atrioventricular valves open. The opening of these valves is characteristically silent. However, when the mitral or tricuspid valve is altered, such as in rheumatic heart disease, it produces an *opening snap* in early diastole (Fig. 2-14). The opening snap of the mitral valve is differentiated from S_3 at the apex because it occurs earlier, is sharper and higher pitched, and radiates more widely.

Third heart sound

S_3 occurs early in diastole during the phase of rapid ventricular filling after S_2 (Fig. 2-14). It is a low-pitched sound heard best with the bell of the stethoscope pressed lightly over the apex and the patient in the left lateral decubitus position (Fig. 2-13, *E*). When S_3 is heard in healthy children and young adults, it is called a *physiologic third heart sound* and usually disappears with age. When an S_3 is heard in an older person with heart disease, it usually indicates myocardial failure and is called a *ventricular gallop*. In patients with cardiac disease, the examiner should search carefully for a ventricular gallop, since it is a key diagnostic sign for congestive heart failure from any cause.

Fourth heart sound

S_4 occurs late in diastole, before S_1, and is related to atrial contraction (Fig. 2-14). It is a low-pitched sound heard best at the apex with the bell (Fig. 2-13, *F*). It is uncommon to hear this sound in normal individuals. S_4, or *atrial gallop*, is associated with increased resistance to ventricular filling and is frequently heard in patients with hypertensive cardiovascular disease, coronary artery disease,

HEART SOUNDS   AREA HEARD BEST

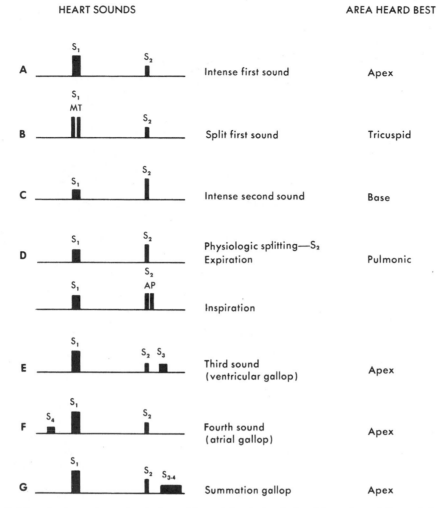

Fig. 2-13 The intensity and splitting of S_1 and S_2, their relationship to S_3 and S_4, and the auscultatory areas where these sounds are heard best. *MP,* Mitral tricuspid; *AP,* aortopulmonic.

myocardiopathy, and aortic stenosis. It is a common finding in patients who have had a myocardial infarction.

Summation gallop

In adults with severe myocardial disease and tachycardia, summation of S_3 and S_4 may occur, producing the so-called summation gallop (Fig. 2-13, *G*).

Murmurs

Murmurs are carefully evaluated and described in a manner that provides maximum information. Murmurs are usually characterized in relation to the following criteria:

1. *Timing.* Does the murmur occur during systole, during diastole, or continuously through both? A murmur may be easily differentiated as systolic or diastolic by palpating the carotid pulse. If the murmur occurs with the pulse, it is systolic; if it does not, it is diastolic. If it occupies all the time period measured, it is described as *holosystolic* (pansystolic) or *holodiastolic* (pandiastolic).

2. *Intensity.* How loud is the murmur? A graded point system is generally accepted to describe the intensity of murmurs, as follows:

Grade 1	Softest audible murmur
Grade 2	Murmur of medium intensity
Grade 3	Loud murmur unaccompanied by thrill
Grade 4	Murmur with thrill
Grade 5	Loudest murmur that cannot be heard with the stethoscope off the chest, thrill associated
Grade 6	Murmur audible with the stethoscope off the chest, thrill associated.

3. *Quality.* What is the tonal characteristic of the murmur? Is it harsh, musical, blowing, or rumbling? The configuration or shape of a murmur further defines its quality. It may be a crescendo (increasing intensity), decrescendo (decreasing intensity), or crescendo-decrescendo (diamond-shaped) type. Fig. 2-15 depicts these configurations.

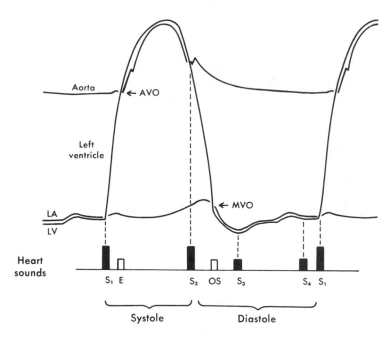

Fig. 2-14 Normal and abnormal heart sounds during a complete cardiac cycle as correlated with left-sided heart pressure waves. Right-sided heart pressures have been omitted for simplification. At the onset of ventricular systole, left ventricular *(LV)* pressure exceeds left atrial *(LA)* pressure to close the mitral valve, producing S_1 (in association with tricuspid valve closure). When LV pressure exceeds aortic pressure, the aortic valve opens *(AVO)*. With valvular disease and hypertension, aortic valve opening may be audible and heard as an early ejection click *(E)*. When aortic pressure exceeds LV pressure, the aortic valve closes to produce S_2 in association with pulmonic valve closure. When LV pressure drops below LA pressure, the mitral valve opens *(MVO)*. With thickening of the mitral valve as a result of rheumatic heart disease, an opening snap *(OS)* is produced in early diastole. During rapid ventricular filling, an S_3, or ventricular gallop, is produced in patients with myocardial failure. Late in diastole an S_4, or atrial gallop, is produced in association with atrial contraction, resulting from increased resistance to ventricular filling.

4. *Pitch*. What is the sound frequency of the murmur? Is it high, medium, or low? If the murmur is heard best with the diaphragm of the stethoscope, it is high pitched. If it is heard best with the bell, it is low pitched. If it is heard equally well with either the bell or the diaphragm, it is medium pitched.
5. *Location*. Over what area on the precordium is the murmur heard best? Is it the aortic area, the pulmonic area, the tricuspid area, or the mitral area?
6. *Radiation*. Is there transmission of the murmur elsewhere in the body? Does it radiate across the chest, into the axilla, into the neck, or down the left sternal border?

In addition, each of these characteristics is further evaluated as it is influenced by the patient's position and respiration. Asking the patient to sit up, exhale, lean forward, and hold the breath may make aortic murmurs easier to hear. The left lateral decubitus position makes mitral murmurs more easily heard.

Systolic murmurs. Systolic murmurs are the most common murmurs and generally are ejection or regurgitant murmurs. *Functional* or innocent systolic murmurs are common in young people and should be distinguished from murmurs that represent valvular heart disease. Functional murmurs occur during ejection, are short (less than two thirds of systole), are grade 2 or less in intensity (they may become inaudible if the patient raises from a supine to a sitting position), and are heard best over the pulmonary outflow tract.

Midsystolic (ejection) murmurs. *Aortic stenosis* and *pulmonic stenosis* produce systolic ejection murmurs that begin after S_1, swell to a crescendo in midsystole, decrease in intensity, and terminate before S_2, generated by closure of the appropriate valve (Fig. 2-15, *A*). The murmur may be harsh or musical and is usually high pitched because of the high velocity of blood flow. Aortic valve murmurs frequently radiate from the second right interspace to the cardiac apex and the carotid arteries. A systolic thrill may be

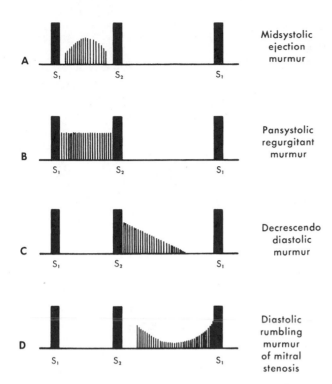

Fig. 2-15 Configuration of murmurs. **A,** Aortic and pulmonic stenosis produce systolic ejection murmurs that begin after S$_1$, swell to a crescendo in midsystole, decrease in intensity (decrescendo), and terminate before S$_2$. **B,** Tricuspid and mitral regurgitation and ventricular septal defects produce pansystolic (holosystolic) murmurs that last throughout ventricular systole; usually no interval can be heard between S$_1$ and S$_2$. **C,** Aortic and pulmonic regurgitation produce murmurs that begin early in diastole, immediately after S$_2$, and then diminish in intensity (decrescendo). **D,** Mitral and tricuspid stenosis produce murmurs that begin during early diastole, have a rumbling or rolling quality, and terminate in late diastole with a crescendo effect.

present. Characteristically, a pulmonic stenosis murmur is heard better at the second left interspace.

Holosystolic (regurgitant) murmurs. Holosystolic murmurs last throughout ventricular systole (Fig. 2-15, *B*), and no interval can be heard between S$_1$ and S$_2$. *Tricuspid* and *mitral regurgitation* and *ventricular septal defects* produce holosystolic murmurs resulting from the backflow of blood from the ventricle (high pressure) to the atrium (low pressure) through an incompetent tricuspid or mitral valve or from a higher-pressure ventricle (left) to a low-pressure ventricle (right). The murmurs may be blowing, musical, or harsh and are often high pitched. The tricuspid regurgitation murmur is best heard along the lower left sternal border, and the intensity commonly increases during inspiration. Mitral regurgitation is best heard at the apex with the patient lying on the left side. It often radiates to the left axilla or back.

Myocardial infarction may produce *papillary muscle rupture,* with subsequent mitral insufficiency and predominantly left-sided heart failure. Abnormalities of the chordae tendineae may produce clicking sounds that occur in the middle of ventricular systole and are referred to as *midsystolic clicks.* These may occur with or without a late systolic murmur.

Diastolic murmurs. Diastolic murmurs generally can be classified into two types: the high-pitched decrescendo murmurs of aortic and pulmonic regurgitation and the lower-pitched murmurs of mitral and tricuspid stenosis.

Murmurs of aortic and pulmonic regurgitation begin early in diastole, immediately after S$_2$, and then diminish in intensity (decrescendo), as shown in Fig. 2-15, *C.* They are high pitched and blowing and may vary in intensity roughly according to the size of the leak. The murmur of aortic regurgitation may be heard best at the second right or third left interspace along the left sternal border with the patient holding the breath in expiration while leaning forward. The murmur of pulmonic regurgitation is heard at the upper left border of the sternum and cannot be distinguished from its aortic counterpart by auscultation alone.

Mitral stenosis characteristically produces a low-pitched, localized apical, diastolic rumble, which may be accentuated in late diastole (Fig. 2-15, *D*), when atrial systole causes increased flow across the narrowed mitral valve. A sharp mitral "opening snap" frequently initiates the murmur in early diastole. In addition, a loud, sharp S$_1$ and accentuation of S$_2$ often accompany mitral stenosis. The murmur of mitral stenosis is usually confined to the apex and may be enhanced by mild exercise or by the patient lying on the left side. The *tricuspid stenosis* murmur is heard near the tricuspid area and is often accentuated along the left sternal border by inspiration.

Continuous murmurs. Murmurs audible in systole and diastole are usually caused by connections between the arterial and venous or systemic and pulmonary circulations. A patent ductus arteriosus produces such a murmur. Table 2-1 summarizes the characteristics of the most common heart murmurs.

Pericardial friction rub. An extracardiac sound that may be detected during auscultation is the pericardial friction rub. It is a sign of pericardial inflammation, and in its complete form, it exhibits three components. One component is associated with ventricular systole; the second is associated with the phase of rapid ventricular filling early in diastole, and the third is associated with atrial systole. If only the systolic component of the rub is present, it may be misinterpreted as a scratchy murmur. With the patient lying flat, the pericardial friction rub is best heard in the third or fourth interspace to the left of the sternum, although the location may be variable. There is little radiation, and the quality of the sound is a leathery, high-pitched, multiphasic, scratchy rub, which sounds like two pieces of sandpaper being rubbed together.

TABLE 2-1 Characteristics of Types of Valvular Heart Disease: Description of Murmurs

Time	Quality	Pitch (Frequency)	Location of Maximum Intensity	Radiation or Transmission	Other Signs	Condition	Causes
Systolic (ejection)	Crescendo-decrescendo (diamond-shaped) Harsh Rough	Variable pitch	Second interspace (aortic area)	Carotid arteries and apex	Slow, rising "anacrotic" Sustained pulse Left ventricle lift Systolic thrill Ejection "click" Diminished aortic closing sound	Aortic stenosis (narrowing of valve)	Rheumatic heart disease Calcification Congenital heart disease
Diastolic	Blowing that is loudest just after S_2, and that diminishes during diastole (decrescendo)	High pitch	Second right interspace; third left interspace or along left sternal border with patient leaning forward and holding breath	—	Wide pulse pressure Left ventricular lift Brisk, quick pulses (water hammer) Tambour aortic closing sound	Aortic regurgitation (blood flowing back from aorta into left ventricle)	Rheumatic heart disease Syphilitic heart disease Calcification Cystic medial necrosis
	Rumbling, presystolic accentuation in sinus rhythm	Low pitch	Apex (well localized), left lateral decubitus position (best)	—	Development of atrial fibrillation (often) Loud S_1 Opening snap	Mitral stenosis (narrowing of valve; blood flowing through valve during diastole)	Rheumatic heart disease Congenital heart disease Tumor (myxoma)
Holosystolic	Blowing	High pitch	Apex, left lateral decubitus position (best)	Axilla and back	S_3 (common)	Mitral regurgitation ("leaky" valve—blood reentering left atrium from left ventricle during systole)	Rheumatic heart disease Congenital heart disease Papillary muscle dysfunction or rupture Chordae tendineae dysfunction or rupture Heart failure associated with left ventricular dilatation from any cause
Variable Late systolic, which can become holosystolic	Crescendo-decrescendo whooping, honking	High	Apex with patient in left lateral decubitus position Murmur earlier in systole caused by decreased venous return (sitting, standing, and performing Valsalva's maneuver) Murmur later in systole caused by increased venous return (squatting, lying down, and elevating legs)	—	Loud mitral component of S_1, early midsystolic or late systolic nonejection click, intermittent atrial and ventricular dysrhythmias	Mitral valve prolapse syndrome— billowing upward and backward of one or both valve leaflets into the left atrium during systole	Marfan's syndrome Rheumatic endocarditis Mitral valve surgery Trauma Lupus erythematosus Congestive cardiomyopathy

Dysrhythmias

Assess the patient for dysrhythmias, including tachydysrhythmias; bradydysrhythmias; atrial, junctional, or ventricular dysrhythmias; first-, second-, or third-degree heart blocks; and premature atrial, junctional, or ventricular beats. Investigate hemodynamic symptoms associated with the dysrhythmia such as hypotension, dizziness, confusion, or decreased cardiac or urinary output.

Cardiac output and cardiac index

Patients in critical care units sometimes require cardiac output monitoring. Normal cardiac output is 5 L/min[4] (see Chapter 1). Also evaluate the cardiac index. The normal cardiac index is 3.5 L/min/m^2 and ranges from 2.5 to 4.5 L/min/m^2. The cardiac index is derived by dividing the cardiac output by the body surface area[8] (see Chapter 1).

Pulmonary artery and pulmonary capillary wedge pressures

Evaluate the patient's pulmonary artery pressure (PAP) and pulmonary capillary wedge pressure (PCWP). Normal PAP is less than 25 mm Hg systolic and 5 to 10 mm Hg diastolic, with a mean PAP of less than 13 mm Hg.[4] Normal PCWP ranges from 4 to 12 mm Hg (see Chapter 3).

Serum enzyme levels

Evaluate the levels of the patient's serum cardiac enzymes, including creatine phosphokinase (CPK), CPK-MB isoenzyme, lactate dehydrogenase (LDH), and LDH isoenzymes,[4,16] (see Chapter 3). Refer to your institution's designated normal values.

Oxygenation
Dyspnea and orthopnea

Explore whether the patient has complaints of dyspnea (see box). Dyspnea is labored or difficult breathing; it accompanies a number of cardiac conditions and is a manifestation of congestive heart failure. It commonly occurs with exertion and may be affected by position. Dyspnea varies in degree; the amount of exertion required to cause it and the amount of rest necessary to relieve it should be quantified carefully. *Paroxysmal nocturnal dyspnea* occurs at night; the patient awakens with a terrifying sensation of suffocating. The distress diminishes after sitting up for a few minutes. *Orthopnea* is associated with congestive heart failure; the patient has difficulty breathing when lying flat in bed and requires two or more pillows for sleep. Thus when evaluating dyspnea, determine when the dyspnea occurs, what precipitates it, what alleviates it, and what body position is associated with it.

Respiratory rate, rhythm, depth, and expansion

Determine the patient's rate, rhythm, and depth of respirations. Under normal conditions, the adult breathes comfortably 16 to 20 times per minute. Observe the depth of breathing to determine whether it is shallow, moderate, or deep. Investigate if the breathing is labored or unlabored and if the patient is expending a great deal of energy to breathe. Observe whether the patient is using accessory muscles to breathe and whether the chest expands symmetrically. Normally the entire rib cage uniformly moves laterally and upward with respiration. Evaluate abnormal breathing patterns such as asymmetric, obstructive, or restrictive breathing. Variations in the normal rate and character of respirations are outlined in the box.

Cough and sputum

If the patient has a cough, observe whether it is productive or nonproductive. Is the patient's cough effort effective or ineffective, and is it weak or strong? What is the color, amount, odor, and consistency of the sputum? Investigate any hemoptysis, or coughing up blood, which may be associated with pulmonary edema or a pulmonary embolus.

Breath sounds

Auscultate the patient's breath sounds on deep inspiration with the mouth open. Auscultation is accomplished in an ordered sequence, beginning with the upper lung fields; one side and then the other are auscultated, and then both are compared down to the level of the diaphragm. All portions of the lung fields—posterior, anterior, and lateral—must be systematically auscultated. The nurse first concentrates on normal breath sounds and then on abnormal sounds.

Normal breath sounds can be categorized as vesicular, bronchial, and bronchovesicular. *Vesicular* breath sounds occur over most of the lungs and have a prominent inspiratory component and a brief expiratory phase. *Bronchial* breath sounds, also called *tracheal breath sounds,* are normally heard over the trachea and main bronchi. These sounds are hollow, tubular, and harsh and are heard best during expiration. *Bronchovesicular* breath sounds are heard over the main stem of the bronchi and represent an intermediate stage between bronchial and vesicular breathing.

Diminished breath sounds occur with bronchial obstruction and with pleural disease associated with the presence of fluid, air, or scar tissue. When airways are narrowed, the breath sounds are characteristically wheezing and whistling in nature, with a prolonged expiratory and a short inspiratory phase, as heard in patients with asthma.

Rales are abnormal sounds that occur when air passes through bronchi that contain fluid of any kind. They are subdivided into crackling sounds, termed *moist rales,* and continuous coarse sounds called *rhonchi.* Rhonchi suggest a pathologic condition in the trachea or larger bronchi, whereas moist medium and fine rales imply bronchiolar and alveolar disease. *Fine rales* are short and high pitched and can be simulated by rubbing a strand of hair between

OXYGENATION HISTORY

Client's Usual Pattern of Respiration

Character of breathing pattern
Presence of allergies?
- Type
- Symptoms
- Frequency of occurrence
- Occurrence of wheezing

Does the Client Smoke or Chew Tobacco?

Number of years of smoking
Number of packs or amount chewed per day

Recent Changes in Breathing Pattern?

Symptoms
Onset (sudden or gradual)
Associated with any other symptoms?
What helps to ease the problem?
What makes it worse?
Is breathing painful?

Past History of Respiratory Problems

Infections
- Type
- Frequency
- Treatment

Cough

Recent or longstanding (how long)?
How often and how much?
Character of the cough (dry, hacking, wet)
Is the cough productive or nonproductive of sputum?
Character of the sputum
Color
Viscosity (fluid, thick, or tenacious)
Amount of sputum (estimate)
Presence of odor

Shortness of Breath (Dyspnea)

Continual or intermittent?
Associated with activity?
What helps to ease the problem?
What makes it worse or better?
Occurrence of any other symptoms?
Affected by different positions?

Stress

Perception of level of stress?
Usual method of coping with stress?
Perception of coping abilities?

Medication

Current listing of prescription and over-the-counter drugs
Purpose for use
Length of time taking medication
Observed side effects

Pulmonary Risk Factors

Family history of hypertension, lung cancer, or other
    cardiopulmonary conditions
Client history of hypertension, lung cancer, or other
    cardiopulmonary conditions

Environmental Influences

Work setting (use of chemicals or gases)
Air pollution
Exposure to radiation

From Bellack JP, Edlund BJ: *Nursing assessment and diagnosis,* ed 2, Boston, 1992, Jones & Bartlett.

the thumb and forefinger next to the ear. *Medium rales* are louder and lower pitched.

In left ventricular failure the presence of rales is one of the earliest physical findings. Rales occur as a result of the transudation of edema fluid into the pulmonary alveoli. At first the alveolar fluid is dependent in location, and rales are present at the base of the lungs. As the failure becomes increasingly severe, the rales become more generalized. The rales of left ventricular failure are typically fine and crepitant, but as failure progresses, they may become moist and coarse.

Pleural friction rub

Inflammation of the visceral and parietal pleurae may result in loss of lubricating fluid so that opposing pleural sur-

faces rub together, producing a low-pitched, coarse, grating sound with respiration. When patients hold their breath, the rub disappears.

Arterial blood gases and oxygen. Evaluate the patient's arterial blood gases. Describe any type of oxygen therapy and the percentage delivered. If the patient is on a mechanical ventilator, describe the type, settings, and the patient's psychologic reaction to the ventilator.

Abdomen
Abdominal physical examination

Inspect the abdomen for rashes, scars, lesions, striae, or dilated veins. Observe if the patient has *ascites* or edema of the abdominal cavity. Note the size, shape, and contour of

VARIATIONS IN RESPIRATION

Tachypnea is rapid shallow breathing that may indicate pain, cardiac insufficiency, anemia, fever, or pulmonary problems.

Bradypnea is slow breathing resulting from opiates, coma, excessive alcohol intake, and increased intracranial pressure.

Hyperventilation is simultaneous rapid, deep breathing found in extreme anxiety states, in diabetic acidosis, and after vigorous exercise.

Cheyne-Stokes respiration is periodic breathing with *hyperpnea* (increased depth of breathing) alternating with *apnea* (cessation of breathing), encountered in cardiac failure and central nervous system disease.

Sighing respiration is a normal respiratory rhythm that is interrupted by a deep inspiration and then by a prolonged expiration accompanied by an audible sigh. This is often associated with emotional depression.

Dyspnea is a conscious difficulty or effort in breathing. *Orthopnea* occurs when the patient assumes an elevated position of the trunk at rest to breathe more comfortably. Dyspnea is a cardinal sign of left ventricular failure and may also occur in certain lung disorders.

Obstructive breathing is air trapping. In obstructive pulmonary diseases such as emphysema and asthma, it is easier for air to enter the lungs than for it to leave. During rapid respiration, sufficient time for full expiration is not available and air becomes trapped in the lungs as airways collapse. The patient's chest overexpands, and breathing becomes more shallow. Expiratory wheezes may be present.

the abdomen. Auscultate the abdomen for bowel sounds and determine their frequency, quality, and pitch. Auscultation is performed before palpation so that bowel sounds are not altered. Use the following code for classifying bowel sounds:

$$
\begin{array}{ll}
0 & = \text{Absent} \\
1+ & = \text{Hypoactive} \\
2+ & = \text{Normal} \\
3+ & = \text{Hyperactive}
\end{array}
$$

Percuss the abdomen to determine liver borders, gastric air bubbles (in left upper quadrant), splenic dullness, air, fluid, or masses. Palpate the abdomen to determine organ enlargement, muscle spasm or rigidity, masses, involuntary guarding, rebound tenderness, or pain.[8,9,17] Determine if the bladder is distended.

Neurologic Functioning

The initial part of the neurologic examination was discussed earlier in this chapter. This section briefly discusses physical examination techniques for motor and sensory function.

Muscle strength

Assess the strength of the upper and lower extremities.[8,9,17] Compare both sides and observe for deficits.

Senses

Evaluate the status of the patient's senses. Observe if the patient has difficulty seeing and determine whether the patient has cataracts, a false eye, contact lenses, or glasses. Assess the ability to hear normal conversation. Determine if the patient wears a hearing aid and whether it improves hearing. Assess the degree of demonstrated coordination while walking or performing other activities (kinesthetics). Does the patient maintain a sense of balance? Inquire about loss or impairment of taste (gustatory). Does the patient describe a metallic or unusual taste? Question the patient regarding any loss in the sense of touch (tactile impairment). Can the patient distinguish among dull, sharp, and light touches? Explore complaints of numbness, tingling, hypersensitivity, or decreased sensation. Query the patients regarding the sense of smell. Is the patient able to recognize the smell of rubbing alcohol after closing the eyes?

Pupils

Assess the pupils for size, shape, and equality. Determine whether the pupillary reaction to light is brisk, sluggish, or nonreactive.[8,17]

Glasgow coma scale

Determine the patient's level of consciousness using the Glasgow Coma Scale. The three categories of this scale—eye opening, best verbal response, and best motor response—are scored and totaled.[8] The patient who is completely awake scores 15.

Reflexes

Assess deep tendon reflexes. Compare the responses on corresponding sides and grade the responses using the following code[8,17]:

$$
\begin{array}{ll}
0 = & \text{No response} \\
1 = & \text{Sluggish or diminished response} \\
2 = & \text{Active or expected response} \\
3 = & \text{Response that is more brisk than usual} \\
4 = & \text{Brisk or hyperactive response}
\end{array}
$$

Physical Integrity

Assessment of physical integrity provides information related to physical growth and the status of mucous membranes and skin.[6] These are indicators of general health and the level of nutrition and hydration.

Height and weight

Determine the patient's height, weight, and ideal body weight. For men, 5 feet equals 106 pounds; for each additional inch, add 6 pounds. For example, for a man 5 feet 10 inches tall, ideal body weight is 166 pounds. For women, 5 feet equals 100 pounds; for each additional inch, add 5 pounds. For example, for a woman 5 feet 4 inches, ideal body weight is 120 pounds.[19]

Tissue integrity

Explore whether the patient has corneal, mucous membrane, integumentary, or subcutaneous tissue damage such as a crushing injury or intravenous infiltration.

Skin integrity

Assess skin integrity in terms of hydration, vascularity, elasticity, texture, turgor, mobility, and thickness. Does the patient have skin rashes, lesions, petechiae, bruises, abrasions, or surgical incisions? Also investigate other causes of disrupted skin surfaces such as invasive hemodynamic lines, stomas, or tubes.[8,17]

Mouth and throat

Assess the condition and function of the mouth, lips, buccal mucosa, teeth, hard and soft palate, and throat. Is the patient able to bite, chew, taste, and swallow? Is there any oral pain or odor?

Physical Regulation

Regulation of physiologic processes should be assessed. This includes an evaluation of body temperature and hematologic and renal functioning.

Temperature

Assess the patient's temperature. Although several routes are used to assess temperature, rectal temperatures are the most accurate. Normal rectal temperatures range from 36.1° C (97° F) to 37.0° C (99.6° F). In the past, rectal temperatures were avoided in patients with acute myocardial infarction as a precaution against vagal stimulation. However, studies suggest that taking rectal temperatures in such patients is no longer contraindicated.[19] Temperature is measured on a Fahrenheit or centigrade scale. The formula for converting centigrade measurement to Fahrenheit and vice versa follows:

$$\text{Fahrenheit} = 1.8\ (°\text{C}) + 32$$

$$\text{Centigrade} = \frac{°\text{F} - 32}{1.8}$$

WBC count and differential

Elevation of the total white blood cell (WBC) count (leukocytes) usually indicates infection. The differential count is performed to determine the percentage of the types of leukocytes in the blood (that is, neutrophils, lymphocytes, monocytes, eosinophils, and basophils). Elevation of the percentage of neutrophils indicates a bacterial infection. Elevation of the lymphocytes and monocytes indicates a bacterial or viral infection.[16,17]

Urine studies

Record the blood urea nitrogen (BUN) and creatinine levels. Assess the specific gravity of the urine and evaluate additional urine studies, such as a urine culture or an acetone, glucose, blood, or protein level test.[15]

Characteristics of urine

Observe the color of the urine. Is there any blood? Determine if the patient has a urinary catheter, including the type, the length of time it has been inserted, and any problems. Determine the patient's 24-hour urinary output or hourly output as indicated.

Other laboratory data

Assess the patient's laboratory data, which may include blood sodium, potassium, chloride, glucose, cholesterol,

---

NURSING DIAGNOSIS DETERMINATION

Nursing diagnoses are statements of the patient's actual or potential health states and focus on human responses or reactions to that state. These human responses may be any observable manifestation, need, condition, concern, event, dilemma, occurrence, or fact within the target area of nursing practice.

Problem Title

The title or label of the nursing diagnosis gives a concise description of the health state of the patient. The title can be derived from the list from the North American Nursing Diagnosis Association (NANDA), or a new diagnostic category may be developed by the nurse. If may be described as actual, possible, or potential. A possible nursing diagnosis indicates that more data must be collected to be certain of the label. A potential diagnosis is a problem that may occur if the nurse does not initiate nursing measures to prevent it. Examples of problem titles are decreased cardiac output, fear, and impaired skin integrity.

Etiology

Etiology refers to the probable cause of the problem. It can be environmental, psychologic, spiritual, physiologic, sociocultural, or developmental. The term *related to* may be used as the connecting link from the title to the etiology (for example, fear related to inadequate knowledge concerning the cardiac catheterization procedure).

Signs and Symptoms

Signs and symptoms are the defining characteristics, derived from the assessment, that support the problem title and etiology. They can be used to evaluate the patient's progress. For example, the patient states that he is fearful because he has never had a cardiac catheterization and does not know what to expect. Assessment indicates that the patient keeps asking patients and staff members questions about the procedure; he is pacing his hospital room and has an increased heart rate.

and triglyceride levels (determine if these were drawn under fasting conditions), hematocrit, and hemoglobin. Laboratory data might also include a blood coagulation profile or drug toxicity screening.

FORMULATING NURSING DIAGNOSES

Nurses systematically collect and organize data about patient problems and form conclusions or judgments appropriate to their domain of expertise. Nursing practice is guided by a holistic framework that reflects the interconnections of the body and mind. Holistic frameworks convey the oneness and unity of the individual. From this framework, the purpose of a nursing diagnosis is to identify human responses to stressors or other factors that adversely affect the attainment of optimum health.[4,6] Thus a *nursing diagnosis* is defined as a judgment about the health of the person based on the data collected (see box).[6]

REFERENCES

1. Dossey BM and others: *Holistic nursing: a handbook for practice,* Rockville, Md, 1988, Aspen.
2. Carpenito LJ: *Nursing diagnoses: application to clinical practice,* ed 4, Philadelphia, 1992, Lippincott.
3. Kim MJ and others: *Pocket guide to nursing diagnoses,* ed 5, St Louis, 1993, Mosby.
4. Guzzetta CE, Dossey BM: *Cardiovascular nursing: holistic practice,* St Louis, 1992, Mosby.
5. Underhill SL and others: *Cardiac nursing,* Philadelphia, 1989, Lippincott.
6. Bellack JP, Edlund BJ: *Nursing assessment and diagnosis,* Boston, 1992, Jones & Bartlett.
7. Lynam MJ: Taking culture into account: a challenging prospect for cardiovascular nursing, *Can J Cardiovasc Nurs* 2:10, 1991.
8. Malasanos L and others: *Health assessment,* ed 4, St Louis, 1990, Mosby.
9. Bates B: *A guide to physical examination,* ed 5, Philadelphia, 1991, Lippincott.
10. Swartz MH: *Physical diagnosis: history and examination,* Philadelphia, 1989, Saunders.
11. Braunwald E: *Heart disease: a textbook of cardiovascular medicine,* ed 4, Philadelphia, 1991, Saunders.
12. Hurst JW and others, editors: *The heart,* ed 8, New York, 1994, McGraw-Hill.
13. Daily EK, Schroeder JS: *Techniques in bedside hemodynamic monitoring,* ed 5, St Louis, 1994, Mosby.
14. Henneman EA, Henneman PL: Intricacies of blood pressure measurement: reexamining the rituals, *Heart Lung* 18:263, 1989.
15. Kinney MK and others, editors: *AACN's clinical reference for critical-care nursing,* ed 3, St Louis, 1993, Mosby.
16. Thompson J and others: *Mosby's clinical nursing,* ed 3, St Louis, 1993, Mosby.
17. Seidel HM and others: *Mosby's guide to physical examination,* ed 3, St Louis, 1995, Mosby.
18. Guzzetta CE: *Nursing process.* In Dossey BM and others: *Critical care nursing: body-mind-spirit,* ed 3, Philadelphia, 1992, Lippincott.
19. Kirchhoff KT: An examination of the physiologic basis for "coronary precautions," *Heart Lung* 10:874, 1981.

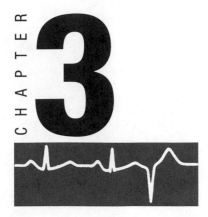

3

Patient Assessment:
Diagnostic Studies

Stephen "Pete" Stribling

As an adjunct to the history and physical examination of the cardiac patient, invasive and noninvasive diagnostic studies reveal valuable information about the status and function of the components of the cardiovascular system. Noninvasive cardiac diagnostic studies do not involve the insertion of vascular devices and include echocardiography and cardiac Doppler studies, exercise and pharmacologic stress testing with or without radionuclide imaging, ambulatory electrocardiogram (ECG) recording, nuclear cardiology tests, and serum enzyme studies. Based on the history, physical examination, and in some situations, noninvasive studies, invasive diagnostic tests may be indicated. These tests would include left ventricular cardiac catheterization with or without ventriculography and coronary angiography, pulmonary artery (PA) pressure monitoring, cardiac electrophysiologic studies, and endomyocardial biopsy.

The applicability of any data from diagnostic studies must be evaluated within the context of the sensitivity, specificity, predictive value, and accuracy of these tests. *Sensitivity* indicates the ability of a test to identify patients with a particular disease (positive test result) from a population, whereas *specificity* is a measure of the frequency with which a test identifies patients without a particular disease (negative test result). A *positive predictive value* is an indication of the percentage of patients with a specific disease in a group

of patients with positive test results. Likewise, *negative predictive value* is an indication of the percentage of patients without disease in a group of patients with negative test results. The diagnostic *accuracy* of a test is the percentage of patients correctly identified by the test and is the function of the sum of the true positives and true negatives divided by the total number of tests. These concepts are represented by the formulas in the box.

The selection and application of invasive and noninvasive diagnostic studies are based on findings in the patient's history and physical examination. In addition, the clinician should remember that not all patients need every test and that no test is completely accurate. Therapeutic decisions should be made with these considerations.

SERUM ENZYME LEVELS IN ACUTE MYOCARDIAL INFARCTION

The most common diagnostic tools used by clinicians to diagnose acute myocardial infarction (MI) involve the analysis of serum enzymes released from the heart muscle after myocardial injury. Three major enzymes that occur with myocardial necrosis are serum glutamic-oxaloacetic transaminase (SGOT), creatine kinase (CK), and lactate dehydrogenase (LDH). CK is present in cardiac and skeletal muscle, as well as in the brain and intestinal tract. Elevation of serum CK levels is seen 4 to 6 hours after the onset of acute MI. Peak levels occur 16 to 30 hours after the on-

---

SENSITIVITY, SPECIFICITY, AND PREDICTIVE VALUE FORMULAS

$$\text{Sensitivity (\%)} = \frac{\text{True positive test results}}{\text{True positive test results } + \text{ False negative test results}}$$

$$\text{Specificity (\%)} = \frac{\text{True negative test results}}{\text{True negative test results } + \text{ False positive test results}}$$

$$\text{Diagnostic accuracy (\%)} = \frac{\text{True positive test results } + \text{ True negative test results}}{\text{Total number of tests performed}}$$

set of an MI and return to normal within 3 to 4 days. Although an elevated total serum CK level is an indicator of an MI, it may be elevated because of treatments such as an intramuscular injection or electrocardioversion, trauma, or a condition such as cerebrovascular accident. Serum CK can be divided into three isoenzymes: CK-MM, found in skeletal muscle; CK-BB, primarily found in brain tissue; and CK-MB, found in cardiac muscle. The level of CK-MB is elevated 3 to 8 hours after an MI, peaks between 10 and 24 hours, and returns to normal after 3 or 4 days. After an acute MI, 5% to 10% of the total serum CK level is CK-MB. If reperfusion of the ischemic myocardium occurs spontaneously or with interventional therapy such as thrombolytic therapy or percutaneous transluminal coronary angioplasty (PTCA), the peak values of total CK and CK-MB occur sooner and may be higher than without reperfusion.[1]

Using high-voltage electrophoresis, CK-MB may be divided into the subforms MB-1 and MB-2. Normally, these subforms are in equilibrium in the plasma, with the ratio of MB-2 to MB-1 being 1:1. After an acute MI, MB-2 is released in minute amounts, with total CK-MB levels remaining within the normal range. However, the ratio of MB-2 to MB-1 may exceed 1.5:1 or greater. This finding, which can be assayed within 6 hours after MI, is diagnostic of myocardial necrosis and may provide an early diagnosis of infarction.[1,2]

Another enzyme released after an MI is LDH, which appears in abnormal amounts in the circulation 24 to 48 hours after the onset of infarction. Peak levels occur in 3 to 6 days and return to normal in 7 to 10 days. LDH is widely distributed throughout body organs such as the heart, kidneys, liver, lungs, and skeletal muscle and red blood cells. As with CK, LDH can be separated into several isoenzymes. Cardiac muscle is particularly rich in one of these isoenzymes, LDH-1. After an MI, LDH-1 levels rise in 8 to 12 hours, peak within 3 to 6 days, and return to normal in 8 to 14 days. Because the levels of LDH-1 are usually lower than those of LDH-2, a value of LDH-1 greater than that of LDH-2 is considered significant and suggests myocardial injury. Because of the relatively late rise and peak of LDH after an MI, serum LDH tests are used in the diagnosis of MI after 48 to 72 hours, whereas CK tests offer an earlier diagnosis. Table 3-1 presents the pattern of cardiac enzyme release after an acute MI.

Serum assays for the proteins troponin-T and myoglobin also offer potential for diagnosis in acute MI. Troponin-T, one of three proteins of the regulatory protein troponin in the myofibril, has isoforms that are cardiac specific. After infarction, troponin-T is elevated for 3½ hours to 10 days, paralleling the initial increase and decrease of CK-MB. Myoglobin, a heme protein, is released earlier from necrotic cells than CK is, and concentrations can increase above normal as early as 1 hour after an MI, with peak levels occurring 4 to 12 hours after infarction.[1]

TABLE 3-1 Cardiac Enzyme Release Patterns After Acute MI			
Enzyme	Elevation	Peak	Return to Normal
Total CK	4-6 hr	16-30 hr	3-4 days
CK-MB	3-8 hr	10-24 hr	3-4 days
Total LDH	24-48 hr	3-6 days	7-10 days
LDH-1	8-12 hr	3-6 days	8-14 days

STRESS TESTING

The exercise stress test is one of the most common non-invasive techniques used to detect coronary artery disease. Cardiovascular responses to physical and emotional stress can result in an increased myocardial oxygen demand. Fixed coronary artery lesions can limit the body's ability to meet this demand with increased coronary arterial blood flow and oxygen supply. The resulting myocardial ischemia is evidenced by symptoms ranging from subtle ECG changes and less serious dysrhythmias to severe angina and ventricular fibrillation. When the exercise stress test is used, an attempt is made to provoke and document, both electrocardiographically and hemodynamically, manifestations of myocardial ischemia, which can then be correlated to the symptoms. Indications for stress testing are many but can be generalized to a few categories: evaluation of chest pain or anginal discomfort, evaluation of dysrhythmias, stratification of high-risk patients (that is, patients who have had an MI), and determination of cardiac reserve and functional capacity.

Exercise stress testing is performed in a controlled environment with appropriate monitoring by trained nurses or physicians. Emergency equipment and medications should be readily available in case the patient has an adverse response to the test. The applicability of stress testing for a particular patient must be determined. Patients who have an acute MI, active unstable angina, resting angina or ECG changes, serious cardiac dysrhythmias, severe left ventricular dysfunction, or significant aortic stenosis are excluded. Special consideration should be given to patients with significant arterial or pulmonary hypertension, less serious dysrhythmias, moderate valvular disease, or moderate left ventricular dysfunction.

Although a stress test can be performed using a bicycle ergometer, a treadmill is more commonly used. Discussion of the protocols for treadmill exercise stress testing is beyond the scope of this text. In general, however, these protocols involve progressive *stages* in which the workload is increased by changing the speed and/or grade of the treadmill. The patient exercises until a target heart rate is achieved, usually about 80% to 85% of the predicted maximum heart rate for the patient's age and sex. The test may be terminated before this target if the patient develops severe chest pain, marked ST-segment changes, hypotension, serious ventricular dysrhythmias, or near-syncope.

Before the stress test is performed, baseline ECG, heart rate, and blood pressure measurements are obtained. Each parameter is monitored at specific intervals throughout exercise and during the recovery phase. In addition, the patient's subjective rating of perceived exertion may be used to quantify effort. A "positive" exercise stress test is an ST-segment depression greater than 1 mm of horizontal or down-sloping that occurs 80 msec after the J point (Fig. 3-1). The magnitude of ST-segment depression and the persistence of ischemic changes during the recovery phase provide an indication of the severity of coronary artery disease.[3] The geographic location of changes on the ECG usually indicates the coronary artery involved; for example, ST-segment changes in the anterior leads of the ECG suggest a left anterior descending coronary artery obstruction.

Stress testing is also useful in the evaluation of patients with known coronary artery disease, such as those who have had an MI, or who have undergone revascularization such as angioplasty, atherectomy, or coronary artery bypass surgery. The exercise stress test can objectively evaluate an individual's functional capacity. This application is especially important for the patient who has angina or valvular heart disease because functional status may determine the timing of medical or surgical intervention. Assessment of functional capacity is also useful in prescribing activity levels and exercise programs for cardiac rehabilitation.

A stress test may be performed to evaluate patients with suspected or known ventricular or supraventricular dysrhythmias. Reduction of vagal tone and an increase in sympathetic activity during exercise contribute to the induction and propagation of dysrhythmias. Exercise stress testing can be used to elicit these dysrhythmias and to evaluate antidysrhythmic therapy. In addition, exercise testing can provide evidence of heart disease because dysrhythmia prevalence, frequency, and complexity are directly related to the type and severity of underlying heart disease.[4]

Exercise stress testing is also used as a prognostic indicator of future cardiac events in patients with stable and unstable coronary syndromes. Occurrence of ischemic

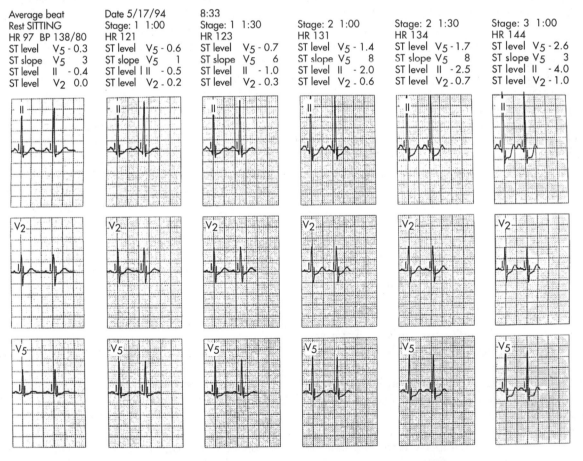

Fig. 3-1   Exercise stress electrograph demonstrating marked, progressive ST-segment depression in leads II, V_2, and V_5 from rest to stage 3 using a Bruce protocol. *HR,* Heart rate; *BP,* blood pressure.   (Courtesy The Heart Center at Baptist, Mississippi Baptist Medical Center, Jackson, Miss.)

changes during exercise testing, both with and without pain, indicates an increased risk of future cardiac death and MI, thus guiding decisions to perform further evaluation.[5]

RADIONUCLIDE IMAGING

Radionuclide imaging of the heart uses radioactive tracers in the assessment of normal and abnormal cardiac function. Techniques used to assess myocardial perfusion and viability, MI location and size, and left ventricular ejection fraction (EF) provide an indicator of overall cardiac function.

Myocardial Perfusion Imaging

Radionuclide imaging with the radioactive tracer thallium-201 used during exercise stress testing provides information regarding the extent and location of myocardial ischemia and potential viability of damaged myocardium. When injected intravenously, thallium-201 is distributed in the myocardium proportional to coronary blood flow and myocardial perfusion. Its uptake by viable myocardial tissue is due to chemical properties similar to those of potassium. In decreased perfusion states such as in ischemic events or in cases of nonviable myocardial tissue, uptake is decreased or absent. This property forms the basis for radionuclide assessment of myocardial perfusion and tissue viability.

During exercise, coronary artery dilatation occurs, and coronary blood flow increases 4 to 5 times that of normal resting values. A fixed coronary artery lesion dilates insufficiently, resulting in a proportionally decreased regional blood flow and thallium-201 uptake by the myocardium. The radiologic documentation of this finding by scintigraphy is termed a *perfusion defect*. This perfusion defect may be the result of exercise-induced ischemia or a previous MI with a nonviable scar. After documentation of a perfusion defect, the patient is re-scanned after a period of time sufficient for the redistribution of thallium-201, usually 2 to 4 hours. During this time, ischemic viable myocardium demonstrates an increase in thallium content despite the presence of a severe coronary artery stenosis. Exercise-induced ischemia typically produces transient perfusion defects immediately after exercise (Fig. 3-2, *A*), whereas myocardial infarction with resulting scar formation results in a perfusion defect that remains during redistribution (Fig. 3-2, *B*).

Thallium-201 myocardial perfusion imaging may also be used to determine the risk of future cardiac events in patients with coronary artery disease. Patients with a large perfusion abnormality (involving more than 15% of the myocardium) demonstrated on exercise SPECT thallium imaging have a 75% event-free survival rate compared with a 95% rate in patients with a small abnormality or no abnormality.[6] In addition, patients with stable chest pain and a fixed perfusion defect demonstrated on dipyridamole thallium imaging have a significantly increased risk of future cardiac events compared with patients with normal scans.[7]

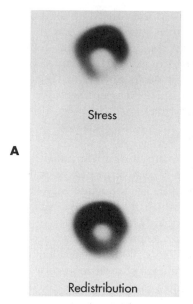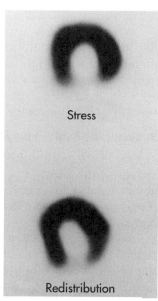

Fig. 3-2 Stress thallium single-photon emission computed tomography (SPECT) myocardial perfusion imaging. **A,** Transient inferior perfusion defect consistent with exercise-induced inferior myocardial ischemia. **B,** Persistent inferior perfusion defect consistent with scar formation after inferior MI.   (Courtesy The Heart Center at Baptist, Mississippi Baptist Medical Center, Jackson, Miss.)

Pharmacologic stress testing with dipyridamole or adenosine may be used with patients unable to exercise sufficiently to reach an adequate heart rate. Dipyridamole and adenosine are potent coronary vasodilators and, when injected intravenously, cause an increase in myocardial blood flow similar to that seen in exercise stress. This increase in coronary blood flow occurs in normal arteries but not in stenotic vessels. The result is a nonhomogeneity of thallium distribution that reflects the pattern of underlying coronary artery disease. Patients who should be considered for pharmacologic stress imaging include those who have severe peripheral vascular disease, significant musculoskeletal disorders (that is, lower-extremity arthritis or amputation), or neurologic disease. Dipyridamole may also be used with patients on β-adrenergic blockers, which attenuate heart rate response in exercise.[8]

MI Imaging

MI imaging uses another radioactive tracer, technetium-99, to localize and size an MI. The technique of technetium-99 imaging involves injection of the radioisotope followed by scanning 4 hours later. During this period, technetium-99 concentrates in necrotic myocardial tissue because of the binding of the radiopharmaceutical to intracellular calcium within damaged myocardial cells. This local concentration and subsequent imaging give the test the name "hot spot" imaging. Infarct imaging with technetium-99 may be useful in clinical settings in which diagnosis of an acute MI is difficult, such as with equivocal serum enzyme levels and ECG findings or age-indeterminate MI. However, the technique's usefulness in the setting of acute MI is limited because optimal uptake does not occur until 2 to 10 days after the event.[8] In addition, this test is not sensitive to small or subendocardial infarctions.

Radionuclide Angiocardiography

One of the most useful applications of nuclear medicine techniques for the patient with cardiac disease is the evaluation of ventricular performance. Radionuclide angiocardiography is a reproducible method of assessing global and regional left ventricular performance.

Global left ventricular systolic pump performance is termed *ejection fraction (EF)*. With radionuclide techniques, the EF is calculated as the percentage of total ventricular radioactive counts ejected from the ventricle during each contraction. A normal EF calculated by this technique is greater than 50%. In addition, regional wall motion can be assessed.

The most commonly used radionuclide technique for assessing ventricular performance is the multiple gated acquisition (MUGA) blood pool imaging. With this technique, the patient's blood cells are tagged with technetium 99. Changes in radioactive counts are therefore proportional to the changes in blood volume of the cardiac chambers during the cardiac cycle. Gating is performed by synchronizing radioactive counting and image acquisition to the patient's ECG, providing a timing reference within the cardiac cycle.

Information is obtained over a period of several hundred heart beats, and the individual beats are then added together and averaged to create a representative cycle of the patient's ventricular performance. Calculations are then performed to determine the percent change of radioactive counts from end-diastole (maximum volume) to end-systole (minimum volume). This percent change is expressed as the EF. Fig. 3-3 shows end-diastolic and end-systolic dimensions of the left ventricle in a MUGA scan. In addition to measuring EF, gated pool blood imaging provides an excellent means of evaluating left ventricular regional wall motion. Thus one can determine whether a segment of the left ventricle is hypokinetic or akinetic or whether a left ventricular aneurysm is present.

Radionuclide angiocardiography with gated blood pool imaging can be used with exercise stress testing using a bicycle ergometer. Patients with normal ventricular performance demonstrate a 5% or greater increase in left ventricular EF during exercise stress. In contrast, most patients with coronary artery disease who develop myocardial ischemia during exercise fail to evidence an increase or demonstrate a decrease in EF during exercise. In addition to an abnormal EF response, the patient with exercise-induced ischemia may also develop abnormalities in regional wall motion that can localize the site of exercise-induced isch-

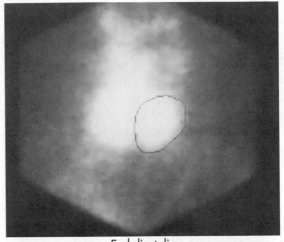

End diastolic

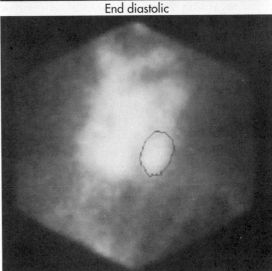

End systolic

Fig. 3-3 MUGA scan of the left ventricle. End-diastolic and end-systolic volumes are outlined with an estimated EF of 60%. (Courtesy The Heart Center at Baptist, Mississippi Baptist Medical Center, Jackson, Miss.)

emia. Therefore MUGA scans with stress provide an alternative to thallium studies for the detection of coronary artery disease. Radionuclide angiocardiography is also useful as a noninvasive test for screening patients who might have left ventricular dysfunction after MI, since patients with large infarctions and a markedly diminished EF are at increased risk for death. Other uses of radionuclide angiocardiography include quantification of left ventricular function or dysfunction before initiation of some antidysrhythmic agents with powerful negative inotropic effects or before and during treatment of cancer with certain chemotherapeutic agents.

OTHER CARDIAC IMAGING TECHNIQUES

Emerging cardiac imaging modalities are adding to the array of techniques that may be used to assess cardiac anatomy and function. Ultrafast computed tomography (cine CT), magnetic resonance imaging (MRI), and positron emission tomography (PET) provide information about internal cardiac anatomy, cardiac tissue characteristics, regional myocardial perfusion, coronary blood flow, myocardial function, and myocardial metabolism.

Cine CT uses ultrafast imaging capabilities to provide high-resolution definition of cardiac structures and function to aid in the assessment of global and regional ventricular performance, measurement of cardiac volumes and mass, and assessment of myocardial perfusion. MRI is particularly useful in evaluating intracardiac thrombi, intracardiac and paracardiac tumors, ischemic heart disease, cardiomyopathy, pericardial disease, congenital heart disease, and thoracic aortic disease. PET imaging involves the use of positron-emitting radiotracers that are distributed within the myocardium in direct proportion to blood flow; PET is used to assess regional blood flow and myocardial perfusion.[9]

AMBULATORY ECG

Ambulatory monitoring, long-term ECG recording, and *Holter monitoring* are synonymous with *ambulatory ECG.* Ambulatory ECG has had widespread application as a noninvasive tool since Holter demonstrated this technique. Lightweight, battery-powered recorders worn continuously for at least 24 hours can collect one- or two-lead ECG data for subsequent analysis. A two-lead system is preferred, since the extra lead is more sensitive in documenting ST-segment abnormalities, identifying aberrant conduction, and screening out artifact. Attached to a belt or shoulder strap, these recorders are used in the hospital, or the patient may be out of the hospital and pursue normal daily activities. A clock on the recorder correlates ECG events with the patient's log of symptoms, activities, and medications.

Computers scan and analyze the record with the technician's input for interpretation. Data are reported by mounting representative printout strips of abnormalities (Fig. 3-4) or those that correspond with patient log entries. A summary of the frequency of ventricular and supraventricular ectopy, heart rate changes, and shifts in the ST segment are displayed (Fig. 3-5). The physician must correlate data from the ambulatory ECG reports with the total patient picture, since it is common for long-term ECG recordings to show abnormalities, even in patients with normal cardiac function. For example, marked sinus bradycardia, sinus pauses, premature atrial and ventricular complexes, transient atrioventricular block, and short runs of atrial tachycardia have been recorded in the normal population.

In general, ambulatory ECG is used to document abnormal cardiac electrical activity and to correlate this activity to patient activity or symptoms. Indications for

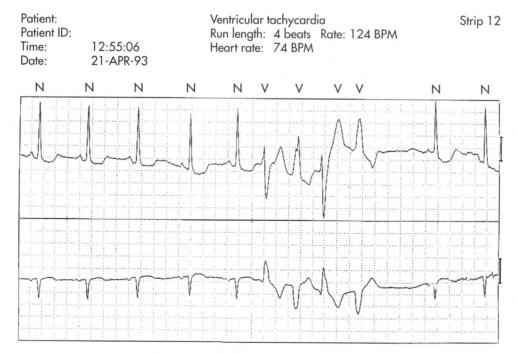

Fig. 3-4 Ambulatory ECG printout showing complex ventricular ectopy. *BPM,* Beats per minute. (Courtesy The Heart Center at Baptist, Mississippi Baptist Medical Center, Jackson, Miss.)

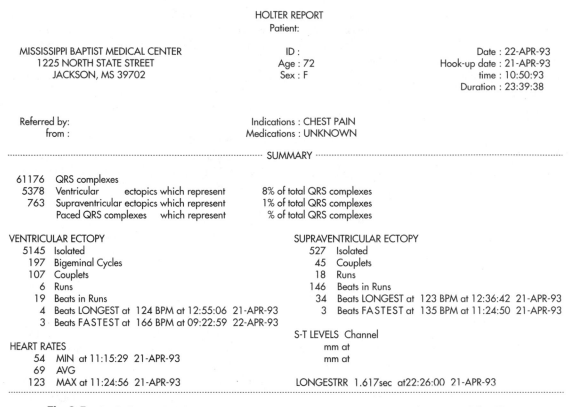

HOLTER REPORT
Patient:

MISSISSIPPI BAPTIST MEDICAL CENTER	ID :	Date : 22-APR-93
1225 NORTH STATE STREET	Age : 72	Hook-up date : 21-APR-93
JACKSON, MS 39702	Sex : F	time : 10:50:93
		Duration : 23:39:38

Referred by:
    from :

Indications : CHEST PAIN
Medications : UNKNOWN

--- SUMMARY ---

61176	QRS complexes	
5378	Ventricular ectopics which represent	8% of total QRS complexes
763	Supraventricular ectopics which represent	1% of total QRS complexes
	Paced QRS complexes which represent	% of total QRS complexes

VENTRICULAR ECTOPY
5145	Isolated
197	Bigeminal Cycles
107	Couplets
6	Runs
19	Beats in Runs
4	Beats LONGEST at 124 BPM at 12:55:06 21-APR-93
3	Beats FASTEST at 166 BPM at 09:22:59 22-APR-93

SUPRAVENTRICULAR ECTOPY
527	Isolated
45	Couplets
18	Runs
146	Beats in Runs
34	Beats LONGEST at 123 BPM at 12:36:42 21-APR-93
3	Beats FASTEST at 135 BPM at 11:24:50 21-APR-93

HEART RATES
54	MIN at 11:15:29 21-APR-93
69	AVG
123	MAX at 11:24:56 21-APR-93

S-T LEVELS Channel
    mm at
    mm at

LONGESTRR 1.617sec at22:26:00 21-APR-93

Fig. 3-5 Ambulatory ECG summary report. *BPM,* Beats per minute. (Courtesy The Heart Center at Baptist, Mississippi Baptist Medical Center, Jackson, Miss.)

ambulatory ECG include evaluating symptoms and documenting suspected cardiac dysrhythmias, documenting myocardial ischemia, diagnosing silent ischemia, and evaluating antidysrhythmic therapy and pacemaker function. Because of the episodic nature of dysrhythmias, detection of complex ventricular dysrhythmias varies with the duration of the recording. Detection of the highest premature ventricular complex grade is determined within 18 to 36 hours in 95% of the population.

Serial ambulatory ECG recordings may be used to judge the efficacy of antidysrhythmic drug therapy. Because of the spontaneous variability in the occurrence of a dysrhythmia, the use of ambulatory ECG in this manner may be limited. An 83% reduction in premature ventricular complexes, a 65% decrease in ventricular tachycardia, and a 75% reduction in ventricular couplets are considered a demonstration of antidysrhythmic drug efficacy rather than spontaneous variability of dysrhythmia occurrence alone.[10]

Although ambulatory ECG recordings are useful in correlating episodes of chest pain with diagnostic ST-segment abnormalities, there are some limitations. First, since only two ECG leads are usually represented, significant ST-segment changes can occur during an episode of chest pain, but ST-T wave changes from the area of the heart involved

may not be recorded. Second, false-positive ST-segment shifts with changes in position, hyperventilation, or heart rate may occur.[11] Despite these limitations in patients with typical effort angina, it is possible that these recordings may be more useful than stress testing for patients with suspected coronary artery spasm. These patients have episodes of chest pain that cannot be induced routinely by stress testing, and ambulatory ECG recording may be useful in screening for ST-segment abnormalities during episodes of spontaneous chest pain.

ECHOCARDIOGRAPHY

Echocardiography is one of the most commonly used noninvasive diagnostic procedures used in the assessment of cardiovascular function. Short pulses of ultrasonic sound are used to visualize the anatomy, motion, and function of the cardiac walls and chambers, cardiac valves, pericardium, and great vessels. Wall thickness and motion, cardiac chamber dimensions, cardiac valvular orifice dimension and leaflet movement, pericardial thickness and fluid volume estimation, great vessel dimensions, and congenital abnormalities may also be evaluated with echocardiography.

Two approaches to echocardiography are transthoracic and transesophageal. In *transthoracic echocardiography,* a transducer is placed onto the external chest wall overlying the precordium to transmit and receive the pulsed, ultrasonic sound waves. A lubricating gel is used to maintain air-free contact with the chest wall and to provide ease of movement of the transducer on the chest wall as cardiac structures are examined. The sound waves are transmitted through the chest wall, reflected off the underlying cardiac structures, and received by the transducer. These reflected pulses are analyzed and displayed by the echocardiograph and recorded on a strip recorder or videotape. *Transesophageal echocardiography* is performed by placing the transesophageal transducer (much like a gastroscope) into the patient's esophagus, orienting it to view the heart, and advancing or withdrawing the transducer to visualize the different cardiac structures and great vessels.

Techniques

There are three techniques by which an echocardiogram can be obtained: M-mode echocardiography; two-dimensional or cross-sectional echocardiography; and Doppler echocardiography. These techniques use the principle of transmission and reflection of high-frequency sound waves to visualize cardiac structures.

M-mode (or motion) echocardiography uses a single ultrasound beam to, over time, record cardiac structures by their distance from the transducer. This beam is swept across the cardiac structures, and the resulting time-motion information is displayed on a strip chart recording with the ECG of the patient. M-mode echocardiography records detailed, subtle motions of cardiac structures and is useful in measuring cardiac chamber dimensions and wall thickness.[12]

Two-dimensional (2D) echocardiography uses a planar beam of ultrasound that can be transmitted by a single crystal that oscillates or rotates throughout a given plane or by a series of crystals, with each crystal transmitting ultrasound through a different point on the chest. The resulting "echo" information is recorded on videotape for further interpretation. Because of the high resolution of cardiac structures and their movements, 2D echocardiography provides detailed information about cardiac anatomy and function and forms the basis for echocardiographic assessment of the heart. 2D echocardiography allows for quantitative measurements of cardiac dimensions, valvular areas, and chamber volumes. In addition, 2D echocardiography provides the framework for cardiac Doppler and color-flow studies.[12]

Doppler echocardiography provides information about the flow of blood within the heart, throughout its chambers, across the valves, and in the great vessels. This information is gained using the principle known as *Doppler shift,* the difference between reflected frequency and transmitted frequency. By identification of this Doppler shift, the forward or backward velocity and the flow characteristics of blood can be determined.

Applications
Normal heart

Figs. 3-6 and 3-7 show normal M-mode and 2D echocardiograms in two patients. Of importance is the relative size and position of the cardiac chambers and the motion of the cardiac valves during systole and diastole.

Cardiac chamber size and functions

The size of the cardiac chambers can be assessed by echocardiography. The diameter of the left ventricle, left atrium, and aortic root can be measured. Measurements of the right ventricle are less reliable because of its shape and the fact that it varies in size with patient position. 2D echocardiography allows a more accurate visualization of the cardiac chambers and valves, their motion during the cardiac cycle, and their spatial relationships. In addition, the aorta, PA, and venae cavae can be visualized.

With 2D echocardiography, segmental wall motion of the left ventricle can be assessed via different views. Ischemic segments may show hypokinesis, akinesis, or dyskinesis. Echocardiography may be performed with exercise to induce wall-motion abnormalities that may not be seen at rest. 2D echocardiography also is useful in identifying the presence of mural thrombi, ventricular aneurysms, and intracardiac masses and the existence and degree of left and right ventricular hypertrophy, dilatation, or both.

Hypertrophic cardiomyopathy is characterized by asymmetric hypertrophy, usually of the interventricular septum. Systolic anterior motion of the anterior leaflet of the mitral valve suggests associated left ventricular outflow tract obstruction, which may be dynamic. Generalized depression of ventricular function suggests cardiomyopathy, diffuse ischemia, a negative inotropic drug effect, or severe valvular disease. Segmental left ventricular wall-motion abnormalities suggest infarction, ischemia, or an infiltrative process.

Valvular functions

Echocardiography can be used to evaluate patients with valvular heart disease. Echocardiography is most commonly used in the diagnosis of mitral valve prolapse, stenosis, or regurgitation as well as aortic stenosis or regurgitation. Pericardial disease can also be evaluated using echocardiography.

Mitral valve

M-mode echocardiographic features of mitral stenosis include a thickened or calcified mitral valve, a decrease in the size of the valvular opening, a decrease in the EF slope of the valve, and parallel motion of the fused mitral leaflets during diastole. Commissural fusion with doming of the leaflets on 2D echocardiography also indicates mitral stenosis. The severity of the mitral valve stenosis can be assessed using 2D echocardiography because the size of the orifice can be measured directly from the image in the short-axis view. Also, changes in the chamber size, such as dilatation

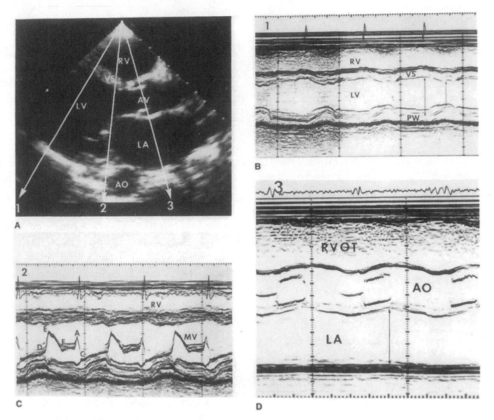

Fig. 3-6   Normal M-mode echocardiogram. **A,** An M-mode cursor is placed along different levels (*1,* ventricular level; *2,* mitral valve level; *3,* aortic valve level) with 2D echocardiogram guidance. **B,** (ventricular), **C** (mitral valve), and **D** (aortic valve), Corresponding M-mode recordings are represented. *RV,* Right ventricle; *LV,* left ventricle; *VS,* ventricular septum; *AV,* aortic valve; *LA,* left atrium; *AO,* aorta; *MV,* mitral valve; *PW,* posterior left ventricular wall; *RVOT,* right ventricular outflow tract.   (From Oh JK and others: *The echo manual,* Boston, 1994, Little, Brown; copyrighted by Mayo Foundation, Rochester, Minn.)

of the left atrium, further suggest the severity of the stenosis. On the other hand, mitral valve regurgitation is not directly assessed with echocardiography. Its presence may be suggested by increases in the size of the left ventricle and left atrium. Hemodynamic assessment of mitral stenosis and evaluation of mitral regurgitation are further discussed in the section related to Doppler echocardiography.

Auscultation of a midsystolic click and a late systolic murmur in an otherwise healthy person suggests mitral valve prolapse. Specific diagnosis of mitral valve prolapse is accomplished with echocardiography. Echocardiographic findings include bowing of the posterior mitral leaflet into the left atrium during systole and abrupt posterior displacement of the posterior mitral leaflet in midsystole.[13]

A flail mitral valve secondary to infective endocarditis or a ruptured chorda tendinea can be identified from the echocardiogram. The flail leaflet may appear to displace posteriorly but to a much greater degree than in mitral valve prolapse. Also, the motion of the mitral valve leaflets may be in an irregular pattern. With 2D echocardiography,

the leaflet may prolapse entirely into the left atrium during systole. Through the use of M-mode echocardiography, various hemodynamic states, such as low cardiac output (CO) and decreased ventricular compliance, may be manifested by a diminished amplitude of the mitral valve opening or by a delayed mitral valve closure.

Aortic valve

Echocardiography is useful in determining whether the aortic valve is tricuspid or bicuspid, thickened, and/or calcified. The severity of aortic stenosis is difficult to determine using 2D or M-mode echocardiography because these modes detect only the presence of thickened aortic cusps and decreased systolic motion of the valve. An indirect estimation of the severity of aortic stenosis can be made by measuring the extent of left ventricular hypertrophy and aortic root dilatation. However, the severity of aortic stenosis can be judged most accurately by Doppler echocardiography.

Aortic regurgitation cannot be directly assessed through echocardiography. Indirectly, the fine fluttering of the

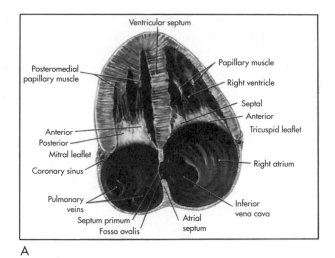

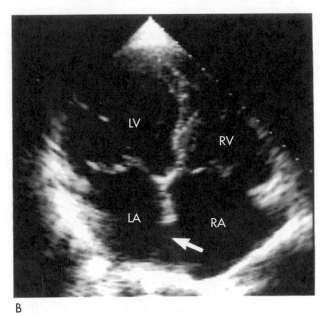

Fig. 3-7 Normal 2D echocardiogram. Schematic representation (**A**) and corresponding 2D echocardiographic image (**B**) of the apical four-chamber view. Arrow is pointing to the atrial septum and indicates an area of "dropout," a technical artifact related to the orientation of the ultrasound beam over the cardiac structure. *LV*, Left ventricle; *RV*, right ventricle; *LA*, left atrium; *RA*, right atrium. (From Oh JK and others: *The echo manual*, Boston, 1994, Little, Brown; copyrighted by Mayo Foundation, Rochester, Minn.)

anterior mitral valve leaflet during diastole caused by the regurgitant jet flowing into the left ventricle indicates aortic regurgitation. Other indirect evidence includes left ventricular dilatation and exaggerated left ventricular wall motion. Premature closure of the mitral valve suggests severe, acute aortic regurgitation. Doppler echocardiography can aid in the quantification of the extent of aortic regurgitation.

Tricuspid and pulmonic valve

The tricuspid and pulmonic valves are not usually as well visualized as the mitral and aortic valves using echocardiography. Tricuspid valve stenosis is identified by noting abnormalities similar to those of mitral stenosis. Tricuspid valve regurgitation manifests predominantly with signs of right ventricular overload, such as right ventricular dilatation and paradoxical septal motion. Pulmonic valve stenosis appears as an early opening of the pulmonic valve caused by the right atrium contracting and ejecting blood into an overloaded right ventricle. Pulmonary hypertension can be diagnosed by a change in the typical contour of the pulmonic valves on an M-mode echocardiogram with notching during systole and the loss of an "a" dip.

Pericardial disease

Pericardial disease can be easily assessed with echocardiography. The existence of a pericardial effusion is determined by the presence of an echo-free space between the pericardium and epicardium. Furthermore, assessment of ventricular wall motion with pericardial effusion yields useful information regarding the possibility of cardiac tamponade. An echocardiogram with a moderately sized pericardial effusion and compression of the right ventricular free wall suggests cardiac tamponade. Collapse of the right atrial wall on the 2D study may also be seen. Constrictive pericarditis is indicated by a thickening of the pericardium and a flat diastolic slope of the posterior left ventricular wall.

Other applications

Echocardiography plays an important role in the assessment of congenital heart disease. The relative spatial arrangement of the cardiac structures and specific chamber abnormalities provide useful information and identification of congenital lesions. Intracardiac masses such as tumors, vegetations, and thrombi are frequently identified through echocardiography. 2D echocardiography is superior to M-mode in these applications.

Stress echocardiography

Stress echocardiography combines exercise or pharmacologic stress testing with echocardiography to provide an alternative means of assessing cardiac function and response to exercise. Images from both studies are displayed side-by-side in a digital format, allowing a more precise comparison of the images. The primary use of stress echocardiography is in assessing regional wall motion and left ventricular function; however, as with standard echocardiographic studies, valvular structure and function, chamber size and wall thickness, and pericardial abnormalities may also be assessed.

Transesophageal echocardiography

Transesophageal echocardiography offers distinct advantages over conventional transthoracic echocardiography. This minimally invasive technique provides more specific pathologic and anatomic information at a higher resolution than the precordial technique because of the proximity of the esophagus to the cardiac structures. Transesophageal echocardiography is useful in evaluating prosthetic valve dysfunction, mitral valve dysfunction, intracardiac masses, thoracic aortic disease, and the immediate efficacy of valvular repair or replacement. In addition, transesophageal echocardiography may be used when precordial echocardiography study data are limited by significant pulmonary disease or when additional detailed information is required.

Doppler Echocardiography

Doppler echocardiography provides data about the flow of blood within the heart, throughout its chambers, across the valves, and in the great vessels. It is a valuable adjunct to the conventional echocardiographic examination for a more complete noninvasive evaluation of cardiac function. Doppler echocardiography provides data that quantify stenotic gradients, intracardiac masses, and blood flow; semiquantitative assessment of valvular regurgitation; and hemodynamic assessment of cardiac function to supplement the anatomic assessment obtained by M-mode and 2D echocardiography.

Doppler echocardiography may use pulsed- or continuous-wave techniques. Each technique can be used independently or with simultaneously interrupted 2D imaging capabilities. With the pulsed-wave Doppler technique, one crystal emits short bursts of ultrasound and receives the ultrasound reflected from moving red blood cells. The pulsed-wave Doppler is combined with 2D echocardiography so that the exact location of the sample volume within the chamber can be visually displayed. Because this sample volume can be positioned in various cardiac chambers and vessels, it can be used to localize abnormal blood flow within cardiac structures. However, a disadvantage of this technique is that high-velocity flow cannot be quantified. Continuous-wave Doppler has one crystal that continuously emits the ultrasound and another that continuously receives the reflected signal. High-velocity flow can be measured, but the location from which the flow is obtained cannot be specified.

The problem of indicating directional flow using Doppler and the 2D echocardiographic image was solved by adding color to the Doppler scan. Color-flow Doppler echocardiographic systems use red Doppler signals to indicate blood flow toward the transducer and blue to indicate flow away from the transducer. With color-flow Doppler superimposed on the 2D echocardiographic image, blood flow through all cardiac chambers throughout the cardiac cycle is seen.

Clinical applications

Doppler echocardiography is used to evaluate valvular stenosis, valvular regurgitation, blood flow, intracardiac pressures, and intracardiac shunts.

Valvular stenosis

The peak gradient and the valvular area across a stenotic valve are obtained by measuring the peak velocity of blood flow across the valve using continuous-wave Doppler techniques. For example, a peak velocity of 4 m/sec in the ascending aorta with aortic stenosis yields a calculated peak pressure gradient of approximately 64 mm Hg across the aortic valve by using the modified Bernoulli equation:

$$P = 4 \times V^2$$

where P is the pressure gradient in millimeters of mercury and V is the peak velocity in meters per second.

Valvular regurgitation

Valvular regurgitation is detected as retrograde flow across the valve. Mapping of the extent of regurgitation flow in the receiving cardiac chamber allows semiquantitative assessment of severity and can be done with pulsed-wave or color-flow Doppler. For example, in patients with mild aortic insufficiency, a turbulent flow is detected in the upper left ventricle during diastole. The farther from the aortic valve that turbulence is detected, the more severe the amount of regurgitation. Mitral, tricuspid, pulmonic, and prosthetic valvular regurgitation can be assessed in the same way.

Cardiac output

Echocardiography can be used to noninvasively estimate CO. Flow is equal to the product of the cross-sectional area of the cylinder and the flow velocity. Through the use of echocardiography to measure the diameter of the main PA, the cross-sectional area of the PA can be calculated. Blood flow velocity through the PA is measured using Doppler echocardiography, and stroke volume is then calculated by multiplying the cross-sectional area of the PA and the velocity of the blood flow through the PA.[14] CO is calculated by multiplying the stroke volume by the patient's heart rate. The following formula represents these calculations:

$$CO = FVI \times PA\ area \times HR$$

where FVI is the flow velocity integral, $PA\ area$ is the PA cross-sectional area, and HR is the heart rate.

Intracardiac pressures

With valvular regurgitation, the peak velocity of abnormal blood flow is proportional to the difference in pressure between the two cardiac chambers. Thus in tricuspid regurgitation, if the pressure in the right atrium has been calculated by clinical estimation of the jugular venous pressure, the pressure in the right ventricle can be derived, and a rough approximation of PA pressure is established, provided that there is no obstruction of the right ventricular outflow tract.

Intracardiac shunts

An intracardiac shunt results in an abnormal velocity and patterns of blood flow on the lower pressure side of the shunt, which usually is seen on a color-flow Doppler scan. In addition, when the amount of blood flow in the PA and aorta is obtained, the ratio of the pulmonic venous systemic flow can be approximated.

In summary, 2D and M-mode echocardiography with Doppler echocardiography provide a sensitive, noninvasive means of assessing cardiac conditions such as valvular heart disease, pericardial disease, congenital heart disease, cardiomyopathy, and coronary artery disease.

BEDSIDE RIGHT-SIDED HEART CATHETERIZATION USING A FLOW-DIRECTED, BALLOON-TIPPED PA CATHETER

Catheterization of the right side of the heart can be performed at the bedside in the intensive care unit with the use of a flow-directed, balloon-tipped PA catheter. Continuous bedside hemodynamic monitoring provides a valuable adjunct to the assessment and management of a variety of cardiovascular disorders. This technique provides continuous monitoring of PA pressures and, in some situations, right ventricular pressures. In addition, CO measurements are obtained using thermodilution catheters. Many catheters allow for continuous measurement of mixed venous oxygen saturation levels or of CO. In general, PA catheterization and bedside hemodynamic monitoring are indicated in any situation in which evaluation and management of intravascular volume and hemodynamic parameters substantially aid in choosing the best therapeutic intervention for the patient. Although it is a relatively noninvasive and low-risk procedure, PA catheter insertion and chronic placement involve risks such as pneumothorax, infection, thrombosis, pulmonary embolism, dysrhythmias, and vascular injury.

PA catheterization involves inserting a balloon-tipped, flow-directed, sterile catheter through a protective sheath using a percutaneous approach or directly into a surgically exposed vein. The catheter is advanced while intravascular pressure is monitored through the central lumen of the catheter. Fig. 3-8 shows a representation of the pressure waveforms seen as the catheter is advanced. When the catheter tip is near the right atrium, the balloon is inflated, and the catheter is advanced farther, carried by blood flow across the tricuspid valve directly into the right ventricle. The catheter is then advanced, with the assistance of blood flow, across the pulmonic valve into the pulmonary artery until the balloon becomes wedged in an arterial branch. Pressure recordings should be obtained in each chamber

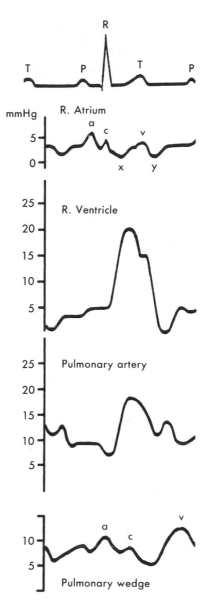

Fig. 3-8 Simultaneous normal right atrial pressure, ventricular pressure, PA pressure, and PCWP tracings related to the electrical cardiac cycle.

as the catheter is being inserted, and PA pressure should be recorded after the balloon is deflated.

Depending on the manufacturer, a PA catheter may have a central lumen that opens at the distal tip of the catheter, a lumen that is used for balloon inflation, and one to three other lumens (right atrial for pressure monitoring and/or infusions and right ventricular for pressure monitoring or temporary pacemaker lead placement). The distal lumen located at the tip of the catheter is first used to record entry pressures and then to record the PA and pulmonary capillary wedge pressure. The pressure obtained through the distal lumen when the balloon is wedged in the PA is referred to as the *pulmonary capillary wedge pres-*

sure *(PCWP)* and reflects the left ventricular end-diastolic pressure *(LVEDP),* provided that there is no obstructive disease in the pulmonary circulation or at the level of the mitral valve. The proximal lumen, located 30 cm from the tip of the catheter, is used to record right atrial pressure, or central venous pressure, and is the injection port in the thermodilution CO procedure. In addition, medication and fluid infusions may be administered through this port. Many catheters have an additional port that opens in the right atrium and is used for medication and fluid administration. Normal pressure values are shown in Table 3-2.

CO can be easily assessed after the thermodilution PA catheter is in position by using the thermodilution technique, which involves the injection of a known volume of fluid at a known temperature into the proximal port. A thermistor located near the catheter tip detects the change in temperature as the fluid flows through the PA. The change in temperature is inversely proportional to the CO; that is, the greater the change in temperature, the lower the CO.

Once the right atrial pressure, PA pressure, PCWP, and CO have been obtained, calculations of stroke volume, systemic vascular resistance, and pulmonary vascular resistance can be made using the formulas shown in Table 3-3. These reflect the hemodynamic status of the patient. Note that cardiac index is calculated by dividing the CO by the body surface area and provides a more accurate assessment of cardiac function for a specific patient.

Elevated left ventricular filling pressures, indicated by an elevated PCWP, suggest heart failure or vascular volume overload, and depressed left ventricular filling pressures suggest volume depletion. Equalization of left and right filling pressures (right atrial pressure = PCWP) suggests filling problems such as cardiac tamponade, constriction, or restrictive cardiomyopathy. A very dominant v wave in the PCWP indicates acute mitral regurgitation or increased LVEDP. Elevated right atrial pressures suggest right ventricular injury from myocardial infarction, and elevated PA pressures may indicate pulmonary hypertension. Additional information can be obtained by measuring oxy-

---

TABLE 3-2   Range of Normal Resting Hemodynamic Values (mm Hg)

Pressures	a Wave	v Wave	Mean	Systolic	End Diastolic
Right atrial	2-10	2-10	0-8	—	—
Right ventricular	—	—	—	15-30	0-8
PA	—	—	9-16	15-30	3-12
PCWP (left atrial)	3-15	3-12	1-10	—	—
Left ventricular	—	—	—	100-140	3-12
Systemic arterial	—	—	90-105	100-140	60-90

TABLE 3-3   Hemodynamic Equations and Normal Values

Value	Equation	Normal Values
Cardiac index (CI)	$CI = \dfrac{CO}{BSA}$	$2\text{-}5 - 4.2 \text{ L/min/m}^2$
Stroke volume (SV)	$SV = \dfrac{CO}{HR}$	$60 - 100 \text{ ml}$
Stroke index (SI)	$SI = \dfrac{SV}{BSA}$	$45 \pm 13 \text{ ml/m}^2$
Systemic vascular resistance (SVR)	$SVR = \dfrac{80\,(MAP - CVP)}{CO}$	$770 - 1500 \text{ dyne-seconds-cm}^2/\text{m}^2$
Pulmonary vascular resistance (PVR)	$PVR = \dfrac{80\,(MPA - PCWP)}{CO}$	$20 - 120 \text{ dyne-seconds-cm}^2/\text{m}^2$

BSA, body surface area; *HR,* heart rate; *MAP,* mean systemic arterial pressure; *CVP,* central venous pressure; *MPA,* mean pulmonary arterial pressure.

gen saturations from the right atrium and PA, looking for a possible oxygen saturation increase, or step up, that is consistent with a left-to-right intracardiac shunt. PA catheters with fiber optics are used to continuously monitor mixed venous oxygen saturation to assess oxygen delivery and consumption.

CARDIAC CATHETERIZATION AND CARDIAC ANGIOGRAPHY

Cardiac catheterization and angiography are the definitive techniques for establishing the cause and severity of cardiac diseases. These techniques provide physiologic data regarding cardiovascular hemodynamics and angiographic evaluation of cardiac chambers and coronary artery anatomy.

Cardiac catheterization involves passing a catheter through a vein or artery to the right or left cardiac chambers so that pressures and oxygen saturations within the chambers can be measured and gradients across stenotic valves can be determined. In addition, radiopaque contrast dye can be injected to visualize the cardiac chambers, great vessels, and coronary arteries. Through the use of these invasive diagnostic techniques, the presence and severity of regional wall-motion abnormalities, valvular disease, and coronary artery disease can be evaluated. Complications of MI, such as acquired ventricular septal defect with a left-to-right shunt, can be detected and quantified through the measurement of oxygen saturations in the right cardiac chambers.

The most commonly performed angiographic procedure in the patient who has known or suspected coronary artery disease is coronary arteriography. With this technique, selective catheterization of the coronary arteries is performed by a brachial arteriotomy (Sones technique) or by a percutaneous femoral arterial puncture (Judkins technique). A percutaneous brachial approach may also be used. Several injections of the right and left coronary artery systems are performed with multiple imaging views to ensure adequate visualization of the proximal and distal portions of both vessels. Angiographic findings of luminal diameter reduction of greater than 50% are considered significant (Fig. 3-9). These lesions may be concentric, eccentric, or tubular, which makes grading their severity difficult at times. Computer-assisted assessment of coronary artery lesions accurately quantifies the extent of obstruction. Cardiac digital subtraction angiography, intracoronary angioscopy, and intravascular ultrasound are techniques being developed to more accurately define coronary artery lesions.

In addition to assessing coronary artery lesions, conditions such as hypertrophic obstructive cardiomyopathy or coronary artery spasm, which can mimic coronary artery disease in clinical presentation, can be diagnosed with cardiac catheterization and coronary angiography. The measurement of pressures in the left ventricular outflow tract reveals subvalvular gradients indicative of outflow obstruction resulting from asymmetric septal hypertrophy in hypertrophic obstructive cardiomyopathy. Vasospastic angina, such as Prinzmetal variant angina, can be diagnosed through the use of coronary angiography with agents such as ergonovine.

Although it is a relatively low-risk procedure, cardiac catheterization can have complications. Death and major

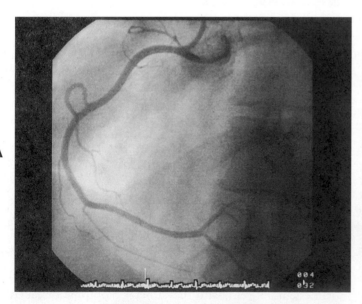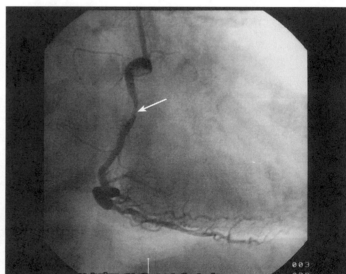

A

B

Fig. 3-9 Coronary angiograms depicting a normal right coronary artery **(A)** and right coronary artery with narrowing *(arrow)* in the proximal portion of the vessel **(B).** (Courtesy The Heart Center at Baptist, Mississippi Baptist Medical Center, Jackson, Miss.)

complications such as MI and cerebrovascular accident during or within 24 hours of catheterization have a reported incidence of 0.2% to 0.4%.[15] More common but less serious complications include nausea and vomiting, a transient fall in blood pressure after the injection of the contrast media, bleeding or hematoma formation at the access site, and compromised distal perfusion. After cardiac catheterization, patients who have had a femoral approach must remain supine with the affected leg immobilized for several hours. In addition, patients who have had catheter-based interventions, such as PTCA or atherectomy, usually have the femoral access sheath left in place and are placed on anticoagulation therapy, thus increasing the chance of hemorrhagic complications. Frequent monitoring of vital signs and venous and arterial access sites must be performed to note any sign of hemorrhage. Also, because the contrast media promotes osmotic diuresis, the patient should receive sufficient oral or intravenous fluids after the procedure.

Traditionally, coronary arteriography has been performed in the patient who has classic angina to delineate the anatomic sites and the degree of coronary artery stenosis before revascularization interventions via aortocoronary bypass grafting or PTCA are considered. Coronary arteriography may be performed with an acute MI or unstable angina. Coronary arteriography also may be indicated for patients with atypical chest pain for whom noninvasive tests such as thallium imaging have been equivocal or nondiagnostic. For the patient who develops myocardial ischemia after coronary artery bypass surgery or catheter revascularization, coronary arteriography may be used to assess the patency of the graft or the status of the lesion or to determine whether stenoses have developed in other coronary vessels.

CARDIAC ELECTROPHYSIOLOGIC STUDIES

Cardiac electrophysiologic studies (EPS) have become widely used in the evaluation and treatment of specific cardiac dysrhythmias since first being described by Scherlag and others in 1969.[16] EPS are used to assess sinus node function, atrioventricular block, supraventricular tachycardias, and ventricular tachycardia and fibrillation. EPS are also used to guide subsequent interventions, such as antidysrhythmic pharmacologic therapy, catheter and surgical ablation of dysrhythmic foci, and implantation of pacemakers, antitachycardia devices, and implantable cardioverter defibrillators as well as to assess the efficacy of these interventions.[17]

EPS are performed in the controlled setting of the cardiovascular catheterization laboratory by a specially trained cardiologist. Patients are generally awake but sedated. The procedure involves inserting four catheters, or electrodes, through a femoral vein and advancing them under fluoroscopy to specific sites within the heart. The electrodes are positioned in the coronary sinus, high right atrium, and right ventricular apex and at the level of the His bundle. With the electrodes in place, electrical activity within the heart can be recorded, and dysrhythmias can be induced with pulses of current using programmed electrical stimulation (PES).[18] Inducing a dysrhythmia and recording the electrical activity allows the cardiologist to accurately characterize and identify the dysrhythmia. The dysrhythmia can then be terminated with rapid programmed pacing or defibrillation and cardioversion.

Indications for EPS include assessment of patients with recurrent supraventricular tachycardia or palpitations, diagnosis of wide-complex tachycardias, identification of a possible cardiac dysrhythmic cause of syncope or near syncope, and mapping of the dysrhythmogenic focus before surgical or catheter ablation.[18] In patients with preexcitation syndromes, such as Wolff-Parkinson-White syndrome, EPS may be used to localize the accessory pathway and guide appropriate therapy.[19]

As an extension of EPS, catheter ablation of the dysrhythmic focus may be performed. Two techniques may be used to destroy or modify the cardiac tissue responsible for the dysrhythmia: high-voltage, direct-current (DC) ablation and radiofrequency (RF) ablation. DC ablation uses a defibrillator to deliver a high-energy electrical impulse through a catheter positioned at the site of the dysrhythmia. With RF ablation, high-frequency, or radiofrequency, currents are delivered through a catheter to the point of the dysrhythmia. RF ablation has become the more common technique; it has several advantages over DC ablation, including the following: general anesthesia is not required, tissue modification is more localized, and there are fewer complications.[20]

ENDOMYOCARDIAL BIOPSY

Endomyocardial biopsy is a procedure that would seem to offer invaluable information in the assessment of underlying cardiac disease. However, the amount of information gathered has not been great, and this technique is indicated in just a few circumstances. The primary indications are monitoring patients after heart transplant for evidence of rejection and guiding the use of immunosuppressive agents in this population. Additional indications include monitoring patients on chemotherapy for signs of cardiac toxicity and detecting or diagnosing infiltrative or inflammatory processes of the myocardium.

The biopsy specimens are usually obtained from the right ventricular endocardium, although specimens may also be obtained from the left ventricle. The right ventricle is preferred because of the venous access and the risk of arterial embolization of left-sided heart biopsies. The procedure may be performed through the right internal jugular or the femoral vein, with the catheter bioptome threaded to the right ventricle with fluoroscopic or echocardiographic guidance. Several specimens are obtained and submitted for examination by a pathologist with expertise in the evaluation of endomyocardial tissue. Contraindications include bleeding disorders, anticoagulant therapy, and the presence of mural thrombi. Because access is through the low-pressure venous system, these procedures are usually done on an outpatient basis. Although complications are rare, perforation, tamponade, dysrhythmias, vascular trauma, pneumothorax, or infection may occur.

REFERENCES

1. Apple FS: Acute myocardial infarction and coronary reperfusion: serum cardiac markers for the 1990s, *Am J Clin Path* 97:217, 1992.
2. Roberts R and others: *Pathophysiology, recognition and treatment of acute myocardial infarction and its complications.* In Schlant RC and others, editors: *Hurst's the heart,* ed 8, New York, 1994, McGraw-Hill.
3. Miranda CP and others: Correlation between resting ST segment depression, exercising testing, coronary angiography, and long-term prognosis, *Am Heart J* 122:1617, 1991.
4. Podrid PJ: *Exercise testing.* In Horowitz LH, editor: *Current management of arrhythmias,* Philadelphia, 1991, Decker.
5. Nyman I and others: The predictive value of silent ischemia at an exercise test before discharge after an episode of unstable coronary artery disease, *Am Heart J* 123:324, 1992.
6. Iskandrian AS and others: Independent and incremental prognostic value of exercise single-photon emission computed tomographic thallium imaging in coronary artery disease, *J Am Coll Cardiol* 22(3):665, 1993.
7. Stratmann HG and others: Prognostic value of dipyridamole thallium-201 scintigraphy in patients with stable chest pain, *Am Heart J* 123:317, 1992.
8. Johnson JL, Pohust GM: *Nuclear cardiology.* In Schlant RC and others: *Hurst's the heart,* ed 8, New York, 1994, McGraw-Hill.
9. Caputo GR, Higgins CB: Advances in cardiac imaging modalities: fast computed tomography, magnetic resonance imaging and positron emission tomography, *Invest Radiol* 25:838, 1990.
10. Hepp RH, Horowitz LN: *Ambulatory electrocardiographic monitoring.* In Horowitz LH, editor: *Current management of arrhythmias,* Philadelphia, 1991, Decker.
11. Knobel SB and others: Clinical competence in ambulatory electrocardiography: a statement for physicians from the AHA/ACC/ACP Task Force on clinical privileges in cardiology, *Circulation* 88(1):337, 1993.
12. Oh JK and others: *The echo manual,* Boston, 1994, Little, Brown.
13. Felner JM, Martin RP: *The echocardiogram.* In Schlant RC and others, editors: *Hurst's the heart,* ed 8, New York, 1994, McGraw-Hill.
14. Gorcsan J and others: Intraoperative determination of cardiac output by transesophageal continuous wave Doppler, *Am Heart J* 123(1):171, 1992.
15. Hillis DL and others: *Cardiac catheterization.* In Kloner RA, editor: *The guide to cardiology,* ed 2, New York, 1990, Le Jacq.
16. Scherlag BJ and others: Catheter technique for recording His bundle activity in man, *Circulation* 39:13, 1969.
17. Akhtar M and others: Clinical competence in invasive cardiac electrophysiological studies: ACP/ACC/AHA Task Force on Clinical Privileges in Cardiology, *J Am Coll Cardiol* 23(5):1258, 1994.
18. Teo WS and others: New directions in cardiovascular mapping and therapy, *Ann Acad Med* 22(2):197, 1993.
19. McComb JM: Clinical cardiac electrophysiology: the last 10 years, *Int J Cardiol* 33:351, 1991.
20. Hindricks G and others: *Catheter ablation.* In Horowitz LH, editor: *Current management of arrhythmias,* Philadelphia, 1991, Decker.

4

Introduction to Electrocardiography

Barbara A. Erickson

The chapter explains the basic principles and use of electrocardiography (ECG) and introduces common ECG findings in patients with cardiac disease. Additional electrocardiographic disorders are presented in Chapter 5.

BASIC CONSIDERATIONS

The ECG is a graphic recording of the electrical activity generated by the functioning heart. The first ECG was introduced by Willem Einthoven, a Dutch physiologist, in 1901. From the monopolar lead recorded by Einthoven's string galvanometer, the ECG's progression has included the unipolar leads added by Frank N. Wilson and his associates in 1933 to the present electrocardiogram, which includes 12 leads. This standard 12-lead ECG may be extended to six additional leads on the right precordium when right ventricular infarction is suspected.

The ECG is one of the most valuable of the diagnostic tools available for the recognition of cardiac diseases or abnormalities. It is especially significant when combined with the total cardiac assessment, which includes a history and physical examination. Changes in the ECG may be in pattern, rhythm, or both. Changes noted on the ECG need to be correlated with clinical findings. Variations from the normal ECG may be found in an individual with a healthy heart. Conversely, cardiac disease may not be reflected by changes in an ECG. Thus a normal ECG does not guarantee a normal heart and vice versa. One of the essential roles of the ECG is in the recognition of cardiac dysrhythmias.

In addition to individual variations, numerous other extrinsic factors may alter the ECG. These include but are not limited to drugs, metabolic changes, electrolyte imbalances, technical factors such as incorrectly applied electrodes, and the patient's age and body build. The ECG's precision of interpretation increases when the greatest amount of clinical information is available. It is essential to compare new with previous tracings.

Standardization

The ECG is recorded on graph paper divided into small and large boxes. The small boxes are 1 mm², and the large boxes, designated by heavy lines, contain 25 small boxes, 5 across and 5 down (Fig. 4-1). Horizontally, the paper measures time, and vertically, it measures voltage. The standard ECG paper moves at 25 mm/sec. Therefore horizontally, each small box is equal to 0.04 second; each large box (5 mm) is equal to 0.20 second (5 × 0.04). Read vertically, the ECG measures voltage or amplitude of the deflections. The exact voltage can be measured because the ECG is set, or standardized, so that 1 mV of electric current causes a deflection 10 mm in amplitude (Fig. 4-2). The deflection may be modified by being set at one-half standard, which means that 1 mV of electric current causes only a 5-mm deflection, or twice standard, which means that 1 mV of electric current causes a deflection of 20 mm. When very large deflections are present, it is advisable to record the ECG at one-half standard; when the deflections are very small, the ECG may be recorded at twice standard. Any change in standardization must be indicated on the ECG.

Deflections

When the amplitude of the deflections inscribed on the ECG are described, the following terms are used: *baseline, wave, segment, interval,* and *complex.* The baseline is the starting or resting line of the ECG. A deflection from the baseline is called a *wave.* A wave above the baseline is considered positive; one below the baseline is considered negative. If the deflection has both positive and negative components, it is called *biphasic* or *diphasic.* A deflection, or wave, that rests on the baseline is called *isoelectric.* A segment is a straight line connecting waves, as in the ST segment. An interval is a wave and a straight line, as in the PR interval. A complex is a group of waves, as in the QRS complex.

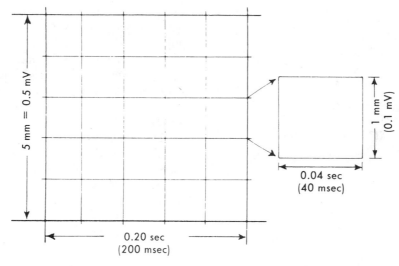

Fig. 4-1   Time and voltage lines of the ECG. The interval between two heavy vertical lines is 0.20 second (200 msec), and between each light line it is 0.04 second (40 msec). The voltage between each heavy horizontal line is 0.5 mV.

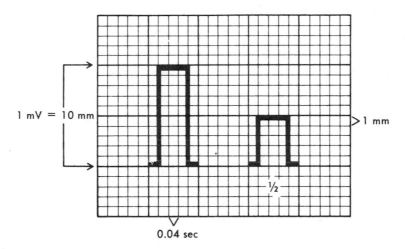

Fig. 4-2   Normal standardization of the ECG. A total of 1 mV causes a deflection of 10 mm. For large ECG deflections the standard must be halved so that 1 mV equals 5 mm. For small ECG deflections the standard may be doubled so that 1 mV equals 20 mm. Changes in standardization must be noted on the ECG recording.

The six major deflections of the normal ECG are designated by the letters P, Q, R, S, T, and U (Fig. 4-3). These waves are produced by the electrical energy caused by the movement of charged particles across the membranes of myocardial cells (depolarization and repolarization).

ELECTROPHYSIOLOGIC PRINCIPLES

The membrane of the myocardial cell is a semipermeable two-layered lipid that is a barrier between two very different solutions. Outside the normal resting cell, the concentration of sodium is very high, and the potassium

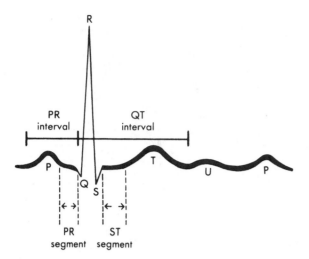

Fig. 4-3   The deflections in a normal ECG are the P wave (atrial depolarization), QRS complex (ventricular depolarization), and T wave (ventricular repolarization). The U wave is sometimes present and follows the T wave. The PR segment is the interval between the end of the P wave and the beginning of the QRS complex. The ST segment is the interval between the end of the QRS complex and the beginning of the T wave. Sometimes, atrial repolarization, the Ta wave, can be recorded (see Fig. 4-7). The PR interval is from the onset of the P wave to the onset of the QRS complex. The QT interval is from the onset of the QRS complex to the end of the T wave.

level is very low. Within this cell, the potassium level is high, and the sodium level is low. The voltage inside a resting (polarized) cardiac cell is negative with respect to the outside of the cell, in large part because of the cell membrane's relative permeability to the potassium ion and impermeability to the sodium ion during diastole. The ratio of extracellular to intracellular potassium concentrations primarily determines the resting potential of the cell; when the cell becomes depolarized, the cell membrane alters its permeability so that it becomes more permeable to sodium ions and less permeable to potassium ions. Sodium ions rush into the cell, making the voltage inside the cell positive with respect to the voltage outside the cell. The channels that permit this rapid entry of sodium ions into the cell are known as *fast channels* or *fast sodium channels*. These events occur in atrial and ventricular muscle and in the His-Purkinje system. In the normal sinus and atrioventricular (AV) nodes, and possibly in other fibers if they become damaged and lose membrane potential, calcium appears to play a prominent role in the depolarization process. Calcium (and possibly sodium in some instances) enters the cell through the "slow channel," producing the slow response. It is called the *slow response* because the time to activate and inactivate the channel (in essence, turn it

on and off) is slow compared with that of the sodium or fast channel, which is active in muscle and in the His-Purkinje fibers (Fig. 4-4).

Understanding these ionic mechanisms is clinically important because of the development of drugs such as verapamil that fairly specifically block the slow channel. These drugs are often called *calcium channel* or *calcium entry blockers*.

The cell in a resting, polarized state can be represented by negative and positive charges lining, respectively, the inside and outside of the cell membrane (Fig. 4-5, *A*). If an electrode of an ECG machine (galvanometer) were attached to this polarized cell, no electrical potential would be registered because no net change in ionic composition would occur. Hence, there would be no voltage shift and no deviation from the isoelectric baseline (Fig. 4-5, *A*).

When a cell or more likely a group of cells is stimulated and the change in membrane permeability permits sodium ions to migrate rapidly into the cell, making the inside positive with respect to the outside depolarization, an electric field is generated between the depolarized and polarized areas of myocardium. The P wave represents atrial depolarization, and the QRS complex represents ventricular depolarization (Fig. 4-5, *B* to *D*).

A slower movement of ions across the membrane restoring the cell to the polarized state is termed *repolarization*. Movement of potassium ions out of myocardial cells primarily accounts for repolarization. In late diastole, after most of the repolarization has occurred, potassium and sodium reverse positions to restore ionic concentrations to the polarized state. The Ta wave, representing atrial repolarization, generally lies buried in the QRS complex and ST segment. The ST segment is an isoelectric line extending from the end of the QRS complex to the beginning of the T wave, during which early ventricular repolarization is beginning very slowly (Fig. 4-5, *E*). The T wave represents ventricular repolarization (Fig. 4-5, *F*).

WAVES AND COMPLEXES
P Wave

As previously mentioned, the P wave represents atrial depolarization and begins as soon as the impulse leaves the sinus (SA) node and initiates atrial depolarization. Because the sinus node is situated in the right atrium, right atrial activation begins first and is followed shortly thereafter by left atrial activation. As left atrial activation begins and before the end of right atrial activation, the two processes overlap. This close overlap results in a gently rounded P wave. As discussed later, the P wave normally may be positive, negative, or diphasic, depending on the lead of the ECG recorded. Whatever the case, the amplitude of the P wave should not exceed 2 or 3 mm in any lead (Fig. 4-6). Although not usually visible on the ECG, the Ta wave of atrial repolarization occurs in a direction opposite to that

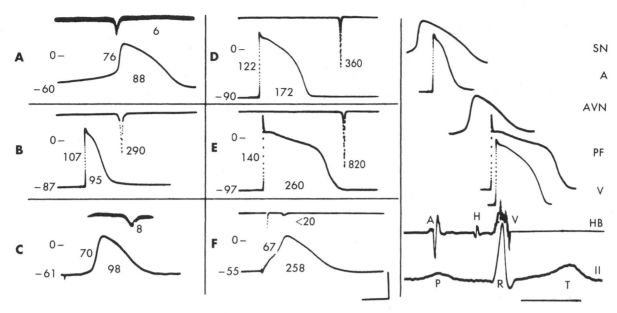

Fig. 4-4 Action potentials recorded from different tissues in the heart *(left)* remounted with a His bundle recording and scalar ECG from a patient *(right)* to illustrate the timing during a single cardiac cycle. In **A** to **F** the top tracing is the rate of change in voltage with respect to time (dV/dt) of phase 0, and the second tracing is the action potential. For each panel the numbers from left to right indicate maximum diastolic potential (mV), action potential amplitude (mV), action potential duration at 90% of repolarization (msec), and maximum rate of rise in volts per second (V/sec) of cardiac action potential (V_{max}) of phase 0. Zero potential is indicated by the short horizontal line next to the zero on the upper left of each action potential. **A,** Rabbit sinoatrial (SA) node. **B,** Canine atrial muscle. **C,** Rabbit AV node. **D,** Canine ventricular muscle. **E,** Canine Purkinje fiber. **F,** Diseased human ventricle. Note that the action potentials recorded in **A, C,** and **F** have reduced resting membrane potentials, amplitudes, and V_{max} compared with the other action potentials. Horizontal calibration on left is 50 msec for **A** and **C,** 100 msec for **B** and **D** through **F.** Vertical calibration on left is 50 mV. Horizontal calibration on right is 200 msec. *SN,* Sinus nodal potential; *A,* atrial muscle potential; *AVN,* AV nodal potential; *PF,* Purkinje fiber potential; *V,* ventricular muscle potential; *HB,* His bundle recording; *II,* lead II. (From Gilmour RF Jr, Zipes DP: *Basic electrophysiology of the slow inward current.* In Antman E, Stone PH, editors: *Calcium blocking agents in the treatment of cardiovascular disorders,* Mt Kisco, NY, 1983, Futura.)

of the P wave and is recorded after the first portion of the P wave and continues through the PR interval. It is usually not identified unless the P wave occurs independently of the QRS complex, as in complete AV block (see Chapter 5). When the P wave is large, the Ta wave is also generally large and may extend beyond the QRS complex, resulting in a distortion of the initial portion of the ST segment. This may cause a depression of the ST segment that may be mistaken to have a pathologic significance. To make a correct interpretation in the setting of a depressed ST segment, the clinician must observe the configuration of the atrial repolarization wave (smooth curve with upward concavity), recognize a similar deviation of the baseline before the QRS is recorded, and recognize a large P wave (Fig. 4-7).

QRS Complex

The QRS complex representing ventricular depolarization may have various components, depending on the lead of the ECG recorded. These components are illustrated in Fig. 4-8 and described as follows:

R wave	The first positive deflection
Q wave	The initial negative deflection before an R wave
S wave	The negative deflection after an R wave
R' wave	The second positive deflection
S' wave	The negative deflection after the R' wave
QS wave	The totally negative deflection

The QRS complexes should be examined for the following:
1. The duration of the complex
2. The amplitude of the components

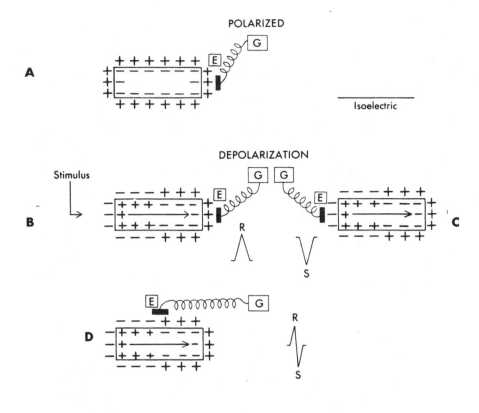

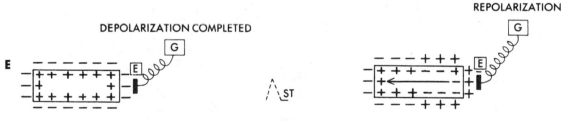

Fig. 4-5 **A,** Schematic illustration of a polarized (resting) myocardial muscle cell maintaining a negative charge on the inside of the cell membrane and a positive charge on the outside of the membrane. An electrode *(E)* facing the right side of the polarized cell and attached to an ECG machine *(G,* galvanometer) records no current, and an isoelectric line results. **B,** The cell is stimulated from the left, and depolarization proceeds from left to right in the direction of the arrow. The depolarized left end of the cell becomes electrically negative, whereas the right end of the cell is still polarized and electrically positive. Now a difference of electric potentials (negative and positive ions) exists, and an electric current is flowing. The electrode facing the positive side of this current and attached to an ECG machine records a positive deflection, and in the case of ventricular depolarization, this deflection is called an *R wave.* **C,** The same myocardial cell is stimulated again from the left; however, the electrode is facing the negative side of the current and therefore records a negative deflection. In the case of ventricular depolarization, this deflection is called an *S wave.* **D,** Once again the cell is activated from the left. The electrode facing the center of the cell first writes a positive and then a negative deflection. In the case of ventricular depolarization, this deflection is called an *RS complex.* **E,** With the completion of depolarization, the outer surface of the myocardial cell becomes electrically negative; the flow of electric current ceases, and the R wave returns to the isoelectric line. The short period after complete ventricular depolarization is recorded as the ST segment. **F,** In **B** through **D,** the myocardial muscle cell was depolarized from left to right. Now the cell returns to the resting state, repolarization, in the opposite direction, from right to left. The right end of the cell becomes positive first, and an electrode facing this site inscribes a positive deflection. In the case of ventricular repolarization, this deflection is termed a *T wave.*

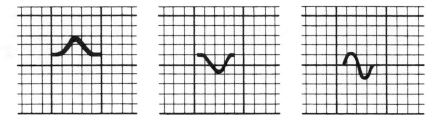

Fig. 4-6   The P wave is gently rounded in contour; may be normally positive, negative, or diphasic in different ECG leads; and should not exceed 2 or 3 mm.

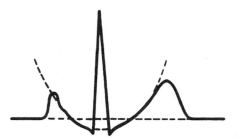

Fig. 4-7   Atrial repolarization as a cause of ST-segment deviation. Note that the PQ (PR) and ST segments can be connected by a smooth curve and that the direction of the deviation is opposite in direction to the P wave.   (Modified from Hurst JW and others: *The heart: arteries and veins,* ed 6, New York, 1984, McGraw-Hill.)

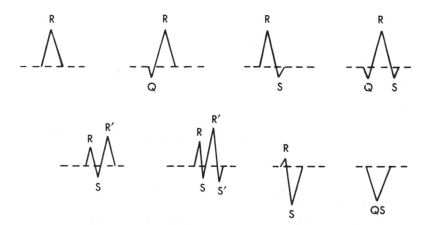

Fig. 4-8   Components of the QRS complex.

3. The general configuration of the complex, including the presence and location of any slurred component (see discussion of bundle branch block and Wolff-Parkinson-White syndrome in Chapter 5)
4. The presence of abnormal Q waves (see the section on myocardial infarction in this chapter)
5. The timing of the intrinsicoid deflections in precordial leads V_1 to V_6

Amplitude

The amplitude of the QRS complex has wide normal limits; however, if the total amplitude (above and below the baseline) is 5 mm or less in all three standard leads, it is considered abnormally low. Such low voltage may be seen in patients who have cardiac failure, diffuse coronary disease, pericardial effusion, myxedema, primary amyloidosis, or other conditions producing widespread myocardial damage. Furthermore, it may be found in patients who have emphysema and generalized edema and who are obese. The minimum normal QRS amplitude in precordial leads varies from right to left across the chest, being generally accepted as 5 mm in leads V_1 and V_6, 7 mm in V_2 and V_5, and 9 mm in V_3 and V_4.

Upper limits for normal QRS voltage (amplitude) have been difficult to set. Diagnostic evaluation is important when QRS amplitudes reach the following upper limits: lead V_1, an R wave of 5 mm; leads V_1 and V_2, an S wave of 30 mm leads; V_5 and V_6, an R wave of 30 mm; and limb leads, an R or S wave of 20 mm.

Intrinsicoid deflection

Ventricular activation time is the interval between the beginning of the QRS complex and the onset of the intrinsicoid deflection. The time of onset of the intrinsicoid deflection is measured from the beginning of the QRS complex to the peak of the R wave, and it is measured in the precordial leads (Fig. 4-9). In right-sided precordial leads (or V_2) the time of onset for the intrinsicoid deflection is normally 0.03 second or less. In left-sided precordial leads (V_5 or V_6) the time of onset is normally 0.05 second or less in adults. If the time of onset for the intrinsicoid deflection exceeds 0.03 or 0.05 second in right- and left-sided leads respectively, it is taken to indicate that the impulse arrived late at the epicardial surface of the ventricle under the electrode. Such delay may be caused by thickening or dilatation of the ventricular wall or a block in the conducting system to the ventricle involved (bundle branch block).

ST Segment

The interval that occurs between the end of the QRS complex and the beginning of the T wave is called the *ST segment*. It represents the time during which the ventricles have been completely depolarized and are beginning ven-

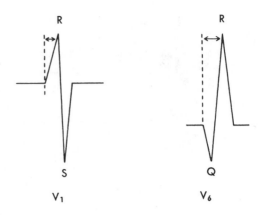

Fig. 4-9   The time of onset of the intrinsicoid deflection is measured from the beginning of the QRS complex to the peak of the R wave.

tricular repolarization. The J point marks the beginning of the ST segment. Usually, the ST segment is isoelectric (see Fig. 4-3), but it may normally deviate from −0.5 to +1.0 mm from the baseline in the standard and unipolar leads (ECG leads are presented in the next section). In some instances, upward displacement of 2 or 3 mm may be normal, provided that the ST segment is concave upward and the succeeding T wave is tall and upright. This is called *early repolarization*. Downward displacement in excess of 0.5 mm generally is abnormal. In all situations, depression caused by a depressed PR segment must be considered. More important are elevated or depressed ST segments that vary temporarily (see discussions of myocardial infarction and pericarditis). Correlation with the clinical condition of the patient is often necessary to determine the significance of ST segment displacement.

Elevation of the ST segment is measured from the upper edge of the isoelectric line to the upper edge of the ST segment; depression is measured from the lower edge of the isoelectric line to the lower edge of the ST segment (Fig. 4-10).

T Wave

The T wave, normally slightly rounded and slightly asymmetric, represents the electric recovery period (repolarization) of the ventricles. Upright T waves are measured from the upper level of the baseline to the summit of the T wave, whereas inverted T waves are measured from the lower level of the baseline to the lowest point of the T wave. Diphasic T waves are measured by adding the amplitudes above and below the baseline. T waves normally do not exceed 5 mm in any standard lead or 10 mm in any precordial lead. T wave contour is often very labile, and as with the ST segment, correlation with the clinical status of the patient, often in serially repeated ECGs, is necessary for correct interpretation.

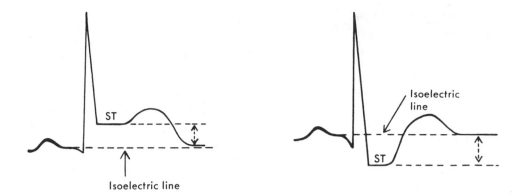

Fig. 4-10   Elevation of the ST segment is measured from the upper edge of the isoelectric line to the upper edge of the ST segment; depression is measured from the lower edge of the isoelectric line to the lower edge of the ST segment.

QT Interval

The QT interval is measured in seconds from the beginning of the Q wave to the end of the T wave. It is the summation of depolarization and repolarization representing electrical systole and diastole. Variations in this interval occur with heart rate, gender, and age. In general the slower the heart rate, the longer the QT interval; the faster the heart rate, the shorter the QT interval. This is due almost solely to a shortening or lengthening of the myocardial refractory period. Women tend to have slightly longer QT intervals than men (Fig. 4-11). The QT interval is preferably determined using a lead showing a QRS complex with an initial q wave (leads I, II, aV_L, V_5, and V_6). When a U wave is present, the dip or notch between the T and U waves is taken as the end of the T wave. A quick method of determining the QT interval is to measure the R-R interval between two consecutive R waves and divide it by 2; the "normal" QT interval should be the result of this quick calculation.

A QT interval corrected for what it would theoretically be at a rate of 60 beats/min is called a *QTc interval*. The most frequently used formula to correct the QT interval for rate is Bazett's, which states: $Qtc = QT/\sqrt{R\text{-}R}$. The QT interval is measured; the R-R interval is measured between two consecutive R waves. Both figures are expressed in seconds. The normal range for the Qtc interval is 0.35 to 0.43 second; an interval of 0.44 second or more is considered prolonged. The Qtc interval may be prolonged by ischemia (acute myocardial infarction), hypocalcemia, hypertrophy, antidysrhythmic drugs (quinidine, procainamide, amiodarone), hypothermia and sympathetic stimulation, such as that associated with a head injury. Hypercalcemia, digitalis effect, hyperthermia, and vagal stimulation shorten the Qtc interval. A prolonged Qtc interval is associated with a higher incidence of ventricular tachycardia and sudden death.

Heart Rate / Minute	Men and Children	Women
40	0.49	0.50
50	0.45	0.46
60	0.42	0.43
70	0.40	0.41
80	0.38	0.39
90	0.36	0.37
100	0.34	0.35
120	0.31	0.32
150	0.28	0.29

Fig. 4-11   Upper limits of the normal QT interval.

U Wave

The U wave is a small wave of low voltage sometimes observed after a T wave and in the same direction as its preceding T wave; that is, when the T wave is upright, the U wave normally will be upright. It is best observed in the chest leads, although it is present but barely detectable in the limb leads.

Relatively little is known about the U wave. Although the cause and clinical significance of the U wave are uncertain, the appearance of U waves or an increase in their magnitude is seen in certain disorders (see discussion of hypokalemia in Chapter 5). The U wave is generally upright in the precordial leads. A negative U wave may occur in patients who have left ventricular hypertrophy, hypertension, or coronary artery disease. An upright (positive) U wave that becomes inverted (negative) during an exercise stress test often indicates the presence of significant coronary artery obstruction in the left main or left anterior descending coronary artery.

ECG LEADS

As previously mentioned, the deflections on the ECG are produced by the electric energy caused by the movement of charged ions across the membranes of myocardial cells (depolarization and repolarization). This movement of charged particles results in a flow of electric current. The pressure behind the flow of electric current is called *electric potential*, and it creates an electric field. This electric field extends to the body surface, where the electric potential can be measured by the ECG.

By convention, 12-lead recordings compose the ECG. Each lead has a positive and a negative pole (electrode), and the location of these poles determines the polarity of the lead. A hypothetic line joining the poles of a lead is known as the *axis* of the lead. Moreover, every lead axis is oriented in a certain direction, depending on the location of the positive and negative electrodes.

A total of 6 of the 12 ECG leads measure cardiac forces in the frontal plane (the standard limb leads [I, II, III] and the augmented leads [aV_R, aV_L, and aV_F]); the remaining six leads (V_1 to V_6) measure the cardiac forces in the horizontal plane.

Standard Limb Leads

The standard (bipolar) limb leads, designated leads I, II, and III, were developed by Willem Einthoven (1860-1927), physiologist and inventor of the string galvanometer. Using the principle that the heart is situated in the center of the electric field it generates, Einthoven placed the electrodes of the three standard leads as far away from the heart as possible (that is, on the extremities—the right arm, left arm, and left leg).* These three electrodes therefore are considered to be electrically equidistant from the heart. Consequently, the heart may be viewed as a point source in the center of an equilateral triangle, whose apices are the right arm, left arm, and left leg. This is called *Einthoven's triangle* (Fig. 4-12, *A*).

The standard bipolar limb leads measure the difference between two recording sites. The actual potential under either of the electrodes is not known, as it is for the unipolar leads. For lead I, the negative electrode is placed on the right arm, and the positive electrode is placed on the left arm. For lead II, the negative electrode is on the right arm, and the positive electrode is on the left leg. For lead III, the left arm electrode is negative, and the left leg electrode is positive (Fig. 4-12, *A*). This is summarized as follows:

Lead	Location
I	Right arm ($-$) to left arm ($+$)
II	Right arm ($-$) to left leg ($+$)
III	Left arm ($-$) to left leg ($+$)

Because of the established relationship of the standard limb leads to each other, the sum of the electric potentials recorded in leads I and III equals the electric potential recorded in lead II at any given instant during the cardiac cycle. This is Einthoven's law, and it applies to a triangle of any shape. Stated mathematically, the law is as follows:

$$\text{Lead I} + \text{Lead III} = \text{Lead II}$$

Einthoven's law may be used to detect errors in electrode placement. Furthermore, it may clarify perplexing findings in another lead. For example, if the deflections of lead II are obscured by muscular or electric interference or by a wandering baseline, the characteristics of the other two leads may be used to determine the presence of a Q-wave or ST-segment deviation in lead II. Einthoven's law also is helpful in evaluating serial tracings. For example, if in a given tracing the T wave in lead I appears to be more negative than in the previous tracing, changes must be present in the T waves of the other two limb leads as well so that T1 + T3 = T2 (Fig. 4-13).

To prevent confusion about polarities, the ECG machine records a positive deflection in the bipolar leads when the left arm is in the positive portion of the electric field in lead I, the left leg is in the positive portion of the electric field in lead II, and the left leg is in the positive portion of the electric field in lead III.

Triaxial reference figure

The three lead axes of the equilateral triangle can be shifted without changing their direction so that their midpoints intersect at the same point. Thus the triaxial reference figure is formed with each of the lead axes separated from one another by 60 degrees (Fig. 4-12, *B*).

Augmented Leads

All augmented (unipolar) leads are called *V leads* and consist of extremity (limb) leads and precordial (chest) leads. The augmented leads aV_R, aV_L, and aV_F use the same electrode locations as the standard limb leads. Therefore the positive electrode is attached to the right arm (aV_R), left arm (aV_L), or left leg (aV_F). The negative electrode, however, is formed by combining leads I, II, and III, whose algebraic sum is zero. Because the electric center of the heart is at zero potential, the augmented leads measure the difference in potential between the limbs and the center of the heart.

The axis for each augmented lead is a line drawn from the extremity, where the positive electrode is placed, to the zero point of the electric field of the heart, which is at the center of the equilateral triangle (Fig. 4-12, *C*). These

---

*The right leg serves as a ground electrode, thereby providing a pathway of least resistance for electric interference in the body. Actually, the ground electrode can be placed at any location on the body.

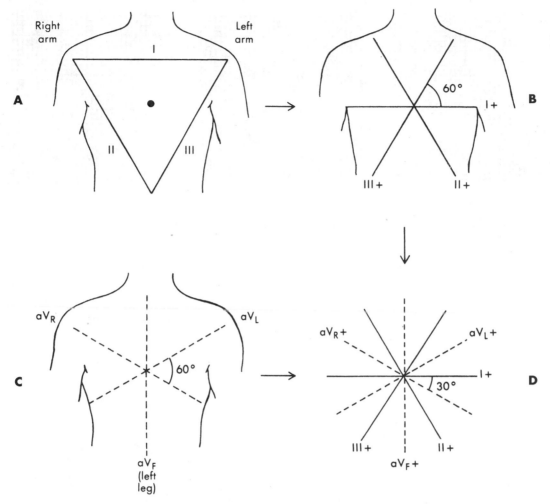

Fig. 4-12 **A,** The Einthoven equilateral triangle showing the axes of bipolar standard limb leads I, II, and III. The heart is at the center or zero point. **B,** The axes of the standard limb leads are shifted to the center of the triangle (zero point of the electric field), forming a triaxial figure. **C,** The axes of the unipolar augmented leads. **D,** The axes of the standard and augmented limb leads are combined to form a hexaxial figure. Each lead is labeled at its positive pole.

three unipolar lead axes also form a triaxial reference system whose axes are 60 degrees apart.

Hexaxial reference figure

When the triaxial figure of the standard leads and the triaxial figure of the augmented leads are combined, they form a hexaxial reference figure in which each augmented lead is perpendicular to a standard limb lead (Fig. 4-12, D). The hexaxial figure is a useful reference for plotting mean cardiac forces in the frontal plane.

Precordial Leads

In the horizontal plane, precordial (unipolar) leads are used to determine how far anteriorly or posteriorly from the frontal plane the electric forces of the heart are directed. The standard precordial ECG consists of six

unipolar leads, V_1 through V_6. In Fig. 4-14, _A,_ the V leads are shown with reference to their electrode positions on the anterior chest wall. These chest electrodes represent a positive pole (unipolar). Any electric force traveling toward one of these leads produces a positive deflection; a force traveling away from it produces a negative deflection. For descriptive purposes, leads V_1 and V_2 are called _right-sided precordial leads,_ leads V_3 and V_4 are called _midprecordial leads,_ and leads V_5 and V_6 are called _left-sided precordial leads._

Precordial reference figure

A transverse representation of the chest wall and the V leads results in the precordial reference figure (Fig. 4-14, _B_). This figure is a useful reference for plotting mean cardiac forces in the horizontal plane.

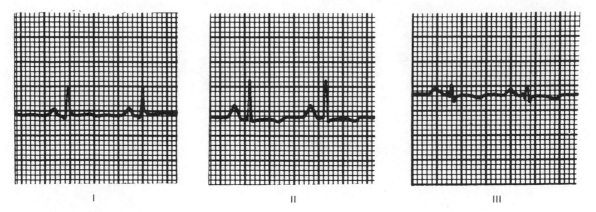

Fig. 4-13 Einthoven's law states that Lead I + Lead III = Lead II. The deflections in the ECG leads demonstrate this law.

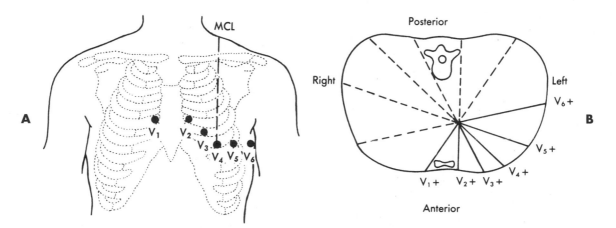

Fig. 4-14 **A,** Electrode positions of the precordial leads: V_1, fourth intercostal space at the right sternal border; V_2, fourth intercostal space at the left sternal border; V_3, halfway between V_2 and V_4; V_4, fifth intercostal space at the midclavicular line; V_5, anterior axillary line directly lateral to V_4; V_6, midaxillary line directly lateral to V_5. *MCL,* Midclavicular line. **B,** The precordial reference figure. Leads V_1 and V_2 are called *right-sided precordial leads;* leads V_3 and V_4 are called *midprecordial leads;* and leads V_5 and V_6 are called *left-sided precordial leads.*

Right precordial leads

Six right precordial (VR) leads provide specific information about right ventricular function. Their placement is comparable to V_3 to V_6 but on the right chest (see Fig. 4-28). If lead $V4_R$ is used to monitor a patient diagnosed with an inferior myocardial infarction, it is possible to predict the occlusion site. If the ST segment is elevated, proximal occlusion of the right coronary artery is suspected. If the ST segment is not elevated but coves to a positive T wave, distal right coronary artery occlusion is suspected. If the T wave is inverted, occlusion of the circumflex artery should be suspected.

Posterior leads

Abnormalities of the posterior wall of the left ventricle may be detected through the use of leads V_7 through V_9. These leads are positioned in the fifth intercostal space: leads V_7 in the posterior axillary line, V_8 in the scapular line, and V_9 in the paravertebral line (Fig. 4-14, *B*).

VECTOR APPROACH TO ECG

The electric potentials generated during the cardiac cycle can be described and measured. To adequately characterize such an electric potential or force, the magnitude and the direction of the force must be specified; this can be done by a vector. Briefly stated, a vector is a quantity of electric force that has a known magnitude and direction. A vector may be illustrated graphically by an arrow; the length of the arrow represents the magnitude of the force, and the direction of the arrow indicates the direction of the force. The arrowhead depicts the location of the positive field.

Representing electric forces of the heart by vectors more easily explains the relationship between the electric activity generated by the heart and the recording of this electric activity by a specific lead. When an electric force (and therefore the vector that represents it) establishes a direction parallel to the lead that records it, this electric force causes the largest deflection to be inscribed by that lead. An electric force perpendicular to the recording lead produces no deflection in that lead. Forces in between these extremes generate deflections according to their directions. The more nearly parallel the force (and vector) to the recording lead, the larger the deflection produced in that lead, and the more nearly perpendicular the force to the recording lead, the smaller the deflection. When the positive and negative forces on a lead are equal, the net area of the deflection is zero. This results in a biphasic or transitional deflection (Fig. 4-15).

Sequence of Electric Events in the Heart

In the normal heart, depolarization of the ventricle is a sequential process. The process can be represented by instantaneous vectors, each of which corresponds to all the heart's electric forces at a given moment. A diagram of successive instantaneous vectors depicting ventricular depolarization is shown in Fig. 4-16, *A.* Initial depolarization passes from left to right across the interventricular septum. During the second phase, depolarization of subendocardial muscle occurs near the apex. The last phase of depolarization occurs in the posterior free wall of the left ventricle.

The deflection recorded by any given lead results from the projection of the cardiac vector generated during depolarization onto the axis of the lead. Thus arrow 1 (Fig. 4-16, *B*), depicting depolarization of the septum, usually causes a small negative deflection in lead I, resulting in a Q wave and a larger positive deflection in lead III, resulting in an R wave. Arrow 2, illustrating depolarization of the apical region of the heart, usually produces a very small positive deflection (R wave) in lead I because of its leftward orientation and an R wave in lead II. Late depolarization of the heart, beginning from right to left in the posterior free wall of the left ventricle, causes a large positive deflection in lead I (the major part of the R wave) and an S wave in lead III. After completion of depolarization of ventricles, the electric wave returns to the baseline. Therefore the three arrows have generated a small initial Q wave followed by a large R wave in lead I and an R wave followed by an S wave in lead III (Fig. 4-16, *D*).

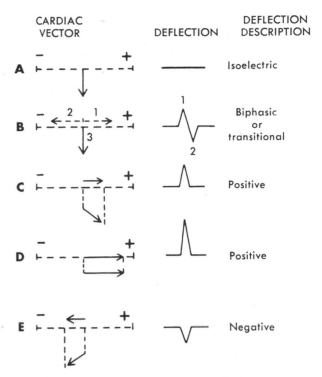

Fig. 4-15 Vectors and their ECG recordings. Each arrow represents the vector generated by an electric force. This force produces an ECG deflection, shown on the right. **A,** Because the vector is perpendicular to the axis of the recording lead, no projection appears on that lead. The absence of a deflection establishes an uninterrupted isoelectric line. **B,** The mean vector (vector 3) is perpendicular to the axis of the recording lead when the positive and negative forces are equal (the net area of the deflection is zero). A biphasic or transitional deflection is recorded because the initial forces moved right (vector 1) at the same distance that the later forces moved left (vector 2). The instantaneous vectors have equal magnitude but opposite direction. **C,** The vector projects on the positive side of the axis of the recording lead to inscribe a small positive deflection. **D,** When the vector is parallel with the lead axis, the projection onto the recording lead has its maximum magnitude. **E,** The vector projects on the negative side of the lead axis, and a small negative deflection is recorded.

As previously discussed, each ECG lead has a different orientation to the heart. Therefore the instantaneous vectors of ventricular depolarization produce a different deflection in each lead. This is also true of ventricular repolarization and atrial depolarization.

In this chapter, detailed consideration is given to the vectors of the QRS complex. However, the positions of the P wave and T wave in the frontal plane are also important. Normally the P wave is upright in leads I and II and may be biphasic, flat, or inverted in lead III; inverted in lead aV_R; upright, biphasic, or inverted in lead aV_L; and upright in lead aV_F.

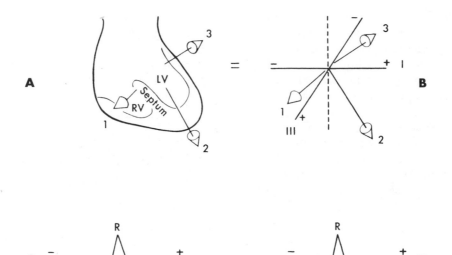

Fig. 4-16 Depolarization of the ventricles illustrated by instantaneous vectors. **A,** Arrow 1 depicts depolarization of the septum from left to right and is directed to the right and somewhat anteriorly. Arrow 2 illustrates depolarization of the apical region of the heart and is directed to the left and inferiorly. Arrow 3 represents depolarization of the posterior aspect of the left ventricle *(LV)* and is directed to the left and posteriorly. *RV,* Right ventricle. **B,** The instantaneous vectors representing ventricular depolarization are inscribed on lead I and III. **C and D,** Arrow 1 causes a small negative deflection in lead I, resulting in a Q wave, and a larger positive deflection in lead III, resulting in an R wave. Arrow 2 produces a small positive deflection (R wave) in lead I and an R wave in lead III. Arrow 3 causes a large R wave in lead I and an S wave in lead III.

Normally the T wave is upright in leads I and II; flat, biphasic, or inverted in lead III; and inverted in lead aV_R. In lead aV_L, the T wave may be upright, flattened, or biphasic, according to the QRS pattern. It may also be inverted, provided that the T wave in lead aV_R is also inverted. In lead aV_F the T wave is usually upright; however, it can be normally flattened, biphasic, or inverted, provided that the T wave in lead aV_R is also inverted.

In the horizontal plane the P wave is normally upright in all precordial leads, but it may be inverted in leads V_1 and V_2 without being abnormal. The normal QRS complex is transitional at some point between leads V_3 and V_4. The precordial transition zone is characterized by the transition from the RS complexes recorded by the leads oriented to the right ventricle to the QR complexes recorded by the leads oriented to the left ventricle (Fig. 4-17). The normal T wave is upright in leads V_2 through V_6. The T wave may be flat or inverted in lead V_1 and still be normal.

Mean Cardiac Vector

The mean cardiac vector, which is the average of all the instantaneous vectors, can be expressed accurately on the hexaxial reference figure. Furthermore, since the hexaxial reference system divides the frontal plane into 30-degree

intervals, the leads have been classified as follows: all degrees in the upper hemisphere of the hexaxial figure are labeled as negative degrees, and all degrees in the lower hemisphere are labeled as positive degrees. Accordingly, beginning at the positive end of the standard lead I axis (labeled 0 degrees and progressing counterclockwise), the leads are successively at −30, −60, −90, −120, −150, and −180 degrees. Progressing clockwise, the leads are successively at +30, +60, +90, +120, +150, and +180 degrees* (Fig. 4-18).

The position of the mean cardiac vector provides information about the electric "position" of the heart, also expressed as the mean electric axis, and it is influenced by the anatomic position of the heart within the chest, the anatomy of the heart itself, and the pathway traveled by the depolarizing wave. If the P vector is projected on the hexaxial figure, the mean electric axis of the P wave in the frontal plane lies approximately along the +60-degree axis (see Fig. 4-18). The mean QRS vector lies normally between 0 and +90 degrees, whereas the mean electric axis

---

*The conventional labeling of the hexaxial reference figure as positive and negative units should not be confused with the positive and negative poles of the lead axis.

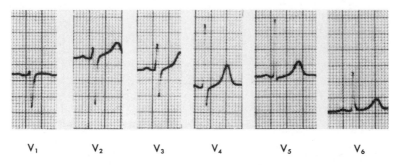

Fig. 4-17 Normal precordial lead ECG.

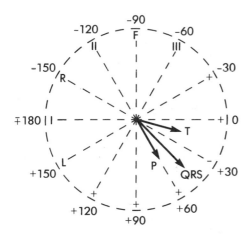

Fig. 4-18 The hexaxial reference system, which is formed by combining standard limb leads, (I, II, III) with augmented leads (aV_R, aV_L, aV_F), divides the frontal plane into 30-degree intervals. The inside of the hexaxial circle represents leads and their positive and negative poles. The outside of the circle is arbitrarily labeled with a negative value for the degrees in the upper hemisphere and a positive value for those in the lower hemisphere. The mean P vector normally lies along +60-degree axis. The mean QRS vector normally lies anywhere between 0 and +90 degrees; in this figure the mean QRS vector lies on +45-degree axis. The mean T vector normally lies between −10 and +75 degrees; in this figure the mean T vector lies on +15-degree axis. The mean frontal plane QRS-complex axis and T-wave axis are usually similarly directed, and the angle between them normally does not exceed 60 degrees.

of the T wave lies between −10 and +75 degrees. The mean frontal plane QRS-complex and T-wave axes are usually similarly directed, and the angle between them normally does not exceed 60 degrees (Fig. 4-18).

Mean QRS Axis

The remainder of this section discusses the significance and determination of the mean electric force, or axis, of the QRS. The principles used to determine the QRS axis

also may be applied to the determination of the P wave and T-wave axis.

Determination of the frontal plane projection of the mean QRS vector

In the standard ECG the average of the electric forces, or axis, can be determined in the frontal or horizontal plane leads. However, for practical purposes the axis is usually determined from leads of the frontal plane, or leads I, II, III, aV_R, aV_L, and aV_F.

The hexaxial reference system (see Fig. 4-18) and the following principles are used to determine the electric axis:

1. An electric force perpendicular to a lead axis will record a small or biphasic complex in that ECG lead.
2. An electric force parallel to a given lead will record its largest deflection in that lead.
3. An electric force going toward a positive electrode will record an upright or positive deflection.

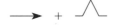

4. An electric force going away from a positive electrode will record a downward or negative deflection.

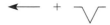

Although there are many methods to determine axes, method A is one of the easiest.

Method A

The frontal plane leads of an ECG (I, II, III, aV_R, aV_L, and aV_F) and the hexaxial reference circle are used to determine the direction of the axes in leads I and aV_F. This indicates the quarter of the hexaxial circle in which the axis falls.

1. Find the *main* direction of the QRS complex in lead I (the algebraic sum of the positive and negative QRS-complex deflections).

a. If positive, or upright, the axis is going toward the positive pole of lead I. Therefore it cannot be in the shaded area of the circle.

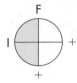

b. If negative, or downward, the axis is going away from the positive pole of lead I. Therefore it cannot be in the shaded area of the circle.

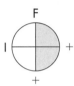

2. Find the *main* direction of the QRS complex in lead aV_F.
   a. If positive, or upright, the axis is going toward the positive pole of lead aV_F or toward the bottom of the hexaxial reference circle. Therefore it cannot be in the shaded area of the circle.

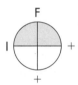

   b. If negative or downward, the axis is going toward the negative pole of lead aV_F or toward the top of the hexaxial reference circle. Therefore it cannot be in the shaded half of the circle.

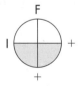

3. Use these two determinations to locate the average electric forces, or axis, in one quarter of the circle and eliminate three fourths of the circle as a possible location.

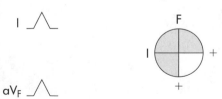

4. After locating the quadrant, identify the one fourth of the circle in which the average electric force is located and determine what other leads are in that quadrant. In this example, other leads in the quadrant are II and aV_R.

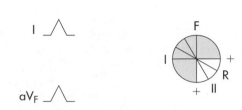

5. Look at the leads in the identified quadrant (that is, I, aV_F, II, and aV_R) and determine in which lead the largest deflection is found. The electric axis is parallel to the lead with the largest deflection. Draw an arrow from the center of the circle along this axis. The tip of the arrow should point toward the outside of the circle.
6. Finally, ensure that the lead axis is perpendicular to the arrow and that it contains the smallest deflection.

Use method A to determine the axis of the QRS complex in the ECG in Fig. 4-19, *A*. To make method A even more precise, note that the lead in which the smallest deflection was found, aV_L, is not an algebraic zero but a negative 3. This implies that the true QRS axis is more toward the negative pole of aV_L, or about +75, rather than +60 as originally calculated (Fig. 4-19, *C*).

Method B

Another way to determine axes is method B (see Fig. 4-19, *D*).
1. Calculate the algebraic sum of the QRS in two leads. (Leads I and III are convenient.)
2. Plot these values on the hexaxial reference system. Perpendicular lines dropped from the plotted points of leads I and III produce a crossing point between the two lines.
3. Find the line formed by connecting the center point of the circle and the plotted crossing point; this is the QRS axis in the frontal plane.

Clinical Significance of Axis

The determination of axis provides one additional piece of ECG information. By itself, the information may not be significant, but combined with the total clinical picture, the axis may clarify a diagnosis. Although there is no universal agreement defining "normal" and "abnormal" axes, the following criteria have been used (Fig. 4-20):
   A. General: convenient and realistic boundaries
   B. Marked left axis between −30 and −90
   C. Extreme left axis or extreme right axis between +180 and −90 (The ECG axis should be interpreted with the patient's clinical background.)

The ECG axis may help determine the presence of normal sinus rhythm when the mean axis of the P wave is within the normal limits of 0 to +90. A wide QRS-T angle almost always means cardiac disease. However, there are a number of causes of axis deviation, some of which are normal variations (see the section on causes of axis deviation).

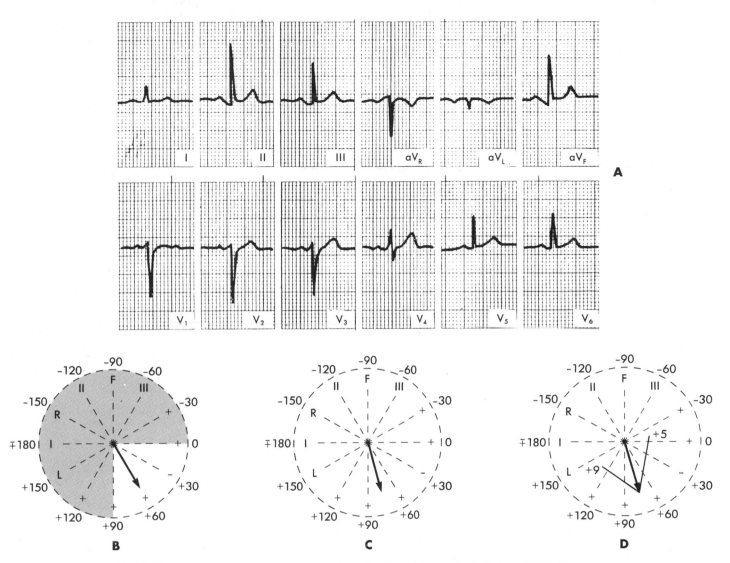

Fig. 4-19 Determination of mean QRS axis in the frontal plane. **A,** A 12-lead ECG. **B,** Method A for axis determination. The QRS axis in lead I is mainly upright; therefore the axis is toward the positive pole of lead I. The QRS axis in lead aV$_F$ is mainly upright; therefore the axis is toward the positive pole of lead aV$_F$. The quadrant in which the axis falls is between 0 and +90, or the unshaded area of circle B. Leads II and aV$_R$ are also found in this quadrant. The largest deflection is found in lead II; the smallest deflection is found in lead aV$_L$. The mean QRS axis is about +60 degrees. **C,** Method A, more precisely used. Because lead aV$_L$ is −3 and not algebraic zero, the true mean QRS axis would be toward the negative pole of lead aV$_L$, or about +75 degrees. **D,** Method B for axis determination. The algebraic sum of lead I is +5; the algebraic sum of lead III is +9. Plot these two values on the hexaxial circle. Perpendicular lines dropped from these plotted points produce a crossing point. The line formed by connecting the center point of the circle and the crossing point is the mean QRS axis in the frontal plane or +75 degrees.

Electric Heart Positions and Electric Axis

There is a close relationship between electric axis and electric heart positions. The electric position is customarily divided into five positions; their corresponding axes are horizontal (−30), semihorizontal (0), intermediate (+30), semivertical (+60), and vertical (+90). Because electric positions give little additional clinical information, they are usually not mentioned on a routine ECG interpretation.

Other terms that may be used are *clockwise* and *counterclockwise rotation*. Clockwise rotation occurs when the

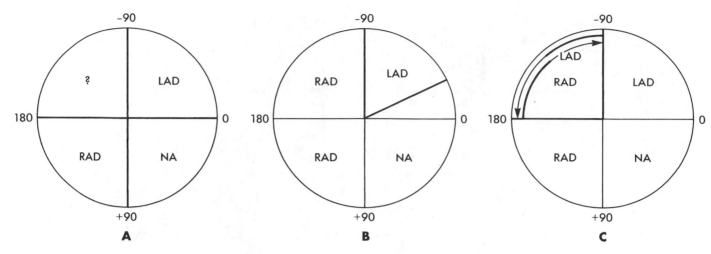

Fig. 4-20 Hexaxial reference circles indicating values for axis deviation. **A,** Convenient and realistic boundaries; 0 to +90, normal axis *(NA)*; 0 to −90, left axis deviation *(LAD)*; +90 to +180, right axis deviation *(RAD)*; +180 to −90, questionable axis *(?)*. (Axis of ventricular ectopy may fall in this quadrant.) **B,** Marked left axis deviation, −30 and −90; right axis, +90 to −90. **C,** Extreme left axis deviation or extreme right axis deviation, +180 to −90.

transitional zone is shifted toward the left precordial leads (V₅ to V₆); it means that there is a posterior axis deviation. Counterclockwise rotation occurs when the transitional zone is shifted toward the right (V₁ to V₂); it means anterior axis deviation. Anterior and posterior axis deviation are not routinely calculated because they are derived by determining electric axis from the horizontal plane in the precordial leads. Horizontal plane axes are not determined for routine ECG interpretation.

CAUSES OF AXIS DEVIATION

Causes of right axis deviation include the following:
Normal variation (that is, youth and thinness)
Mechanical shifts associated with inspiration or emphysema
Right ventricular hypertrophy
Right bundle branch block
Left posterior hemiblock
Dextrocardia
Left ventricular ectopic rhythms
Right ventricular ectopic rhythms (some)
Pulmonary embolism and/or infarction
Causes of left axis deviation include the following:
Normal variation (that is, older adulthood and obesity)
Mechanical shifts associated with expiration, a high diaphragm from pregnancy, ascites, and abdominal tumors
Left anterior hemiblock
Left bundle branch block
Endocardial cushion defects and/or other congenital lesions

Wolff-Parkinson-White syndrome
Hyperkalemia
Right ventricular ectopic rhythms

Determination of the Horizontal Plane Projection of the Mean QRS Vector

1. The clinician should identify the precordial lead with the transitional QRS deflection in Fig. 4-21, *A*.
2. Lead V₄ is transitional.
3. The QRS vector is perpendicular to the transitional lead (V₄).
4. The vector should be directed toward the positive sides of the leads with positive deflections and on the negative sides of the leads with negative deflections, as shown in Fig. 4-21, *C*.
5. When the horizontal plane direction of the mean QRS is noted, an arrowhead may be placed on the mean QRS frontal plane vector to indicate the vector's anterior or posterior direction, as shown in Fig. 4-21, *B*.

LEFT VENTRICULAR ENLARGEMENT

It is not usually possible in the ECG to differentiate ventricular dilatation and hypertrophy. The term *hypertrophy* is commonly used; however, this presentation will use *enlargement*, since it includes dilatation and hypertrophy.

Hypertension, aortic valvular disease, mitral insufficiency, coronary artery disease, and congenital heart disease (for example, patent ductus arteriosus and coarctation of the aorta) commonly produce left ventricular enlargement. Under these circumstances the wall of the left ventricle is

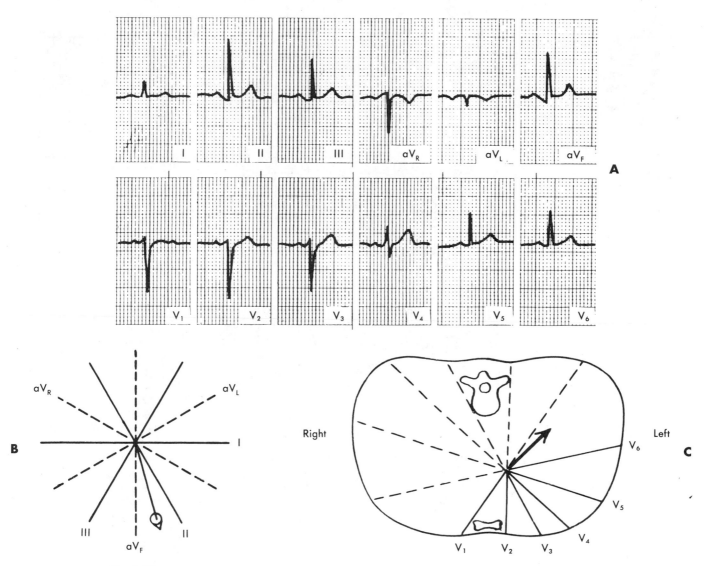

Fig. 4-21   Determination of the mean QRS vector in the frontal and horizontal planes. **A,** A 12-lead ECG. **B,** The mean QRS vector in the frontal plane is located at +70 degrees. The arrowhead indicates that the mean QRS vector points posteriorly in the horizontal plane. **C,** The horizontal plane projection of the mean QRS is drawn in a posterior direction on the precordial reference figure. This calculation gives information for the direction of the arrowhead in the frontal plane (**B**).

thicker or more dilated than normal. Furthermore, this increase in muscle mass results in increased voltage of the QRS deflections that represent left ventricular potentials. Accordingly, the QRS interval may increase in duration to the upper limits of normal, the intrinsicoid deflection may be somewhat delayed over the left ventricle, and the voltage of the QRS complex will increase, producing deeper S waves over the right ventricle (leads V_1 and V_2) and taller R waves over the left ventricle (leads V_5, V_6, I, aV_L).

Leads oriented to the left ventricle may also demonstrate a strain pattern (that is, depressed ST segments and inverted T waves). The mechanism of strain (a useful, non-committal term) is not understood. However, it develops in patients who have long-standing left ventricular enlargement and intensifies when dilatation and failure set in. Myocardial ischemia and slowing of intraventricular conduction are some of the important factors that probably contribute to the pattern.

In general, the voltage criteria proposed for the diagnosis of left ventricular enlargement are unreliable. However, the best approach so far is the Estes scoring system, which is as follows (Fig. 4-22):

1. An R wave or S wave in a limb lead of 20 mm or more; an S wave in lead V_1, V_2, or V_3 of 25 mm or

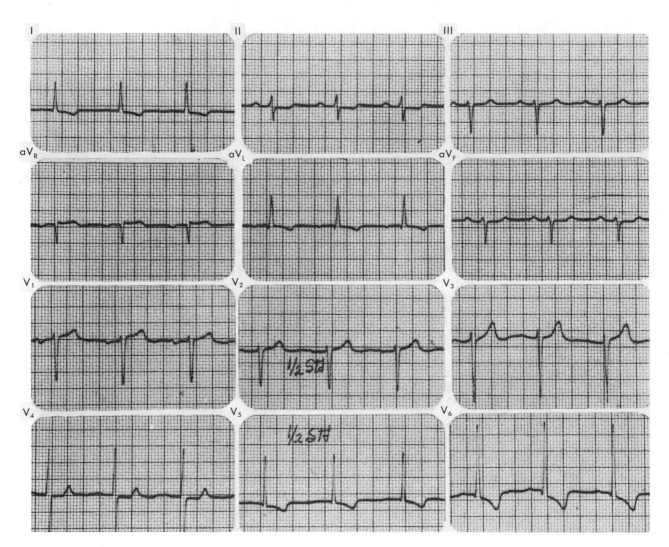

Fig. 4-22 Left ventricular enlargement. This tracing illustrates left ventricular hypertrophy (enlargement) using the Estes criteria: an S wave in lead III of 20 mm or more or an R wave in lead V_4 of 25 mm or more, which equal a score of 3; ST shift (without digitalis), which equals a score of 3; left axis deviation of -60, which equals a score of 2. Total score equals 8. Right bundle branch block and left anterior hemiblock are also present.

more; an R wave in lead V_4, V_5, or V_6 of 25 mm or more, which equals a score of 3

2. Any ST-segment shift opposite to the mean QRS vector (without digitalis), which equals a score of 3, and typical "strain" segments in the T wave (with digitalis), which equals a score of 1

3. Left axis deviation of -15 degrees or more, which equals a score of 2

4. A QRS interval of 0.09 second or more, which equals a score of 1, and intrinsicoid deflection in leads V_5 to V_6 of 0.05 second or more, which equals a score of 1

5. Left atrial enlargement, which equals a score of 3

Definite left ventricular enlargement is present with a score of 5 or more. Probable left ventricular enlargement is present if the score is 4.

Left ventricular enlargement may be present without concomitant left axis deviation. Left axis deviation supports the diagnosis of left ventricular enlargement only when the voltage criteria are fulfilled. The voltage criteria just listed, however, include a small percentage of false-positive and false-negative diagnoses. Before an ECG diagnosis of left ventricular enlargement is made, it is wise to evaluate factors such as body build, the thickness of the chest wall, and the presence of complicating disease. Echocardiography has eliminated many uncertainties about the presence of ventricular enlargement.

LEFT ATRIAL ENLARGEMENT

Left atrial abnormality occurs frequently but not always in left ventricular enlargement. For example, left atrial enlargement caused by mitral stenosis is not associated with left ventricular enlargement unless there is mitral insufficiency or concomitant aortic valvular disease.

The following criteria are used in the ECG diagnosis of left atrial enlargement (Fig. 4-23):

1. The duration of the P wave is often widened to 0.12 second or more. (Normal P wave duration is 0.11 second.)

2. The contour of the P wave is notched and slurred in leads I and II (P mitrale). (Notching per se is not abnormal unless the P wave shows increased voltage, duration, or both or the summits are more than 0.03 second apart.)

3. The right precordial leads (V_1 and V_2) reflect diphasic P waves with a wide, deep, negative terminal component. The duration (in seconds) and amplitude (in millimeters) of the terminal component are measured and the algebraic product determined. A negative value greater than -0.03 second is considered abnormal.

4. The mean electric axis of the P wave may be shifted left, to between $+45$ and -30 degrees.

RIGHT VENTRICULAR ENLARGEMENT

Right ventricular enlargement is commonly seen with mitral stenosis, some forms of congenital heart disease, and chronic diffuse pulmonary disease such as pulmonary hypertension, emphysema, and bronchiectasis. For right ventricular enlargement to become evident electrocardiographically in the adult, however, the right ventricle must enlarge considerably, since the normal adult ECG reflects left ventricular predominance. This accounts for the relative frequency of a normal ECG in right ventricular enlargement.

Most of the criteria for diagnosing right ventricular enlargement focus on the QRS pattern in the right precordial leads. As the right ventricle enlarges, the height of the right precordial R waves increases, with a concomitant decrease in the depth of the S wave. When right ventricular

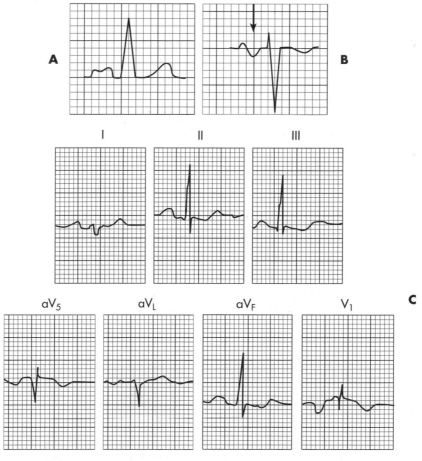

Fig. 4-23 Left atrial enlargement. **A,** Wide, humped P wave produced in at least one of the extremity leads (P mitrale pattern). **B,** Wide, biphasic (initially positive and then negative) P wave may be produced in lead V_1. **C,** Example of broad, humped P waves in a patient with left atrial enlargement.

enlargement becomes fully developed, the normal precordial pattern is completely reversed so that tall R waves (QR or RS) are recorded in lead V_1 with deep S waves (RS) in lead V_6.

Prolongation of the QRS interval does not develop unless an intraventricular conduction defect develops with the enlarged right ventricle. However, the time of onset of the intrinsicoid deflection may be delayed in the right precordial leads because the vectors representing activation of the right ventricle usually occur later in the QRS interval than they normally do; these vectors are also increased in magnitude.

Right axis deviation is the most common sign of right ventricular enlargement. However, the diagnosis of right ventricular enlargement should not be made on this finding alone unless other causes for right axis deviation have been ruled out. Furthermore, right ventricular enlargement may occur without abnormal right axis deviation.

A right ventricular strain pattern is manifested in ST-segment and T-wave alterations, with T-wave changes similar to those seen in left ventricular enlargement. The ST segment is depressed and the T wave is inverted in the right-sided precordial leads and often in leads II, III, and aV_F. This is a nonspecific abnormality.

Right bundle branch block is seen in right ventricular enlargement, especially of the volume-overload variety. In the younger person, right ventricular enlargement is commonly associated with complete or incomplete right bundle branch block. In the older age group (at least 40 years old), coronary artery disease is the most common cause. The surface ECG is less useful than the vectorcardiogram in the assessment of the degree of right ventricular enlargement in cases of incomplete or complete right bundle branch block. Further elaboration on the vectorcardiogram is beyond the scope of this presentation; refer to other textbooks on this subject. See Chapter 5 for a discussion of right bundle branch block.

A summary of the features of right ventricular enlargement follows; these should be compared with the example in Fig. 4-24.

1. Reversal of precordial lead pattern with tall R waves over the right precordium (leads V_1 and V_2) and

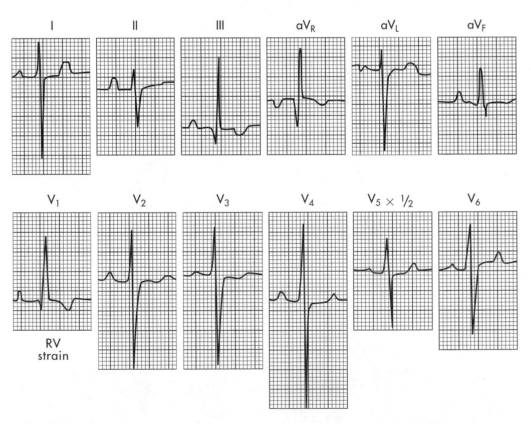

Fig. 4-24 Right ventricular enlargement. Reversal precordial pattern with a tall R wave over the right precordium (leads V_1 to V_2) and a deep S wave over the left (leads V_5 to V_6), QRS interval within normal limits, right axis deviation, and ST-segment depression with upward convexity and inverted T waves in the right precordial leads (V_1 to V_2) and in leads III and aV_R. Note the peaked P waves in leads II, III, and V_1 resulting from right atrial enlargement. *RV strain*, Right ventricular strain.

deep S waves over the left precordium (leads V_5 and V_6); the R to S ratio in lead V_1 greater than 1.0
2. Duration of QRS interval within normal limits (if there is no right bundle branch block)
3. Late intrinsicoid deflection in leads V_1 and V_2
4. Right axis deviation
5. Typical strain ST-segment and T-wave patterns in leads V_1, V_2, II, III, and aV_F

RIGHT ATRIAL ENLARGEMENT

In the presence of right ventricular enlargement, it is not unusual to find an enlarged right atrium. Moreover, right atrial enlargement is often an indirect sign of right ventricular enlargement.

The following criteria are used in the ECG diagnosis of right atrial enlargement (Fig. 4-25):
1. The duration of the P wave is 0.11 second or less.
2. The contour of the P wave is tall, is peaked (P pulmonale), and measures 2.5 mm or more in amplitude in leads II, III, and aV_F.

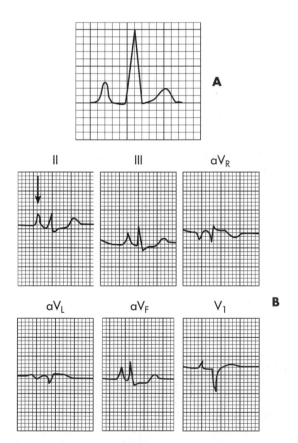

Fig. 4-25 Right atrial enlargement. **A,** Tall, narrow P waves indicate right atrial enlargement (P pulmonale pattern). **B,** Note tall P waves, seen here in leads II, III, aV_F, and V_1 in a patient with right atrial enlargement.

3. The right precordial leads reflect diphasic P waves, often with increased voltage of the initial component.
4. The mean electric axis of the P wave may be shifted right to +70 degrees or more.

Abnormal P waves may occur in healthy patients. For example, acceleration of the heart rate alone may cause peaking and increased voltage of the P wave. Conversely, normal P waves may be identified in atrial disease.

MYOCARDIAL INFARCTION

For diagnosis of myocardial infarction, the ECG should be used to confirm the clinical impression. Because the ECG may not be diagnostic in many instances, a patient suspected clinically of having myocardial infarction should be treated accordingly, regardless of what the ECG shows.

Only Q wave changes (necrosis) are diagnostic of infarction, but changes in the ST segments (injury) and T waves (ischemia) may be suspicious and provide presumptive evidence. These changes are illustrated in Fig. 4-26.

Q Wave

The Q wave is one of the most important and sometimes most difficult feature to interpret in the assessment of myocardial infarction on the ECG. For example, with normal intraventricular conditions, small Q waves are present in leads V_5, V_6, aV_L, and I, particularly with a horizontal heart position or left axis deviation. Furthermore, with a vertical heart position or right axis deviation, small Q waves may be present in leads II, III, and aV_F. Finally, deep, wide Q waves or QS complexes are normally present in lead aV_R and may be present in lead V_1.

Major importance is placed on the development of *new* Q waves in ECG leads where they previously were not present. Accordingly, the appearance of abnormal Q waves must be considered in light of the overall picture, considering that pathologic Q waves have the following features:
1. They are 0.04 second or longer in duration.
2. They are usually greater than 4 mm in depth.
3. They appear in leads that do not normally have deep, wide Q waves; leads V_1 and aV_R normally record Q waves. Pathologic Q waves are usually present in several leads oriented in similar directions (for example, leads II, III, and aV_F or I and aV_L).

Vector Abnormalities

In acute myocardial infarction, electric and anatomic death of the myocardium occurs in the region of the infarct; hence the initial forces of depolarization tend to point away from the infarcted area, producing Q waves in the ECG leads facing the involved site. The mean T vector also tends to point away from the site of infarction, presumably because of electric ischemia in the tissues around the infarct. The ST vector represents the effect of injury current. When the injury current is in the epicardial layers of the myocardium, as in myocardial infarction and peri-

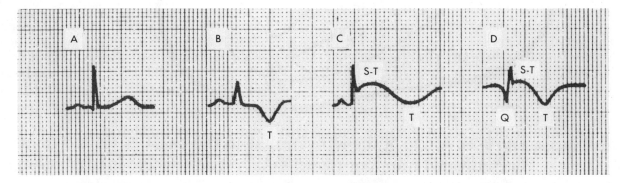

Fig. 4-26 ECG wave changes indicative of ischemia, injury, and necrosis of the myocardium. **A,** Normal left ventricular wave pattern. **B,** Ischemia indicated by inversion of the T wave. **C,** Ischemia and current of injury indicated by T-wave inversion and ST-segment elevation. The ST segment may be elevated above or depressed below the baseline, depending on whether the tracing is from a lead facing toward or away from the infarcted area and depending on whether epicardial or endocardial injury occurs. Epicardial injury causes ST-segment elevation in the leads facing the epicardium. **D,** Ischemia, injury, and myocardial necrosis. The Q wave indicates necrosis of the myocardium.

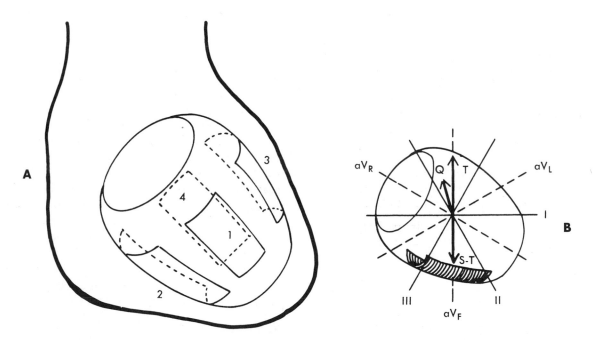

Fig. 4-27 **A,** Lie of the left ventricle in the chest as viewed frontally. The left ventricle has been divided into four topographic regions where infarctions may occur: *1,* anterior, *2,* diaphragmatic or inferior, *3,* lateral, and *4,* posterior (pure). **B,** Vectors of a diaphragmatic myocardial infarction. Hexaxial reference figure is superimposed on the left ventricle as viewed in **B.** The mean vector for the initial 0.04 second of the QRS complex points *away* from the infarcted area and indicates the dead zone. This produces Q waves in the leads "looking at" the infarction. The mean T vector indicates the ischemic zone around the infarct and points *away* from the infarcted area. The ST vector indicates the injury zone, and in the event of myocardial infarction, the ST vector points *toward* the injured area. In this example of a diaphragmatic myocardial infarction, leads II, III, and aV$_F$ exhibit the Q waves, ST-segment elevation, and T-wave inversion shown in Fig. 4-26, *D.*

carditis, the ST segment is elevated in leads facing the injury, and the ST vector points toward the injured area. When the injury current is located in the subendocardial layers, as in angina pectoris, coronary insufficiency, and subendocardial infarction, the ST segment is depressed in leads facing the injury, and the ST vector points away from the site of injury (Fig. 4-27). ST displacement in subendocardial infarction persists longer than that of angina pectoris and coronary insufficiency.

Thus with an acute myocardial infarction the ST vector is opposite in direction to the Q vector and the mean T vector, resulting in ST-segment elevation in leads that have Q waves and inverted T waves. The relationship of these three vectors to one another is diagrammed in Fig. 4-27, B.

According to data obtained from animal studies, loss of resting membrane potential in the ischemic cells occurs first and is responsible for T-Q–segment depression in the scalar ECG. Reduction in action potential duration and amplitude follows and causes ST-segment elevation. Delayed repolarization in the ischemic area results in T-wave inversion.

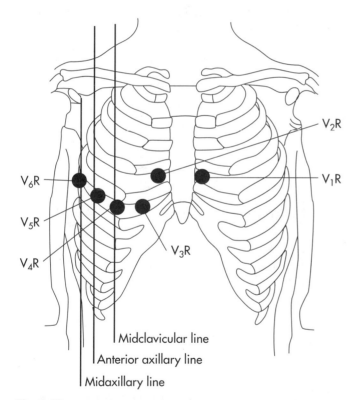

Fig. 4-28 Lead placement for right precordial leads. The six right precordial *(VR)* leads provide specific information about right ventricular function in a patient diagnosed with myocardial infarction of the inferior wall. If the ST segment is elevated in V_4R, proximal occlusion of the right coronary artery should be considered. If the ST segment is not elevated but coves to a positive T wave, distal occlusion of the right coronary artery should be considered. If the T wave is inverted, occlusion of the circumflex artery should be considered.

Localization of Infarction

Localization of infarcts may be important for several reasons, including prognosis. Localization is based on the principle that diagnostic ECG signs of myocardial infarction (see Fig. 4-26) occur in leads whose positive terminals face the damaged surface of the heart. To facilitate localization, the left ventricle has been divided into four topographic regions where infarctions may occur (see Fig. 4-27, *A*). Although these locations represent electric rather than anatomic sites of infarction, anatomic correlations occur with reasonable frequency, particularly for the first myocardial infarction.

An anterior infarction produces characteristic changes in leads V_1, V_2, and V_3; a diaphragmatic or inferior infarction affects leads II, III, and aV_F; and a lateral infarction involves leads I, aV_L, V_5, and V_6. In strictly posterior infarction, there are no leads whose positive terminals are directly over the infarct. However, the changes of the electric field produced by any infarction still apply; hence in a purely posterior infarction the initial forces of the QRS complex and the T wave point anteriorly away from the site of the infarct, and the ST segment is directed posteriorly. This is recognized in the ECG as tall, broad initial R waves; ST-segment depression; and tall, upright T waves in leads V_1 and V_2. In other words, a mirror image of the typical infarction pattern of an anterior myocardial infarction is recorded. Stated another way, infarction of the true posterior surface of the heart must be inferred from reciprocal (opposite) changes occurring in the anterior leads. Infarction of the right ventricle may also occur in inferior infarctions. In addition to the ST-segment elevations in leads II, III, and aV_F seen in inferior infarction, ST-segment elevation in leads V_1 and V_4R may be seen. Placement of right chest leads is shown in Fig. 4-28. Locations of myocardial infarction are summarized in Table 4-1.

Although diagnostic signs of myocardial infarction appear in leads facing the infarcted heart surface, reciprocal

TABLE 4-1	Location of Myocardial Infarction
Area of Infarction	**Leads Showing Wave Changes**
Anterior	V_1, V_2, V_3
Diaphragmatic or inferior	II, III, aV_F
Lateral	I, aV_L, V_5, V_6
Posterior (pure)	V_1 and V_2: tall, broad initial R wave; ST-segment depression; tall, upright T wave
Right ventricular	II, III, aV_F and V_1 and V_4R

TABLE 4-2   Time Relationships in the Evolution and Resolution of a Myocardial Infarction

ECG Abnormality	Onset	Disappearance
ST-segment elevation	Immediately	1 to 6 weeks
Q waves of greater than 0.04 second	Immediately or in several days	Years to never
T-wave inversion	6 to 24 hours	Months to years

changes occur concomitantly in leads facing the diametrically opposed surface of the heart. These changes include the absence of a Q wave; some increase of the R wave; a depressed ST segment; and an upright, tall T wave.

Therefore reciprocal changes in an anterior infarction occur in leads II, III, and aV_F. In a diaphragmatic or inferior infarction, reciprocal changes occur in lead I, lead aV_L, and some of the precordial leads. In lateral wall infarction, lead V_1 may show reciprocal changes.

Frequently the localization of an infarction is not as strict as described. If the anterior and lateral walls of the left ventricle are involved in the process, it is called an *anterolateral infarction*. If the limb leads indicate an inferior infarction and diagnostic changes are also present in leads V_5 and V_6, it is called an *inferior infarction with lateral extension*, or an *inferolateral infarction*.

Evolution of a Myocardial Infarction

The evolution of a myocardial infarction is a sequential process, and it is important to record the time relationships in the diagnosis. Within the first few hours after infarction, sometimes referred to as the *hyperacute state*, elevated ST segments and tall (hyperacute), upright T waves appear in leads facing the infarction. Q waves may appear early or may not develop for several days. Within several days of the infarct the ST segment begins to return to baseline, whereas the T waves develop progressively deeper inversion. After weeks or months the T waves become shallower and may finally return to normal. The Q waves are most likely to remain as a permanent record of the myocardial scar (Fig. 4-29). Persistent ST-segment elevation (beyond 6 weeks) suggests the possibility of ventricular aneurysm (Table 4-2). The different locations of myocardial infarction in different stages of clinical evolution are shown in Figs. 4-29 to 4-33.

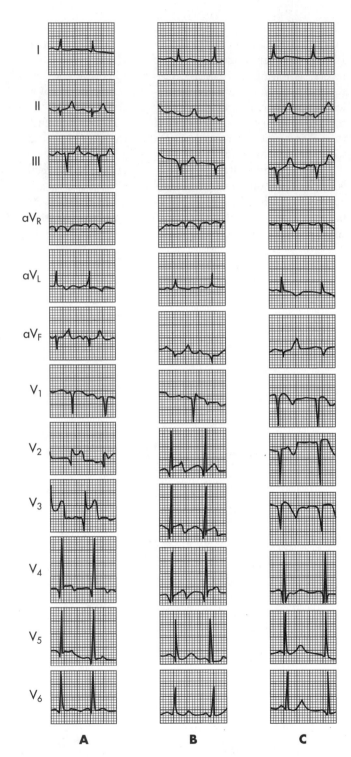

Fig. 4-29 Evolutionary changes in anteroseptal myocardial infarction reflected in Leads V_2 to V_4. **A,** At admission, hyperacute phase is reflected by ST elevations. **B,** At 24 hours, there are Pardee T waves. **C,** At 48 hours, there are pathologic Q waves.

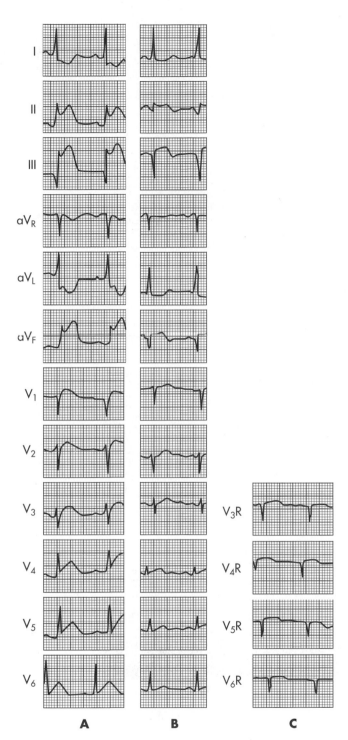

Fig. 4-30 Evolutionary changes in inferior and right ventricular myocardial infarction. **A,** At admission—acute phase. **B,** At 12 hours. **C,** Right chest leads demonstrating right ventricular infarction.

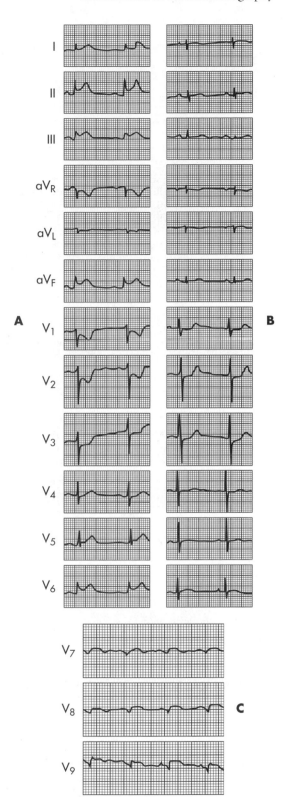

Fig. 4-31 Evolutionary changes in inferior and posterior myocardial infarction. **A,** Acute inferior and apical injury. **B,** At 24 hours. Note tall R wave in lead V_1 not present in **A,** suggesting posterior myocardial infarction. **C,** Posterior infarction confirmed.

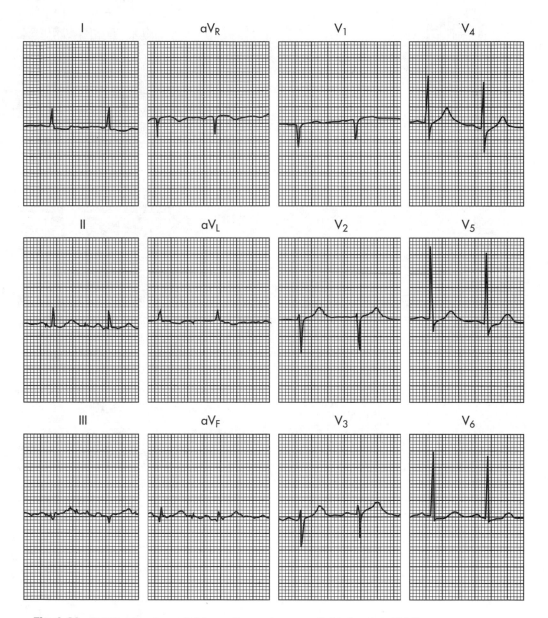

Fig. 4-32   ECG subendocardial (non-Q-wave) myocardial infarction. ECG may appear normal. Myocardial infarction is diagnosed by abnormal cardiac enzyme levels.

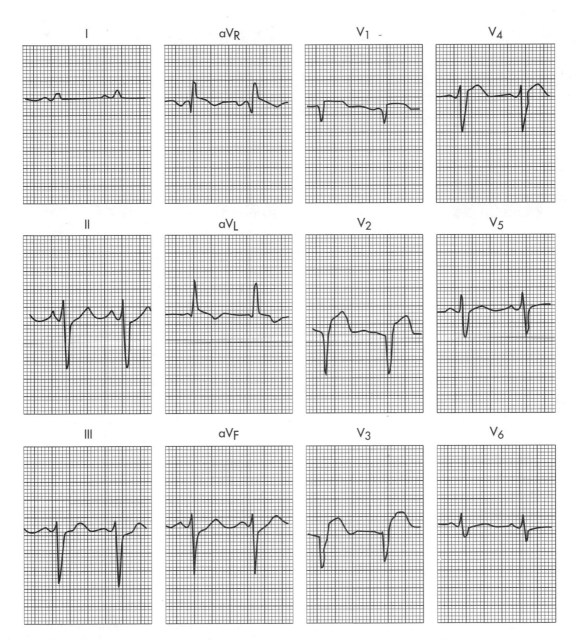

Fig. 4-33 ECG 8 weeks after anteroseptal myocardial infarction. Persistent ST-segment elevation beyond 2 weeks after myocardial infarction may indicate the development of ventricular aneurysm. This complication is most frequently associated with anteroseptal myocardial infarction.

SUGGESTED READINGS

Advanced Skills: *Deciphering difficult ECGs,* Springhouse, Penn, 1993, Springhouse.

Braunwald E, editor: *Heart disease: a textbook of cardiovascular medicine,* ed 4, Philadelphia, 1992, Saunders.

Chung EK: *Principles of cardiac arrhythmias,* ed 4, Baltimore, 1989, Williams & Wilkins.

Constant J: *Essentials of bedside cardiology,* ed 4, Boston, 1993, Little, Brown.

Grauer K: *A practical guide to ECG interpretation,* St Louis, 1992, Mosby.

Schlant RC and others: *Hurst's the heart,* ed 8, New York, 1995, Mc-Graw-Hill.

Sweetwood HM: *Clinical electrocardiography for nurses,* Rockville, Md, 1989, Aspen.

Zipes DP: *Progress in cardiology,* Philadelphia, 1988, Lea & Febiger.

Dysrhythmias

Barbara A. Erickson

NORMAL CARDIAC CYCLE

Before electrocardiographic (ECG) interpretation of cardiac dysrhythmias is discussed, a review of the normal electric events that occur during a cardiac cycle, as well as a discussion of basic electrophysiologic principles, is necessary.[1] During normal sinus rhythm, the cardiac impulse originates in the sinus node and then travels to the right and left atria via the Bachmann bundle, which is a division of the anterior internodal pathway. The impulse transmission is so rapid that activation of the left atrium occurs almost simultaneously with that of the right. Sinus node discharge and conduction from the sinus node to the atria are not recorded from the body surface, and therefore these events are not seen on the ECG. In response to the sinus node impulse, the atria depolarize and generate the P wave; atrial repolarization (Ta wave) is generally obscured by the QRS complex and is therefore not usually seen. Impulse conduction through the right atrium probably occurs via three internodal tracts—the anterior, the middle (Wenckebach), and the posterior (Thorel)—and eventually reaches the AV node and bundle of His. However, the functional importance of these pathways in providing specialized tracts for conduction is unsettled. Most experts agree that these pathways are not analogous to the specialized conducting pathways in the ventricles (for example, the bundle branches and Purkinje fibers, which are discrete histologically identifiable tracts of tissue). However, preferential internodal conduction (more rapid conduction velocity between nodes in some parts of the atrium compared with other parts) probably does exist and may be caused by fiber orientation, size, geometry, or other factors rather than by specialized tracts located between the sinoatrial (SA) and atrioventricular (AV) nodes.

The speed at which the impulse travels (conduction velocity) becomes reduced as the impulse traverses the AV node but once again accelerates through the bundle of His, bundle branches, and Purkinje fibers. The Purkinje fibers distribute the impulse rapidly and uniformly over the ventricular endocardium, finally depolarizing the ventricular myocardium (Fig. 5-1). The surface ECG records only ventricular muscle depolarization (the QRS complex) and repolarization (the T wave), atrial depolarization (the P wave), and sometimes repolarization (the Ta wave). Activity from the SA and AV nodes, bundle of His, bundle branches, and Purkinje fibers is not recorded in the ECG. Special intracardiac electrodes can be used to record activity from some of these structures and are discussed briefly later in this chapter.

It has been postulated that the bundle branches are composed of three divisions, called *fascicles*,[2] that are formed by the right bundle branch and two divisions of the left bundle branch (the anterosuperior and posteroinferior divisions). The term *hemiblock* has been used to describe block in one of these fascicles.[2] A more accurate term is *fascicular block*. Although a number of careful anatomic and pathologic studies of human hearts have failed to substantiate the anatomic separation of the left bundle branch into two distinct and specific divisions, the fascicular block concept has been used to explain observed ECG and clinical entities (see section on bundle branch block) (Fig. 5-2).

The electric pattern of a typical cardiac cycle is displayed in Fig. 5-3 and is discussed in Table 5-1 (see also Chapter 4).

DETERMINATION OF HEART RATE

Several methods are available for determining the heart rate from an ECG recording. When the atrial and ventricular rates are different, as in third-degree AV block, atrial and ventricular rates should be determined separately.

Five possible methods for determining heart rate follow:
1. 6-second interval method (Figs. 5-3 and 5-4): This method is the easiest and most practical. It is accurate for regular and irregular rhythms.
   a. The clinician counts the cardiac waves (that is, P waves and/or QRS complexes) in a 6-second interval and multiplies it by 10.
   b. The ECG paper is marked at the top into 3-second intervals. If these marks are absent, there are 15 large ECG squares in a 3-second interval.

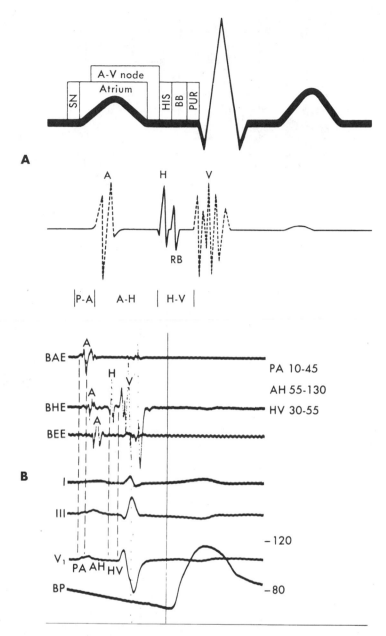

Fig. 5-1 **A,** Schematic illustration of a cardiac cycle demonstrating the normal ECG *(top)* and an intracardiac recording *(bottom)*. The diagram illustrates the approximate time of activation of various structures in the specialized conduction system. Conduction has reached the Purkinje fibers just before the onset of the QRS complex. *SN,* Sinus node; *HIS,* bundle of His; *BB,* bundle branches; *PUR,* Purkinje fibers; *A,* low right atrial deflection; *H,* bundle of His deflection; *RB,* right bundle branch deflection; *V,* ventricular septal muscle depolarization; *P-A,* interval from the onset of the P wave in the surface tracing to the onset of the low right atrial deflection, serving as a measure of intraatrial conduction; *A-H,* measurement of conduction across the AV node; *H-V* measurement of conduction through the bundle of His distal to the recording electrode, the bundle branches, and the Purkinje system up to the point of ventricular activation. **B,** Electrophysiologic and blood pressure recordings during one cardiac cycle. *BAE,* Bipolar high right atrial electrogram; *BHE,* bipolar His electrogram; *BEE,* bipolar esophageal electrogram. Normal intervals in milliseconds to the right.   (Top panel of **A** modified from Hoffman BF, Singer DH: Effects of digitalis on electrical activity of cardiac fibers, *Prog Cardiovasc Dis* 7:226, 1964.)

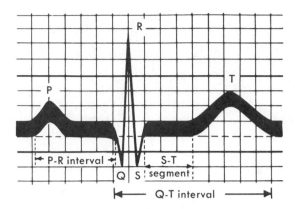

Fig. 5-2   Electric pattern of cardiac cycle (see Table 5-1).

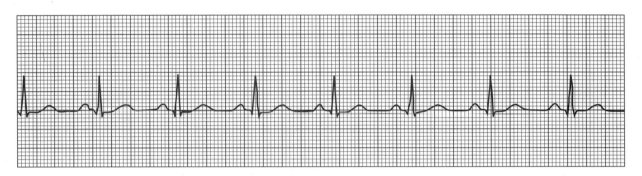

Fig. 5-3   Calculation of atrial and ventricular rates. Heart rate is almost 80 beats/min, determined by dividing the time interval between consecutive P waves and/or consecutive R waves by 1 second, by dividing 5 large squares into 300 or 25 small squares into 1500, or by multiplying the number of complexes occurring in a 6-second strip by 10. See Table 5-2.

TABLE 5-1	Definition and Significance of ECG Intervals*	
Description	**Duration**	**Significance of Disturbance**
PR interval: from beginning of P wave to beginning of QRS complex; represents time taken for impulse to spread through atria, AV node and bundle of His, bundle branches and Purkinje fibers, to point immediately preceding ventricular activation	0.12 to 0.20 second	Disturbance in conduction usually in AV node, bundle of His, or bundle branches but can be in atria
QRS interval: from beginning to end of QRS complex; represents time taken for depolarization of both ventricles	0.06 to 0.10 second	Disturbance in conduction in bundle branches, ventricles, or both
QT interval: from beginning of QRS complex to end of T wave; represents time taken for entire electric depolarization and repolarization of ventricles	0.36 to 0.44 second	Disturbances usually affecting repolarization more than depolarization such as drug effects, electrolyte disturbances, and rate changes

*Heart rate influences the duration of these intervals, especially that of the PR and QT intervals.

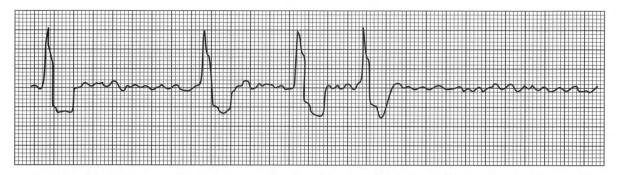

Fig. 5-4   Calculation of the rate of an irregular rhythm. Heart rate is 40 beats/min, determined by multiplying 4 (the number of R waves occurring in a 6-second strip) by 10.

2. 1500 small squares method (see Fig. 5-3): At the standard ECG paper speed of 25 mm/sec, 1500 mm (or 1500 small squares) run under the ECG stylus in 1 minute. This method is accurate only with regular rhythms. For irregular rhythms, the lowest and highest rates are calculated.
   a. The number of small squares between the cardiac waves (that is, P waves and/or QRS complexes) are counted.
   b. The number 1500 is divided by the number of small squares between the cardiac waves.
   c. The result gives the rate of occurrence of the wave per minute.
3. 300 large squares method (see Fig. 5-3): At the standard ECG paper speed of 25 mm/sec, 300 mm (or 300 large squares) run under the ECG stylus in 1 minute. This method is accurate only with regular rhythms. For irregular rhythms, the lowest and highest rates are calculated.
   a. The number of large squares between the cardiac waves (that is, P waves and/or QRS complexes) is counted.
   b. The number 300 is divided by the number of large squares between the cardiac waves.
   c. The result gives the rate of occurrence of the wave per minute.
4. Quick-glance method (Fig. 5-5): This method illustrates a simple way of approximating heart rate. Although it is not exact, it permits a quick method of determining rate if it is over 100 beats/min but less than 150 beats/min.
   a. The number of large squares between waves is determined. (For convenience, a wave that coincides with a heavy line is selected.)
      1. If 1 large square, the rate is 300 (300 ÷ 1).
      2. If 2 large squares, the rate is 150 (300 ÷ 2).
      3. If 3 large squares, the rate is 100 (300 ÷ 3).
      4. If 4 large squares, the rate is 75 (300 ÷ 4).
      5. If 5 large squares, the rate is 60 (300 ÷ 5).
      6. If 6 large squares, the rate is 50 (300 ÷ 6).
      7. If 7 large squares, the rate is 42 (300 ÷ 7).
      8. If 8 large squares, the rate is 38 (300 ÷ 8).
   b. The clinician memorizes the resulting mnemonic, "300, 150, 100, 75, 60, 50, 42, 38."
   c. Using the mnemonic, the clinician selects the wave and goes to the next occurrence of the wave (see Fig. 5-5).
5. Precalculated table method (Table 5-2): This method is most accurate for regular rhythms. For irregular rhythms, the highest and lowest rates are calculated.
   a. The number of small squares between cardiac waves is counted.
   b. This number is found on the table.
   c. The rate is read from the column to the right of this number in the table.

ELECTROPHYSIOLOGIC PRINCIPLES

Certain specialized cells, such as those in the sinus node, some parts of the atria, AV node, and His-Purkinje system, are able to discharge spontaneously; they do not require an external or propagated stimulus to fire. This property, known as *automaticity* (also called *diastolic depolarization*), creates the potential for these cells to depolarize the rest of the heart. Normally the sinus node functions as the pacemaker, since it spontaneously discharges at a rate of 60 to 100 beats/min, which is faster than these other latent pacemakers.

If a latent pacemaker possessing the property of automaticity discharges more rapidly than the sinus node, it may depolarize the atria, ventricles, or both. This may occur in two ways. If the SA node discharges more slowly than the discharge rate of the latent pacemaker or if the sinus impulse is blocked before reaching the latent pacemaker site (see Fig. 5-13), the latent pacemaker may passively escape sinus domination and discharge automatically at its own intrinsic rate. Such escape beats are slower than normal, since the AV junction and bundle branch–Purkinje system (two probable escape focus sites)

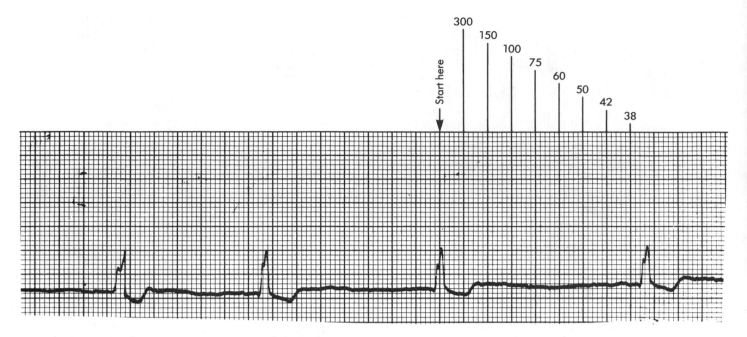

Fig. 5-5   Quick-glance method of calculating heart rate. Determine the number of large squares between waves. (For convenience, select a wave that coincides with a heavy line.) Count the number of large squares between waves. If it is 1 large square, the rate is 300. If it is 2 large squares, the rate is 150. If it is 3 large squares, the rate is 100. If it is 4 large squares, the rate is 75. If it is 5 large squares, the rate is 60. If it is 6 large squares, the rate is 50. If it is 7 large squares, the rate is 42. If it is 8 large squares, the rate is 38. Memorize the resulting mnemonic, "300, 150, 100, 75, 60, 50, 42, 38."

TABLE 5-2   Determination of Heart Rate from the ECG

Time (Second)	No. of Small Squares	Rate (Beats/Min)	Time (Second)	No. of Small Squares	Rate (Beats/Min)
0.10	2.5	600	0.60	15.00	100
0.12	3.0	500	0.64	16.00	94
0.15	3.75	400	0.70	17.50	86
0.16	4.0	375	0.72	18.00	83
0.20	5.0	300	0.76	19.00	79
0.24	6.0	250	0.80	20.00	75
0.26	6.5	230	0.84	21.00	71
0.28	7.0	214	0.88	22.00	68
0.30	7.5	200	0.92	23.00	65
0.32	8.0	188	0.96	24.00	63
0.34	8.5	176	1.00	25.00	60
0.36	9.0	167	1.08	27.00	56
0.38	9.5	158	1.14	28.50	53
0.40	10.0	150	1.20	30.00	50
0.42	10.5	143	1.40	35.00	43
0.44	11.0	136	1.50	37.50	40
0.46	11.5	130	1.60	40.00	38
0.48	12.0	125	1.80	45.00	33
0.50	12.5	120	2.00	50.00	30
0.52	13.0	115	2.50	62.50	25
0.56	14.0	107	3.00	75.00	20

generally beat at 40 to 60 beats/min and 30 to 40 beats/min, respectively. However, if a latent pacemaker abnormally accelerates its discharge rate and actively usurps control of the heartbeat from the sinus node, a premature beat results. This may happen in the atria, ventricles, or AV junction. A series of these premature beats produces a tachycardia. A shift in the normal manner of atrial or ventricular activation, such as that produced by a shift in pacemaker focus, is reflected by a change in P-wave or QRS-complex contour.

Automatic discharge of a pacemaker focus is not sufficient to depolarize a cardiac chamber; the impulse must also be conducted from its site of origin to the surrounding myocardium. The heart possesses the property of excitability, which enables it to be depolarized by a stimulus; this is an integral part of the propagation or conduction of the impulse from one fiber to the next. Many factors influence the level of excitability, but the most important in the normal state is the length of time that the heart is restimulated after depolarization. Cardiac tissue requires a recovery period after depolarization. If a stimulus occurs too early, the heart has had insufficient time to recover, and it will not respond to the stimulus no matter how intense it is (absolute refractory period, excitability zero). A slightly later stimulus allows more time for recovery (relative refractory period, excitability improving), and a still later stimulus finds the heart completely recovered (no longer refractory, full excitability).

If conduction becomes unevenly depressed, with block in some areas and not in others, some regions of the myocardium (unblocked areas) must necessarily be activated (and recover) earlier than others. Under appropriate circumstances, when the block is in only one direction (unidirectional), this uneven conduction may allow the initial impulse to reenter areas previously unexcitable but that have now recovered. If the reentering impulse is then able to depolarize the atria, ventricles, or both, a corresponding premature extrasystole results; maintenance of the reentrant excitation establishes a tachycardia. A special form of reentry may produce echo or reciprocal beats (see Fig. 5-54, D). Thus disorders of impulse formation (automaticity) or conduction (unidirectional block and reentry) or at times combinations of both may initiate dysrhythmias.

Only indirect evidence exists to enable a clinical classification of dysrhythmias according to electrophysiologic mechanisms. In addition, a dysrhythmia may be initiated and perpetuated by different mechanisms. For example, spontaneous diastolic depolarization (automaticity) may trigger a premature atrial or ventricular systole that initiates a dysrhythmia caused by reentry. Also, studies on parasystole,[3] a type of automaticity, and reflection,[4] a form of reentry, is causing clinicians to rethink many clinical definitions (see box). Thus the clinical classification of *dysrhythmias* according to mechanism remains speculative. Antidysrhythmic agents specifically indicated to treat one mechanism or another do not yet exist.[5]

PROBABLE ELECTROPHYSIOLOGIC MECHANISM RESPONSIBLE FOR VARIOUS CARDIAC DYSRHYTHMIAS

Automaticity

Escape beats—atrial, junctional, or ventricular
Atrial rhythm
Atrial tachycardia with or without AV block
Junctional rhythm
Nonparoxysmal AV junctional tachycardia
Accelerated idioventricular rhythm
Parasystole

Reentry

AV nodal reentry
AV reciprocating tachycardia using an accessory (WPW) pathway
Atrial flutter
Atrial fibrillation
Ventricular tachycardia
Ventricular flutter
Ventricular fibrillation

Automaticity or Reentry

Premature systoles—atrial, junctional, or ventricular
Flutter and fibrillation
Ventricular tachycardia

Depolarization of cells in the atria, ventricles, and His-Purkinje system depends on a rapid movement of sodium into the cell. Such an event is called the *fast response*. In the sinus and AV nodes, depolarization depends primarily on intracellular movement of calcium and is called the *slow response*.[6] The slow response may play a role in the genesis of certain cardiac dysrhythmias and is affected by a specific class of drugs called *calcium entry blockers* such as verapamil, diltiazem, and nifedipine.[7]

DYSRHYTHMIA ANALYSIS

For proper analysis (see box), each dysrhythmia must be approached in a systematic manner. A suggested guide follows:

1. What is the rate? Is it too fast or too slow? Are P waves present? Are atrial and ventricular rates the same?
2. Are the P-P and R-R intervals regular or irregular? If irregular, are they consistent, repeating irregularities?
3. Are a P wave and therefore atrial activity related to each ventricular complex? Does the P wave precede or follow the QRS complex? Is the PR or RP interval constant?
4. Are all P waves and QRS complexes identical and normal in contour? What is the lead being recorded so that the significance of changes in P or QRS contour or amplitude can be determined?

CLASSIFICATION OF NORMAL AND ABNORMAL CARDIAC RHYTHMS

Rhythms Originating in the Sinus Node

Sinus rhythm
Sinus tachycardia
Sinus bradycardia
Sinus dysrhythmia
Sinus arrest
Sinus exit block
Sinus nodal reentry

Rhythms Originating in the Atria

Wandering pacemaker between sinus node and atrium or AV junction
Premature atrial complex
Intraatrial reentry
Atrial flutter
Atrial fibrillation
Atrial tachycardia (with or without block)
Multifocal atrial tachycardia

Rhythms Originating in the AV Junction (AV Node–Bundle of His)

Premature AV junctional complex
AV junctional escape complexes
AV junctional rhythm
AV nodal reentry
AV reciprocating tachycardia using accessory (WPW) pathway

Rhythms Originating in the Ventricles

Ventricular escape complexes
Premature ventricular complex
Ventricular tachycardia
Idioventricular tachycardia (accelerated idioventricular rhythm)
Ventricular flutter
Ventricular fibrillation

AV Block

First-degree
Second degree
   Type I (Wenckebach)
   Type II
Third-degree (complete)

Bundle Branch Block

Right
Left
Fascicular blocks (hemiblocks)

Parasystole

Atrial
Junctional
Ventricular

From Zipes DP: *Specific arrhythmias: diagnosis and treatment.* In Braunwald E, editor: *Heart disease: a textbook of cardiovascular medicine,* Philadelphia, 1984, Saunders.

---

5. Are the PR, QRS, and QT intervals normal?
6. Are premature complexes present? If so, are they atrial, junctional, or ventricular? Is there a constant coupling interval between the premature complex and the normal complex? Is there a constant interval between premature complexes?
7. Are escape beats present? If so, are they atrial, junctional, or ventricular in origin?
8. What is the dominant rhythm?
9. Considering the clinical setting, what is the significance of the dysrhythmia?
10. How should the dysrhythmia be treated?

THERAPY OF DYSRHYTHMIAS (TABLE 5-3)
General Therapeutic Concepts

The therapeutic approach[10,11] to a patient who has a cardiac dysrhythmia begins with an accurate ECG interpretation of the dysrhythmia and continues with determination of the cause of the dysrhythmia (if possible), the nature of the underlying heart disease (if any), and the consequences of the dysrhythmia for the individual. Thus one cannot treat dysrhythmias as isolated events without knowing the clinical situation; patients who have dysrhythmias, not dysrhythmias themselves, are treated.

Electrophysiologic and Hemodynamic Consequences

The ventricular rate and duration of a dysrhythmia, its site of origin, and the cardiovascular status of the patient primarily determine the electrophysiologic and hemodynamic consequences of a particular rhythm disturbance. Electrophysiologic consequences, often influenced by underlying heart disease such as acute myocardial infarction, include the development of serious dysrhythmias as a result of rapid and slow rates, initiation of sustained dysrhythmias by premature complexes, and degeneration of rhythms such as ventricular tachycardia into ventricular fibrillation. The hemodynamic performance of the heart and circulation may be altered by extremes of heart rate or by loss of atrial contribution to ventricular filling. Rapid rates greatly shorten the diastolic filling time, and particularly in diseased hearts, the increased heart rate may fail to compensate for the reduced stroke output; blood pressure and cardiac output decline. Dysrhythmias such as NPJT (see Fig. 5-51) that prevent sequential AV contraction mitigate the hemodynamic benefits of the atrial booster pump, whereas atrial fibrillation causes complete loss of atrial contraction and may reduce cardiac output.

Slowing the ventricular rate

When a patient develops a tachydysrhythmia, slowing the ventricular rate is the initial and frequently the most important therapeutic maneuver. Because medical therapy frequently involves a time-consuming and potentially dangerous biologic titration of drugs such as digitalis or quinidine, electric DC cardioversion may be preferable, depending on the clinical situation. Therapy may differ radically for the very same dysrhythmia in two different patients because the consequences of the tachycardia on the individual differ. For example, a supraventricular tachycardia at 200 beats/min may produce little or no symptoms in a healthy young adult and therefore require little or no therapy; the same dysrhythmia may precipitate pulmonary edema in a patient with mitral stenosis, syncope in a patient with aortic stenosis, shock in a patient with an acute myocardial infarction, or hemiparesis in a patient with cerebrovascular disease. In these situations the tachycardia requires prompt electric conversion.

Etiology

The etiology of the dysrhythmia may markedly influence therapy. Electrolyte imbalance (potassium, magnesium, calcium), acidosis or alkalosis, hypoxemia, and many drugs produce dysrhythmias. Because heart failure can cause dysrhythmias, digitalis may effectively suppress dysrhythmias during heart failure when all other agents are unsuccessful, or it may prevent more severe dysrhythmias by reversing early congestive heart failure. Similarly, a dysrhythmia secondary to hypotension may respond to leg elevation or vasopressor therapy. Mild sedation or reassurance may be successful in treating some dysrhythmias related to emotional stress. Precipitating or contributing disease states such as infection, hypovolemia, anemia, and thyroid disorders should be diagnosed and treated. Aggressive management of premature atrial or ventricular complexes that often presage or precipitate the occurrence of sustained tachydysrhythmias may prevent later occurrence of more serious tachydysrhythmias.

Risks of therapy

Since therapy always involves some risk, one must decide, particularly as the therapeutic regimen escalates, whether the risks of not treating the dysrhythmia continue to outweigh the risks of therapy. The antidysrhythmic agents[7,10,12] lidocaine, procainamide, quinidine, propranolol, disopyramide, and phenytoin exert negative inotropic effects on the myocardium, and when given parenterally, they may produce hypotension. Antidysrhythmic agents may slow conduction velocity, depress the activity of normal (sinus) and abnormal (ectopic) pacemaker sites, and cause dysrhythmias. Doses of all drugs may need to be adjusted according to the size of the patient, routes of excretion or degradation, presence of impaired organ function (heart, liver, kidney), degree of absorption if given orally, adverse side effects, interaction with other drugs, electrolyte imbalance, and hypoxemia.

The remainder of this chapter is devoted to a discussion of cardiac dysrhythmias (see Table 5-3). The systematic approach, previously discussed in the section on dysrhythmia analysis, is used.

Normal Sinus Rhythm

In adults, normal sinus rhythm (Fig. 5-6 on p.98) is arbitrarily limited to rates of 60 to 100 beats/min. The P wave is upright in leads I and II and negative in lead aV_R, with a vector in the frontal plane between 0 and +90 degrees. In the horizontal plane the P vector is directed anteriorly and slightly leftward and may therefore be negative in leads V_1 and V_2 but positive in lead V_3. The P-P interval characteristically varies slightly but by less than 0.16/sec/cycle. The PR interval is between 0.12 and 2.0 seconds and may vary slightly with rate. The QRS duration is 0.06 to 0.20 second, and the QT duration is 0.36 to 0.44 second. The sinus node responds readily to autonomic stimuli; parasympathetic (cholinergic) stimuli slow and sympathetic (adrenergic) stimuli speed the rate of discharge. The resulting rate depends on the net effect of these two opposing forces.

Sinus Tachycardia

The conduction pathway in sinus tachycardia (Figs. 5-7 and 5-8 on p. 99) is the same as that in normal sinus rhythm, but because of enhanced discharge of the sinus node from vagal inhibition, sympathetic stimulation, or both, the sinus rate is between 100 and 180 beats/min. It may be higher with extreme exertion and in infants. It has a gradual onset and termination, and the P-P interval may vary slightly from cycle to cycle. P waves have a normal contour but may develop larger amplitudes and become peaked. Carotid sinus massage and the Valsalva or other vagal maneuvers gradually slow sinus tachycardia, which then accelerates to its previous rate. More rapid sinus rates may fail to slow in response to a vagal maneuver.

Significance

Sinus tachycardia is the normal physiologic response to stressors such as fever, hypotension, thyrotoxicosis, anemia, anxiety, exertion, hypovolemia, pulmonary emboli, myocardial ischemia, congestive heart failure, and shock. Inflammation such as pericarditis may produce sinus tachycardia. Sinus tachycardia is usually of no physiologic significance; however, reduced cardiac output, congestive heart failure, and dysrhythmias may result in patients with organic myocardial disease. Since heart rate is a major determinant of oxygen requirements, angina or perhaps an increase in the size of an infarction may accompany persistent sinus tachycardia in patients with coronary artery disease.

Treatment

Therapy should be directed toward correcting the underlying disease state that caused the sinus tachycardia. Elimination of tobacco, alcohol, coffee, tea, or other stimulants (for example, sympathomimetic vasoconstrictors in nose drops) may help. If sinus tachycardia is not secondary to a correctable physiologic stress, treatment with sedatives, reserpine, or clonidine is occasionally useful. The

Text continued on p. 99.

TABLE 5-3   Cardiac Dysrhythmias*

Type of Dysrhythmia	P Waves			QRS Complexes		
	Rate	Rhythm	Contour	Rate	Rhythm	Contour
Sinus rhythm	60-100	Regular†	Normal	60-100	Regular	Normal
Sinus bradycardia	<60	Regular	Normal	<60	Regular	Normal
Sinus tachycardia	100-180	Regular	May be peaked	100-180	Regular	Normal
AV nodal reentry	150-250	Very regular except at onset and termination	Retrograde; difficult to see; lost in QRS complex	150-250	Very regular except at onset and termination	Normal
Atrial flutter	250-350	Regular	Sawtooth	75-175	Generally regular in absence of drugs or disease	Normal
Atrial fibrillation	400-600	Grossly irregular	Baseline undulations; no P waves	100-160	Grossly irregular	Normal
Atrial tachycardia with block	150-250	Regular; may be irregular	Abnormal	75-200	Generally regular in absence of drugs or disease	Normal
AV junctional rhythm	40-100§	Regular	Normal	40-60	Fairly regular	Normal
Reciprocating tachycardia using an accessory (WPW) pathway	150-250	Very regular except at onset and termination	Retrograde; difficult to see; follows the QRS complex	150-250	Very regular except at onset and termination	Normal
Nonparoxysmal AV junctional tachycardia (NPJT)	60-100§	Regular	Normal	70-130	Fairly regular	Normal

*In an effort to summarize these dysrhythmias in a tabular form, generalizations have to be made, especially under therapy. Particularly, acute therapy to terminate a tachycardia may be different from chronic therapy to prevent a recurrence. Some of the exceptions are indicated by the footnotes, but the reader is referred to the text for a complete discussion.

†P waves initiated by sinus node discharge may not be precisely regular because of sinus dysrhythmia.

‡Often, carotid sinus massage fails to slow a sinus tachycardia.

Ventricular Response to Carotid Sinus Massage	Physical Examination			Treatment
	Intensity of S_1	Splitting of S_2	A Waves	
Gradual slowing and return to former rate	Constant	Normal	Normal	None
Gradual slowing and return to former rate	Constant	Normal	Normal	None, unless symptomatic; atropine, isoproterenol
Gradual slowing‡ and return to former rate	Constant	Normal	Normal	None, unless symptomatic; treatment of underlying disease
Abrupt slowing caused by termination of tachycardia or no effect	Constant	Normal	Constant cannon A waves	Vagal stimulation, verapamil, digitalis, propranolol, DC shock, pacing
Abrupt slowing and return to former rate; flutter remains	Constant; variable if AV block changing	Normal	Flutter waves	DC shock, digitalis, quinidine, propranolol, verapamil, pacing
Slowing; gross irregularity remains	Variable	Normal	No A waves	Digitalis, quinidine, DC shock, verapamil, propranolol
Abrupt slowing and return to former rate; tachycardia remains	Constant; variable if AV block changing	Normal	More A waves than CV waves	Stopping digitalis if toxic; digitalis if not toxic; possibly verapamil, quinidine
None; may be slight slowing	Variable‖	Normal	Intermittent cannon waves‖	None, unless symptomatic; atropine
Abrupt slowing caused by termination of tachycardia or no effect	Constant but decreased	Normal	Constant cannon waves	See paroxysmal supraventricular tachycardia above
None; may be slight slowing	Variable‖	Normal	Intermittent cannon waves‖	None, unless symptomatic; stopping digitalis if toxic

§An independent atrial dysrhythmia may exist, or the atria may be captured retrogradely.
‖Constant if atria are captured retrogradely.
¶Atrial rhythm and rate may vary, depending on whether sinus bradycardia or tachycardia, atrial tachycardia, or something else is the atrial mechanism.
#Regular or constant if block is unchanging.

Continued.

TABLE 5-3   Cardiac Dysrhythmias—cont'd

Type of Dysrhythmia	P Waves			QRS Complexes		
	Rate	Rhythm	Contour	Rate	Rhythm	Contour
Ventricular tachycardia	60-100§	Regular	Normal	110-250	Fairly regular; possibly irregular	Abnormal, >0.12 second
Accelerated idioventricular rhythm	60-100§	Regular	Normal	50-110	Fairly regular; possibly irregular	Abnormal, >0.12 second
Ventricular flutter	60-100§	Regular	Normal; difficult to see	150-300	Regular	Sine wave
Ventricular fibrillation	60-100§	Regular	Normal; difficult too see	400-600	Grossly irregular	Baseline undulations; no QRS complexes
First-degree AV block	60-100¶	Regular	Normal	60-100	Regular	Normal
Type I second-degree AV block	60-100¶	Regular	Normal	30-100	Irregular#	Normal
Type II second-degree AV block	60-100¶	Regular	Normal	30-100	Irregular#	Abnormal, >0.12 second
Complete AV block	60-100§	Regular	Normal	<40	Fairly regular	Abnormal, >0.12 second
Right bundle branch block (RBBB)	60-100	Regular	Normal	60-100	Regular	Abnormal, >0.12 second
Left bundle branch block (LBBB)	60-100	Regular	Normal	60-100	Regular	Abnormal, >0.12 second

| Ventricular Response to Carotid Sinus Massage | Physical Examination | | | Treatment |
	Intensity of S_1	Splitting of S_2	A Waves	
None	Variable‖	Abnormal	Intermittent cannon waves‖	Lidocaine, procainamide, direct current (DC) shock, quinidine
None	Variable‖	Abnormal	Intermittent cannon waves‖	None, unless symptomatic; lidocaine, atropine
None	None	None	Cannon waves	DC shock
None	None	None	Cannon waves	DC shock
Gradual slowing caused by sinus showing	Constant, diminished	Normal	Normal	None
Slowing caused by sinus slowing and an increase in AV block	Cyclic decrease and then increase after pause	Normal	Normal; increasing AC interval; A waves without C waves	None, unless symptomatic; atropine
Gradual slowing caused by sinus slowing	Constant	Abnormal	Normal; constant AC interval; A waves without C waves	Pacemaker
None	Variable‖	Abnormal	Intermittent cannon waves‖	Pacemaker
Gradual slowing and return to former rate	Constant	Wide	None	None
Gradual slowing and return to former rate	Constant	Paradoxical	Normal	None

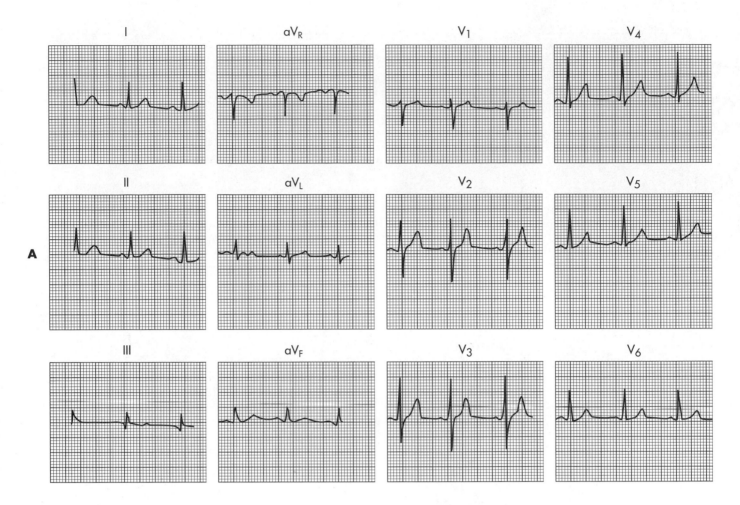

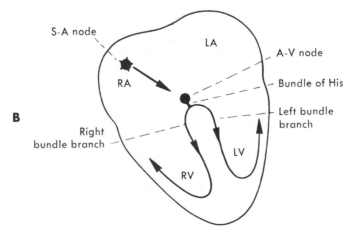

Fig. 5-6 **A,** Normal sinus rhythm. The ECG is normal. **B,** Schematic illustration. *RA,* Right atrium; *LA,* left atrium; *LV,* left ventricle; *RV,* right ventricle.

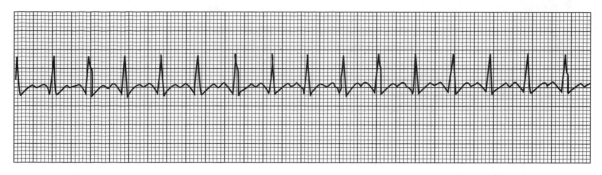

Fig. 5-7 Sinus tachycardia.
Rate   170 beats/min.
Rhythm   Regular.
P waves   Normal; precede each QRS complex with regular contour at fixed interval.
PR interval   0.16 second.
QRS complex   Normal, 0.08 second. Upright QRS-T complex.

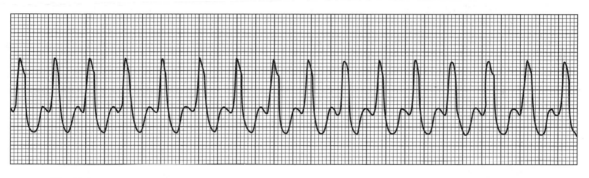

Fig. 5-8 Sinus tachycardia.
Rate   170 beats/min.
Rhythm   Regular.
P waves   Normal; precede each QRS complex with regular contour at fixed interval.
PR interval   0.12 second.
QRS complex   0.12 second. Broad QRS complex reflective of bundle branch block. Inverted
                  T waves.

only medication that consistently slows a sinus tachycardia directly is propranolol (10 to 60 mg 4 times daily administered orally). Drugs that block the slow inward current, such as verapamil, may also slow the rate of sinus node discharge.

Sinus Bradycardia

In sinus bradycardia (Figs. 5-9 and 5-10), impulses travel down the same pathway as in sinus rhythm, but the sinus node discharges at a rate less than 60 beats/min. P waves have a normal contour and occur before each QRS complex, with a constant PR interval exceeding 0.12 second. Sinus dysrhythmia is frequently present.

Significance

Sinus bradycardia results from excessive vagal tone, decreased sympathetic tone, or both. Eye surgery, meningitis, intracranial tumors, cervical and mediastinal tumors, and certain disease states such as myocardial infarction, myxedema, obstructive jaundice, and cardiac fibrosis may produce sinus bradycardia. In most instances, sinus bradycardia is a benign dysrhythmia and may be beneficial by producing a longer period of diastole and increased ventricular filling. It occurs commonly in well-trained athletes and during sleep, vomiting, or vasovagal syncope and may be produced by carotid sinus stimulation or by the administration of parasympathomimetic drugs. Sinus bradycardia

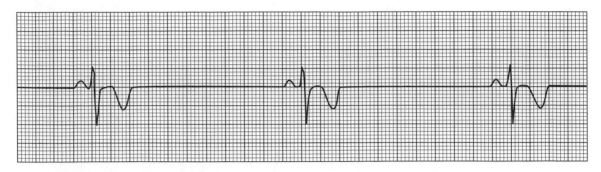

Fig. 5-9 Sinus bradycardia.
Rate   30 beats/min.
Rhythm   Regular.
P waves   Normal; precede each QRS complex with regular contour at fixed interval.
PR interval   0.16 second.
QRS complex   0.10 second. Biphasic QRS complex with T-wave inversion.

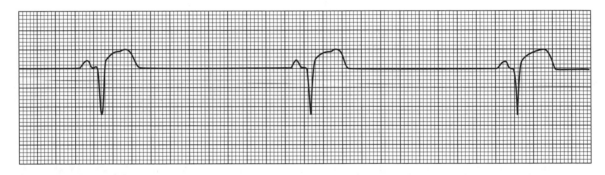

Fig. 5-10 Sinus bradycardia with ST-segment elevation.
Rate   30 beats/min.
Rhythm   Regular.
P waves   Normal; precede each QRS complex with regular contour at fixed interval.
PR interval   0.16 second.
QRS complex   0.08 second. QS complex with ST-segment elevation.

occurring with myocardial infarction, more commonly diaphragmatic or posterior, may compromise optimal myocardial function and predispose to premature systoles and sustained tachydysrhythmias. Sinus bradycardia may be beneficial in some patients who have acute myocardial infarction because it reduces oxygen demands, may help minimize the size of the infarction, and may lessen the frequency of some dysrhythmias. Patients with acute myocardial infarction who have sinus bradycardia generally have lower mortality rates than patients who have sinus tachycardia.

Treatment

Treatment of sinus bradycardia is needed only when symptoms such as chest pain, dyspnea, lightheadedness, hypotension, or ventricular ectopy occur. If an acute myocar-

dial infarction is asymptomatic, it is probably best not to try to speed the sinus rate. If the cardiac output is inadequate or if dysrhythmias are associated with the slow rate, atropine (0.5 mg intravenously as an initial dose, repeated if necessary to a total dosage of 2.0 mg) or isoproterenol (2 to 10 μg/minute intravenously) is usually effective.[3] These drugs should be used cautiously, with care taken not to produce too rapid a rate. In patients who have symptoms as a result of chronic sinus bradycardia, electric pacing may be needed, since few if any drugs successfully speed sinus node discharge chronically without producing side effects.

Sinus Dysrhythmia

Sinus dysrhythmia (Figs. 5-11 to 5-13) is characterized by a phasic variation in cycle length exceeding 0.16 second during sinus rhythm. It is the most frequent form of dys-

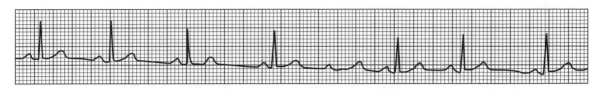

Fig. 5-11 Respiratory sinus dysrhythmia. The phasic variation in heart rate corresponds to respiratory rate. Monitor lead.

Rate	80 beats/min.
Rhythm	Irregular with repetitive variation in cycle length according to respiratory cycle. Increased rate with inspiration and decreased rate with expiration.
P waves	Precede each QRS complex.
PR interval	0.16 second.
QRS complex	Normal, 0.06 second.

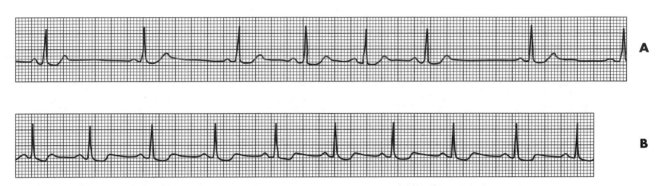

Fig. 5-12 Nonrespiratory sinus dysrhythmia. In this instance the dysrhythmia was caused by digitalis toxicity **(A)**. One week after discontinuation of digitalis, the nonrespiratory sinus dysrhythmia disappeared **(B)**.

Rate	**A,** Increases and decreases independent of respiration (47 to 80 beats/min); **B,** constant rate (78 beats/min).
Rhythm	**A,** Irregular with a repetitive phasic variation in cycle length that continues during breath-holding. **B,** Regular.
P waves	Precede each QRS complex with a normal, fairly constant contour.
PR interval	0.12 second.
QRS complex	Normal, 0.06 second.

rhythmia and occurs as a normal phenomenon. The P waves do not vary in morphology, and the PR interval exceeds 0.12 second and remains unchanged, since the focus of discharge is fixed within the sinus node. Occasionally the pacemaker focus may wander within the sinus node, producing P waves of slightly different contour (but not retrograde) and a changing PR interval (but not less than 0.12 second). Sinus dysrhythmia commonly occurs in youth or older adulthood, especially in patients with slower heart rates or after enhanced vagal tone from digitalis or morphine administration.

Sinus dysrhythmia appears in two basic forms. In the respiratory form the P-P interval cyclically shortens during inspiration as a result of reflex inhibition of vagal tone, en-

hancement of sympathetic tone, or both. Breath-holding eliminates the cycle length variation. Nonrespiratory sinus dysrhythmia is characterized by a phasic variation unrelated to the respiratory cycle. In both forms, impulses are generated in the sinus node and travel over the normal pathway to the AV node.

Significance

Symptoms produced by sinus dysrhythmias are rare, but on occasion, palpitations or dizziness may be experienced if the pauses between beats are excessively long. Marked sinus dysrhythmia can produce a sinus pause sufficiently prolonged to induce syncope if it is not accompanied by an escape rhythm.

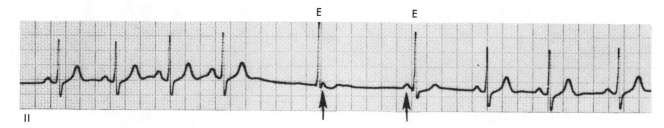

Fig. 5-13 Respiratory sinus dysrhythmia. The first four P waves are fairly regular; the PR interval is 0.16 second and constant. Then the sinus node slows, and the next two P waves occur much later *(arrows)*. The marked sinus node slowing allows a latent pacemaker, possibly located in the bundle of His or high in the fascicles, to escape sinus domination, depolarize automatically, and discharge the ventricles (*E*, Junctional escapes). A slight change in QRS contour is apparent in these beats. The sinus node then speeds up to resume control. This slightly complex dysrhythmia is completely normal in an otherwise healthy person.

Rate	Increases with inspiration and decreases with expiration (55 to 80 beats/min).
Rhythm	Irregular with a repetitive phasic variation in cycle length.
P waves	Normal, fairly constant contour.
PR interval	0.16 second during sinus-conducted beats.
QRS complex	Normal, 0.08 second during sinus-conducted beats.

Treatment

Treatment is usually unnecessary. Increasing the heart rate by exercise or drugs abolishes sinus dysrhythmia. Individuals with symptomatic dysrhythmias may experience relief from feelings of palpitations through the use of sedatives, tranquilizers, atropine, ephedrine, or isoproterenol administration, as in the treatment of sinus bradycardia.

Sinus Arrest

Failure of sinus node discharge results in the absence of atrial depolarization and periods of ventricular asystole if escape beats produced by latent pacemakers do not discharge. Sinus arrest (Figs. 5-14 and 5-15) may be produced by involvement of the sinus node or the sinus node artery by acute myocardial infarction, digitalis toxicity, excessive vagal tone, or degenerative forms of fibrosis. It may occur as a side effect of therapy with certain drugs such as amiodarone.

Significance

Transient sinus arrest may have no clinical significance by itself if latent pacemakers promptly escape to prevent ventricular asystole (Fig. 5-14). Prolonged ventricular asystole results if the latent pacemakers fail to escape. Other dysrhythmias may be precipitated by the slow rates (Fig. 5-15).

Treatment

Atropine (0.5 mg intravenously initially, repeated if necessary to a total dosage of 2.0 mg) or isoproterenol (2 to 10 μg/min intravenously) may be tried as the first therapeutic approach.[3] If these drugs are unsuccessful, atrial or ventricular pacing may be required. In patients who have a chronic form of sinus node disease characterized by marked sinus bradycardia or sinus arrest (sick sinus syndrome), permanent pacing is often necessary. Sometimes, sinus bradycardia alternates with supraventricular tachycardia (bradycardia-tachycardia syndrome). This condition is best treated by a combination of drugs to slow the ventricular rate during the supraventricular tachycardia and implantation of a permanent demand pacemaker to prevent the slow rate when the tachycardia terminates.

Sinus Exit Block

Sinus exit block (Figs. 5-16 and 5-17) is a conduction disturbance during which an impulse formed within the sinus node is blocked from depolarizing the atria. Sinus exit block is indicated on the ECG by the absence of the normally expected P waves. The length of the pause between P waves is a multiple of the basic P-P interval, approximately 2 but less commonly 3 or 4 times the normal P-P interval (type II exit block). Type I (Wenckebach) sinus exit block may also occur, in which case the P-P interval progressively shortens before the pause and the duration of the pause is less than two P-P cycles.

Significance

Sinus exit block may be caused by excessive vagal stimulation, by acute infections such as diphtheria or rheumatic carditis, by atherosclerosis involving the sinus nodal artery,

V$_1$

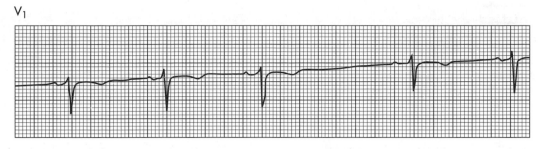

Fig. 5-14 Sinus arrest. Normal sinus rhythm interrupted by a pause.

Rate   70 beats/min.
Rhythm   Regular, interrupted by pause.
P waves   Normal, constant contour.
PR interval   0.16 second.
QRS complex   0.10 second.

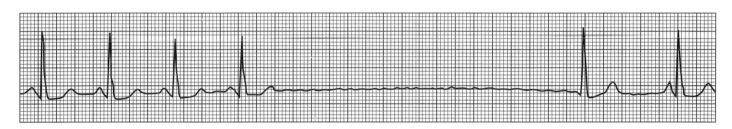

Fig. 5-15 Sinus arrest with asystole. Sinus arrest lasting 4 seconds and terminated with a junctional escape beat.

Rate   Varying.
Rhythm   Irregular.
P waves   Normal before sinus arrest.
PR interval   0.16 before sinus arrest.
QRS complex   0.08 second.

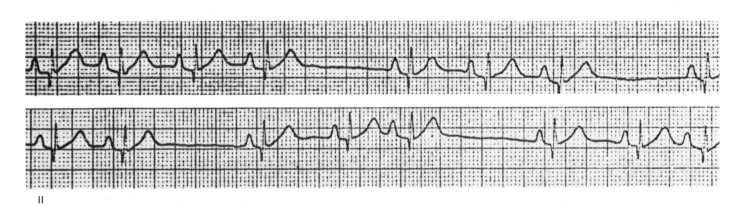

II

Fig. 5-16 Sinus exit block (type II). The longer P-P intervals are approximately twice the shorter P-P intervals, indicating an intermittent 2:1 sinus exit block of the type II variety.

Rate   Varying, slow (43 to 68 beats/min).
Rhythm   Irregular; pauses twice as long as the shorter intervals.
P waves   Contour normal, precede each QRS complex; intermittent loss of P wave.
PR interval   0.16 second.
QRS complex   Normal, 0.08 second.

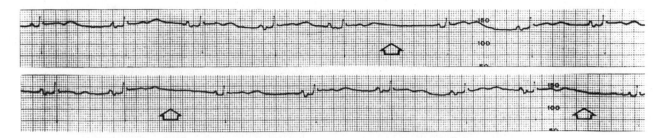

Fig. 5-17   Sinus exit block, type I (Wenckebach block). The following characteristics of this tracing suggest the diagnosis of a Wenckebach exit block from a sinus node. The P-P intervals progressively shorten until a pause in atrial activity occurs, as depicted by the arrows; the duration of the pause is less than twice the shortest P-P interval; the P-P interval after the pause exceeds the P-P interval preceding the pause, which is the shortest P-P interval. Monitor lead.

Rate	Varying from 33 to 50 beats/min.
Rhythm	The four features previously mentioned.
P waves	Biphasic but fairly constant contour; intermittent loss of P waves, producing a pause *(arrows)*.
PR interval	0.24 second.
QRS complex	0.07 second.

or by fibrosis involving the atrium. Occlusion of the sinus nodal artery caused by acute myocardial infarction may result in an atrial infarction and produce sinus exit block. Medications such as quinidine, procainamide, amiodarone, and digitalis may lead to sinus exit block. Sinus exit block is usually transient and often of no clinical importance except to prompt a search for the underlying cause. Syncope may result if the sinus exit block is prolonged and unaccompanied by an AV junctional or ventricular escape rhythm. Digitalis produces type II sinus exit block but not type I AV block.

Treatment

Therapy for symptomatic sinus exit block is directed toward increasing sympathetic tone and decreasing parasympathetic tone. Thus atropine and isoproterenol are useful, as described in the section on sinus bradycardia. If the clinical situation demands therapy and pharmacologic measures are not effective, atrial or ventricular pacing may be indicated.

Wandering Pacemaker

Wandering pacemaker (Figs. 5-18 and 5-19), a variant of sinus dysrhythmia, involves the passive transfer of the dominant pacemaker focus from the sinus node to latent pacemakers with the next highest degree of automaticity in other atrial sites or in the AV junctional tissue. Thus only one pacemaker is operative at a time. As with other forms of sinus dysrhythmia, the change occurs in a gradual fashion over the duration of several beats. The ECG displays a cyclic increase of the R-R interval, a PR interval that gradually shortens and may become less than 0.12 second, and

a change in P-wave configuration until it becomes negative in lead I or II or becomes buried in the QRS complex. A slight change in QRS configuration may occur because of aberrant conduction. Generally these changes occur in reverse as the pacemaker shifts back to the sinus node. Rarely a wandering pacemaker may appear without changes in rate.

Significance

Wandering pacemaker is a normal phenomenon often seen in very young persons, in older adults, and particularly in athletes. Persistence of an AV junctional rhythm for long periods, however, usually indicates underlying heart disease.

Treatment

Treatment of a wandering pacemaker usually is not indicated. Sympathomimetic agents such as ephedrine or isoproterenol or parasympatholytic agents such as atropine can be used if necessary (see section on sinus bradycardia).

Premature Atrial Complexes

Premature atrial complexes (Figs. 5-20 to 5-24) are the most common cause of an intermittent pulse. They may originate in any area of the heart, most frequently in the ventricles, less often in the atria and AV junctional region, and rarely in the sinus node. Although premature complexes arise in normal hearts, they are more often associated with organic disease, particularly in older patients.

The diagnosis of premature atrial complexes is indicated by a premature P wave and a PR interval greater than 0.12 second. Although the contour of the premature P wave

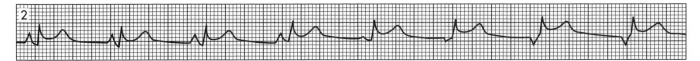

Fig. 5-18 Wandering atrial pacemaker. The strip begins with sinus rhythm; by the end of the strip, the rhythm has changed to a junctional rhythm with retrograde P waves preceding the QRS complex.

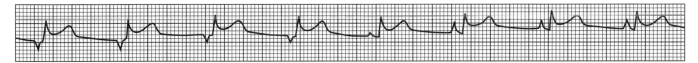

Fig. 5-19 Wandering atrial pacemaker. The strip is continuous from Fig. 5-18. The strip begins with junctional rhythm, but by the end, normal sinus rhythm has resumed.

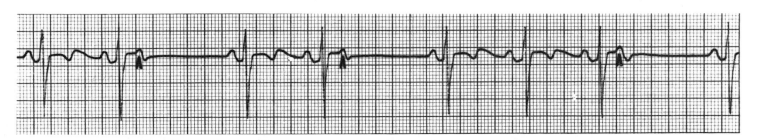

Fig. 5-20 Premature atrial complexes, blocked and hidden in the T wave. The deformed T waves *(arrows)* indicate a nonconducted premature atrial complex that blocks within the AV node or bundle of His. The premature atrial complex discharges the sinus node and delays its return so that the P-P interval from the premature atrial complex to the next sinus P wave exceeds the normal sinus P-P interval. A noncompensatory pulse follows the blocked premature atrial complexes. Monitor lead.

Rate	67 beats/min during sinus rhythm.
Rhythm	Varying because of premature atrial complexes.
P waves	Premature atrial complexes are hidden within and deform the T waves.
PR interval	Of normal sinus beats, 0.18 second.
QRS complex	0.10 second.

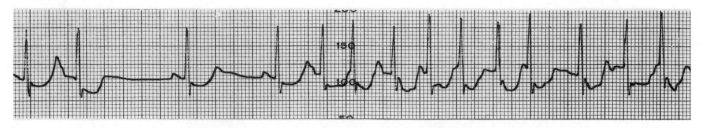

Fig. 5-21 Premature atrial complex precipitating atrial flutter-fibrillation. A premature atrial complex is hidden within the T wave of the first QRS complex and occurs again in the T wave of the fourth QRS complex. This premature atrial complex precipitates atrial flutter-fibrillation. Monitor lead.

Rate	Varying.
Rhythm	Varying because of premature atrial complexes and atrial flutter-fibrillation.
P waves	Premature atrial complexes hidden in the T waves.
PR interval	Of normally conducted beats, 0.14 second.
QRS complex	0.08 second.

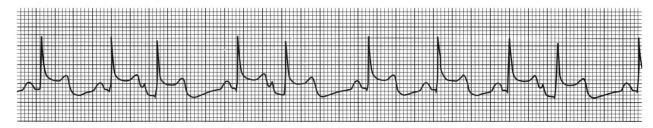

Fig. 5-22 Premature atrial complexes. Third, fifth, and ninth complexes represent premature atrial complexes. Monitor lead.

Rate	80 beats/min.
Rhythm	Varying because of premature atrial complexes.
P waves	Precede each QRS complex.
QRS interval	0.06 second, biphasic QRS complex with T inversion.

may resemble the normal sinus P wave, it generally is different. Variations in the basic sinus rate may make the diagnosis of prematurity difficult at times, but differences in the contour of the P wave are usually quite apparent and indicate a different focus of origin. When a premature atrial complex occurs early in diastole, conduction may not be completely normal. The AV junction may still be refractory from the preceding beat and prevents propagation of the impulse (blocked premature atrial complex) or causes conduction to be slowed in the AV junction (prolonged PR interval) or ventricle (functional bundle branch block). As a rule, a short RP interval produced by an early premature atrial complex close to the preceding QRS complex is followed by a long PR interval. On occasion, when the AV

junction has sufficiently repolarized to conduct normally, the supraventricular QRS complex may be aberrant in configuration because the ventricle has not completely repolarized (see section on supraventricular dysrhythmias with abnormal QRS complexes and Figs. 5-23 and 5-24).

The length of the pause after any premature beat or series of premature beats is determined by the interaction of several factors. If the premature atrial complex occurs when the sinus node is not refractory, the impulse may conduct to the sinus node, discharge it prematurely, and cause the next sinus cycle to begin from that point. The interval between the two normal beats flanking a premature atrial complex that has reset the timing of the basic sinus rhythm is less than twice the normal cycle, and the pause after the

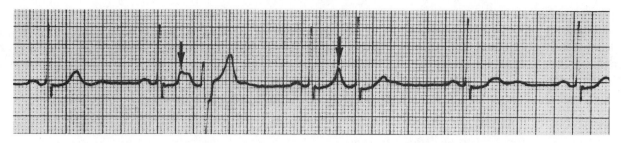

Fig. 5-23 Premature atrial complexes with and without aberrancy. The first premature atrial complex *(arrow)* occurs at a shorter RP interval than the second premature atrial complex *(arrow)* and conducts with a bundle branch block contour (probably RBBB in this monitor lead). The first premature atrial complex conducts with aberrancy, whereas the second does not because the first reaches the bundle branch system before complete recovery of repolarization.

Rate	50 beats/min during the normally conducted complexes.
Rhythm	Irregular because of the premature atrial complexes.
P waves	Normal for the normally conducted sinus beats; premature atrial complexes deform the T waves.
PR interval	Of premature atrial complexes, prolonged because the AV node or bundle of His has incompletely recovered. PR interval of first premature atrial complex is approximately 0.26 second, and that of the second premature atrial complex is approximately 0.22 second. The PR interval of normally conducted sinus beats is 0.19 second.
QRS complex	Of normally conducted beats, 0.07 second; of aberrantly conducted QRS complex, 0.12 second.

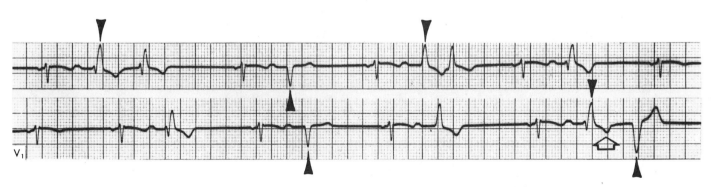

Fig. 5-24 Premature atrial complexes that produce functional right and functional left bundle branch block. Upright arrowheads point to QRS complexes that conduct with complete or incomplete functional left bundle branch block; inverted arrowheads point to some of the QRS complexes that conduct with functional right bundle branch block. The latter have monophasic and triphasic contours. The deformed T waves (*open arrow* at the end of the last strip) indicate a premature atrial complex. They occur singly and in pairs.

Rate	Varying because of premature atrial complexes.
Rhythm	Irregular because of premature atrial complexes.
P waves	During sinus rhythm, normal; P waves of premature atrial complexes are hard to discern because they occur in the preceding T wave.
PR interval	Of normal sinus beats, 0.12 second; of premature atrial complexes, prolonged and of differing durations because of differences in RP intervals.

premature atrial complex is said to be *noncompensatory.* The interval after the premature atrial complex is generally slightly longer than one sinus cycle, however. Less commonly the premature atrial complex may find the sinus node refractory, in which case the timing of the basic sinus rhythm is not altered, and the interval between the two normal beats flanking the premature atrial complex is twice the normal P-P cycle. The interval after this premature atrial discharge is therefore said to be a *full compensatory pause.* A compensatory pause is one of sufficient duration to make the interval between the two normal beats on each side of the premature beat equal to twice the basic cycle length. However, sinus dysrhythmia may lengthen or shorten this pause.

Significance

Premature atrial complexes may occur in a variety of situations (for example, during infection, inflammation, or myocardial ischemia), or they may be provoked by a variety of medications, by tension states, or by tobacco and caffeine. Premature atrial complexes may precipitate or presage the occurrence of a sustained supraventricular tachycardia.

Treatment

In the absence of organic heart disease, treatment may not be necessary, unless the patient complains of symptoms such as palpitations or has recurrent tachycardias or an excessive number of premature atrial complexes. If treatment is indicated (for example, in acute myocardial infarction),

initial therapy should probably be with digitalis with quinidine or procainamide if digitalis alone is not successful. Sedation and omission of alcohol, caffeine, smoking, or other stimulants (for example, amphetamines, cocaine) may help some patients.

AV Nodal Reentry

The tachycardias formerly called *paroxysmal atrial* and *junctional tachycardias* are caused most commonly by AV nodal reentry or reentry over an accessory pathway. They are often called, nonspecifically, *paroxysmal supraventricular tachycardia* when the mechanism responsible for the tachycardia cannot be determined with certainty (Figs. 5-25 to 5-28). In this section, AV nodal reentry is examined. Reentry over an accessory pathway is dealt with in the section on preexcitation syndrome.

AV nodal reentry is characterized by a rapid, regular tachycardia of sudden onset and termination that occurs at rates generally between 150 and 250 beats/min. Uncommonly the rate may exceed 250 beats/min. Unless aberrant ventricular conduction exists, the QRS complex is normal in contour and duration. The retrograde P wave is usually lost within the QRS complex. AV nodal reentry is most commonly caused by reentry within the AV node, anterogradely over a slowly conducting pathway and retrogradely over a more rapidly conducting pathway (Fig. 5-28).

AV nodal reentry recorded at the onset begins abruptly, usually after a premature atrial complex that conducts with a prolonged PR interval; the abrupt termination is some-

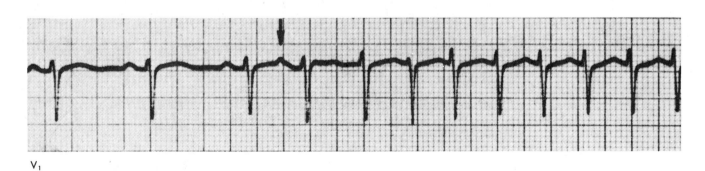

V₁

Fig. 5-25 Paroxysmal supraventricular tachycardia. Three sinus beats are interrupted by a premature atrial complex *(arrow)*, which conducts with PR prolongation and initiates the supraventricular tachycardia.

Rate	Sinus rhythm, 83 beats/min; paroxysmal supraventricular tachycardia, 190 beats/min.
Rhythm	Regular during sinus rhythm and during paroxysmal supraventricular tachycardia.
P waves	Seen in first four beats but not afterward.
PR interval	Normal during sinus beats, 0.16 second; slightly prolonged (0.20 second) during premature atrial complex.
QRS complex	Normal, 0.08 second.

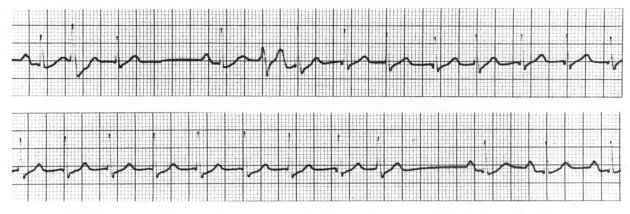

Fig. 5-26 Initiation of paroxysmal supraventricular tachycardia after a premature ventricular complex and spontaneous termination of paroxysmal supraventricular tachycardia. *Top,* Paroxysmal supraventricular tachycardia begins after the fifth QRS complex, which is a premature ventricular complex. Two interpretations are possible. The first possibility is that the normally conducted sinus complex occurs in the T wave of the premature ventricular complex and conducts with a prolonged PR interval (the premature ventricular complex is interpolated) and initiates paroxysmal supraventricular tachycardia. The second possibility is that the premature ventricular complex conducts retrogradely to the atrium and initiates the paroxysmal supraventricular tachycardia in that manner. *Bottom,* the paroxysmal supraventricular tachycardia terminates spontaneously with a slight pause. Monitor lead.

Rate	During paroxysmal supraventricular tachycardia, 120 beats/min.
Rhythm	Fairly regular during paroxysmal supraventricular tachycardia.
P waves	Cannot be seen during paroxysmal supraventricular tachycardia.
PR interval	Cannot determine during paroxysmal supraventricular tachycardia.
QRS complex	Normal, 0.07 second.
Dysrhythmia	Probably AV nodal reentry.

times followed by a brief period of asystole, which results in part from tachycardia-induced depression of sinus nodal automaticity. The R-R interval may shorten during the first few beats at the onset or lengthen during the last few beats before termination of the tachycardia. Variation in cycle length is usually caused by variation in AV nodal conduction time. The mechanism of the tachycardia is reentry within the AV node (see Fig. 5-91).

Significance

AV nodal reentry may occur at any age and is often unassociated with underlying heart disease. The dysrhythmia may be related to specific inciting causes such as overexertion, emotional stimuli, and coffee and smoking, although this is often difficult to prove. It may follow a specific pattern, or its onset may be unrelated to any particular event.

Symptoms frequently accompanying the attack range from feelings of palpitations, nervousness, or anxiety to angina, frank heart failure, or shock, depending on the duration and rate of the AV nodal reentry and the presence of organic heart disease. The AV nodal reentry may cause syncope because of the rapid ventricular rate, reduced cardiac output, and cerebral circulation or because of asystole when the AV nodal reentry terminates. The prognosis for patients without heart disease is usually quite good.

Treatment

Treatment of the acute attack depends on the clinical situation, the way in which the AV nodal reentry is tolerated, the natural history of the attacks in the patient, and the presence of associated disease. For some patients, rest, reassurance, and sedation may be all that are required to abort an attack. Treatment options follow:

1. For stable patients, simple vagal maneuvers, including carotid sinus massage, the Valsalva maneuver, gagging, or activation of the "diving reflex" by facial immersion in ice water (in the absence of ischemic heart disease) serve as the first line of therapy and terminate AV nodal reentry by prolonging AV nodal refractoriness or leave it unaffected (actually, slight slowing may occur during vagal stimulation). These maneuvers should be retried after each pharmacologic approach.

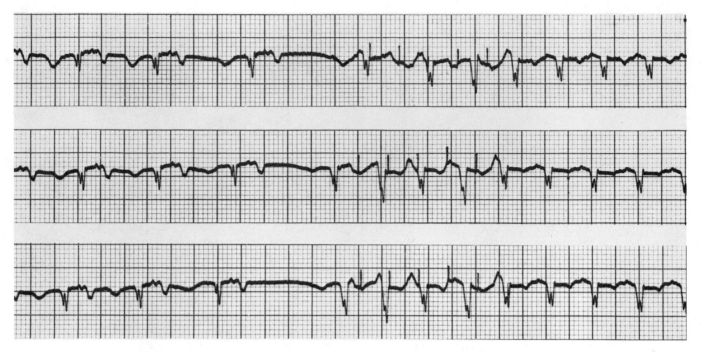

Fig. 5-27   Pacing-induced termination of paroxysmal supraventricular tachycardia. The patient had recurrent episodes of paroxysmal supraventricular tachycardia that were easily terminated by rapid atrial pacing. Pacing stimuli can be seen before the onset of sinus rhythm in the midportion of each monitor lead tracing.

Rate	During paroxysmal supraventricular tachycardia, 150 beats/min.
Rhythm	During paroxysmal supraventricular tachycardia, regular.
P waves	Not seen during paroxysmal supraventricular tachycardia. P waves during sinus rhythm are abnormal with a low-amplitude biphasic component after an initial positive component.
PR interval	During sinus rhythm, 0.24 second; during paroxysmal supraventricular tachycardia, cannot be discerned.
QRS complex	0.08 second.
Dysrhythmia	AV nodal reentry documented by invasive electrophysiologic study.

2. Verapamil, a calcium antagonist (5 to 10 mg intravenously), terminates AV nodal reentry successfully in about 2 minutes in over 90% of instances. A second injection may be administered in 15 to 20 minutes if necessary. It has become the preferred treatment if the simple vagal maneuvers fail.[13-15]

3. If signs or symptoms of cardiac decompensation (such as chest pain, dyspnea, hypotension, or congestive heart failure) occur, synchronized cardioversion is the treatment of choice. DC shock, synchronized to the QRS complex to avoid precipitating ventricular fibrillation, successfully terminates AV nodal reentry with energies in the range of 10 to 50 joules; higher energies may be required in some instances. Short-acting barbiturates such as sodium methohexital (Brevital), 50 to 120 mg given intravenously at 50 mg/30 sec, may be used to provide anesthesia, or diazepam (Valium), 5 to 15 mg given intravenously at 5 mg/min, may be used to provide sedation and amnesia. Doses must be individualized and in general should be reduced for patients who have heart failure, hypotension, or liver disease. During DC cardioversion, a physician skilled in airway management should be in attendance, an intravenous route established, and all equipment and drugs necessary for emergency resuscitation immediately accessible. Oxygen (100%) is administered throughout the procedure using manually assisted ventilation if necessary. If DC shock becomes necessary in patients who have received large amounts of digitalis, the clinician should begin with 1 to 5 joules and gradually increase the energy level in increments of approximately 25 to 50 joules as long as premature ventricular systoles do not result. If premature ven-

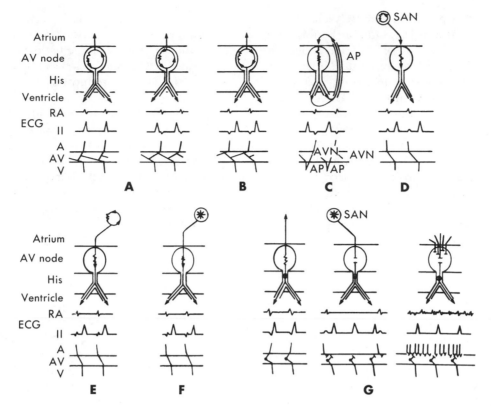

Fig. 5-28 Diagrammatic representation of various tachycardias. In the top portion of each example is a schematic representation of the presumed anatomic pathways. In the lower portion the ECG presentation in the explanatory ladder diagram is depicted. **A,** AV nodal reentry. *Left,* Reentrant excitation is confined to the AV node with retrograde atrial activity occurring with ventricular activity because of anterograde conduction over the slow AV nodal pathway and retrograde conduction over the fast AV nodal pathway. *Right,* Atrial activity occurs slightly later than ventricular activity because of a retrograde conduction delay. **B,** Atypical AV nodal reentry as a result of anterograde conduction over a fast AV nodal pathway and retrograde conduction over a slow AV nodal pathway. **C,** Concealed accessory pathway *(AP).* Reciprocating tachycardia is caused by anterograde conduction over the AV node and retrograde conduction over the accessory pathway. Retrograde P waves occur after the QRS complex. **D,** Sinus nodal reentry. The tachycardia occurs as a result of reentry within the sinus node, which then conducts to the rest of the heart. *SAN,* SA node. **E,** Atrial reentry. Tachycardia is caused by reentry with the atrium, which then conducts to the rest of the heart. **F,** Automatic atrial tachycardia. Tachycardia is result of automatic discharge in the atrium, which then conducts to the rest of the heart. It is difficult to distinguish this tachycardia from tachycardia caused by atrial reentry. **G,** NPJT. Various presentations of this tachycardia are depicted with retrograde atrial capture, AV dissociation with the sinus node in control of the atria, and AV dissociation with atrial fibrillation. (From Zipes DP: *Specific arrhythmias: diagnosis and treatment.* In Braunwald E, editor: *Heart disease: textbook of cardiovascular medicine,* ed 3, Philadelphia, 1988, Saunders.)

tricular systoles occur but can be suppressed with lidocaine or phenytoin, the next higher energy level may be tried.

4. Cholinergic drugs, particularly edrophonium chloride (Tensilon), a short-acting cholinesterase inhibitor, may terminate AV nodal reentry when administered initially at a dose of 3 to 5 mg intravenously and, if unsuccessful, repeated at a dose of 10 mg intra-

venously. Its action is rapid in onset and short in duration, with minimal side effects. Edrophonium chloride should be used cautiously or not at all in patients who are hypotensive or who have lung disease, especially asthma.

5. Pressor drugs may terminate AV nodal reentry by inducing reflex vagal stimulation mediated via baroreceptors in the carotid sinus and aorta when

the systolic blood pressure is acutely elevated to levels of about 180 mm Hg. One of the following drugs, diluted in 5 to 10 ml of 5% dextrose and water, may be given over 1 to 3 minutes: phenylephrine hydrochloride (Neo-Synephrine), 0.5 to 1.0 mg; methoxamine hydrochloride (Vasoxyl), 3 to 5 mg; or metaraminol (Aramine), 0.5 to 2.0 mg. Pressor drugs should be used cautiously or not at all in older patients or in patients with organic heart disease, significant hypertension, hyperthyroidism, or acute myocardial infarction. This potentially dangerous and almost always uncomfortable procedure is rarely needed any longer, unless the patient is also hypotensive. Other, safer procedures are preferred.

6. If these approaches are unsuccessful, intravenous administration of digitalis may be attempted next, using one of the following short-acting digitalis preparations: ouabain, 0.25 to 0.50 mg intravenously followed by 0.1 mg every 30 to 60 minutes if needed, keeping the total dosage less than 1.0 mg within 24 hours; digoxin (Lanoxin), 0.5 to 1.0 mg intravenously followed by 0.25 mg every 2 to 4 hours, with a total dosage less than 1.5 mg within 24 hours; or deslanoside (Cedilanid-D), 0.8 mg intravenously, followed by 0.4 mg every 2 to 4 hours, restricting the total dosage to less than 2.0 mg within 24 hours. Oral administration of digitalis to terminate an acute attack is generally not indicated. Vagal maneuvers, previously ineffective, may terminate AV nodal reentry after digitalis administration and therefore should be repeated.

7. Propranolol (Inderal), given intravenously at 0.5 to 1 mg/min for a total dose of 1 to 3 mg, may be tried if digitalis administration is unsuccessful. Propranolol must be used cautiously, if at all, in patients who have heart failure or chronic lung disease because its adrenergic β-receptor blocking action depresses myocardial contractility and may produce bronchospasm. Before administration of digitalis or propranolol, it is advisable to reassess the clinical status of the patient and consider whether DC cardioversion may be advisable. DC shock administered to patients who have received excessive amounts of digitalis may be dangerous and result in serious postshock ventricular dysrhythmias.

8. In the event that digitalis has been given in large doses and DC shock is contraindicated, right atrial pacing may restore sinus rhythm, presumably by prematurely depolarizing one of the pathways required for continued reentry (see Fig. 5-27). In some patients, right atrial pacing may precipitate atrial fibrillation; however, because the latter is generally accompanied by a slower ventricular rate, the patient's clinical status improves.

9. Procainamide (Pronestyl), quinidine, or disopyramide (Norpace) may be required to terminate AV nodal reentry in some patients. Unless contraindicated, DC cardioversion should be used before these agents, which are more often administered to prevent recurrences.

Prevention of recurrences is often more difficult than terminating the acute episode. Smoking, alcohol, or excessive fatigue, if identified as precipitating factors, should be avoided. Initially, one must decide whether the frequency and severity of the attacks warrant drug prophylaxis. For example, an attempt should probably not be made to suppress AV nodal reentry occurring twice yearly in an otherwise healthy patient.

1. If drug prophylaxis is indicated, digitalis is the initial drug of choice. The speed at which digitalization is achieved is determined by the clinical situation. Using digoxin, rapid oral digitalization can be accomplished in 24 to 36 hours with an initial dose of 1.0 to 1.5 mg, followed by 0.25 to 0.5 mg every 6 hours for a total dose of 2.0 to 3.0 mg. A less rapid oral regimen digitalizes in 2 to 3 days with an initial dose of 0.75 to 1.0 mg, followed by 0.25 to 0.5 mg every 12 hours for a total dose of 2.0 to 3.0 mg. Alternatively, digoxin administered as a maintenance dose of 0.125 to 0.5 mg achieves digitalization in about 1 week. Because of its shorter half-life, digoxin may provide more effective control when administered twice daily. Digitoxin, which has a longer duration of action, may be used instead of digoxin. Oral digitalization with digitoxin may be accomplished in 24 to 36 hours with an initial dose of 0.5 to 0.8 mg, followed by 0.2 mg every 6 to 8 hours until a total dose of 1.2 mg is reached. A slower approach involves administering 0.2 mg 3 times daily for 2 to 3 days. Complete digitalization can also be accomplished in about 1 month by simply giving a maintenance dose of 0.05 to 0.2 mg daily.

2. If digitalis alone is unsuccessful, the clinician can then add quinidine, 200 to 400 mg every 6 hours, or propranolol (Inderal), 10 to 40 mg every 6 hours. Verapamil (80 to 120 mg every 6 to 8 hours) with digitalis may be very effective.

3. If a combination of digitalis and quinidine or digitalis and propranolol is unsuccessful, concomitant administration of all three drugs may be tried. If this regimen also fails, empiric trials with other antidysrhythmic agents such as procainamide or disopyramide may be warranted. Flecainide or amiodarone is often effective in patients with supraventricular tachycardia but is investigational for that purpose.

4. For many patients, pacemaker implantation is an acceptable treatment. Rapid atrial pacing promptly terminates AV nodal reentry, restoring sinus rhythm immediately or sometimes after a transient episode of

atrial fibrillation. Some pacemaker units need to be activated by the patient when AV nodal reentry occurs; other units discharge automatically when they detect the onset of AV nodal reentry. Such pacing devices can be combined with drug therapy.

5. Ablation of the AV node–bundle of His area by a catheter or surgical techniques may be indicated to eliminate episodes of the tachycardia. Such an approach may make the patient pacemaker dependent if complete AV heart block results.

Preexcitation Syndrome

Ventricular preexcitation[1,8,16] (Figs. 5-29 to 5-38) exists when the atrial impulse activates the whole or some part of ventricular muscle earlier than would be expected if the atrial impulse reached the ventricles by way of the normal specialized conduction system only. Four basic features typify the usual ECG of a patient with the preexcitation (Wolff-Parkinson-White [WPW]) syndrome: (1) PR interval less than 0.12 second during sinus rhythm; (2) QRS complex duration greater than 0.12 second with a slurred, slow-rising onset of the R-wave upstroke in some leads (delta [δ] wave) and a usually normal terminal QRS portion; (3) secondary ST-T–wave changes that are usually directed opposite the major delta and QRS vectors; and (4) paroxysmal tachydysrhythmias in many patients (the exact percentage varies widely, from 4% to 80%, and depends on the patient population studied). The explanation for those ECG findings is the presence of a rapidly conducting muscular accessory pathway connection that bypasses the AV node by communicating directly from atrium to ventricle.

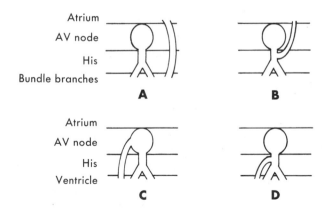

Fig. 5-29 Schematic representation of accessory pathways. **A,** The usual AV connection, often called a *Kent bundle.* **B,** Atriohisian bypass tract in which the connection is from the atrium to the bundle of His, thus bypassing the AV node. **C,** Nodoventricular connection from the AV node to the ventricle. **D,** Fasciculoventricular connection from the bundle of His or bundle branches to the ventricle.   (From Zipes DP: *Specific arrhythmias: diagnosis and treatment.* In Braunwald E, editor: *Heart disease: a textbook of cardiovascular medicine,* ed 3, Philadelphia, 1988, Saunders.)

Other patients may possess variants of the preexcitation syndrome that are explained by the presence of bypass tracts between the AV node and ventricle (nodoventricular) or between the fascicles and ventricle (fasciculoventricular). Patients who have a short PR interval (less than 0.12 second) and a normal QRS complex with supraventricular tachycardias most often do not have a bypass tract from atrium to the bundle of His (so-called Lown-Ganong-Levine syndrome). These patients may simply possess an AV node that conducts rapidly and also have episodes of supraventricular tachycardia (see Fig. 5-29).

The site of the accessory pathway can be determined by a careful analysis of the spatial direction of the δ wave in maximally preexcited QRS complexes (see Fig. 5-34), as well as from electric recordings made directly on the heart using catheters during an electrophysiologic study or at the time of open heart surgery. Once identified, the accessory pathway can be interrupted surgically or by other ablation techniques.

Because of the accessory pathway, two parallel routes of AV conduction are possible: one subject to physiologic delay over the AV node and the other passing directly without delay over the accessory pathway from atrium to ventricle. This produces the typical QRS complex that is a fusion beat caused by depolarization of the ventricle, in part by the wavefront traveling over the accessory pathway and in part by the wavefront traveling over the normal AV node–bundle of His route. The δ wave represents ventricular activation from input over the accessory pathway. The extent of contribution to ventricular depolarization by the wavefront over each route depends on the relative activation time of each wavefront.

The usual tachycardia is characterized by anterograde conduction over the normal pathway and retrograde conduction over the accessory pathway, which results in a normal QRS complex at rates of 150 to 250 beats/min. Because the reentrant loop involves atria and ventricles, the tachycardia is called an *AV reciprocating tachycardia (AVRT).* In contrast to most patients who have AV nodal reentry, the retrograde P wave during AVRT occurs in the ST segment.

The rhythm of AVRT may change spontaneously into atrial flutter or atrial fibrillation, and patients with preexcitation syndrome may have other types of tachycardia. Patients who have atrial fibrillation almost always have AVRT that can be induced during electrophysiologic study. Atrial fibrillation presents a potentially serious risk because of the possibility for rapid conduction over the accessory pathway and rapid ventricular rates. On occasion, ventricular fibrillation may result.

Significance

The reported incidence of preexcitation syndrome averages about 1.5 in 1000 persons, although the actual incidence is unknown. It occurs in all age groups and more of-

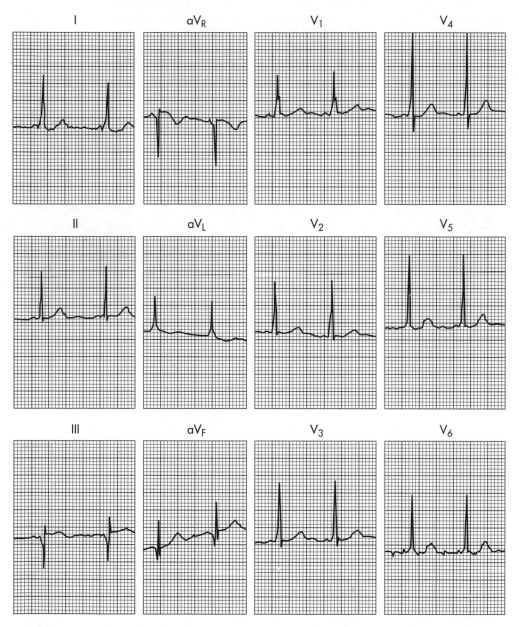

Fig. 5-30   Twelve-lead ECG illustrating preexcitation syndrome. Preexcitation syndrome may be classified according to position (see Fig. 5-34) or into a classification type. This ECG represents type A, with a positive QRS complex in lead V_1. The bypass fibers in type A usually bridge the posterior aspects of the right or left atrium and ventricle.

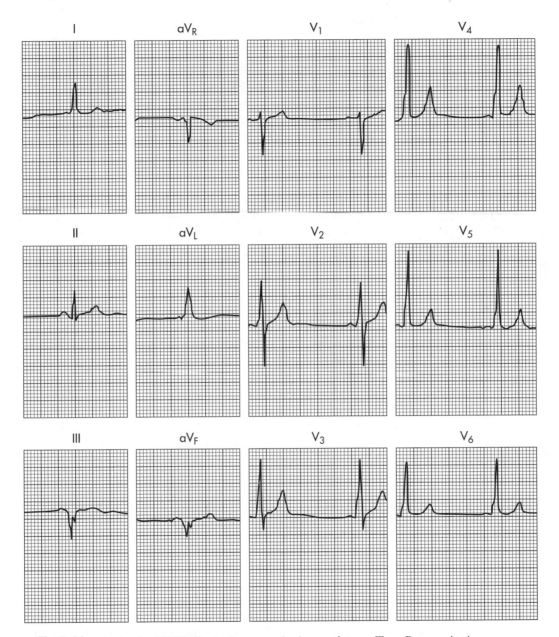

Fig. 5-31 Twelve-lead ECG illustrating preexcitation syndrome. Type B preexcitation syndrome with a negative QRS complex in lead V_1. The bypass fibers in type B usually connect the anterior or lateral aspects of the right atrium.

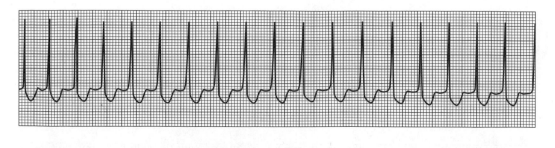

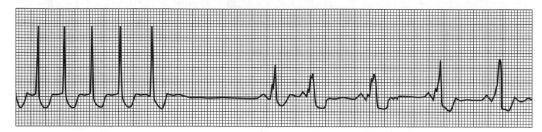

Fig. 5-32   Onset of paroxysmal atrial tachycardia in a patient with preexcitation syndrome. Paroxysmal atrial tachycardia is terminated in the bottom strip by pressure on the carotid sinus.

ten (60% to 70%) in men. Two thirds of patients with the short PR interval and normal QRS complex are women. Patients may seek help because of recurrent supraventricular tachycardia, atrial fibrillation with a rapid ventricular response, heart failure, syncope, or symptoms related to associated cardiac anomalies; the symptoms may be discovered during examination for noncardiac-related reasons. Of adults with preexcitation syndrome, 60% to 70% have normal hearts; a higher proportion of children have heart disease. A variety of acquired and congenital cardiac defects, including Ebstein anomaly, cardiomyopathies, and mitral valve prolapse, have been reported.

Of patients with preexcitation syndrome who have recurrent tachydysrhythmias, 80% have AVRT, 15% to 30% have atrial fibrillation, and 5% have atrial flutter. Ventricular tachycardia rarely occurs, and most reports have misdiagnosed as ventricular tachycardia the aberrant QRS complexes caused by anomalous conduction. Recognition of the preexcitation syndrome is clinically important, since the tachydysrhythmias at times do not respond to conventional therapy and may be associated with very rapid ventricular rates. For example, digitalis may accelerate the ventricular rate in some patients who have atrial fibrillation and preexcitation syndrome. The anomalous complexes may mask or mimic myocardial infarction, bundle branch block, or ventricular hypertrophy, and the presence of preexcitation syndrome may call attention to an associated cardiac defect.

The prognosis is excellent in patients without tachycardia or an associated cardiac anomaly. In most patients with recurrent tachycardia the prognosis is good, but sudden unexpected death can occur, especially when the ventricular rate during atrial fibrillation is rapid or when associated congenital defects are present. Ventricular fibrillation has been documented in humans and in dogs with preexcitation syndrome and is probably caused by extremely rapid ventricular rates, which are permitted by the bypass during atrial flutter or fibrillation that exceeds the ability of the ventricle to follow in an organized fashion. Consequently, fragmented, disorganized ventricular activation results and leads to ventricular fibrillation. Alternatively, bypassing the AV nodal delay, supraventricular discharge may activate the ventricle during the vulnerable period of the antecedent T wave and precipitate ventricular fibrillation.

Treatment[7,9,16]

Patients with ventricular preexcitation who have none or only occasional episodes of tachydysrhythmias unassociated with significant symptoms do not require electrophysiologic evaluation or therapy. However, if the patient has frequent episodes of tachydysrhythmias and/or the dysrhythmias cause significant symptoms, therapy should be instituted.

Drugs that increase the refractory period, slow conduction, or cause block in one of the reentrant pathways may suppress reciprocating tachycardia. Verapamil, propranolol, and digitalis prolong conduction time and refractoriness in the AV node. Verapamil and propranolol do not directly affect conduction in the accessory pathway, whereas digitalis has variable effects. However, because digitalis has

Reciprocating tachycardias

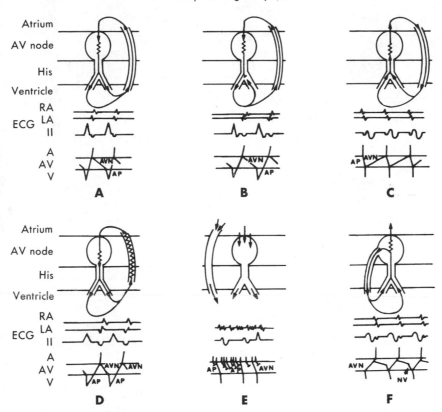

Fig. 5-33 Schematic diagram of tachycardia associated with accessory pathways *(AP)*. **A,** Usual (orthodromic) form of tachycardia with anterograde conduction over the AV node–bundle of His route and retrograde conduction over the accessory pathway (left-sided, as depicted here by left atrial activation preceding right atrial activation). *AVN,* AV node; *RA,* right atrial; *LA,* left atrial. **B,** Usual (orthodromic) form of tachycardia and functional bundle branch block on the same side as the accessory pathway. **C,** Unusual (antidromic) form of tachycardia with anterograde conduction over the accessory pathway and retrograde conduction over the AV node–bundle of His route. **D,** Orthodromic tachycardia with a slowly conducting accessory pathway. **E,** Atrial fibrillation conducting over the accessory pathway and the AV node. **F,** Nodoventricular *(NV)* tachycardia with anterograde conduction over a portion of the AV node and a nodoventricular pathway and retrograde conduction over the AV node.   (From Zipes DP: *Specific arrhythmias: diagnosis and treatment.* In Braunwald E, editor: *Heart disease: a textbook of cardiovascular medicine,* ed 3, Philadelphia, 1988, Saunders.)

been reported to shorten refractoriness in the accessory pathway and speed the ventricular response in some patients with atrial fibrillation, it is advisable not to use digitalis as a single drug in patients with preexcitation syndrome who have or may develop atrial flutter or atrial fibrillation. Since atrial flutter or fibrillation often develops during the reciprocating tachycardia, the caveat about digitalis probably applies to all patients who have tachycardia and preexcitation syndrome.

Drugs (see box on p. 121) that prolong the refractory period in the accessory pathway (for example, quinidine)

should be used to treat atrial flutter or fibrillation. Lidocaine does not prolong refractoriness of the accessory pathway when the effective refractory period is less than 300 msec. Verapamil and lidocaine given intravenously may increase the ventricular rate during atrial fibrillation in preexcitation syndrome.

Termination of the acute episode of AVRT—suspected electrocardiographically by a normal QRS complex, regular R-R intervals at rate of about 200 beats/min, and a P wave in the ST segment—should be approached as for AV nodal reentry. For atrial flutter or fibrillation, drugs that

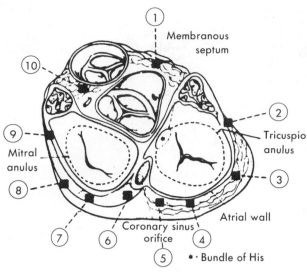

1 Right anterior paraseptal   6 Left posterior paraseptal
2 Right anterior   7 Left posterior
3 Right lateral   8 Left lateral
4 Right posterior   9 Left anterior
5 Right paraseptal   10 Left anterior paraseptal

Delta wave polarity

	I	II	III	aVR	aVL	aVF	V1	V2	V3	V4	V5	V6
①	+	+	+(±)	-	±(+)	±(+)	+	±	±	+(±)	+	+
②	+	+	-(±)	-	+(±)	±(-)	±	+(±)	+(±)	+	+	+
③	+	±(-)	-	-	+	-(±)	±	±	±	+	+	+
④	+	-	-	-	+	-	±(+)	±	+	+	+	+
⑤	+	-	-	-(+)	+	+	+	±	+	+	+	+
⑥	+	-	-	-	+	-	+	+	+	+	+	+
⑦	+	-	-	±(+)	+	-	+	+	+	+	+	-(±)
⑧	-(±)	±	±	±(+)	-(±)	±	+	+	+	+	-(±)	-(±)
⑨	-(±)	+	+	-	-(±)	+	+	+	+	+	+	+
⑩	+	+	+(±)	-	±	+	±(+)	+	+	+	+	+

± · Initial 40 msec delta isoelectic
+ · Initial 40 msec delta positive
- · Initial 40 msec delta negative

Fig. 5-34 In this schematic representation *(top)*, sites of the potential position of the accessory pathways are indicated by filled boxes numbered 1 through 10. δ Wave polarity in the 12-lead ECG for each of the 10 sites is depicted in the table at the bottom.   (From Gallagher JJ and others: The preexcitation syndrome, *Prog Cardiovasc Dis* 20:285, 1978.)

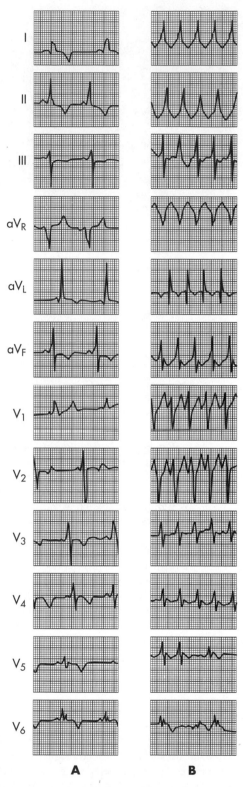

A   B

Fig. 5-35 Preexcitation syndrome. Twelve-lead ECG of patient with type B preexcitation syndrome. **A,** ECG taken during normal sinus rhythm. **B,** ECG taken during tachycardia.

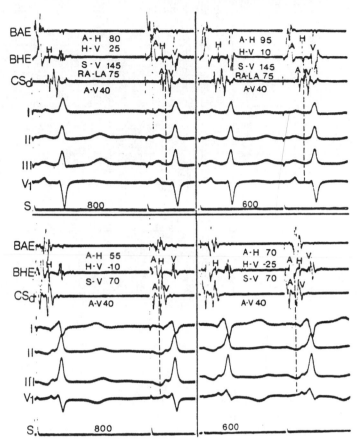

Fig. 5-36 Influence of pacing site and cycle length on the degree of preexcitation. In this patient with a left anterolateral accessory pathway (site *9* in Fig. 5-34), pacing the high right atrium at a cycle length of 800 msec *(top left panel)* produced an atriohisian *(A-H)* interval of 80 msec and a His-to-ventricle *(H-V)* interval of 25 msec. The interval from the stimulus to the onset of ventricular activity *(S-V)* was 145 msec, and the right-to-left atrial activation time was 75 msec. The interrupted line indicates the onset of the δ wave. Little preexcitation is seen in the ECG because the fairly rapid AV conduction time over the normal pathway allows much of the ventricle to be activated normally before the impulse traveling from the right to left atrium and then over the accessory pathway can depolarize the ventricles. Shortening the pacing cycle length to 600 msec *(top right panel)* without changing the pacing site lengthened the A-H interval by 15 msec and shortened the H-V interval by 10 msec. The other intervals remained the same, and the QRS complex changed very slightly. The coronary sinus is paced at a cycle length of 800 msec *(bottom left panel)*. Even though the A-H interval shortens to 55 msec because of coronary sinus pacing, the S-V shortens to 70 msec, bundle of His activation follows the onset of ventricular depolarization by 10 msec, and the QRS complex becomes more aberrant. By pacing at a site near the atrial insertion of the accessory pathway, conduction rapidly reaches the ventricle over the accessory pathway to activate more of the ventricle than when pacing the right atrium at the same cycle length. Shortening the pacing cycle length to 600 msec *(bottom right panel)* lengthens the A-H interval 15 msec, and bundle of His activation begins 25 msec after the onset of the QRS complex. S-V and A-V intervals remain unchanged, and the QRS complex becomes ever more aberrant. *BAE,* Bipolar atrial electrode; *BHE,* bipolar His electrode; *CSd,* coronary sinus. (From Zipes DP: *Specific arrhythmias: diagnosis and treatment.* In Braunwald E, editor: *Heart disease: a textbook of cardiovascular medicine,* ed 3, Philadelphia, 1988, Saunders.)

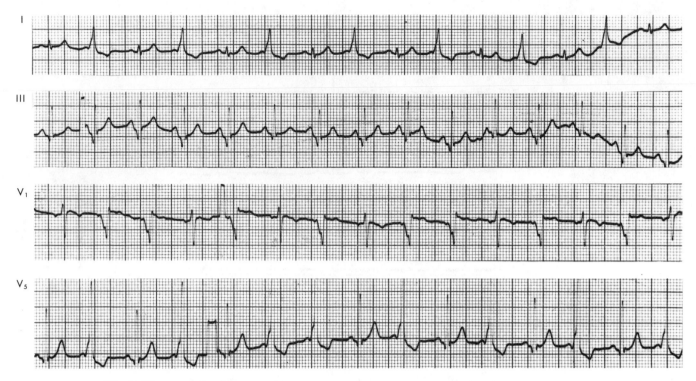

Fig. 5-37 Alternating conduction over the accessory pathway in preexcitation syndrome during normal sinus rhythm. Almost throughout the recording, the QRS complexes alternate between conduction over the accessory pathway and conduction over the normal pathway. Occasionally two consecutive beats conduct over the accessory pathway. Conduction over the accessory pathway is characterized by a short PR interval, δ wave, prolonged QRS duration, and secondary T-wave changes. Such intermittent conduction over an accessory pathway suggests that its refractory period is prolonged and implies that extremely rapid rates during atrial flutter or atrial fibrillation, as seen in Fig. 5-38, would not occur.

Rate	105 beats/min.
Rhythm	Regular.
P waves	Normal.
PR interval	Alternating between 0.08 and 0.12 second.
QRS complex	Normal, 0.06 second during conduction over the AV node; abnormal, 0.12 second during conduction over the accessory pathway.

prolong refractoriness in the accessory pathway—often coupled with drugs that prolong AV nodal refractoriness (for example, quinidine and propranolol) or a drug that affects both pathways (for example, encainide or amiodarone)—must be used. In some patients, particularly those with a very rapid ventricular response during atrial fibrillation, electric cardioversion should be the initial treatment of choice.

For long-term therapy to prevent a recurrence, drugs are selected on the basis of their effects on the AV node or accessory pathway. Invasive electrophysiologic studies are often necessary.

Surgical ablation of the accessory pathway may be required, particularly when symptomatic tachydysrhythmias are recurrent or incompletely controlled by drugs or are associated with rapid ventricular rates. Improved surgical techniques now permit surgery as a logical therapy for a young person who would otherwise face many years of drug management. For symptomatic drug-refractory, recurrent tachycardia, surgery to interrupt the accessory pathway has been extremely useful.[7]

Some patients who have supraventricular tachycardia without overt evidence of preexcitation syndrome may have an accessory pathway that conducts only retrogradely (concealed preexcitation syndrome).[16] The surface ECG during AVRT may provide some clues about the presence of a concealed accessory pathway by demonstrating the retrograde P wave to be in the ST segment (rather than simultaneous with the QRS complex, as in AV nodal reentry) and, if the accessory pathway is left-

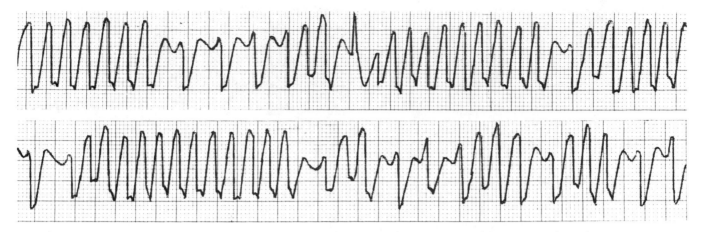

Fig. 5-38   Atrial fibrillation with an extremely rapid ventricular response in a patient who has preexcitation syndrome. In this monitor lead the extremely rapid ventricular rates and gross irregularity of the R-R intervals (ventricular tachycardia can also be irregular; see Fig. 5-57) suggest the diagnosis of atrial fibrillation in a patient who has preexcitation syndrome. The atrial fibrillatory impulses conduct to the ventricle over the accessory pathway, bypassing the AV node.

Rate	Atrial, indeterminate; ventricular, 150 to 350 beats/min.
Rhythm	Irregular.
P waves	Cannot be seen.
PR interval	Cannot be determined.
QRS complex	Difficult to determine but approximately 0.12 to 0.14 second.

DRUG THERAPY IN PREEXCITATION SYNDROME

Affects AV Node

Digitalis
Propranolol
Verapamil
Vagal stimulation

Affects Accessory Pathway

Quinidine
Procainamide
Disopyramide

Affects Both

Flecainide
Encainide
Amiodarone

---

sided, a negative P wave in lead I. Naturally, the short PR interval, δ wave, and prolonged QRS duration during sinus rhythm are not present.

Atrial Flutter

Atrial flutter (Figs. 5-39 to 5-42) is an atrial tachydysrhythmia characterized electrocardiographically by identically recurring, regular, sawtooth-shaped flutter waves and evidence of continual electric activity (lack of an isoelectric interval between flutter waves), often best visualized in Leads II, III, aV_F, or V_1. Commonly the flutter waves appear inverted in these leads; less commonly they are upright (positive). In most instances, reentry in the atria causes atrial flutter. If the AV conduction ratio remains constant, the ventricular rhythm is regular; if the ratio of conducted beats varies (usually the result of a Wenckebach AV block), the ventricular rhythm is irregular. Impure flutter (flutter-fibrillation) occurring at a faster rate than pure flutter shows variability in the contour and spacing of the flutter waves and may represent dissimilar atrial rhythms (that is, fibrillation in one atrium or part of the atrium and a slower, more regular rhythm in the opposite atrium).

The atrial rate during atrial flutter is usually 250 to 350 beats/min; antidysrhythmic drugs such as quinidine or procainamide may reduce the rate to 200 beats/min. In untreated atrial flutter the ventricular rate is usually half the atrial rate (that is, 150 beats/min). A significantly slower ventricular rate (in the absence of drugs) suggests abnormal AV conduction. Atrial flutter in children, in patients who have preexcitation syndrome or hyperthyroidism, and occasionally in otherwise normal adults may conduct to the ventricle in a 1:1 fashion, producing a ventricular rate of 300 beats/min. When the atrial flutter rate has been slowed by drugs, 1:1 conduction to the ventricle may also occur.

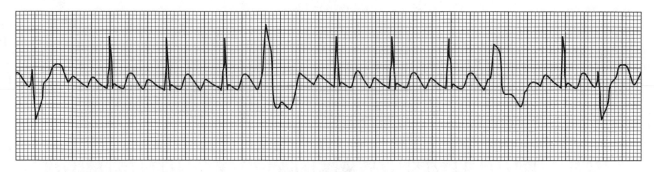

Fig. 5-39 Atrial flutter. The conduction ratio is 3:1 (that is, three flutter waves to one QRS complex) and is a less common conduction ratio than 2:1 or 4:1. Monitor lead.

Rate	Atrial, 300 beats/min; ventricular, 100 beats/min. Multiform premature ventricular contractions.
Rhythm	Atrial, regular; ventricular, regular.
P waves	Flutter waves with regular oscillations resembling a sawtooth pattern are apparent.
PR interval	Flutter-R interval is constant.
QRS complex	0.12 second.

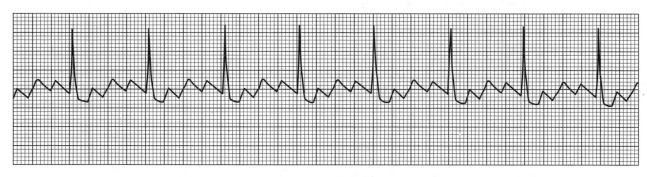

Fig. 5-40 Atrial flutter rate slowed by an antidysrhythmic agent. The atrial flutter in this patient had a rate of 300 beats/min before therapy but was slowed by the antidysrhythmic agent amiodarone. The lead is monitored.

Rate	Atrial, 3000; ventricular, 75.
Rhythm	Atrial, regular; ventricular, regular.
P waves	Flutter waves are apparent.
PR interval	The flutter-R interval varies as the conduction ratio varies.
QRS complex	Normal, 0.08 second.

Significance

Atrial flutter is a less common tachydysrhythmia than atrial fibrillation. Although paroxysmal atrial flutter usually indicates cardiac disease, it may occur in normal hearts. Chronic, or persistent, atrial flutter rarely occurs in the absence of underlying heart disease. Atrial flutter usually responds to carotid sinus massage with a decrease in ventricular rate in stepwise multiples, reversing to the former ventricular rate at the termination of carotid massage. The ratio of conducted atrial impulses to ventricular responses is most often of an even number (for example, 2:1 or 4:1). Sinus rhythm rarely follows carotid sinus massage. By enhancing the sympathetic tone, lessening the parasympathetic tone, or both, exercise may reduce the AV conduction delay and increase the ventricular rate.

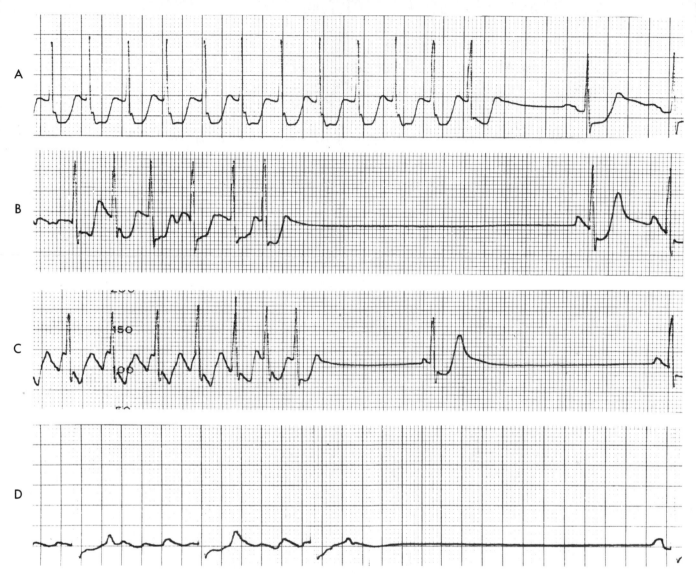

Fig. 5-41   Termination of multiple supraventricular tachycardias. **A,** Paroxysmal supraventricular tachycardia abruptly terminates with only a short pulse before restoration of sinus rhythm. **B** and **C,** Atrial flutter-fibrillation and pure atrial flutter, respectively, terminate on separate occasions in the same patient. In **B,** a fairly long period of asystole results before restoration of the first sinus beat, whereas the lengthy pause is interrupted by an escape beat in **C. D,** Termination of atrial flutter-fibrillation in another patient results in a long period of asystole before the first sinus beat occurs. The long pauses in **B, C,** and **D** are consistent with sick sinus syndrome and episodes of bradycardia-tachycardia. The leads are monitored.

Rate	158 **A;** varying ventricular rate, approximately 150 in **B;** 136 in **C;** 48 in **D.**
Rhythm	Atrial and ventricular rhythm, regular in **A;** atrial and ventricular rhythm, irregular in **B;** atrial rhythm, regular, and ventricular rhythm, irregular, in **C;** atrial rhythm and ventricular rhythm, irregular in **D.**
PR interval	Not measurable.
QRS complex	Normal in all panels.

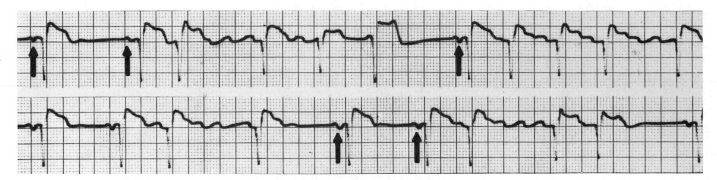

Fig. 5-42 Intermittent atrial flutter. Atrial flutter starts and stops intermittently throughout this continuous recording. The lead is monitored.

Rate and rhythm	Atrial and ventricular rate and rhythm vary.
P waves	Precede same QRS complexes. Atrial flutter waves precede other QRS complexes. Several P waves indicated by arrows.
PR interval	0.14 second when it can be measured.
QRS complex	0.08 second.

Treatment

Treatment for atrial flutter, which is aimed at slowing the ventricular rate, is as follows:

1. Synchronous DC cardioversion is the preferred initial treatment for atrial flutter, since it promptly and effectively restores sinus rhythm with an initial energy of 25 joules. If DC shock results in atrial fibrillation, a second shock of 100 joules may be used to restore sinus rhythm, or depending on the clinical circumstance, the atrial fibrillation may be left untreated. The untreated fibrillation usually reverts to atrial flutter or sinus rhythm.

2. If the patient's heart cannot be cardioverted or the DC cardioversion is contraindicated (for example, after administering large amounts of digitalis), rapid atrial pacing can effectively terminate atrial flutter in many patients.

3. If the patient's heart cannot be cardioverted or if atrial flutter recurs at frequent intervals, therapy with a short-acting digitalis preparation such as digoxin should be prescribed. The dosage of digitalis necessary to slow the ventricular response varies and at times may result in toxic levels because it is often difficult to slow the ventricular rate during atrial flutter. Frequently, atrial fibrillation develops after digitalization, and it may revert to normal sinus rhythm on withdrawal of digitalis; occasionally, normal sinus rhythm may occur without intervening atrial fibrillation.

4. Verapamil (in an initial bolus of 5 mg intravenously with a repeat dose of 10 mg intravenously in 15 to 20 minutes followed by a constant infusion at a rate of 0.005 mg/kg/min) may be used to slow the ven-

tricular response. Peak therapeutic effects occur within 3 to 5 minutes of bolus injection.[13] Verapamil less commonly restores sinus rhythm in patients who have atrial flutter.

5. If the atrial flutter persists after digitalization, quinidine (200 to 400 mg orally every 6 hours) is used to restore sinus rhythm. Large doses of quinidine, formerly used to terminate atrial flutter before the development of DC cardioversion, are no longer warranted. If atrial flutter persists after digitalis and quinidine administration, termination may be attempted with DC cardioversion, and the patient may be maintained on digitalis and quinidine after reversion to sinus rhythm. Sometimes, treatment of the specific, underlying disorder (for example, thyrotoxicosis) is necessary to effect conversion to sinus rhythm.

6. In certain instances, atrial flutter may continue, and if the ventricular rate can be controlled with digitalis, conversion may not be indicated. Quinidine maintenance therapy should be discontinued if flutter remains. Quinidine and procainamide should not be used unless digitalization has occurred. Both drugs have a vagolytic action and also directly slow the atrial rate. These two effects may facilitate AV conduction sufficiently to result in a 1:1 ventricular response to the atrial flutter, unless digitalis has been administered previously.

7. Propranolol effectively diminishes the ventricular response to atrial flutter and may be used with digitalis when the ventricular rate has not decreased after digitalization. Propranolol does not appear to affect the atrial rate during atrial flutter.

8. Uncommonly, atrial flutter may be resistant to cardioversion as well as to the AV blocking effects of digitalis. Rapid atrial pacing on a temporary or permanent basis may be used to convert flutter to fibrillation with a decrease in ventricular rate.

9. Rarely, neostigmine (Prostigmin), 0.25 to 0.5 mg subcutaneously, or edrophonium (Tensilon), 0.25 to 2.0 mg/min in an intravenous solution, may be administered over a few days to control the ventricular rate.

Prevention of recurrent atrial flutter is often difficult to achieve but should be approached as outlined for the prevention of paroxysmal supraventricular tachycardia caused by AV nodal reentry. If recurrences cannot be prevented, therapy is directed toward a controlled ventricular rate when the flutter does recur, with digitalis alone or combined with propranolol or with verapamil given orally.

Atrial Fibrillation

Atrial fibrillation (Figs. 5-43 and 5-44) is characterized by a total disorganization of atrial activity without effective atrial contraction. The ECG reveals small deflections appearing for the most part as irregular baseline undulations of variable amplitude and contour at a rate of 305 to 600 beats/min. The ventricular response is totally irregular, and if the condition is untreated, the rate is usually between 100 and 160 beats/min. Carotid sinus massage slows the ventricular rate, but the ventricular rhythm remains completely irregular. The conversion of atrial flutter to atrial fibrillation is usually accompanied by a slowing of the ven-

tricular rate because more atrial impulses become blocked at the AV node. As a result, it is generally easier to slow the ventricular rate with digitalis during atrial fibrillation than during atrial flutter. When the ventricular rhythm becomes regular in atrial fibrillation, four explanations are possible: conversion to sinus rhythm, conversion to atrial flutter, development of atrial tachycardia, or development of an independent junctional or ventricular rhythm (or tachycardia) controlling the ventricles and giving rise to AV dissociation. In the last two instances, digitalis intoxication must be suspected. After a period of regularization, a ventricular rhythm that becomes irregular again after administration of an excessive amount of digitalis may be caused by an exit block, generally of the Wenckebach type, from the junctional or ventricular focus.

Because irregular ventricular cycle lengths cause changes in ventricular refractoriness (long cycles lengthening refractoriness and short cycles shortening refractoriness), when a short ventricular cycle follows a long ventricular cycle, aberrant ventricular conduction may occur, generally of RBBB configuration. This is called the *Ashman phenomenon* (see Figs. 5-103 and 5-109).

Significance

Like other tachydysrhythmias, atrial fibrillation may be chronic or intermittent; the former is almost always associated with underlying heart disease, whereas the latter may occur in clinically normal patients. Underlying heart disease is more frequent in atrial fibrillation than in atrial flutter. The dysrhythmia is commonly seen in rheumatic mi-

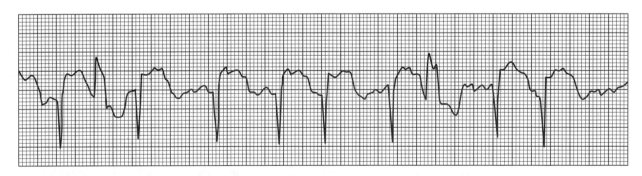

Fig. 5-43 Atrial fibrillation. Atrial activity is present as the undulating wave. Note that the premature ventricular complex follows the longest R-R cycle. This conforms to a phenomenon known as the *rule of bigeminy* (that is, ventricular ectopy during atrial fibrillation more commonly follows the long R-R cycles). The premature ventricular complex would have to be differentiated from aberrant supraventricular conduction. Monitor lead.

Rate	Atrial, cannot be determined accurately; ventricular, average of 90 beats/min.
Rhythm	Atrial and ventricular, irregularly irregular.
P waves	Only the fibrillatory waves of atrial fibrillation can be seen.
PR interval	Not measurable.
QRS complex	0.08 second; premature ventricular contractions, 0.14 second.

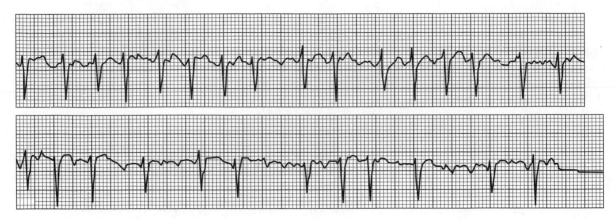

Fig. 5-44   Intermittent, "coarse" atrial flutter-fibrillation. The fibrillatory waves are more coarse than usual, and the flutter waves are irregularly spaced. The ventricular rate is not controlled. The strips are continuous. The lead is monitored.

Rate	Atrial, varying; ventricular, 280.
P waves	Undulating baseline indicates flutter-fibrillation.
PR interval	Not measurable.
QRS complex	0.08 second.

tral stenosis, thyrotoxicosis, cardiomyopathy, hypertensive heart disease, pericarditis, and coronary heart disease.

Approximately 30% of patients who have atrial fibrillation have systemic or pulmonary emboli. Such a catastrophe is most common in rheumatic mitral valvular disease. Of the emboli that occur with mitral stenosis, 90% occur in patients who have atrial fibrillation.

Treatment

It is of paramount importance to search for a precipitating cause of atrial fibrillation in the patient who has it for the first time. Thyrotoxicosis, mitral stenosis, acute myocardial infarction, pericarditis, and other known associated causes should be considered. Atrial fibrillation may also occur after coronary artery bypass graft surgery.

1. Initial therapy is determined by the patient's clinical status. The primary therapeutic objective is to slow the ventricular rate, and the secondary objective is to restore atrial systole. DC cardioversion may accomplish both. If the sudden onset of atrial fibrillation with a rapid ventricular rate results in acute cardiovascular decompensation, DC cardioversion is the preferred treatment, beginning with 100 joules.

2. In the absence of hemodynamic decompensation the patient may be given digitalis to maintain an apical rate of 60 to 80 beats/min at rest and 100 beats/min after slight exercise. The speed, route, dosage, and type are determined by the degree of cardiovascular compensation (see the section on treatment of AV nodal reentry). The ventricular rate cannot be slowed sufficiently by digitalis in some patients, and digitalis toxicity may result before the

ventricular rate is slowed. In such cases, complicating factors such as pulmonary emboli, atelectasis, myocarditis, infection, congestive heart failure, and hyperthyroidism should be excluded and treated if found. If some instances,[11] verapamil may be useful (see section on atrial flutter).

3. Digitalis and propranolol or digitalis and verapamil may be used to slow the ventricular rate when digitalis alone fails. Occasionally, conversion of atrial fibrillation to normal sinus rhythm may result from one of these combinations or from digitalis alone.

4. Often the use of quinidine to maintain a controlled ventricular rate, together with digitalis administration,[1] is necessary to convert atrial fibrillation to sinus rhythm medically. Because of the availability and safety of the electric cardioverter, it is preferable not to administer the large doses of quinidine that were used formerly to produce drug reversion to normal sinus rhythm. Rather, maintenance doses in the range of 1.2 to 2.4 g/day should be administered for a few days before the DC cardioversion. During this time, 10% to 15% of patients establish normal sinus rhythms. If sinus rhythm does not occur, DC cardioversion is carried out. Digitalis may not have to be discontinued before cardioversion if the patient has not received an excessive amount of digitalis. Pretreatment with quinidine establishes an effective tissue concentration, determines whether the drug will be tolerated, improves chances of maintaining normal sinus rhythm after cardioversion, and reduces the number of shocks. Successful establishment of normal sinus rhythm by electric DC cardioversion

occurs in over 90% of patients; with maintenance quinidine therapy, approximately 30% to 50% of patients continue to have normal sinus rhythm for 12 months. In patients who do not tolerate quinidine, disopyramide or procainamide may be tried. Amiodarone is very effective in maintaining sinus rhythm.

Certain patients should not be considered for cardioversion. These are patients who have (1) known sensitivity or intolerance to quinidine or other antidysrhythmic agents (according to some studies,[7] the recurrence rate of atrial fibrillation is higher in the absence of prophylactic quinidine administration),[7] (2) repetitive paroxysmal atrial fibrillation that cannot be prevented by drugs,[7] (3) digitalis intoxication,[7] (4) numerous conversion procedures without clinical improvement or preservation of sinus rhythm,[7] (5) difficult-to-control atrial tachydysrhythmias that finally result in atrial fibrillation with clinical improvement and stability of dysrhythmia,[7] (6) cardiac surgery planned in the near future,[7] (7) a high degree of partial or complete AV block and thus a slow ventricular response, and (8) sick sinus syndrome (see Fig. 5-41).

Many older patients in the last two groups tolerate the atrial fibrillation well because the ventricular rate is slow, and they often do not require treatment with digitalis unless the ventricular rate increases or congestive heart failure develops. These patients may demonstrate serious supraventricular and ventricular dysrhythmias after cardioversion because concomitant sinus node disease is manifested. A related group of patients may have supraventricular tachycardias that alternate with bradycardias; these patients represent a subgroup of the sick sinus syndrome called *bradycardia-tachycardia syndrome*. Usually, these patients are best treated with a ventricular pacemaker to correct the slow rates and digitalis to control the ventricular rates during the supraventricular tachycardia.[17]

In general, all other patients in whom improved circulatory hemodynamics are desirable may be considered candidates for electric cardioversion. Failure to maintain normal sinus rhythm after electric reversion is related to the duration of atrial fibrillation, the functional classification of the patient, and the cause of the underlying heart disease. The likelihood of establishing and maintaining sinus rhythm should be weighed against the risks of cardioversion or other forms of therapy. The presence of multiple factors that adversely affect maintenance of sinus rhythm militates against cardioversion attempts.

Anticoagulation before cardioversion is indicated in patients with a high risk of emboli (that is, those who have mitral stenosis, recent onset of atrial fibrillation, recent or recurrent emboli, or enlarged hearts).[18,19] The incidence of embolization during conversion to normal sinus rhythm is 1% to 3%. Some experts suggest anticoagulation for patients for 2 weeks before elective cardioversion of atrial fibrillation present for more than 1 to 2 weeks, if no contraindications to anticoagulation exist, and continuation of anticoagulation for 2 additional weeks. However, few controlled studies exist to definitively establish that approach.

Atrial Tachycardia With and Without AV Block

The atrial rate is usually between 150 and 200 beats/min, with a range similar to AV nodal reentry, 150 to 250 beats/min. When caused by digitalis excess, the atrial rate is generally less than 200 beats/min and may increase gradually as the digitalis is continued. The PR interval also may gradually lengthen until Wenckebach second-degree AV block develops. On occasion the degree of AV block (Figs. 5-45 and 5-46) may be more advanced. Frequently other manifestations of digitalis excess, such as premature ventricular complexes, coexist. In nearly 50% of cases of atrial tachycardia with block the atrial rate is irreg-

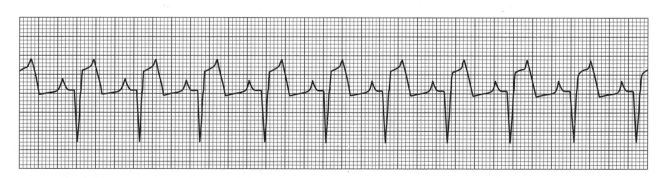

Fig. 5-45   Atrial tachycardia with 2:1 block. Alternate P waves are in the T wave.

Rate	Atrial, 180 beats/min; ventricular, 90 beats/min.
Rhythm	Atrial and ventricular, regular.
P waves	Seen clearly before QRS complex; others hidden in T wave.
PR interval	0.16 second for the conducted beats.
QRS complex	0.08 second.

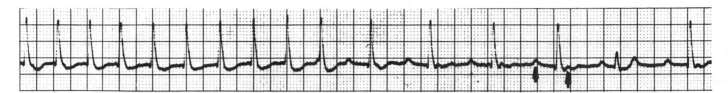

Fig. 5-46   Atrial tachycardia with 1:1 conduction becoming 2:1 conduction during carotid sinus massage. At the left portion of the ECG, P waves can be seen to conduct to each QRS complex. Carotid sinus massage performed at the large arrow precipitates 2:1 conduction. Clear atrial activity can be seen (arrows) as 2:1 conduction occurs. Monitor lead.

Rate	Atrial, 150 beat/min; ventricular, 150 beats/min in left portion and 75 beats/min in right portion.
Rhythm	Atrial, regular; ventricular, regular.
P waves	Can be seen in the ST segment in the left portion of the tracing and are quite clear in the right portion of the tracing.
PR interval	Difficult to measure in the left portion of the tracing, but P waves conduct with a PR interval of 0.25 second in the right portion of the tracing.
QRS complex	0.09 second.

ular, whereas in AV nodal reentry the atrial rate is generally exceedingly regular. Characteristic isoelectric intervals between P waves, in contrast to atrial flutter, are usually present in all leads. However, at rapid atrial rates the distinction between atrial tachycardia with block and atrial flutter may be quite difficult. As in atrial flutter, carotid sinus massage slows the ventricular rate by increasing the degree of AV block but does not terminate the tachycardia.

Significance

Atrial tachycardia with block occurs most commonly in patients who have significant organic heart disease such as coronary artery disease or cor pulmonale. It is associated with digitalis excess in 50% to 75% of such patients. A different type of atrial tachycardia, multifocal atrial tachycardia, is characterized by atrial rates of 100 to 250 beats/min and marked variations in R-wave morphology and the P-P interval; it is associated with a high mortality rate, and it is rarely produced by digitalis. Verapamil may be effective therapy.

Treatment

If the ventricular rate is within a normal range and the condition is asymptomatic, often no therapy at all is necessary.

1. Very slow ventricular rates may respond to atropine (0.5 mg intravenously, repeated as needed to a total dose of 2.0 mg[13]) or, rarely, they may require ventricular pacing.
2. Atrial tachycardia with block in a patient who is not taking digitalis may be treated with digitalis to slow the ventricular rate.
3. If atrial tachycardia with block remains after digitalization, quinidine given orally, disopyramide, or procainamide may be added. Amiodarone is commonly used but has not been approved by the Food and Drug Administration for this purpose.
4. The rhythm may resist termination by pharmacologic means, and if digitalis excess is not the cause, DC cardioversion may be tried.
5. If atrial tachycardia with or without block appears in a patient receiving digitalis, it should be assumed initially that the digitalis is responsible for the dysrhythmia, especially if the patient recently has received diuretics, the serum potassium level is low, the digitalis dose has been increased, quinidine has been added to the therapeutic regimen, or multiple premature ventricular complexes are also present. In such patients, initial therapy includes omission of digitalis and potassium-depleting diuretics (discontinuation of quinidine if it has been started recently) and the administration of potassium chloride, orally (30 to 45 mEq initially, repeated if necessary in 1 hour) or intravenously (0.5 mEq/min in 5% dextrose and water during constant ECG monitoring, for a total of 30 to 60 mEq initially). A gradual slowing of the atrial rate with a decrease in AV block usually occurs if the dysrhythmia is caused by digitalis. In the presence of advanced AV block, potassium as well as other antidysrhythmic agents must be given with great caution and under constant ECG monitoring. Renal dysfunction, acidosis, and excess digitalis predispose to the development of hyperkalemia, and therefore potassium must be administered cautiously;

the ECG and serum potassium and blood urea nitrogen levels are frequently checked.

6. Verapamil (5 mg intravenously) may be given; then verapamil (10 mg intravenously) may be repeated in 15 to 20 minutes if needed.

7. Propranolol (0.5 to 1 mg/min intravenously for a total dose of 0.5 to 3 mg) or phenytoin (50 to 100 mg intravenously every 5 minutes until the tachycardia terminates; the patient develops signs of toxicity such as nystagmus, vertigo, or nausea; or a total dose of 1 g is given) may be quite useful for digitalis-induced dysrhythmias, including atrial tachycardia with block. The latter agent, since it does not appear to slow AV conduction, may be particularly useful.

8. If these agents are not effective, further short-acting digitalis preparations may be given cautiously, assuming that the development of atrial tachycardia with block was not caused by digitalis.

Premature AV Junctional Complexes

Rhythms formerly called *nodal, coronary nodal,* and *coronary sinus complexes* are now termed *AV junctional complexes* (Fig. 5-47). This term, which includes the AV nodal–bundle of His area, is preferred to terms that imply a more exact site of impulse origin because the exact location at which the impulse originates often cannot be determined from the surface ECG. A premature AV junctional complex arises in the AV junction and spreads in an anterograde and retrograde fashion. If unimpeded in its course, the impulse discharges the atrium to produce a premature retrograde P wave and a QRS complex with a supraventricular contour. Retrograde atrial activation generally results in a negative R wave in leads II, III, aV_F, and V_6, with positive P waves in leads I, aV_L, aV_R, and V_1. The retrograde P wave may occur before, be buried in, or less commonly follow the QRS complex. The site at which the impulse originates, as well as the relative speeds of anterograde and retrograde conduction, determines the relationship of the P wave to the QRS complex. A compensatory pause commonly follows a premature AV junctional complex, but if the atrium and sinus node are discharged retrogradely, a noncompensatory pause results.

Significance and treatment

Premature AV junctional complexes usually do not cause symptoms and are rarely of any consequence. If symptoms occur, this dysrhythmia has the same significance and treatment as premature atrial contractions.

AV Junctional Rhythms

An AV junctional escape beat occurs when the rate of impulse formation of the primary pacemaker (usually the sinus node) becomes less than that of the AV junctional pacemaker or when impulses from the primary pacemaker do not penetrate to the region of the escape focus (AV block). The interval from the last normally conducted beat to the escape beat therefore exceeds the normal R-R interval and is a measure of the initial rate of discharge of the AV junctional focus. The inherent discharge rate of the AV junctional escape focus (usually 40 to 60 beats/min) determines when the junctional escape beat occurs. A continued series of AV junctional escape beats is called an *AV junctional rhythm* (Figs. 5-48 to 5-50). An AV junctional escape rhythm is usually fairly regular. Intervals between subsequent escape beats after the initial escape beat may gradually shorten as the rate of discharge of the escape focus increases (rhythm of development). The configuration of the QRS complex may differ from the normal sinus-initiated QRS complex; usually, it maintains the same contour as the normally conducted QRS. The atria may be under retrograde control of the AV junctional pacemaker, or they may discharge independently (see section on AV dissociation).

Significance

An AV junctional escape beat or rhythm may be a normal phenomenon resulting from the effects of vagal tone on higher pacemakers, or it may occur during pathologic slow sinus discharge and heart block. The escape beat or rhythm serves as a safety mechanism that assumes control of the cardiac rhythm because of the default of the primary pacemaker; this prevents the occurrence of complete ventricular asystole.

Treatment

Treatment, if indicated, lies in increasing the discharge rate of higher pacemakers or improving conduction with atropine or isoproterenol. Rarely, pacing may be needed. An AV junctional escape beat should not be suppressed.

Nonparoxysmal AV Junctional Tachycardia

Accepted terminology confers the label of *tachycardia* to rhythms that exceed 100 beats/min. However, since rates greater than 60 to 70 beats/min represent, in effect, a tachycardia for the AV junctional tissue, the term *nonparoxysmal AV junctional tachycardia (NPJT)* (Figs. 5-51 and 5-52), although not entirely correct, has been generally accepted when the rate of junctional discharge exceeds 60 to 70 beats/min.[16] NPJT usually has a more gradual onset and termination than AV nodal reentry, with a ventricular rate commonly between 70 and 130 beats/min. The rate sometimes may be slowed by vagal maneuvers, as in sinus tachycardia, and the rhythm may not always be entirely regular. Although retrograde atrial activation may occur, more commonly the atria are controlled by an independent sinus or atrial focus resulting in AV dissociation.

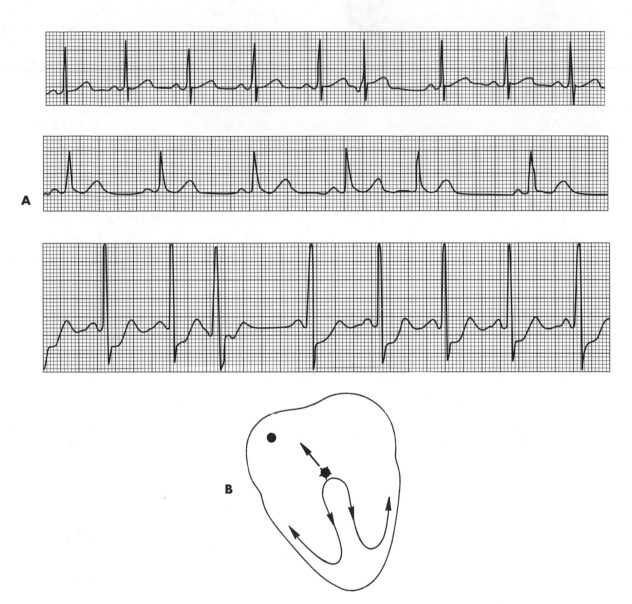

Fig. 5-47   A, Premature AV junctional complexes seen in the top, middle, and bottom tracings were formerly called *upper, middle,* and *lower nodal premature complexes,* respectively, because the retrograde P wave was inscribed before, during, and after the QRS complex. Since not only the site of origin, but also the relative speeds of anterograde and retrograde conduction determine the P-QRS complex relationships during a premature AV junctional complex, it is best to use the nonspecific term *premature AV junctional complex* for all three types. Note that the QRS complex maintains an almost identical contour to the normally conducted beats. Slight QRS aberration occurs in the middle recording. Monitor lead from three different patients. *Arrows,* P waves. **B,** Schematic illustration.

Rate	Determined by basic rate and number of premature complexes.
Rhythm	Irregular because of premature complexes.
P waves	Atria discharged in a retrograde direction, producing negative (inverted) P waves in lead II. P waves occur before *(top tracing),* during *(middle tracing),* and after *(bottom tracing)* the QRS complex, depending on the site of origin of the premature complex and the status of anterograde and retrograde conduction.
QRS complex	Normal.

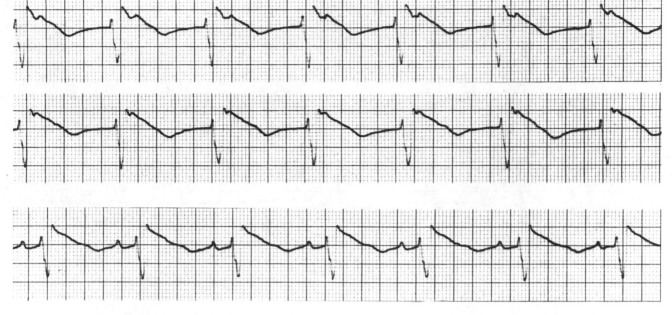

Fig. 5-48 AV junctional rhythm. The top tracings are a continuous recording, whereas the bottom tracing is recorded some time later. In the top two tracings, isorhythmic AV dissociation is present. P waves are in the ST segment and gradually move into the QRS complex. (Compare the QRS-P relationship in the first complex in the top strip with the last complex in the second strip.) In the top strip, sinus slowing initially allowed the escape of the junctional rhythm (not shown). Monitor lead.

Rate	*Top strips,* atrial, 60 beats/min; ventricular, 58 beats/min. *Bottom strip,* atrial and ventricular, 57 beats/min.
Rhythm	Atrial, regular; ventricular, regular.
P waves	Normal.
PR interval	*Top strips,* varying; *bottom strip,* regular (0.22 second).
QRS complex	0.10 second (appears prolonged in this monitor lead but was normal by 12-lead ECG).

Significance

The distinction between NPJT and AV nodal reentry is etiologically and therapeutically quite important. NPJT occurs most commonly in underlying heart disease such as inferior wall infarction and acute rheumatic myocarditis and after open-heart surgery. Probably the most important cause is excessive digitalis, which only rarely produces AV nodal reentry. It is especially important to recognize slowing and regularization of the ventricular rhythm caused by NPJT as an early sign of digitalis intoxication in a patient who has atrial fibrillation.

Treatment

The treatment is as follows:

1. If the ventricular rate is rapid, the cardiovascular status is compromised, and the patient is not taking digitalis, digitalization should be the first measure.
2. Uncommonly in an emergency or if the dysrhythmia does not respond to digitalization and is clearly not induced by digitalis, electric DC cardioversion may be used with initial energies of 75 to 100 joules.
3. However, if the patient tolerates the dysrhythmia well, careful monitoring and attention to the underlying heart disease is usually all that is needed. The dysrhythmia usually abates spontaneously.
4. If digitalis toxicity is the cause, the drug must be immediately stopped. Potassium may be given (see section on treatment of atrial tachycardia with block). The ECG should be monitored, since the blocking effects of potassium administration and digitalis are additive in the AV junctional tissue and advanced AV heart block may result. The rate of potassium administration is important, since a rapid infusion of the potassium, especially in a potassium-depleted patient, may result in transient cardiac arrest or depression of AV conduction.
5. Lidocaine, propranolol, phenytoin, or verapamil also may be tried.

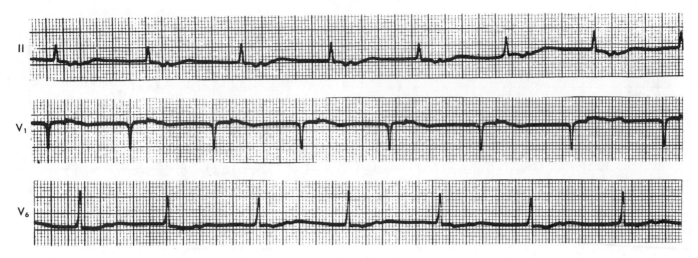

Fig. 5-49 AV junctional rhythm. The patient has an AV junctional rhythm with 1:1 retrograde capture. Thus AV dissociation is not present.

Rate   Atrial and ventricular, 55 beats/min.
Rhythm   Regular.
P waves   Retrograde.
RP interval   0.18 second.
QRS complex   0.06 second.

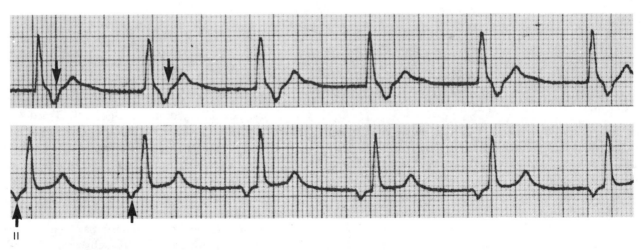

Fig. 5-50 AV junctional rhythm with a changing P-QRS relationship. In the top tracing, retrograde atrial activity follows the QRS complex; in the bottom tracing, retrograde atrial activity *(arrows)* precedes the QRS complex. Thus with the same AV junctional rhythm in the same patient, atrial activity first followed and then preceded the QRS complex.

Rate   Atrial, 65 beats/min; ventricular, 65 beats/min.
Rhythm   Regular.
P waves   Inverted; follow QRS complex in top tracing; precede QRS complex in
              bottom tracing.
PR interval   0.12 second, *bottom*.
RP interval   0.12 second, *top*.
QRS complex   Generally normal, 0.08 second.

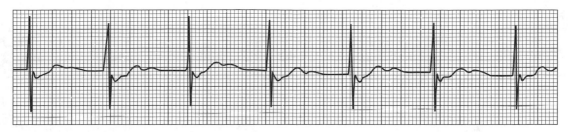

Fig. 5-51 NPJT. This may also be called *accelerated junctional rhythm* because its rate is faster than the inherent rate of junction tissue (40 to 60 beats/min), and yet it is much slower than paroxysmal junctional tachycardia (140 to 220 beats/min).

Rate   About 70 beats/min.
Rhythm   Regular captures.
P waves   Inverted and after the QRS complex.
PR interval   Not able to measure.
QRS complex   0.06 second.

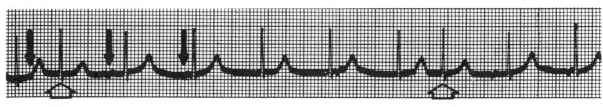

Lead I

Fig. 5-52 NPJT. Atrial activity *(black arrows)* can be seen as small, inverted P waves that occur regularly throughout the QRS complex and that are uninfluenced by ventricular activity. The ventricular rhythm is regular except for intermittent atrial captures indicated by the unfilled large arrowheads.

Rate   Atrial, 72 beats/min; ventricular, 79 beats/min
Rhythm   Atrial, regular; ventricular, irregular because of intermittent atrial captures.
P waves   Abnormal.
PR intervals   Prolonged during ventricular captures.
QRS complex   0.06 second.

Ventricular Escape Beats

A ventricular escape beat (Fig. 5-53) results when the rate of impulse formation of supraventricular pacemakers (sinus node and AV junctional) becomes less than that of potential ventricular pacemakers or when supraventricular impulses do not penetrate to the region of the escape focus because of SA or AV block. The inherent rate of discharge of ventricular escape pacemakers is usually 20 to 40 impulses/min. A continued series of ventricular escape beats is called a *ventricular escape rhythm*. The ventricular rhythm is usually fairly regular, although the rhythm may accelerate for a few complexes shortly after its onset (rhythm of de-velopment). The duration of the QRS complexes is prolonged to greater than 0.12 second because the origin of ventricular discharge is located in the ventricles. Sometimes, the escape focus may shift from one to another portion of ventricle and may generate QRS complexes with different contours and rates.

Significance

The presence of ventricular escape beats indicates significant slowing of supraventricular pacemakers or a fairly high degree of SA or AV block and would therefore generally be considered abnormal.

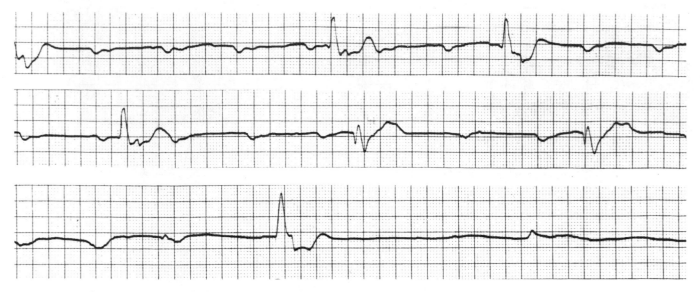

Fig. 5-53 Ventricular escape beats occurring in a dying patient. Ventricular escape beats occur with changing contour and at irregular intervals. AV block is also present, since the P waves do not appear to conduct to the ventricles. The changing QRS contour may be caused by shifting pacemakers or changing activation sequence.

Rate	Varying.
Rhythm	Atrial and ventricular, varying.
P waves	Can be seen in the top strip and then more intermittently in the second and third strips.
PR interval	Varying.
QRS complex	Varying but approximately 0.16 second.

Treatment

Depending on the cause, atropine, isoproterenol, or pacing generally represent the therapeutic approach.

Premature Ventricular Complexes

A premature ventricular complex (Figs. 5-54 to 5-56) is characterized by the premature occurrence of a QRS complex that is initiated in the ventricle and that has a contour different from the normal supraventricular complex and a duration usually greater than 0.12 second. The T wave is generally large and opposite in direction to the major deflection of the QRS complex. The QRS complex generally is not preceded by a premature P wave but may be preceded by a sinus P wave occurring at its expected time. However, these criteria may be met by a supraventricular complex or rhythm that conducts aberrantly through the ventricle; in fact, aberrant supraventricular conduction may mimic all the manifestations of ventricular dysrhythmia except ventricular fibrillation.

Retrograde transmission to the atria from premature ventricular complex occurs more frequently than has often been affirmed but still probably does not occur commonly. The retrograde P wave produced in this fashion is often obscured by the distorted QRS complex. Usually a fully compensatory pause follows a premature ventricular complex. If the retrograde impulse discharges the sinus node prematurely and resets the basic timing, it may produce a pause that is not fully compensatory. A compensatory pause results when the premature complex does not alter the discharge rate or rhythm of the sinus node so that a P wave occurs at its normal time. The P wave does not reach the ventricle, since the AV node is refractory because of (concealed) retrograde penetration into the AV node by the premature junctional or ventricular complex. Therefore the R-R interval produced by the two QRS complexes on either side of the premature complex equals twice the normally conducted R-R interval. A compensatory pause occurs more commonly with ventricular and AV junctional premature complex, but the presence of a compensatory pause is not invariably diagnostic of the site of origin of the premature complex.

The normal sinus P wave after a premature ventricular complex may conduct to the ventricles with a long PR interval, in which case a pause does not follow the premature ventricular complex; in this case the premature complex is said to be *interpolated*. A ventricular fusion beat (the simultaneous activation of one chamber by two foci) represents a blend of the characteristics of the normally con-

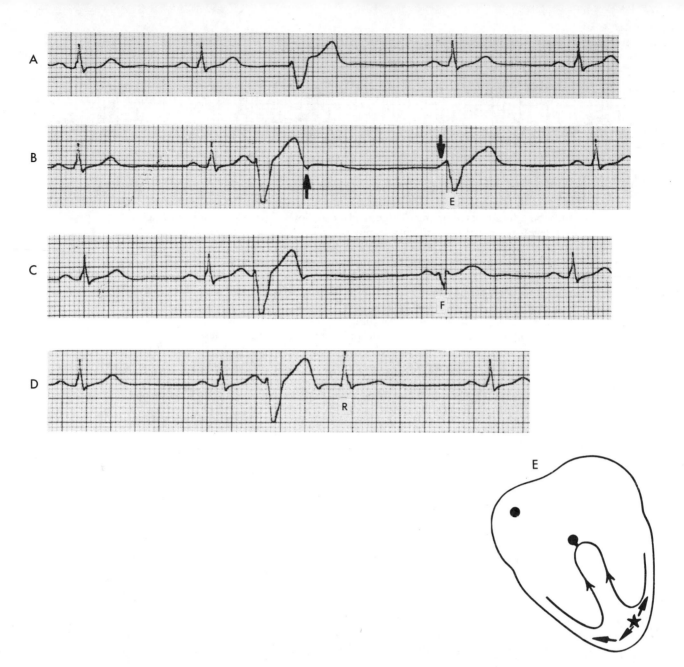

Fig. 5-54 Premature ventricular complexes. All four tracings were recorded from the same patient. **A,** A relatively late premature ventricular complex is followed by a full compensatory pause. Sinus slowing makes the pause after the ventricular complex slightly greater than compensatory, but its characteristics are essentially the same; that is, the interval between the two normal QRS complexes flanking the premature ventricle complex is twice the basic R-R interval. **B,** An earlier premature ventricular complex in the same patient retrogradely discharges the atrial impulse *(ascending arrow)*. This resets the sinus node, and a ventricular escape beat *(E)* occurs before the next P wave *(descending arrow)* can conduct to the ventricles. **C,** The sequence is the same as in **B,** except that the atrial rate is faster. This permits the P wave after the premature ventricular complex and retrograde P wave to partially depolarize the ventricles at the same time the ventricular escape beat occurs, resulting in a fusion beat *(F)*. **D,** The sequence is the same as in **C,** except that after the impulse from the ventricle retrogradely discharges the atria, it returns to the ventricles to produce a ventricular echo, or reciprocal beat *(R)*. **E,** Schematic illustration.

Rate	Determined by basic rate and number of ventricular complexes.
Rhythm	Irregular because of premature complexes.
P waves	Generally normal; may be captured retrogradely; often lost in QRS complex or T wave of premature ventricular complex.
PR interval	Determined by whether P wave is blocked, conducted with a prolonged PR interval, or retrogradely activated.
QRS complex	0.14 second.

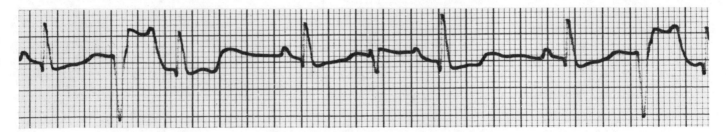

Fig. 5-55 Interpolated premature ventricular complexes. The second, fifth, and eighth QRS complexes are premature ventricular complexes. The sinus P wave that follows these complexes conducts to the ventricle with a long PR interval. Thus the normally expected compensatory pause is not present. The premature ventricular complex does not replace a normally conducted complex (see Fig. 5-54, *A*) but occurs in addition to the normally conducted complex. The PR interval after the premature ventricular complex is prolonged because of incomplete recovery of the AV node because of partial retrograde penetration by the interpolated premature ventricular complex. Monitor lead.

Rate and rhythm	Varying because of the premature ventricular complexes.
P waves	Normal.
PR interval	0.16 second for the normally conducted beats; 0.20 to 0.25 second after the interpolated premature ventricular complexes.
QRS complex	0.09 second for normal beats; 0.12 second for premature ventricular complexes.

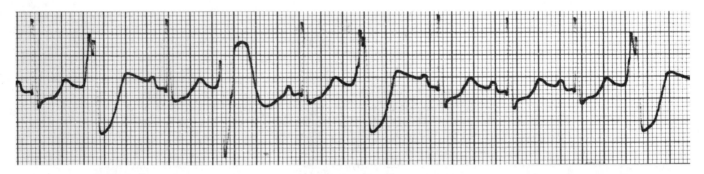

Fig. 5-56 Multiform premature ventricular complexes. Each sinus beat is followed by premature ventricular complexes that have two contours, one predominantly positive and the other predominantly negative. These premature ventricular complexes of different contours are more properly called *multiform* rather than *multifocal*, since it cannot be certain whether more than one focus is active or whether different activation sequences are emerging from the same focus. Monitor lead.

Rate	100 beats/min but varying.
Rhythm	Varying because of premature ventricular complexes.
P waves	Normal preceding the normally conducted beats.
PR interval	0.14 second preceding the normally conducted beats.
QRS complex	0.09 second for the normally conducted beats, 0.16 second for the premature ventricular complexes.

ducted beat and the beat originating in the ventricles, indicating that the ventricle has been depolarized from both atrial and ventricular directions. Atrial fusion beats may occur during ectopic atrial discharge and represent a blend of the characteristics of the sinus-initiated and ectopic atrial P waves. Whether a compensatory or noncompensatory pause, a retrograde atrial excitation, an interpolated complex, a fusion complex, or an echo beat (see Fig. 5-54) occurs is merely a function of how well the AV junction conducts and the timing of the events taking place.

The term *bigeminy* refers to pairs of beats or two complexes and may be used to indicate couplets of normal and ectopic ventricular complex. Premature ventricular complexes may have differing contours and often are called *multifocal*. More properly, they should be called *multiform*, since it is not known from a surface ECG recording that there are multiple foci discharging.

Significance

The frequency of premature ventricular complexes increases with age. The presence of premature complexes may be manifested by palpitations or discomfort in the chest or neck; this is caused by the greater than normal contractile force of the postectopic beats or the feeling that the heart has stopped during the long pause after the premature complexes. Long runs of premature complexes in patients who have heart disease may produce angina or hypotension. Frequent interpolated premature complexes represent a doubling of the heart rate and may compromise hemodynamic status. In the absence of underlying heart disease, premature complexes may have no significance and may not require suppression. Premature ventricular complexes and complex ventricular dysrhythmias occurring in healthy patients with no symptoms portend no increased risk of death, and their long-term prognosis is similar to that of the healthy U.S. population. Ventricular ectopy recorded after myocardial infarction represents an independent risk factor for subsequent death. However, it has not been demonstrated that the premature ventricular complexes or complex ventricular dysrhythmias play a precipitating role in the genesis of sudden death; they may be simply a marker of heart disease. Nor has it been shown unequivocally that antidysrhythmic therapy given to suppress the premature ventricular complexes or complex ventricular dysrhythmias reduces the incidence of sudden death in these patients.

Most of the drugs used to suppress premature complexes may also produce them on certain occasions. This is especially true of the digitalis preparations. On the other hand, digitalis may be effective in controlling premature atrial and ventricular complexes, especially those related to the presence of congestive heart failure. In patients suffering from acute myocardial infarction, it has been commonly held that so-called warning dysrhythmias (premature ventricular complexes occurring close to the preceding T wave; greater than five or six per minute; bigeminal, multiform, or occurring in salvos of two, three, or more) may presage or precipitate ventricular tachycardia or fibrillation. However, it has been demonstrated that about half of the patients who develop ventricular fibrillation have no warning dysrhythmias, and half of those who do have warning dysrhythmias do not develop ventricular fibrillation.

Treatment

In the hospitalized patient with or without acute myocardial infarction, lidocaine given intravenously is the initial drug of choice when suppression of premature ventricular complexes is deemed necessary.

Immediate suppression[13]

1. Lidocaine (1 mg/kg) is given as an intravenous bolus. If ectopy is not suppressed, lidocaine (0.5 mg/kg every 2 to 5 minutes) is given until there is no ectopy or until 3 mg/kg is given. Lidocaine produces less hypotension and negative inotropic effects than procainamide or quinidine in doses having equivalent antidysrhythmic effects. It is ideal for use in patients who have renal disease, since less than 10% is excreted unaltered in the kidney and the rest is metabolized by the liver. In patients exhibiting allergic reactions to quinidine or procainamide, lidocaine is useful, since there appears to be no cross-sensitivity.
2. If maximum doses of lidocaine are unsuccessful, procainamide is administered intravenously (20 mg/min) until there is no ectopy or up to 1 g is given. Toxic effects include hypotension and QRS widening. If this is successful, procainamide may then be given as a continuous intravenous infusion of 1 to 4 mg/min.[13]
3. If ectopy is still unsuppressed and if it is not contraindicated, bretylium given intravenously (5 to 10 mg/kg over 8 to 10 minutes) may be tried.[13]
4. If ectopy is still unsuppressed, overdrive pacing may be considered.

Maintenance[13]

Once ectopy is suppressed, it is maintained as follows:
1. If the lidocaine bolus is successful, start a lidocaine drip:

Bolus dose	Drip rate
1 mg/kg	2 mg/min
2 mg/kg	3 mg/min
3 mg/kg	4 mg/min

2. After a procainamide bolus is used, a procainamide drip at 1 to 4 mg/min is started. The blood level is checked.
3. After the bretylium bolus, a bretylium drip at 2 mg/min is started.

Long-term suppression

1. Oral maintenance therapy can be achieved with procainamide (375 to 500 mg every 3 to 4 hours) to produce therapeutic blood levels of 4 to 8 mg/L or with quinidine sulfate (200 to 400 mg every 6 hours) to produce serum levels of 3 to 6 mg/L. A long-acting procainamide preparation can be given at a dose of 750 to 1000 mg every 6 hours.
2. Disopyramide (Norpace), 100 to 250 mg every 6 hours, may be useful at serum concentrations of 2 to 5 µg/ml.
3. Tocainide (Tonocard), 400 to 600 mg every 8 to 12 hours achieving serum concentrations of 4 to 10 µg/ml, may be effective, particularly if lidocaine has successfully suppressed the dysrhythmia.
4. Flecainide (Tambocor) is given in doses of 100 to 200 mg every 12 hours to produce serum concentrations in the range of 0.6 µg/ml and may be useful.
5. Amiodarone (Cordarone) is generally given in a loading dose of 800 to 1600 mg/day for 1 to 2 weeks and then at maintenance doses of 400 to 800 mg/day (or less); the dose is titrated to the lowest effective amount. Therapeutic serum concentrations range between 1 and 3.5 µg/ml.
6. Mexiletine (Mexitil) may be tried in doses of 250 to 400 mg every 8 hours to achieve plasma concentrations of 1 to 2 µg/ml.
7. Propranolol or phenytoin may be tried if the above drugs fail (see section on treatment of ventricular tachycardia).

Ventricular Tachycardia

Ventricular tachycardia (Figs. 5-57 to 5-59) is usually an ominous finding indicating the presence of significant underlying cardiac disease. In many instances the responsible electrophysiologic mechanism is probably reentry.[1] Although ventricular tachycardia occurs most commonly in acute myocardial infarction and coronary artery disease, this dysrhythmia also occurs in a variety of other cardiac diseases, including cardiomyopathy, mitral valve prolapse, prolonged QT syndrome, and other problems. It has been reported in patients who have no evidence of structural heart disease.

The ECG diagnosis of ventricular tachycardia is suggested when a series of three or more bizarre, premature ventricular complexes occur that have a duration exceeding 0.12 second, with the ST-T vector pointing opposite to the major QRS deflection. The ventricular rate is between 110 and 250 beats/min, and the R-R interval may be exceedingly regular, or it may vary. Atrial activity may be independent of ventricular activity (AV dissociation), or the atria may be depolarized by the ventricles in a retrograde fashion (in which case AV dissociation is not present). Ventricular tachycardia may be sustained (defined in the electrophysiology laboratory as lasting longer than 30 seconds or requiring termination because of hemodynamic deterioration) or nonsustained (lasting less than 30 seconds), and the patient's prognosis as well as the electrophysiologic mechanism may differ for the two forms. One type of nonsustained ventricular tachycardia is characterized by repetitive bursts of premature ventricular complexes separated by a series of sinus beats. Another type of ventricular tachycardia that may be sustained or nonsustained is called *torsades de pointes* and is characterized by a QRS contour that gradually changes its polarity from negative to positive or vice versa over a series of beats. It often occurs in QR prolongation.[8]

The distinction between supraventricular and ventricular tachycardia may be difficult at times because the features of both dysrhythmias frequently overlap, and under

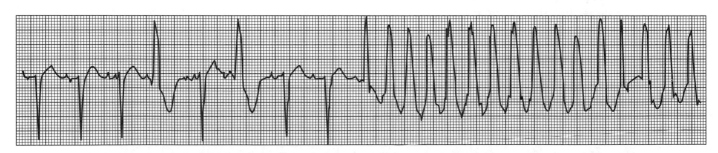

Fig. 5-57 Ventricular tachycardia. Ventricular tachycardia preceded by sinus rhythm and premature ventricular complexes. The strips are continuous.

Rate	Atrial, cannot be determined; ventricular, varying.
Rhythm	Atrial, cannot be determined; ventricular, irregular.
P waves	Can be seen occasionally.
PR interval	0.20 second for normally conducted beats.
QRS complex	0.08 second for normally conducted beats, 0.12 second for ventricular tachycardia.

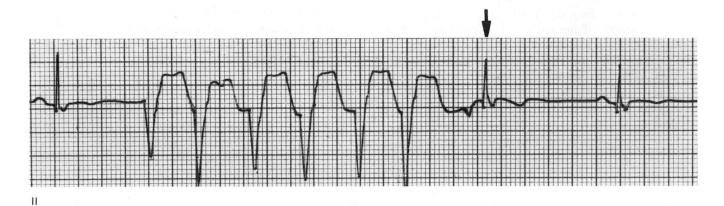

II

Fig. 5-58   Ventricular tachycardia ending with a ventricular echo. Six beats of ventricular tachycardia occur after the first sinus beat. The last ventricular tachycardia beat conducts retrogradely to the atrium (note the small, negative P wave in lead II), which then returns to reexcite the ventricle (*Arrow,* Ventricular echo).

Rate	Atrial, 55 to 75 beats/min; ventricular approximately 150 beats/min.
Rhythm	Atrial, cannot be determined during ventricular tachycardia; regular during sinus rhythm. Ventricular, slightly irregular during ventricular tachycardia.
P waves	Normal during sinus-conducted beats; retrograde P wave after the last ventricular tachycardia beat.
PR interval	0.16 second during sinus rhythm. RP interval after the last ventricular tachycardia beat, 0.52 second.
QRS complex	0.08 second during sinus rhythm and 0.10 second during ventricular tachycardia.

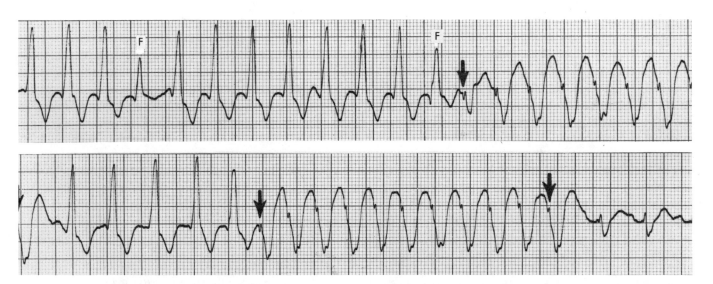

Fig. 5-59   Termination of ventricular tachycardia by rapid ventricular pacing. Intermittent fusion beats *(F)* in the top strip support the diagnosis of ventricular tachycardia. Between the first and second arrows, competitive ventricular pacing is performed at a rate of 166 beats/min, but the ventricular tachycardia continues. Between the third and fourth arrows, competitive ventricular pacing is performed at a rate of 176 beats/min, and after cessation of pacing, sinus rhythm occurs. Monitor lead.

Rate	Atrial, cannot be determined; ventricular, 136 beats/min.
Rhythm	Atrial, cannot be determined; ventricular, fairly regular.
P waves	Cannot be seen.
PR interval	Cannot be determined.
QRS complex	0.13 second.

certain circumstances a supraventricular tachycardia can mimic the criteria established for ventricular tachycardia. Ventricular complexes with abnormal configurations indicate only that conduction through the ventricle is not normal; they do not necessarily indicate the origin of impulse formation or the reason for the abnormal conduction (see section on supraventricular dysrhythmia with abnormal QRS complex).

The presence of fusion and capture beats provides evidence in favor of ventricular tachycardia. Fusion beats indicate simultaneous activation of the ventricles by two separate impulses (suggesting that one of the impulses arose in the ventricles), whereas capture beats signal supraventricular control of the ventricles, generally at a rate faster than the ventricular tachycardia. This proves that normal ventricular conduction can occur at cycle lengths equal to or shorter than the tachycardia in question, again implying that the origin of the wide QRS complexes lies in the ventricles rather than in aberrant supraventricular conduction.

Significance

Symptoms occurring during ventricular tachycardia depend on the ventricular rate, the duration of the tachydysrhythmia, and the severity of the underlying heart disease. The location of impulse formation and therefore the wave in which the depolarization wave spreads across the myocardium may also be important because it influences the ventricle's contraction. The immediate significance of ventricular tachycardia to the patient relates to the hemodynamic dysfunction it produces and the possible development of ventricular fibrillation.

A premature ventricular or, rarely, an atrial complex can initiate ventricular tachycardia or ventricular fibrillation when the premature complex occurs during the vulnerable period of the antecedent T wave. The vulnerable period represents an interval of 20 to 40 msec located near the apex of the T wave during which the heart, when stimulated, is prone to develop ventricular tachycardia or fibrillation (see section on ventricular fibrillation). The stimulus may be from an intrinsic source such as a spontaneous premature complex or from an extrinsic source such as a pacemaker or DC shock. During the interval of the vulnerable period, maximum electric nonuniformity in the ventricular muscle is present; that is, ventricular muscle fibers are at varying stages of recovery of excitability. Some fibers may have completely repolarized, others may have only partially repolarized, and still others may be completely refractory. Therefore stimulation during this period establishes nonuniform conduction with some areas of slowed conduction or actual block and sets the stage for repetitive ventricular discharge possibly caused by reentrant excitation. Equally important, however, is that ventricular tachycardia or fibrillation may begin without preexisting or precipitating premature ventricular complexes or may be ushered in

by a late premature ventricular complex. In fact, the majority of recorded episodes of ventricular tachycardia begin with a late premature ventricular complex that occurs after the vulnerable period has ended.

Treatment

The treatment for ventricular tachycardia is as follows[21]:

1. Striking the patient's chest, sometimes called *thump-version,* may terminate ventricular tachycardia by mechanically inducing a premature ventricular complex that presumably interrupts the reentrant pathway necessary to support the ventricular tachycardia. It is a simple treatment to try initially. Stimulation at the time of the vulnerable period during ventricular tachycardia may provoke ventricular fibrillation.

2. Acute termination of ventricular tachycardia that does not cause any hemodynamic decompensation may be achieved medically by administering lidocaine intravenously in an initial bolus of 1.5 mg/kg of body weight. Lidocaine may be given in doses of 0.5 mg/kg every 8 minutes until ventricular tachycardia resolves, up to 3 mg/kg.[13] The dosage should be reduced in patients who have liver disease, heart failure, or shock. If lidocaine abolishes the ventricular tachycardia, a continuous intravenous infusion of 1 to 4 mg/min can be given. Other infusion schedules also are effective.[7]

3. If maximum doses of lidocaine are unsuccessful, procainamide administered intravenously (20 mg/min until termination of the tachycardia occurs, toxic effects such as QRS widening or significant hypotension result, or up to 1000 mg is administered) may be tried. If successful, procainamide may then be given as a continuous intravenous infusion (1 to 4 mg/min, titrated to the patient's response).[13]

4. When first-line antidysrhythmic agents such as lidocaine or procainamide have failed, bretylium is given intravenously (5 mg/kg) over several minutes and may be increased to 10 mg/kg 15 to 30 minutes later. Doses may be repeated at 15- to 30-minute intervals, not to exceed a total of 40 mg/kg. A continuous infusion at 1 to 2 mg/min can be initiated.

5. If the dysrhythmia does not respond to medical therapy, electric DC cardioversion may be used. Ventricular tachycardia that precipitates hypotension, shock, angina, or congestive heart failure should be treated promptly with DC cardioversion. Cardioversion is started with 50 joules. If it is unsuccessful, the joules are increased progressively to 100, 200, and 360. If the dysrhythmia is recurrent, lidocaine is given, and cardioversion is performed again, starting at the energy level previously successful. Then procainamide or bretylium intravenous infusions are given.[13] Digitalis-induced ventricular tachycardia is best treated

medically. After reversion of the dysrhythmia to a normal rhythm, it is essential to institute measures to prevent a recurrence.

6. In patients who have recurrent ventricular tachycardia, a pacing catheter can be inserted into the right ventricle, and single, double, or multiple stimuli can be introduced competitively to terminate the ventricular tachycardia (Fig. 5-59). This procedure incurs the risk of accelerating the ventricular tachycardia to ventricular flutter or ventricular fibrillation. A catheter electrode is available through which synchronized cardioversion can be performed. In the awake, conscious patient, shocks of 0.25 joules that successfully terminate ventricular tachycardia can be delivered through this catheter electrode.[20]

7. A search for reversible conditions contributing to the initiation and maintenance of ventricular tachydysrhythmias should be made and the conditions corrected if possible. For example, ventricular dysrhythmia related to hypotension or hypokalemia may at times be terminated by vasopressors or potassium, respectively. Slow ventricular rates that are caused by sinus bradycardia or AV block may permit the occurrence of premature ventricular complexes and ventricular tachydysrhythmias that can be corrected by administration of atropine (0.5 to 1.0 mg intravenously), temporary administration of isoproterenol (1 to 2 μg/min in an intravenous drip), or temporary transvenous pacing.

8. Intermittent ventricular tachycardia interrupted by one or more supraventricular beats generally is best treated medically. Lidocaine or procainamide should be tried. If they prove unsuccessful, other class I agents (quinidine, mexilitine, and flecainide) may be tried.

Prevention of recurrences may be difficult at times:

1. Initial preventive drug therapy for recurrent ventricular dysrhythmias in the ambulatory patient should be with quinidine, procainamide, disopyramide, flecainide, or tocainide. Amiodarone is reserved for patients in whom these other drugs fail to work or for those who cannot tolerate them. Procainamide is given as a loading dose of 0.5 to 1 g orally followed by 375 to 500 mg 3 to 6 times daily. Because procainamide has a shorter duration of action than quinidine, the long-acting preparation must be used when giving procainamide at 6-hour intervals to provide therapeutic blood levels (4 to 8 mg/L) for the entire 6-hour period. Hard-to-control dysrhythmias may reflect poor absorption of the drug or nontherapeutic blood levels between two widely spaced doses.

2. Alternatively, quinidine may be used (200 to 400 mg 4 times daily) to achieve therapeutic blood levels of 3 to 6 mg/L.

3. If quinidine is unsuccessful, disopyramide (100 to 250 mg every 6 hours), flecainide (50 to 300 mg every 12 hours), or tocainide (400 to 600 mg every 8 to 12 hours) may be tried. After a loading dose of 800 to 1600 mg/day for 1 to 2 weeks, amiodarone is given at a maintenance dose of 400 to 800 mg/day, working down to the lowest effective dose daily.

4. After an initial approach with these drugs, phenytoin or propranolol may be tried; these drugs are often not very effective in preventing recurrences of ventricular tachydysrhythmias.

5. Combinations of drugs with different mechanisms of action may be successful and allow the clinician to use low doses of both agents rather than high or toxic doses of one drug. For example, propranolol (40 mg daily) combined with average doses of quinidine or procainamide may be efficacious. Similarly, procainamide or quinidine might be effectively combined with amiodarone.

6. Administration of potassium to maintain serum potassium levels of 5 mEq/L or more, in addition to antidysrhythmic agents, may be helpful on occasion.

7. Ventricular or atrial pacing, combined with antidysrhythmic agents if necessary, may be tried empirically; if it is successful, permanent pacing may be instituted. Generally, unless initiation of the ventricular tachycardia is related to significant bradycardia, such as ventricular rates of 30 to 40 beats/min caused by complete AV block, attempts at rapid "overdrive" pacing are often ineffective in the long term.

8. Surgery may be used in selected patients to treat ventricular tachycardia. Multiple surgical techniques are available and include a single ventriculotomy in some patients, cryosurgery, and encircling endocardial ventriculotomy to isolate the dysrhythmogenic area or endocardial resection to remove the dysrhythmogenic area (preferably directed by electrophysiologic mapping techniques) in patients who have ventricular tachycardia related to coronary artery disease (Fig. 5-60). If the surgery alone fails to eliminate recurrences of the dysrhythmias, it may make previously ineffective drug regimens efficacious. Coronary bypass surgery alone, without electrophysiologic mapping and myocardial resection, in patients who do not have ventricular tachycardia definitely associated with ischemia (for example, ventricular tachycardia induced by stress testing) has not been very successful.

9. A number of new antidysrhythmic agents offer promise to control recurrent, life-threatening ventricular tachydysrhythmias.[22]

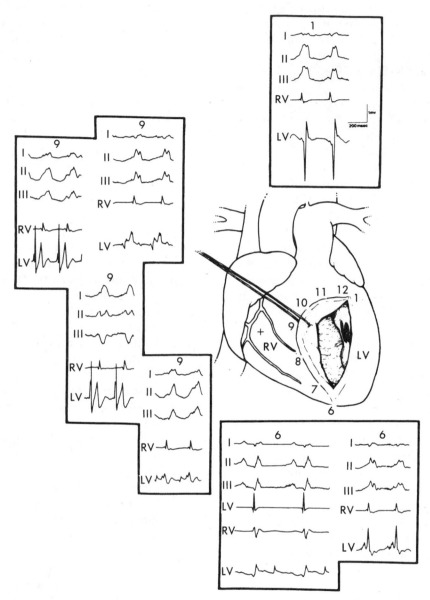

Fig. 5-60 Partial activation map during ventricular tachycardia; tracings have been redrawn for clarity. Left ventricular aneurysm is opened and numbered in a clockwise fashion. Left ventricular endocardial recordings *(LV)* from a handheld exploring electrode are shown in the inserts for sites *1, 6,* and *9.* A stationary right ventricular epicardial electrode *(RV)* was sewn in place (+ on right ventricle). Ventricular tachycardia with four different contours (see surface leads, insert *9*) was initiated. Left ventricular endocardial recordings at site *9* showed earliest activation during each ventricular tachycardia. Left ventricular recordings at site *6* (right portion of insert *6*) show activation starting later than the left ventricular recordings at site *9* but before the left ventricular recording at site *1*, which is relatively normal and late in the QRS complex. However, during sinus rhythm (left portion of insert *6*), recording at site *6* shows a split, late potential. Endocardial resection was carried out between sites *6* and *9*, with elimination of ventricular tachycardia.   (From Braunwald E, editor: *Heart disease: a textbook of cardiovascular medicine,* ed 3, Philadelphia, 1988, Saunders.)

10. Implantable electric devices that competitively pace, synchronously cardiovert, or defibrillate may be very effective in some patients.

Evaluation of therapy

Evaluating the adequacy of drug therapy in patients who have widely spaced episodes of ventricular tachycardia is difficult because there is no adequate end point to judge therapy until the patient has another spontaneous recurrence. Because of this, many groups have taken a more aggressive approach. The patient undergoes a control electrophysiologic study, during which the ventricular tachycardia is initiated and a variety of electrophysiologic and hemodynamic parameters are assessed. Then the patient is treated with a drug, and the electrophysiologic study is repeated. If the drug prevents reinduction of the ventricular tachycardia, there is a high likelihood that the drug will also prevent spontaneous recurrences. If the drug fails to prevent reinitiation of the tachycardia, in many instances the drug may still be successful clinically by slowing the rate of the ventricular tachycardia, converting a sustained form to a nonsustained episode, or preventing a recurrence.[23]

Torsades de Pointes

The term *torsades de pointes* refers to a ventricular tachycardia characterized by QRS complexes of changing amplitude and morphology that appear to twist around the isoelectric line and occur at rates of 200 to 250 beats/min (Fig. 5-61). The peaks of the QRS complexes appear successively on one side of the isoelectric baseline and then the other, giving the typical twisting appearance with continuous and progressive changes in QRS contour and amplitude. Torsades de pointes connotes a syndrome charac-

terized by prolonged ventricular repolarization with corrected QT intervals generally exceeding 500 msec. The U wave also may be prominent, but its role in this syndrome and in the long QT syndrome is not clear. Patients experience recurrent episodes of ventricular tachycardia often precipitated by a late premature complex. Tachycardia may terminate with progressive prolongation of cycle lengths and larger, more distinctly formed QRS complexes.

Rarely, ventricular fibrillation supervenes. Of interest is the fact that changes in cycle length that occur immediately before the onset of torsades de pointes often show a long T–short R-R cycle sequence. A pause in the supraventricular rhythm caused by sinus bradycardia or the compensatory pause after a premature ventricular complex is followed by the next sinus beat that has a premature ventricular complex in its T wave. The premature ventricular complex appears to initiate torsades de pointes.

Significance

Conditions that can prolong the QT interval may be associated with torsades de pointes. These include bradycardia; SA block; cardiac drug therapy (especially quinidine, procainamide, disopyramide, and amiodarone); electrolyte imbalances (especially hypokalemia and hypomagnesemia); myocardial infarction, angina, and other ischemic heart conditions; subarachnoid hemorrhage; tricyclic antidepressants and phenothiazines; vagal response; and congenital QT prolongation.

Treatment

Treatment of ventricular tachycardia that has a polymorphic pattern depends on whether the QT interval is prolonged. Thus it is important to restrict the definition of *torsades de pointes* to the typical electrocardiographic mor-

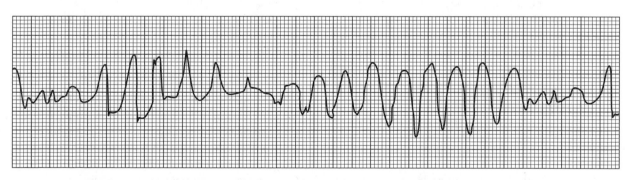

Fig. 5-61 Long QT interval and torsades de pointes. The ventricular complexes appear to twist or spiral around the isoelectric line. It may be seen in a patient with long QT interval.

Rate	Atrial, 60 beats/min; ventricular, irregular.
Rhythm	Atrial, regular; ventricular, irregular.
P waves	Not visible.
PR interval	Not visible.
QRS complex	0.18 second.
Dysrhythmia	Torsades de pointes.

phology that occurs in the setting of a long QT and/or long QT-U wave. In patients with torsades de pointes, administration of antidysrhythmic agents such as quinidine, disopyramide, and procainamide tends to increase the abnormal QT interval and worsen the dysrhythmia. Treatment includes the following:

1. Temporary ventricular or atrial pacing should be instituted. Pacing at rapid rates suppresses the ventricular tachycardia, which often does not recur after cessation of pacing. Isoproterenol can be tried until pacing is instituted.
2. Magnesium sulfate given intravenously has been reported to suppress torsades de pointes in a small number of patients. The dosage is 2 g intravenous push over 1 to 2 minutes, with an intravenous infusion of 1 to 2 g/hr for 4 to 6 hours.
3. The cause of the long QT interval and torsades de pointes should be determined and corrected if possible.
4. Antidysrhythmic drugs that do not prolong the QT interval, such as lidocaine, mexiletine, or tocainide, may be tried.

Long QT Syndrome

Long QT syndrome exists when a QT interval is abnormally prolonged (greater than 0.44 second after correction for rate) or when the QT-U pattern appears abnormal in configuration. The nature of the U wave and its relationship to the long QR syndrome are not clear. Notched, bifid, and sinusoidal T waves may occur.

Significance

Repolarization abnormalities can be divided into two groups: (1) a primary or idiopathic group that includes a congenital, often familial disorder sometimes but not always associated with deafness and (2) an acquired group caused by various drugs such as quinidine, disopyramide, procainamide, phenothiazines, and tricyclic antidepressants; metabolic abnormalities such as hypokalemia; central nervous system lesions; autonomic nervous system dysfunction; coronary artery disease with myocardial infarction; and other problems. Patients with symptomatic long QT syndrome develop a type of ventricular tachycardia, torsades de pointes. Since sudden death may occur in this group of patients, it is obvious that the ventricular dysrhythmia becomes sustained and probably results in ventricular fibrillation in some. Patients with congenital long QT syndrome who are at increased risks for sudden cardiac death include those who have family members who died suddenly at an early age and those who have experienced syncope.

Treatment

Treatment options follow:
1. For patients who do not have syncope, complex ventricular dysrhythmias or a family history of sudden cardiac death, no therapy is recommended.

2. In patients with asymptomatic complex ventricular dysrhythmias or a family history of premature sudden cardiac death, β blockers at maximally tolerated doses are recommended.
3. In patients with syncope, β blockers at maximally tolerated doses, at times combined with phenytoin and phenobarbital, are suggested.
4. In patients who continue to have syncope despite triple drug therapy, left-sided cervicothoracic sympathetic ganglionectomy that interrupts the stellate ganglion and the first three or four thoracic ganglia has been proposed.
5. Implantable automatic defibrillators may be needed in the patient with symptoms who has not responded to other therapy.

Accelerated Idioventricular Rhythm

The ventricular rate, commonly between 50 and 110 beats/min, usually hovers within 10 beats of the sinus rate so that control of the cardiac rhythm may be passed back and forth between these two competing pacemaker sites. Consequently, long runs of fusion beats often appear at the onset and termination of the dysrhythmia as the pacemakers vie for control of ventricular discharge. Because of the slow rates, capture beats are common. The onset of this dysrhythmia is generally gradual (nonparoxysmal) and occurs when the rate of ectopic ventricular discharge exceeds the sinus rate because of sinus slowing or SA or AV block (Figs. 5-62 and 5-63). The ectopic mechanism may also begin after a premature ventricular complex, or the ectopic ventricular rate may simply accelerate sufficiently to overtake the sinus focus. The slow rate and nonparoxysmal onset usually avoid the problems initiated by excitation during the vulnerable period, and consequently, precipitation of more rapid ventricular dysrhythmias is rarely seen. Termination of the rhythm generally occurs gradually as the dominant sinus rhythm accelerates or the ectopic ventricular rhythm decelerates. Occasionally, an accelerated idioventricular rhythm may be present in a patient who also has a more rapid ventricular tachycardia at other times.

Significance

The dysrhythmia occurs as a rule in heart disease such as acute myocardial infarction or as an expression of digitalis toxicity. Generally it is transient and intermittent, with episodes lasting a few seconds to a minute, and does not appear to seriously affect the course or prognosis of the disease. Suppressive therapy is usually unnecessary because the ventricular rate is commonly less than 100 beats/min. Basically, five conditions exist during which therapy may be considered: (1) when AV dissociation results in loss of sequential AV contraction and, with it, the hemodynamic benefits of atrial contraction; (2) when accelerated idioventricular rhythm occurs with more rapid forms of ventricular tachycardia; (3) when accelerated idioventricular rhythm begins with a premature ventricular

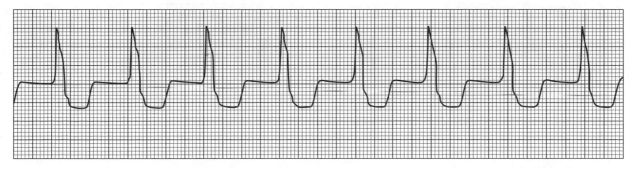

Fig. 5-62 Accelerated idioventricular rhythm.

Rate	75 beats/min.
Rhythm	Regular.
P waves	Not visible.
PR interval	Not visible.
QRS complex	0.12 second.

complex that initiates more rapid ventricular tachycardia; (4) when the ventricular rate is too rapid and produces symptoms; and (5) if ventricular fibrillation develops. The last appears only rarely.

Treatment

Treatment for accelerated idioventricular rhythm follows:

1. The best initial therapeutic approach would appear to be close observation, rhythm monitoring, and care for the underlying heart disease.
2. Digitalis administration should be discontinued if the drug is implicated in the genesis of the dysrhythmia.
3. Atropine (0.5 mg intravenously initially and repeated if necessary) may be used to speed the sinus rate and capture the ventricles. Rarely, pacing may be considered to speed the basic heart rate and suppress the accelerated idioventricular rhythm.
4. Lidocaine or other antidysrhythmic drugs may be given to suppress the ectopic ventricular focus.

Ventricular Flutter and Ventricular Fibrillation

Ventricular flutter and ventricular fibrillation (Figs. 5-64 to 5-66) represent severe derangements of the heartbeat that usually terminate fatally within 3 to 5 minutes unless they are promptly stopped. Ventricular flutter resembles a sine wave with regular, large oscillations occurring at a rate between 150 and 300 beats/min but usually exceeding 200 beats/min. Ventricular fibrillation is recognized by the presence of irregular undulations of varying contour and amplitude. Distinct QRS complexes, ST segments, and T waves are absent. The difference between rapid ventricular tachycardia and ventricular flutter may be difficult to discern and is usually of academic interest only.

Significance

Ventricular fibrillation occurs in a variety of clinical situations but is most commonly associated with coronary heart disease, acute myocardial infarction, and cardiomyopathy. The dysrhythmia occurs frequently as the terminal event in a variety of diseases. It may also be seen during cardiac pacing, cardiac catheterization, an operation, anesthesia, drug toxicity (for example, antidysrhythmic drugs), and hypoxia. It may occur after electric shock administered during cardioversion or accidentally by improperly grounded equipment. Premature stimulation during the vulnerable period (R-on-T phenomenon; see section on ventricular tachycardia) may precipitate ventricular tachycardia, flutter, or fibrillation, particularly when the electric stability of the heart has been altered by the ischemia of an acute myocardial infarction, for example. In many patients, sustained ventricular tachycardia may precede ventricular fibrillation.[23] However, ventricular fibrillation may occur without antecedent or precipitating ventricular tachycardia or premature ventricular complexes. Experimentally, it may occur when a previously occluded coronary artery undergoes sudden restoration of flow. Clinically, this condition may be replicated by streptokinase infusion or percutaneous transluminal coronary angioplasty that restores flow to an occluded coronary artery or possibly when coronary spasm relaxes. Conceivably, the latter event could result in ventricular fibrillation without myocardial infarction.

Ventricular flutter or fibrillation results in faintness followed by loss of consciousness, seizures, apnea, and if the rhythm continues untreated, death. The blood pressure is unobtainable, and heart sounds are usually absent. The atria may continue to beat at an independent rhythm or may be retrogradely captured for a time. Eventually, electric activity of the heart is completely absent.

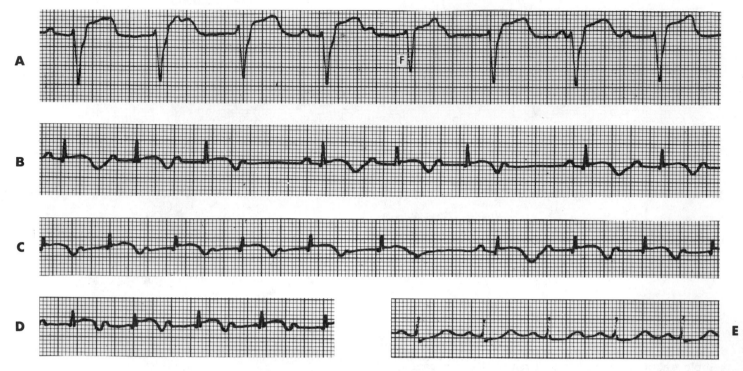

Fig. 5-63 Accelerated idioventricular rhythm and second-degree AV block. This series of tracings was recorded over several days in a patient who had an acute inferior myocardial infarction. **A,** An accelerated idioventricular rhythm occurs at 70 beats/min. Note that the fusion QRS complex *(F)* in the midportion of the strip is preceded by a long PR interval. The long PR interval suggests the presence of an AV conduction disturbance, but its exact degree cannot be determined from this ECG. Thus incomplete AV dissociation is present, caused by a combination of accelerated idioventricular rhythm and AV block. **B,** The accelerated idioventricular rhythm has stopped, but Wenckebach second-degree AV block is still present with a conduction ratio of 4:3. **C,** The Wenckebach second-degree AV block is still present, but the conduction ratio has increased significantly. **D,** On the following day the second-degree AV block has disappeared and is now replaced by first-degree AV block. **E,** Finally, after several days the first-degree AV block is barely present. **A,** Monitor lead. **B-E,** Lead II.

Rate	**A,** Atrial, 88 beats/min; ventricular, 70 beats/min. **B,** Atrial, 87 beats/min; ventricular, varying. **C,** Atrial, 86 beats/min; ventricular, varying. **D,** Atrial and ventricular, 88 beats/min. **E,** Atrial and ventricular, 88 beats/min.
Rhythm	**A,** Atrial and ventricular, regular. **B,** Atrial, regular; ventricular, irregular. **C,** Atrial, regular; ventricular, irregular. **D,** Atrial and ventricular, regular. **E,** Atrial and ventricular, regular.
P waves	Normal in all traces.
PR interval	**A,** Not measurable. **B** and **C,** Progressively increasing. **D,** Regular at 0.3 second. **E,** Regular at 0.20 second.
QRS complex	**A,** 0.12 second. **B** to **E,** 0.06 second.

Many patients who suffer ventricular fibrillation out of the hospital have been resuscitated. It is interesting that only 20% to 30% of them develop a myocardial infarction, and those who have a myocardial infarction experience a 2% to 3% recurrence rate of ventricular fibrillation in the first year. However, patients who are resuscitated from out-of-hospital ventricular fibrillation but do not develop a myocardial infarction have a 1-year recurrence rate of almost 25%.

Treatment

Ventricular flutter and ventricular fibrillation are totally unphysiologic life-threatening dysrhythmias for which immediate electric (nonsynchronized) DC cardioversion, using 200 to 400 joules, is the only reliable treatment. When ventricular tachycardia produces the same hemodynamic response as ventricular flutter or fibrillation, it also must be terminated immediately by DC shock. A sharp blow to the chest may terminate some forms of ventricular tachydys-

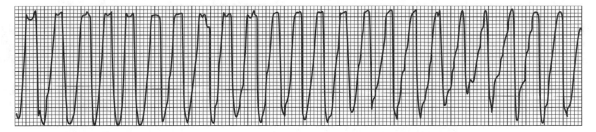

Fig. 5-64 Ventricular flutter. During ventricular flutter, ventricular depolarization and repolarization appear as a sine wave with regular oscillations. The QRS complex cannot be distinguished from the ST segment or T wave. Monitor lead is continuous recording.

Rate   Ventricular, 230 beats/min.
Rhythm   P waves cannot be seen; ventricular, fairly regular.
PR interval   Not measurable.
QRS complex   0.18 second.

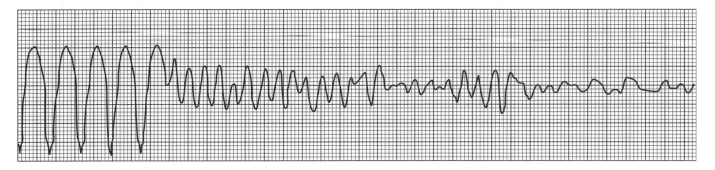

Fig. 5-65 Ventricular tachycardia to fibrillation. The ECG demonstrated the development of a rapid ventricular tachycardia that progressed promptly to ventricular fibrillation. Ventricular fibrillation at its onset may appear fairly regular.

Rate   Ventricular rate during ventricular tachycardia, 180 beats/min.
Rhythm   During rapid ventricular tachycardia, grossly irregular.
P waves   Not visible.
PR interval   Not visible.
QRS complex   Cannot be measured accurately during ventricular tachycardia or fibrillation.

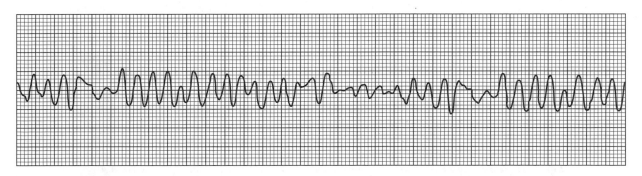

Fig. 5-66 Ventricular fibrillation. In this monitor lead the irregular, undulating baseline without any electric evidence of organized ventricular activity is characteristic of ventricular fibrillation.

Rate   Cannot be determined.
Rhythm   Grossly irregular.
P waves   Cannot be seen.
PR interval   Cannot be determined.
QRS complex   Cannot be measured.

rhythmias (thumpversion), but it should only be used in a witnessed arrest.

Termination of ventricular flutter or fibrillation within 30 to 60 seconds prevents the biochemical derangements accompanying ventricular fibrillation, eliminates the need for endotracheal intubation, and significantly increases the success rate of such procedures.

In an unwitnessed arrest, cardiopulmonary resuscitation (CPR) should be initiated and continued until a defibrillator is available. Defibrillation is started at 200 joules. If it is unsuccessful, joules are progressively increased to 300 and then 360. If it is still unsuccessful, CPR is resumed, and intravenous access is established. Epinephrine (1:10,000, 0.5 to 1 mg intravenous push) is administered. If possible, the patient's trachea is intubated. Defibrillation with up to 360 joules is performed. If ventricular fibrillation is still present, lidocaine (1.5 mg/kg intravenous push) is given. Defibrillation with up to 360 joules is performed. If ventricular fibrillation continues, bretylium (5 mg/kg intravenous push) should be considered. Administration of bicarbonate should also be considered. (Ideally, bicarbonate is given according to blood gas levels.) Defibrillation up to 360 joules is performed. Bretylium (10 mg/kg intravenous push) is given. Defibrillation up to 360 joules is performed. Lidocaine or bretylium administration is repeated; defibrillation up to 360 joules is performed.[13]

The DC shock may cause the asystolic heart to begin discharging and terminate ventricular fibrillation if the latter is present. After a successful cardioversion, measures must be taken to prevent a second episode of ventricular fibrillation, including monitoring of the cardiac rhythm, and administration of lidocaine, procainamide, or bretylium.

Atrioventricular Block[24]

The conduction of an impulse may be slowed or completely blocked at sites along the conduction pathway. If the site of conduction impairment is in the AV node, bundle of His, or surrounding tissue, the resultant conduction abnormality is called an *AV block*. AV blocks are further described as first degree, second degree (type I and type II), or third degree based on several criteria.

First-degree AV block

During first-degree heart block (Figs. 5-67 and 5-68), every atrial impulse is conducted to the ventricles, producing a regular ventricular rhythm. However, the duration of AV conduction is abnormally prolonged, and this is manifested by a PR interval exceeding 0.20 second in the adult. PR intervals as long as 1.0 second have been recorded.

Significance

First-degree AV block is a common conduction disturbance that may occur in healthy or diseased hearts. It is common in older individuals without clinical evidence of heart disease. It may be a precursor to more advanced degrees of block. Acute first-degree block is commonly caused by digitalis toxicity, acute myocardial infarction (inferior), or myocarditis.

Treatment

Generally no therapy is required. If digitalis, quinidine, or procainamide is implicated, the offending drug must be stopped or its dosage reduced.

Second-degree AV block

Failure of some atrial impulses to conduct to the ventricles at a time when physiologic interference would not be expected constitutes second-degree AV block (Figs. 5-69

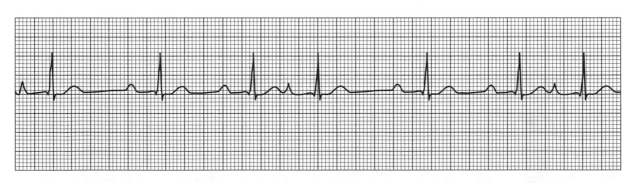

Fig. 5-67   First-degree AV block. In this monitor lead, the clinician cannot be certain of the type of intraventricular conduction delay. The prolonged AV conduction time may be caused by conduction delay within the AV node and/or His-Purkinje system (see section on the bundle of His).

Rate	60 beats/min.
Rhythm	Regular.
P waves	Have normal contour and precede each QRS complex.
PR interval	Prolonged, 0.24 second.

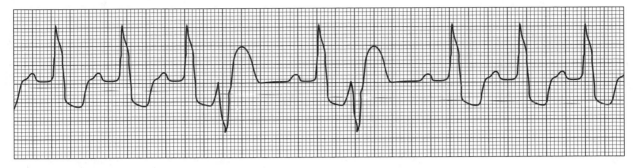

Fig. 5-68 First-degree AV block. Premature ventricular complexes occur in a patient with first-degree AV block.

Rate	85 beats/min.
Rhythm	Regular, for the most part; irregularities caused by premature ventricular complexes.
P waves	Normal.
PR interval	0.28 second.

to 5-73). The nonconducted P wave may be intermittent, frequent, or infrequent; may occur at regular or irregular intervals; and may be preceded by fixed or lengthening PR intervals. A distinguishing feature is that conducted P waves relate to a QRS complex with recurring PR intervals; that is, the association of P waves with QRS complexes is not random. The two types of second-degree AV block can be distinguished with an acceptable degree of accuracy by analysis of the PR intervals.

Second-degree AV block (Mobitz type I)

In a classic type I (Wenckebach) second-degree AV block (Figs. 5-69 to 5-70) a gradual lengthening of the PR interval occurs because of lengthening AV conduction time, until an atrial impulse is nonconducted, so a P wave is not followed by a QRS complex. Then the sequence begins again. The blocked P wave may occur occasionally or frequently, regularly or irregularly. The ratio of atrial impulses to ventricular responses is frequently 5:4, 4:3, 3:2, or 3:1. The duration of the QRS complex may be normal or prolonged. Type I second-degree AV block occurs most commonly in the AV node. Because the increment in conduction time is greatest in the second beat of the type I group and then decreases progressively over succeeding cycles, the interval between successive R-R cycles before the nonconducted P wave progressively decreases, the duration of the pause produced by the nonconducted P wave is less than twice the shortest cycle, and the duration of the R-R cycle after the pause exceeds that preceding the pause.

In atypical type I block (which occurs commonly) the increment in AV conduction time may increase in the last beat so that the last R-R cycle preceding the blocked P wave lengthens rather than shortens.

Significance. Of the second-degree blocks, type I is the most common, is usually transitory, and rarely progresses to complete heart block. It produces little or no clinical symptoms.

Treatment. Generally no therapy is required. Treatment may be necessary for patients who have symptoms of type I block with very slow ventricular rates. This may be more common in older patients. Atropine (in 0.5 mg increments intravenously) or isoproterenol (1 or 2 µg/min) may be tried initially, with care taken not to produce a sinus tachycardia in patients who have an acute myocardial infarction. If there is no response or if the block remains for prolonged periods, pacemaker therapy may be used. Digitalis, if implicated, must be stopped.

Second-degree AV block (Mobitz type II)

In type II second-degree AV block (Figs. 5-72 and 5-73) a P wave is blocked without progressive antecedent PR prolongation and occurs almost always in bundle branch block. The PR interval of the conducted atrial impulses may be prolonged or normal, but it usually remains fairly constant. The pause caused by the nonconducted P wave is equal to or may be slightly less than twice the normal R-R interval. Sinus dysrhythmia, premature beats, AV junctional escape beats, or changes in neurogenic influences may disturb the timing of the expected pauses. Type II AV block almost always occurs in the His-Purkinje system.

Significance. Type II second-degree block is less common and frequently progresses to complete heart block. Clinical symptoms such as dizziness or faintness may occur with frequent nonconducted P waves.

Treatment. If type II block develops with an acute myocardial infarction, temporary transvenous pacing is necessary because this form of block often precedes the occurrence of sudden third-degree AV block with ventricular asystole and Adams-Stokes syncope. Before pacemaker insertion, isoproterenol given intravenously, (2 to 10 µg/min titrated to patient response) may be used temporarily. By increasing the atrial rate without decreasing the AV block, atropine given intravenously, (0.5 to 1 mg) may cause more P waves to block and reduce the ventricular rate. Pa-

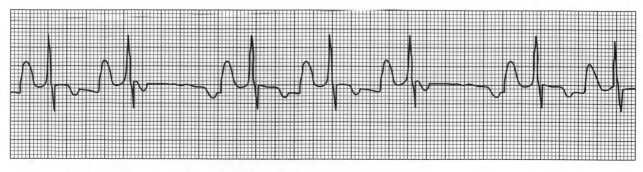

Fig. 5-69   Second-degree AV block (type I). 4:3 conduction ratio.

Rate	Atrial, 80 beats/min; ventricular, varying.
Rhythm	Atrial, regular; ventricular, varying.
P waves	More numerous than QRS complexes but are related to ventricular beats in a consistent, repetitive fashion.
PR interval	Progressive PR prolongation preceding the nonconducted P wave. Finally, one P wave is blocked, and the cycle then repeats.
QRS complex	0.08 second.

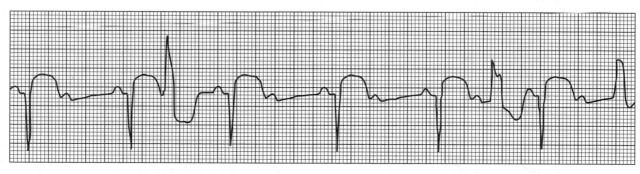

Fig. 5-70   Second-degree AV block (type I). 2:1 conduction occurs. Since 2:1 conduction can occur with type I or type II second-degree heart block, sometimes the two cannot be readily differentiated. However, a normal QRS complex is an indicator of type I second-degree AV heart block. Multiform premature ventricular complexes are also present.

Rate	Atrial: 110 beats/min.
Rhythm	Atrial, regular; ventricular, varying, depending on the degree of AV block.
P waves	Normal.
PR interval	Progressive increase in PR interval until one P wave fails to conduct.
QRS complex	Normal, 0.07 second.

tients who have no symptoms (for instance, with syncope or presyncope) and who do not have acute myocardial infarction should receive permanent pacemakers. For patients with no symptoms, many physicians recommend permanent pacemaker implantation prophylactically, since the natural history of type II AV block is to progress to complete AV block.

Third-degree AV block

Third-degree (complete) AV block (Figs. 5-74 to 5-76) occurs when no P waves are conducted to the ventricles. The atria and ventricles are controlled by independent pacemakers, and as such, third-degree AV block constitutes one form of complete AV dissociation. The atrial pacemaker may be of sinus, ectopic atrial, or (uncommonly)

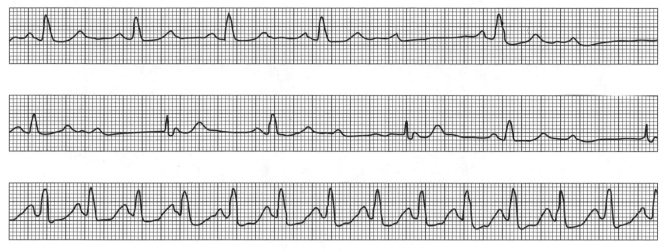

Fig. 5-71 2:1 anterograde AV block, 1:1 retrograde ventriculoatrial conduction. In the top tracing, alternate P waves conduct to the ventricles. In the lower tracing (same patient), ventricular pacing (*upright arrow,* pacemaker artifact) establishes a 1:1 retrograde atrial conduction beginning with the fourth-paced QRS complex. *Inverted arrow,* Retrograde atrial activation.

Rate	Atrial, 68 in the top tracing; 70 in the bottom tracing; ventricular, 34 in the top tracing, 70 in the bottom tracing.
Rhythm	Atrial, regular; ventricular, regular.
P waves	Top tracing, normal; bottom tracing, normal and retrograde.
PR interval	Top tracing, 0.20 second; conduction of alternate P waves.
RP interval	Bottom tracing, 0.16 second
QRS complex	Top tracing, 0.08 second; bottom tracing, 0.14 second.

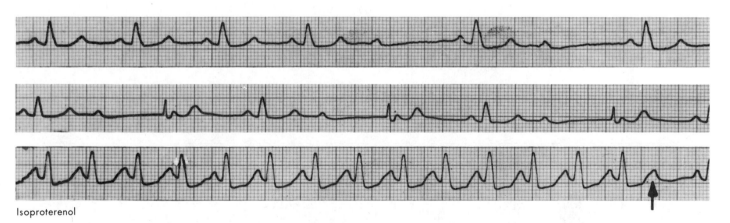

Isoproterenol

Fig. 5-72 Second-degree AV block (type II). LBBB is present in this recording of lead I. Sudden failure of AV conduction results without antecedent PR prolongation. In the second strip the escape beats interrupt the pause produced by the blocked P wave. In the bottom strip, isoproterenol infusion has increased the atrial rate and conduction ratio significantly. Only one nonconducted P wave occurs *(arrow).*

Rate	Atrial, 62 beats/min in the top strip, 71 beats/min in the middle strip, and 122 beats/min in the bottom strip; ventricular, varying.
Rhythm	Atrial, regular; ventricular, varying, depending on the degree of AV block.
P waves	Normal.
PR interval	Normal and constant at 0.19 second in the top and middle strips and difficult to measure in the bottom strip.
QRS complex	Prolonged to 0.12 second with an LBBB contour.

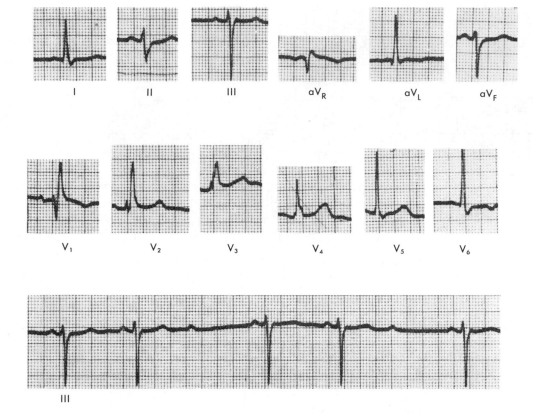

Fig. 5-73   Second-degree AV block (type II). The 12-lead ECG indicates the presence of left anterior fascicular block and RBBB. In the rhythm recording (lead III), sudden failure of AV conduction results without antecedent PR prolongation.

Rate	62 beats/min.
Rhythm	Atrial, regular; ventricular, varying, depending on the degree of AV block.
P waves	Normal.
PR interval	Normal, constant (0.14 second) or may be prolonged, constant; sudden failure of conduction.
QRS complex	Prolonged, 0.12 second.

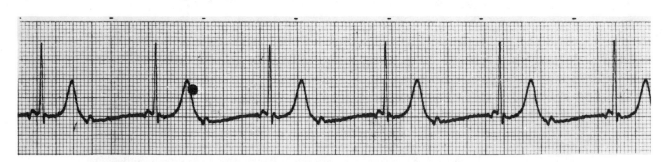

Fig. 5-74   Congenital third-degree AV block in a 7-year-old child.

Rate	Atrial, 95 beats/min; ventricular, 48 beats/min.
Rhythm	Atrial, slightly irregular, possibly caused by ventriculophasic sinus dysrhythmia.
P waves	Vary in contour.
PR interval	There is no consistent PR interval indicating that the atrial and ventricular impulses are not related.
QRS	Normal; 0.06 second.
Dysrhythmia	Third-degree AV block.

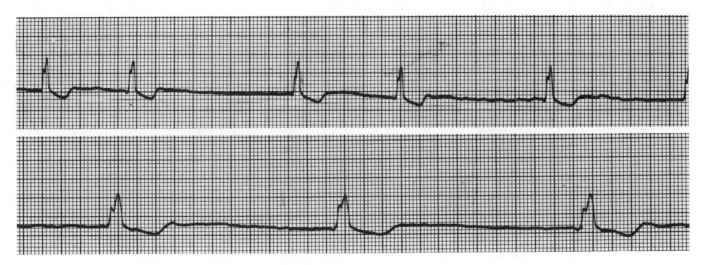

Fig. 5-75   Atrial fibrillation in an older man with third-degree AV block.

Rate	20 to 70 beats/min.
Rhythm	Irregular.
P waves	Irregular baseline indicating atrial fibrillation.
PR interval	Not measurable.
QRS interval	0.10 second in top strip, 0.14 second in bottom strip.
Dysrhythmia	The underlying atrial rhythm is atrial fibrillation. In the bottom strip, there is complete AV dissociation (as a result of third-degree AV block) manifested by ventricular escape beats while the atrial continued to fibrillate.

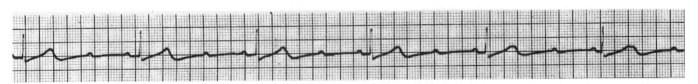

Fig. 5-76   Third-degree AV block. This tracing was recorded from an 80-year-old man who had recurrent syncope caused by an acquired third-degree AV block. The ECG is uncommon, since the QRS complexes are normal in this monitor lead and suggest that the site of block is AV nodal or, more likely, intrahisian. Congenital third-degree AV block has this appearance, although with a faster ventricular rate. Bundle of His recording would be necessary to establish site of block.

Rate	Atrial, 107 beats/min; ventricular, 36 beats/min.
Rhythm	Atrial, regular; ventricular, regular.
P waves	Normal.
PR interval	Totally variable.
QRS complex	Normal, 0.06 second.

junctional origin (tachycardia, flutter, or fibrillation). The ventricular focus may be above or below the bundle of His bifurcation, depending on the site of the block. In congenital third-degree AV block, the block is usually at the level of the AV node, proximal to the bundle of His. The escape focus is supraventricular and as such is more stable and faster than that which occurs with distal His block. The usually regular rhythm may vary because of premature ventricular beats, a shift in pacemaker site, or an irregularly discharging pacemaker focus. The QRS complex is normal, and Adams-Stokes syncope occurs less often. In acquired third-degree AV block, the ventricular rate is 30 to 40 beats/min because the site of the block is distal to the bundle of His and consequently the escape focus is in the bundle branch–Purkinje system (Fig. 5-62). Less commonly, block within the bundle of His may occur (Fig. 5-76).

Significance

In the adult, drug toxicity (predominantly digitalis) and degenerative heart disease are the most common causes of acquired AV heart block. The degenerative process produces partial or complete anatomic or electric disruption within the AV nodal region, the bundle of His, or both bundle branches. Multiple factors may contribute to this degenerative process. They include fibrosclerosis of the cardiac skeleton, fibrosis of the conduction system, coronary artery disease, myocarditis, and cardiomyopathies. Cardiac surgery has become an infrequent but still important cause of heart block. Less commonly, electrolyte disturbances; endocarditis; myocarditis; tumors; Chagas disease; syphilitic gummas; rheumatoid nodules; myxedema; infiltrative processes such as amyloidosis, sarcoidosis, and scleroderma; and other systemic illnesses may lead to AV heart block. Calcium deposition in the region of the aortic and mitral valves may extend to involve the conduction pathways. Digitalis excess produces type I not type II second-degree AV block.

AV heart block occurring during a myocardial infarction may be divided into two groups: that which occurs during an anterior or anteroseptal infarction and that which occurs during a diaphragmatic (inferior) infarction. When an anterior wall infarction produces AV block, it is usually the result of extensive necrosis of the summit of the interventricular septum, which spares the AV node and bundle of His but inflicts severe damage to the bundle branches. Consequently, the block is apt to be distal to the bundle of His (type II) and associated with RBBB and a form of fascicular block. Third-degree AV block may develop, during which the ventricular rate is less than 40 beats/min, asystole and syncope occur more commonly, and the mortality rate is 75% or higher. Death results from pump failure or shock because of the large size of the infarction.

When AV block results from diaphragmatic infarction, the type I second-degree block usually occurs in the region of the AV node because of inflammation or edema that results from the ischemia or infarction of neighboring myocardium. The ventricular pacemaker, located in the region of the AV node or bundle of His, is faster and more stable, and the block is usually transient, without residua. Advanced block and syncope are uncommon, and the mortality rate in patients without associated heart failure does not appear to be increased. Some overlap occurs between these two divisions.

Atropine, isoproterenol, and exercise normally shorten the PR interval as the atrial rate increases; when the atrial rate is increased by atrial pacing, the PR interval lengthens. Steroids and thyroid hormones tend to improve AV conduction, which may lengthen during adrenal insufficiency or myxedema. In patients with type II second-degree AV block occurring in the His-Purkinje system, an increase in the atrial rate after atropine, isoproterenol, or exercise may not concomitantly improve AV conduction and may result in a greater number of blocked P waves.

Symptoms during second-degree AV block are infrequent unless periods of third-degree AV block occur. The slow ventricular rate during complete heart block may not maintain circulation effectively and may result in angina, congestive heart failure, or syncope. Ventricular asystole may occur, or the slow rate may initiate premature ventricular systoles or tachydysrhythmias.

Treatment

If third-degree AV block develops with acute myocardial infarction, temporary transvenous pacing is necessary. Atropine (0.5 mg intravenous push) may be used and repeated as needed to a total dose of 2.0 mg before insertion of the pacemaker. Pacemaker insertion is preferable to repeated doses of atropine.[13]

Asymptomatic patients with chronic stable third-degree AV block may need no specific therapy, although many physicians recommend prophylactic pacemaker implantation for them to prevent an Adams-Stokes attack. In patients with symptoms of congestive heart failure or Adams-Stokes syncope caused by ventricular asystole, severe ventricular bradycardia, and ventricular tachydysrhythmias occurring as a result of the AV block, long-term drug therapy is generally unreliable, and permanent pacemaker implantation is indicated. It has been suggested that patients who develop transient high-degree AV block during myocardial infarction and survive should receive prophylactic permanent pacemaker implantation even though the block resolves.[25]

Bundle Branch Block

Anatomic or functional discontinuity in one of the bundle branches (Figs. 5-77 and 5-78) may prevent or slow conduction so that the ventricle on the affected side becomes activated late because this ventricle, normally supplied by the blocked bundle branch, must be activated by impulses traveling through the ventricular wall and interventricular septum from the unaffected side. Conduction along this circuitous route proceeds more slowly, and therefore the QRS complex becomes widened to 0.10 to 0.12 second (incomplete) or more than 0.12 second (complete RBBB or LBBB). Transient bundle branch block may occur as a result of tachycardia, bradycardia, pulmonary embolism, anemia, infection, myocardial ischemia or infarction, congestive heart failure, metabolic derangements, hypoxia, and other causes. The following criteria are helpful in diagnosing bundle branch block:

1. QRS complex of 0.12 second
2. Supraventricular rhythm
3. PR interval of 0.12 second
4. Wide QRS complex with an M-shape or rSR′ pattern (When the M shape is in lead V_1, RBBB should be considered; when it is in lead V_6, LBBB should be considered.)

LBBB

In complete LBBB (Fig. 5-77) the QRS complex becomes prolonged more than 0.12 second, with the major slowing occurring in the middle and terminal forces. The initial forces are deformed and prevent the development of the normal septal Q wave in lead I or V_6. Initial R waves in leads V_1 to V_3 are small or absent, followed by deep, large, slurred S waves and large, prolonged R waves in leads V_5 and V_6.

Significant mean axis deviation is usually absent. The ST-segment and T-wave shift are characteristically 180 degrees opposite the major QRS deflection.

Significance

LBBB is often associated with serious heart disease such as coronary artery disease, valvular heart disease, and hypertension. Although both RBBB and LBBB can occur in patients without apparent heart disease, LBBB correlates significantly with cardiomegaly and suggests a more serious prognosis. The conduction defect caused by LBBB alters the initial QRS vector, often obscuring the normal ECG signs of an acute myocardial infarction.[24]

Treatment

The cause and not the response to LBBB is treated.

RBBB

In uncomplicated complete RBBB (Fig. 5-78) the QRS complex is 0.11 second or wider. The initial and middle forces of the vector loop are in a normal direction, and the terminal force is directed to the right and anteriorly. These changes produce large S waves in leads I, II, V_5, and V_6, often a terminal R wave in lead III, and R′ in leads V_1 and V_2. Incomplete RBBB is associated with the same ECG pattern, but the QRS complex is 0.10 second or less.

Significance

In a young individual, right ventricular hypertrophy may produce RBBB; in an older patient, coronary artery disease is a more likely cause. Early supraventricular complexes that are conducted aberrantly through the ventricle are more likely to develop RBBB than LBBB, presumably be-

cause the right bundle branch takes longer to repolarize than the left bundle branch. The initial forces in RBBB are not altered, and therefore the ECG signs of myocardial infarction are not obscured.

Treatment

There is no treatment for RBBB itself, but the cause is treated. According to ECG concepts, the left bundle branch divides into two subdivisions or fascicles:

1. The anterior (superior), which traverses the base of the anterior papillary muscle of the left ventricle
2. The posterior (inferior), which traverses the posterior papillary muscle

When the two subdivisions are intact, the impulse is transmitted simultaneously down both fascicles and gives a resultant force (*3* in Fig. 5-79) of its vectors (*1*) and (*2*). The term *hemiblock* is used when one of the subdivisions is blocked.

Left anterior hemiblock

Left anterior hemiblock occurs if the anterior (superior) division is blocked. The vector *1* is no longer present, and the left ventricle is activated by the posterior division, vector *2*. The ECG manifestations include left axis deviation, a small q wave in lead I, a small r wave in lead III, and a normal QRS complex when not accompanied by RBBB (Fig. 5-79, *B* and *D*).

Left posterior hemiblock

Left posterior hemiblock occurs if the posterior (inferior) division is blocked. The vector (*2*) is no longer present, and the left ventricle is activated by the anterior division vector (*1*). The ECG manifestations include right axis deviation, a small r wave in lead I, a small q wave in lead III, normal QRS duration, and no evidence of right ventricular hypertrophy (Figs. 5-79, *C*, and 5-80).

Significance

Left anterior hemiblock is more common than left posterior hemiblock because the posterior branch is shorter and thicker and less influenced by the stresses of the outflow tract. The posterior branch also has a double blood supply. Chronic hemiblock may be seen in older adults without demonstrable heart disease. Acute hemiblock is nearly always caused by an anterior myocardial infarction. Less common causes include cardiomyopathies, a calcified aorta, and hypercalcemia. Two large groups of patients develop ventricular conduction disorders because of a sclerodegenerative process limited to the conduction system (Lenègre disease) or fibrosclerosis of structures adjacent to the conduction system (Lev disease). Patients with Lenègre disease appear to be younger and more prone to developing AV block than those with Lev disease.

Bifascicular block

Bifascicular block occurs when two fascicles are blocked simultaneously: RBBB and left anterior hemiblock occur

Text continued on p. 160.

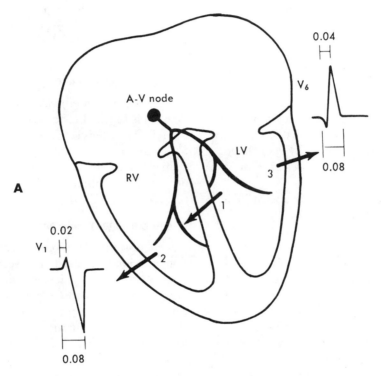

Fig. 5-77   A, Normal intraventricular conduction. Intrinsicoid deflection (interval from the onset of QRS complex to the peak of the R wave, upper brackets) is usually about 0.02 second in right precordial leads and 0.03 to 0.04 second in the left precordial leads. The intrinsicoid deflection prolongs during bundle branch block. *RV,* Right ventricle; *LV,* left ventricle.

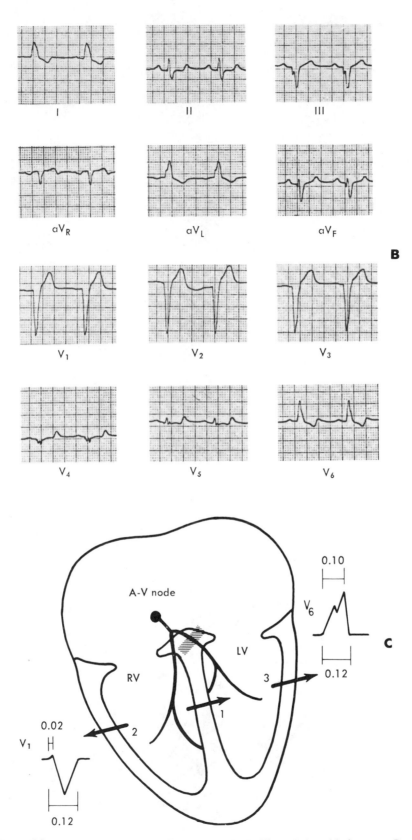

Fig. 5-77, cont'd **B,** Twelve-lead ECG illustrating LBBB. The axis is −30 degrees. **C,** Schematic illustration.

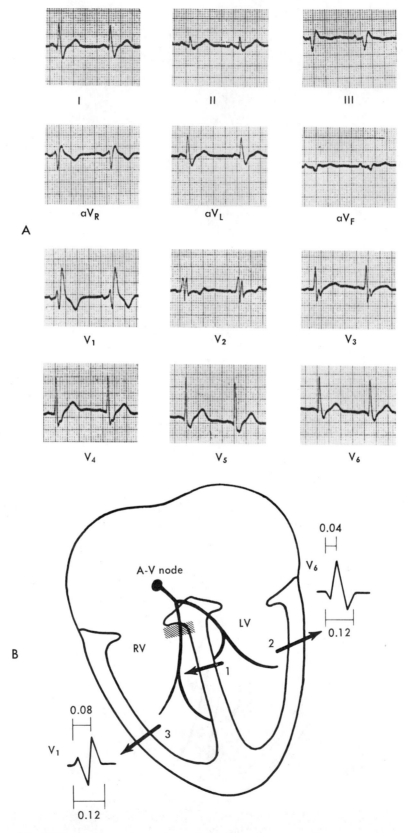

Fig. 5-78 **A,** Twelve-lead ECG illustrating RBBB. **B,** Schematic illustration.

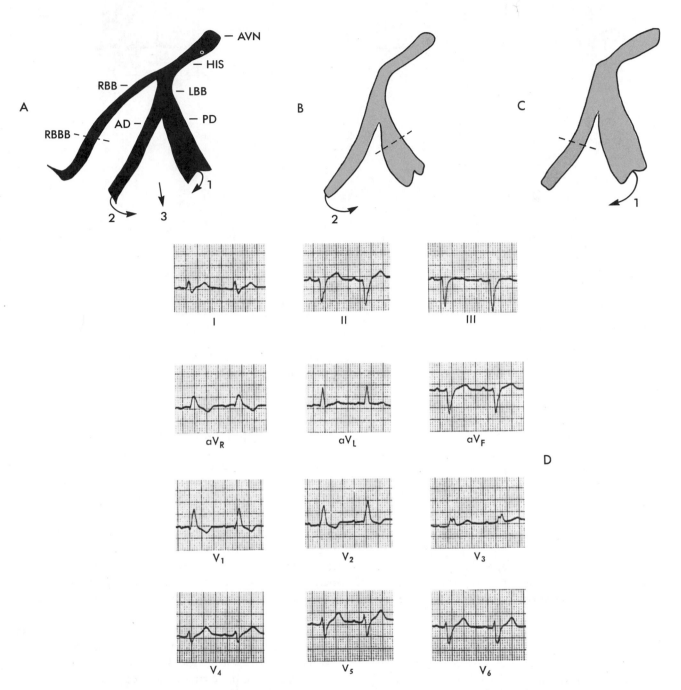

Fig. 5-79 **A,** Schematic illustration of the trifascicular nature of ventricular conduction. *AVN,* Atrioventricular node; *HIS,* bundle of His; *RBB,* right bundle branch; *LBB,* main portion of left bundle branch; *AD,* anterior (superior) division (fascicle) of left bundle branch; *PD,* posterior (inferior) division (fascicle) of left bundle branch. When both divisions of the left bundle are activated simultaneously (vectors *1* and *2*), the resultant force produces vector *3.* **B,** When the anterior (superior) division is blocked, the impulse must travel through the intact posterior division. Left axis shift occurs. **C,** When the posterior (inferior) division is blocked, the impulse must travel through the intact anterior division. Right axis shift occurs. **D,** Twelve-lead ECG illustrating RBBB and left anterior hemiblock. See also Fig. 5-72.

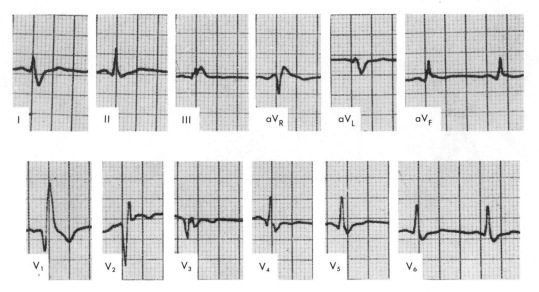

Fig. 5-80 Twelve-lead ECG illustrating RBBB and left posterior fascicular block. The abnormal Q waves in leads V₁ to V₄ indicate an anteroseptal myocardial infarction.

most commonly. RBBB and left posterior hemiblock occur less commonly.

Significance

Chronic bifascicular block is often asymptomatic. If symptoms occur, they may include dizziness, syncope, hypotension, or congestive heart failure because of a slow heart rate and decreased cardiac output. Acute bifascicular block may occur with an acute myocardial infarction, especially anterior infarction, and may precede more advanced forms of heart block.

Treatment

Asymptomatic chronic bifascicular block may not require any treatment. Pacemaker implantation is the treatment of choice if the condition becomes symptomatic. In acute bifascicular block, the patient's heart should be paced regardless of symptoms because complete AV block is likely to occur.

Parasystole

Premature complexes that lack a fixed relationship to the preceding complex (varying coupling intervals) may result from parasystole (Fig. 5-81). As classically defined, a *parasystolic focus* is a protected pacemaker focus that discharges at a fixed rate. Parasystolic discharge becomes manifest when the area in which the parasystolic focus originates has recovered excitability. The parasystolic focus may then depolarize the atrium or ventricle to produce a premature complex. The resulting P wave or QRS complex has a configuration different from that of the dominant rhythm, depending on the site of origin. Although the dominant rhythm may be discharged by the parasystolic focus, the dominant rhythm does not depo-

larize the parasystolic focus because the latter is protected by a unidirectional entrance block; that is, impulses may exit from the parasystolic focus to discharge the surrounding myocardium, but no impulse may enter the parasystolic focus and discharge it. For learning purposes, it can be thought of as a fixed-rate pacemaker that does not sense spontaneous complexes and that is not reset by them but does cause depolarization of the rest of the heart. The manifest parasystolic rate may be much less than the actual rate because of exit block from the parasystolic focus. That is, the parasystolic focus may discharge at more rapid rates than are apparent in the ECG because many of the discharges fail to exit and depolarize the surrounding myocardium. Exit block from the parasystolic focus may produce irregular spacing of the interectopic intervals. However, since the rate of discharge of the parasystolic focus is constant, the interectopic intervals between parasystolic impulses reduce to a common denominator. Premature complexes that are caused by a parasystolic focus ordinarily have no fixed relationship to the basic rhythm and often result in the production of fusion beats.

Parasystole should be suspected when the following criteria are met: varying coupling intervals, constant shortest interectopic intervals, and frequent appearance of fusion beats.[26]

Significance

Atrial and junctional parasystole may occur in patients without clinical evidence of heart disease. Ventricular parasystole generally manifests in patients with heart disease; it is rarely if ever caused by digitalis excess.

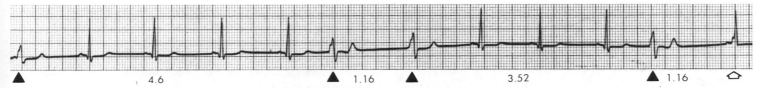

Fig. 5-81 Ventricular parasystole. The parasystolic ventricular beats are indicated by the solid triangles and the open arrow. The interval between parasystolic ventricular complexes is 1.16 seconds. The intervals of 4.6 and 3.52 seconds are 4 times and 3 times, respectively, the interectopic interval of 1.16 seconds. Note that the coupling interval varies and that a fusion beat (next to last QRS complex, indicated by open arrow) is also present. Ventricular refractoriness prevents emergence of the parasystolic ventricular rhythm during the long intervals in which it is absent. This tracing was recorded from an otherwise healthy 15-year-old boy.

Rate	65 beats/min, with some variation; parasystolic rate, 63 beats/min.
Rhythm	Atrial and ventricular rhythms during normally conducted beats, regular; parasystolic ventricular interval, regular.
P waves	Normal.
PR interval	0.11 second during the normally conducted beats.
QRS complex	Of normally conducted beats, 0.09 second; parasystolic ventricular beats, 0.12 second.

Treatment

The therapeutic approach is basically the same as that discussed for premature atrial, junctional, and ventricular complexes. Parasystole is a benign rhythm disorder.

AV DISSOCIATION

As the words imply, *AV dissociation* means that the atria and ventricles are dissociated; they are controlled by separate pacemakers for one or more beats. Used generically the term indicates nothing about the nature of atrial or ventricular activity, except that these chambers are beating independently for a time. It is as if the term described a "symptom" without indicating what caused it. The atria may be fibrillating, fluttering, or responding to an ectopic tachycardia or sinus impulses; the ventricles may be controlled by AV junctional or ectopic ventricular beating. The only fact conveyed is that whatever controls one chamber does not also control the other during the period of AV dissociation.

AV dissociation is never a primary disturbance of rhythm but rather a consequence of a more basic disorder; for the term to be used properly, the causes producing AV dissociation must also be described. Examples can be found throughout this chapter; some of them are as follows:

1. Slowing of the primary pacemaker to allow the escape of a subsidiary (latent) focus. In Fig. 5-13, sinus node slowing allows two ventricular beats to escape under the control of a separate focus while the sinus node still controls the atria. During these two beats, AV dissociation exists.

2. Accelerated discharge of subsidiary focus. In Fig. 5-51, accelerated AV junctional discharge results in an NPJT without retrograde atrial capture. Since the atria remain under sinus domination, separate pacemakers control atria and ventricles, resulting in AV dissociation. Fig. 5-135 presents a similar example, called *isorhythmic AV dissociation* because atria and ventricles maintain similar rates and rhythms. AV dissociation may also occur during ventricular tachycardia if retrograde atrial capture does not ensue (see Figs. 5-57 to 5-62).

3. AV block. In Fig. 5-73, AV block reduces the number of effective (conducted) atrial impulses; this allows the escape of a subsidiary focus to produce AV dissociation. When AV block results in AV dissociation, the atrial rate generally exceeds the ventricular rate (see Fig. 5-162).

4. Combinations of *1, 2,* or *3* may initiate AV dissociation, as, for example, when digitalis causes both first-degree AV block and NPJT or when acute myocardial infarction produces AV block and an accelerated idioventricular rhythm (Fig. 5-63).

In all these examples but for diverse reasons, the ventricular rate either exceeds or becomes equal or nearly equal to the effective (conducted) atrial rate. It is this fact that allows AV dissociation to occur.

The preceding discussion makes it apparent that the presence or absence of AV dissociation depends on the rate and temporal relationships of the two pacemakers and the intactness of AV and VA conduction. If the atrial pacemaker captures control of the ventricle, or vice versa, AV dissociation would be terminated during that period of capture (incomplete AV dissociation).

SUPRAVENTRICULAR DYSRHYTHMIA WITH ABNORMAL QRS COMPLEXES

Wide, bizarre QRS complexes may occur during isolated supraventricular beats or sustained supraventricular rhythms (Figs. 5-82 to 5-85). The term *aberrant ventricular conduction* is commonly applied to such complexes. Thus QRS contours that display prolonged abnormal configuration indicate that conduction through the ventricle is abnormal; they do not necessarily mean that the impulse originated in the ventricles.[28] The presence of fusion and capture complexes strongly supports the diagnosis of ven-

tricular tachycardia or accelerated ventricular rhythm. However, ECG manifestations of ventricular tachycardia, including the presence or absence of AV dissociation and complexes that appear to represent capture or fusion beats, may be mimicked under certain circumstances by supraventricular dysrhythmias.

Intraventricular conduction defects, bundle branch blocks, and anomalous pathway conduction may initiate abnormal ventricular depolarization with widened QRS complexes. Also, premature supraventricular stimulation may conduct to the ventricles before ventricular repolarization has been completed, causing the impulse to conduct aberrantly. The resulting widened QRS complex may display characteristic features that distinguish it from beats arising in the ventricles during a true ventricular tachycar-

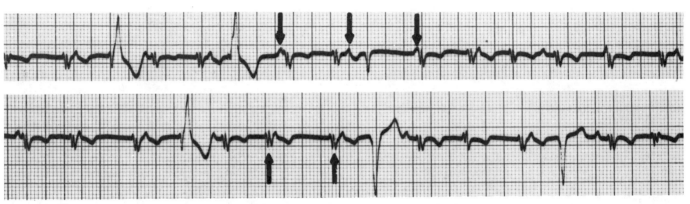

Continuous V₁

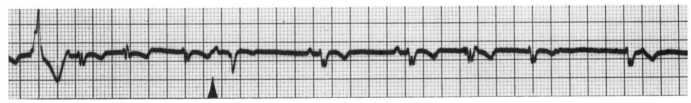

Carotid sinus massage V₁

Fig. 5-82   NPJT with intermittent atrial captures producing functional RBBB and functional LBBB. The NPJT discharges at a slightly irregular rate and accounts for the W-shaped QRS complex, *(upright arrows)*. Intermittent sinus captures (P waves indicated by inverted arrows) shorten the cardiac cycle and result in a normal, W-shaped QRS complex, functional RBBB, or functional LBBB. Carotid sinus massage (in the bottom tracing at the arrowhead) slows both the sinus and junctional discharge rates. This tracing was recorded from a 13-year-old boy with no heart disease other than the cardiac dysrhythmia. Therapy with digitalis slowed the junctional rate sufficiently so that the patient's condition remained asymptomatic with resting rates of 70 to 80 beats/min and a normal response to exercise.

Rate	Atrial and ventricular, approximately 88 beats/min but varying.
Rhythm	Irregular; incomplete AV dissociation.
P waves	Normal.
PR interval	0.14 second when premature capture does not occur.
QRS complex	Normal, functional RBBB and functional LBBB with a duration of 0.12 second.

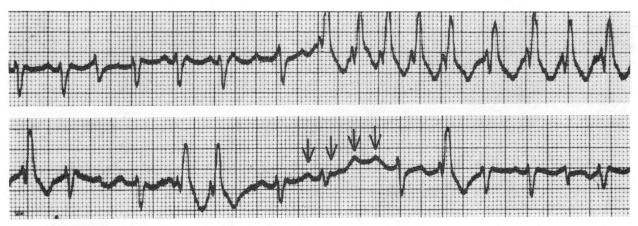

V₁—continuous

Fig. 5-83   Functional RBBB. At first glance the tracing appears to be sinus rhythm interrupted by a burst of ventricular tachycardia and intermittent premature ventricular systoles. Closer inspection reveals flutter waves *(arrows)* when the ventricular rate slows slightly and suggests that the widened QRS complexes may be aberrantly conducted supraventricular beats. These beats conform in all respects to criteria established to differentiate supraventricular aberration from ventricular tachycardia (see text). The patient required digitalis to slow the ventricular rate rather than lidocaine to suppress ectopic ventricular discharge.

Rate	Atrial, 280 beats/min; ventricular, 90 to 200 beats/min.
Rhythm	Atrial, regular; ventricular, irregularly irregular.
P waves	Flutter waves *(arrows)* can be seen when the ventricular rate slows and can be marched out with regularity.
PR interval	Flutter-R interval varies.
QRS complex	Varying contour between normal and functional RBBB.

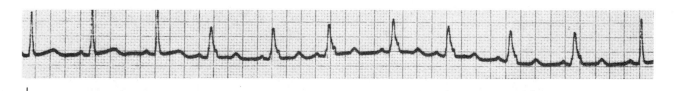

I

Fig. 5-84   Rate-dependent aberrancy of the LBBB type. Gradual acceleration of the sinus rate results in a functional LBBB that remains until the sinus rate slows sufficiently at the end of the tracing. This type of aberrancy is much more commonly of the LBBB rather than the RBBB type and is more apt to be associated with cardiac disease than functional RBBB.

Rate	60 to 78 beats/min.
Rhythm	Slightly irregular.
P waves	Normal.
PR interval	Normal and constant, 0.14 second.
QRS complex	Varies between normal and functional LBBB.

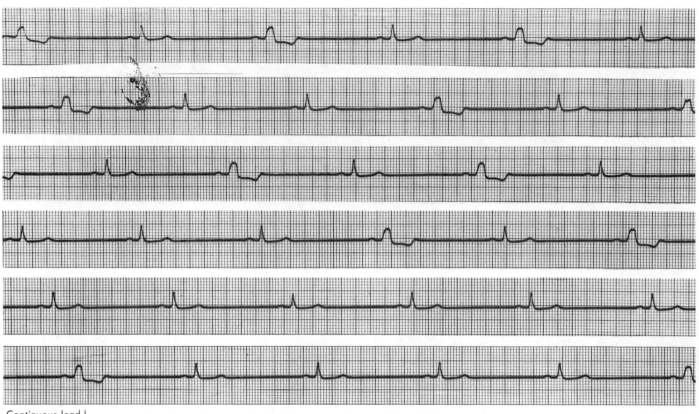

Continuous lead I

Fig. 5-85   Bradycardia-dependent LBBB. In this unusual tracing the patient has a sinus bradycardia. When the sinus cycle increases, the P wave conducts with a LBBB. Shorter sinus cycles are ended with a normally conducted QRS complex. Very small changes in the sinus rate account for these differences.

Rate	34 to 38 beats/min.
Rhythm	Fairly regular.
P waves	Normal and precede each QRS complex.
PR interval	0.19 second.
QRS	Normal and LBBB, 0.14 second.

dia. The following analysis may be helpful in distinguishing aberrant ventricular conduction initiated by a supraventricular impulse from ventricular tachycardia.

Identification of Atrial Activity

During sinus rhythm or an ectopic supraventricular rhythm, identification of distinct atrial activity initiating ventricular depolarization, regardless of how deformed the QRS complex may appear, establishes the diagnosis of supraventricular rhythm with QRS aberration. A casual relationship between the P wave and QRS complex may be demonstrated in one or more of the following ways, depending on the nature of the supraventricular rhythms:

1. P waves with a normal contour precede and maintain a constant relationship to each QRS complex during sinus rhythm.

2. Interventions that alter the sinus rate, such as carotid sinus massage or exercise, secondarily alter the ventricular rate in exactly the same manner and maintain the same or nearly the same PR interval. This indicates that ventricular activation follows as a consequence of atrial discharge. Atrial pacing can be used to alter the atrial rate during a tachycardia characterized by wide QRS complexes, and a diagnosis of ventricular tachycardia is considered likely when fusion and capture complexes result.

3. When atrial flutter, atrial fibrillation, or atrial tachycardia exists, carotid sinus massage or administration of digitalis, verapamil, or edrophonium chloride (Tensilon) produces characteristic slowing of the ventricular response (and at times normalizes the QRS complex); during AV nodal reentry or AVRT,

the rhythm may remain unchanged or terminate and allow sinus rhythm to resume.

4. Atrial and ventricular rhythms may be so related as to suggest dependency of the latter on the former (for example, during typical AV Wenckebach cycles).

5. When atria and ventricles are dissociated, finding ventricular captures that have the same contour as the QRS of the tachydysrhythmia in question indicates a supraventricular rhythm.

6. Bursts of an intermittent tachycardia, always initiated by a premature atrial complex, provide indirect evidence supporting a supraventricular diagnosis. However, it is important to remember that under certain circumstances a premature atrial complex can initiate a ventricular tachycardia.

7. During retrograde atrial capture, the RP interval is of too short a duration to be explained by retrograde conduction from a ventricular focus (about 0.10 second or less).

8. If the rate and rhythm of abnormal QRS complexes are the same as the rate and rhythm of a known supraventricular tachycardia, this provides some support in favor of aberration.

9. The presence of AV dissociation during a wide QRS tachycardia is much more consistent with ventricular than supraventricular tachycardias.

Analysis of QRS Contours and Intervals

The following clues suggest aberrant ventricular conduction initiated by a supraventricular impulse:

1. The contour of the QRS complex is a triphasic rsr′ in lead V_1. RBBB patterns occur more frequently than LBBB patterns because at a slower heart rate, the right bundle branch appears to require more time to repolarize than the left. Therefore premature discharge is more likely to encounter a refractory right bundle branch and produce RBBB.

2. Monophasic or diphasic complexes in lead V_1 or an LBBB pattern favor the diagnosis of ventricular tachycardia, as does a frontal QRS axis that is directed superiorly and to the right.

3. Faster rates speed repolarization, whereas slower rates retard it; the refractory period is proportional to the preceding cycle length. Therefore the heart takes longer to repolarize after a long cycle than it does after a short cycle. Because of this, when an early beat follows a long cycle, the early beat may encounter refractory tissue and conduct aberrantly. A comparison of such long-short cycle sequences aids in determining aberrant conduction.

4. During atrial flutter or fibrillation or a series of premature atrial complexes, aberrantly conducted beats persist in runs rather than maintain a bigeminal pattern and then lack a compensatory pause after their termination.

5. The initial vectors of aberrant and normal beats are similar during functional RBBB, since RBBB preserves the normal initial forces.

6. Aberrantly conducted supraventricular QRS complexes are not wildly bizarre or lengthened; most of the QRS prolongation occurs in the latter portion of the beat. QRS complexes with a duration exceeding 0.14 second are more likely to indicate ventricular tachycardia.

7. A fixed coupling interval between the normal and aberrant beats is absent during atrial flutter or atrial fibrillation. Conversely, fixed coupling during atrial flutter or fibrillation favors ventricular ectopy.

8. The aberrant beats are not excessively premature.

9. During a narrow QRS-complex supraventricular tachycardia (excluding atrial flutter and atrial fibrillation), the presence of alteration of QRS morphology favors the presence of a retrograde accessory pathway in the tachycardia circuit (that is, AVRT associated with preexcitation syndrome).[29]

10. The QRS configuration appears the same as that resulting from known supraventricular conduction at similar rates. Conversely, if the QRS contour is the same as that resulting from known ventricular conduction, the tachycardia is probably ventricular in origin.

11. Vagal maneuvers remain a most important differentiating point, since vagal discharge does not usually affect ventricular tachycardia, whereas it slows the ventricular rate in most supraventricular mechanisms. However, ventricular tachycardia terminated by vagal discharge has been reported.

12. The presence of fusion and capture beats (see p. 134) provides the most important evidence in favor of ventricular tachycardia. None of the aforementioned features can be used to unequivocally establish the diagnosis of ventricular tachycardia, and in many instances, invasive electrophysiologic studies must be performed.

Esophageal Pill Electrode

When wide, bizarre QRS complexes are present, a 12-lead ECG recorded from an esophageal electrode facilitates differential diagnosis.[30] The esophageal pill electrode affords a simple and precise method for obtaining such an ECG. This electrode is a disposable bipolar electrode housed in a gelatin capsule. Two thin, threadlike wires emerge from the electrode and facilitate its placement, attachment to the ECG, and ultimate retrieval. The capsule is easily swallowed by the patient. Optimum position within the esophagus is verified when maximum atrial voltage appears on the ECG. This simple device permits differentiation of supraventricular and ventricular dysrhythmias when a conclusive diagnosis cannot be made from the 12-lead ECG alone.

Moreover, the same electrode can also be used for therapeutic pacing after a definite diagnosis of a supraventricular tachydysrhythmia has been made. The pill electrode may be used for atrial or ventricular pacing, although success with atrial pacing has been more uniform than that with ventricular pacing.[31, 32]

ELECTROLYTE DISTURBANCES[33]
Potassium

During induced hyperkalemia in animals, the ECG correlates closely with the potassium blood level (Figs. 5-86 and 5-87). The T wave peaks when potassium concentration reaches about 5.5 mEq/L; the corrected QT interval is normal or shortens initially but may prolong as the QRS complex widens. The QRS complex may widen when the external potassium concentration exceeds 6.5 mEq/L; at about 7.0 mEq/L, P-wave amplitude diminishes, and P-wave and PR-interval duration are prolonged. At about 8.0 to 9.0 mEq/L, the P wave frequently disappears. Sometimes ST-segment deviation, both elevated and depressed, occurs and simulates an injury pattern. Clinically occurring potassium alterations do not correlate as well as during these experimental changes in animals, probably because the patient has multiple abnormalities that may influence the ECG differently. For example, in some studies, fewer than 25% of patients with hyperkalemia developed the characteristic tall, narrow, peaked T waves. It is believed that the extracellular potassium concentration accounts for the ECG patterns rather than changes in total body or intracellular potassium concentration.

During hypokalemic states, the ST segment becomes depressed, the U wave is exaggerated, and the T-wave amplitude is decreased without changing the duration of QT interval (as long as it can be measured accurately). Actually, the QU interval becomes prolonged. The P and QRS amplitude and duration may increase, and the PR interval may be prolonged. Clinical hypokalemia does not normally slow AV conduction significantly; however, isolated cases have been reported demonstrating varying degrees of PR prolongation. Intraventricular conduction in adults seldom lengthens by more than 20 msec, but it may be more prolonged in children.

Spontaneous hyperkalemia rarely if ever produces more advanced AV block than simple PR prolongation; large doses of potassium administered rapidly may produce further advanced forms of AV block, however. Often the P wave disappears, which precludes the diagnosis of AV block. As the plasma potassium level continues to rise to 6.5 to 7.0 mEq/L, slowed intraventricular conduction results, manifested by uniform widening of the QRS complex. Areas of intraventricular block may occur and lead to ventricular fibrillation.

Potassium may potentiate the slowing effects of digitalis on AV conduction, particularly if the plasma potassium level rises rapidly. However, if AV conduction is also hampered by a rapid atrial rate, slowing the atrial rate with potassium may improve AV conduction and offset any direct depressing effects of potassium. Fortunately, administration of potassium to patients with digitalis-induced dysrhythmias suppresses ectopic discharge at a much lower blood potassium level than that which further depresses AV conduction.

Low blood potassium levels encourage spontaneous ectopic pacemaker discharge, presumably by enhancing automaticity and also possibly by slowing dominant pacemakers or producing conduction defects. Low potassium levels may initiate ventricular fibrillation in humans. Reduced potassium concentration may precipitate dysrhythmias in animals and humans receiving digitalis at plasma potassium levels that ordinarily do not produce ectopic beating in the absence of digitalis. Possibly the synergistic effects of digitalis and reduced potassium on automaticity and conduction make animals and humans receiving digitalis particularly prone to dysrhythmias precipitated by hypokalemia.

The antidysrhythmic effects of potassium administration may suppress varied rhythms, regardless of cause and the presence or absence of hypokalemia. Digitalis-induced ectopic discharge generally responds to potassium therapy at sufficiently low doses to avoid further AV conduction delay. Many believe that potassium remains the drug of choice for ectopic rhythms produced by excessive digitalis. Animals and humans with elevated potassium levels may tolerate large doses of digitalis without developing ectopic dysrhythmias, whereas reduced potassium levels predispose to ectopic activity in animals or patients who have received digitalis. Also, a low level of potassium may worsen the depression of AV conduction produced by digitalis.

Sodium

In general the magnitude of sodium change necessary to produce ECG alterations is not compatible with life, making clinical ECG manifestations of sodium derangements rarely if ever seen.

Calcium

In the ECG, a low calcium level (Fig. 5-88) prolongs the duration of the ST segment and QT interval without prolonging the duration of the T wave, although the T wave may reverse polarity. An elevated calcium level shortens the ST segment and QT interval; the QRS duration may be prolonged during severe hypercalcemia, and AV block may develop. A high calcium level opposes the effects of a high potassium level, whereas a low calcium level opposes the effects of low potassium. If the calcium level varies in a direction opposite that of the potassium level, the effects of the latter are enhanced.

INVASIVE ELECTROPHYSIOLOGIC STUDIES[23]

Invasive electrophysiologic studies (Figs. 5-89 to 5-92) permit the direct study and manipulation of the electric ac-

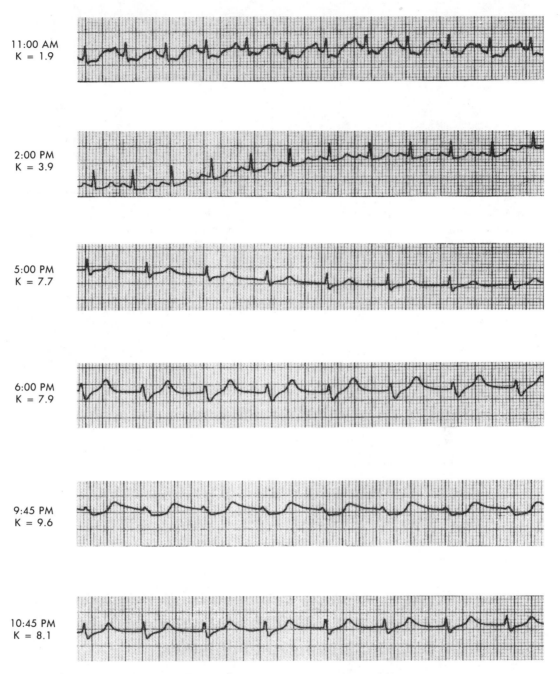

11:00 AM
K = 1.9

2:00 PM
K = 3.9

5:00 PM
K = 7.7

6:00 PM
K = 7.9

9:45 PM
K = 9.6

10:45 PM
K = 8.1

Fig. 5-86 Serial ECG tracings in a patient with marked changes in the serum potassium level. In the 11 AM tracing the depressed ST segment and low-amplitude T wave blending into a probable U wave (this cannot be seen with clarity because of the superimposed P waves) indicate the presence of hypokalemia. After administration of potassium, the 2 PM tracing becomes relatively normal. Continued potassium administration results in hyperkalemia with the disappearance of atrial activity on the ECG and some prolongation of the QRS complex. By 7 PM the QRS complex is more prolonged, and by 9:45 PM the QRS complex is greatly prolonged. Secondary ST-T wave changes are present. Improvement follows the administration of bicarbonate, glucose, and insulin at 10:45 PM with reduction in the serum potassium level; improvement in the ECG results. *K*, Potassium level.

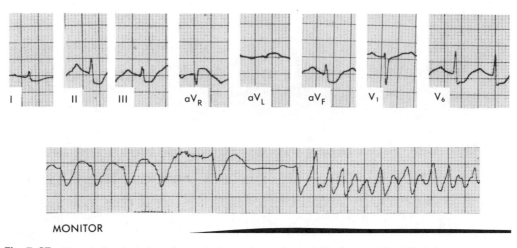

MONITOR

Fig. 5-87   Hypokalemia-induced ventricular tachycardia and fibrillation. The ECG demonstrates the characteristic changes of hypokalemia: depressed ST segment, low-amplitude T wave, and large U wave blending into the following P wave. In the monitor lead a ventricular tachycardia briefly stops and then degenerates into ventricular fibrillation that was reversed with DC shock.

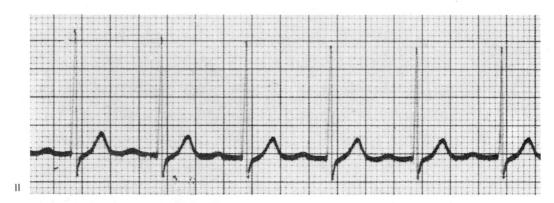

II

Fig. 5-88   The effects of hypercalcemia on the ECG. The serum calcium level is 14.0/100 ml. The ST segment and QT interval are shortened, and the PR interval is slightly prolonged (0.22 second).

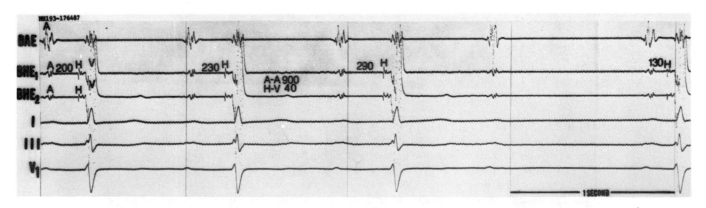

Fig. 5-89   Type I second-degree AV nodal block. Simultaneous recordings of electrograms from the high right atrium *(BAE)* and bundle of His *(BHE₁, BHE₂)* and scalar leads I, III, and V₁ are displayed during normal sinus rhythm. The PR interval progressively lengthens until the fourth P wave fails to conduct. The conduction delay is caused by AH-interval prolongation that increases from 200 msec in the first beat shown (not the first beat in this Wenckebach series) to 290 msec just before the block. The AH interval then shortens to 130 msec in the first beat of the next Wenckebach series. The nonconducted P wave blocks proximal to the bundle of His.

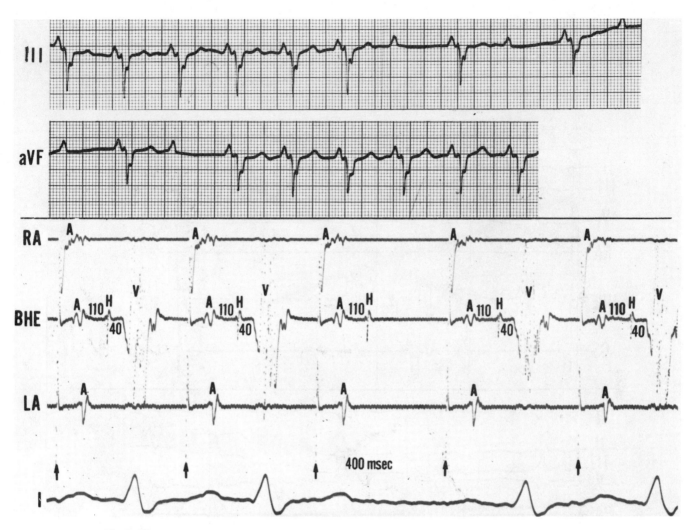

Fig. 5-90 Type II second-degree AV block. The scalar recordings in the top portion of the figure (leads III and aV$_F$) demonstrate type II second-degree AV block characterized by a fixed PR interval preceding the nonconducted P wave. During the electrophysiologic study *(bottom)*, right atrial pacing at a cycle length of 400 msec resulted in a fixed AH interval of 110 msec and HV interval of 40 msec. The third P wave *(A)* blocked distal to the bundle of His recording site, characteristic of type II second-degree AV block. *LA,* Left atrial electrogram; *arrows,* stimuli delivered to right atrium.

tivity of the heart by using electrodes placed inside the cardiac chambers.[34] The technique to record bundle of His activation involves passing an electrode catheter, which is introduced percutaneously into the femoral vein, in a cephalad direction up the inferior vena cava and positioning the catheter tip near the septal leaflet of the tricuspid valve. The bundle of His potential appears as a well-defined, most often bipolar spike between the low right atrial and ventricular electrograms. The interval between the earliest onset of the surface P wave or a high right atrial deflection and the low right atrial deflection (P wave–A wave [PA] interval) is a measure of intraatrial conduction. The atriohisian (AH) interval is a measurement of conduction across the AV node and varies in duration from 55 to 130

msec, depending on the cycle length and autonomic influences. The interval from the bundle of His to the ventricle (HV interval) is determined by the interval between the bundle of His deflection and the earliest ventricular activity recorded in any lead. This interval is a measure of conduction through the bundle of His distal to the recording electrode, the bundle branches, and the Purkinje system to the point of ventricular activation. In contrast to a relatively wide range of values for the AH interval, the HV interval is fairly constant, measuring 30 to 55 msec, with an average value of 45 msec. In some patients, discharge of the right bundle branch may be recorded.

The ability to separate AV nodal and His-Purkinje conduction has enhanced understanding of normal and ab-

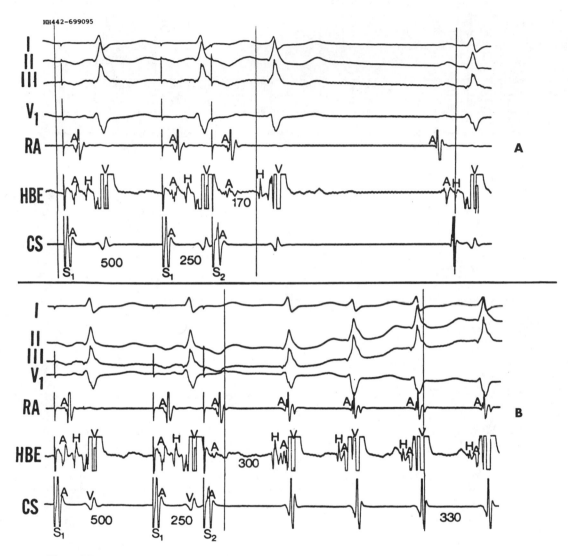

Fig. 5-91   Precipitation of AV nodal reentrant, supraventricular tachycardia. **A,** Recordings were obtained simultaneously from scalar leads I, II, III, and V₁ and intracavitary recordings from the right atrium *(RA)*, bundle of His area *(HBE)*, and coronary sinus *(CS)*. The coronary sinus was stimulated at a fixed cycle length of 500 msec (S₁ to S₁) and then stimulated prematurely (S₂) at a cycle length of 250 msec. The AH interval lengthened slightly to 170 msec, but tachycardia did not result. **B,** Premature stimulation at the same coupling interval produced an AH interval of 300 msec and precipitation of a supraventricular tachycardia caused by AV nodal reentry at a cycle length of 330 msec (rate: 182 beats/min). Findings are consistent with "dual AV nodal" pathways.

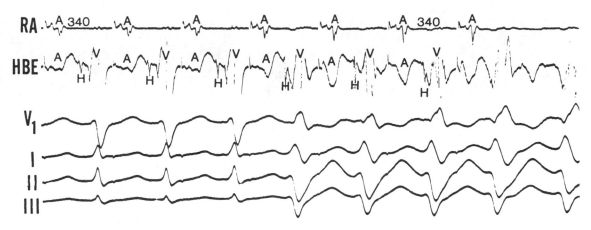

Fig. 5-92 Precipitation of ventricular tachycardia during right atrial pacing. In the left portion of the tracing the right atrium *(RA)* was paced at a cycle length of 340 msec. After the third normally conducted QRS complex, ventricular conduction becomes abnormally prolonged. The HV interval shortens, AV dissociation results, and the ventricular tachycardia continues after cessation of atrial pacing *(top right)*. These findings are consistent with a ventricular tachycardia initiated during atrial stimulation. The tracing was recorded in an 18-year-old man who had exercise-induced ventricular tachycardia. *HBE,* His bundle area.

normal AV conduction. Abnormal AV conduction may be caused by prolongation of PA, AH, or HV intervals or all three. In addition, intra-His block has been demonstrated. During type I second-degree AV block in a patient with a normal QRS complex, the conduction disturbance occurs at the AV node, proximal to the bundle of His (Fig. 5-89). Type II second-degree AV block in a patient with a bundle branch block virtually always results distal to the bundle of His (Fig. 5-90). Thus in type I second-degree AV block the blocked P wave is not followed by a His spike, whereas in type II second-degree AV block the blocked P wave is followed by a His spike.

Insertion of two to five electrode catheters permits recording and stimulating from multiple atrial and ventricular sites and has been useful in differentiating ventricular tachycardia and aberrant ventricular conduction, in understanding the nature of many supraventricular and ventricular tachycardias and other dysrhythmias, in evaluating patients with the preexcitation syndrome or AV block, and in other areas as well, such as in initiating tachydysrhythmias in susceptible patients (Figs. 5-91 and 5-92). Significantly, adequacy of therapy can be judged by precipitating the tachycardia in a control state and then attempting to restart it during therapy. Catheters are used for therapy to ablate sites important for the genesis and/or maintenance of the dysrhythmia as well as for diagnostic purposes. Although areas of application of these electrophysiologic studies are still evolving, fairly definitive indications can be stated.

Artifacts (Figs. 5-93 and 5-94)

Electronic instrumentation has provided vast dividends to the care of patients with heart disease. However, because practice now relies so heavily on various types of monitoring devices, the clinician must constantly be alert and recognize artifacts that mimic dysrhythmias. A tracing that resembles ventricular fibrillation must be artifactual if the patient is sitting up in bed in no distress and reading a newspaper. The cardinal rule is to treat the patient and not the monitor.

DYSRHYTHMIA TEST SECTION

It is suggested that the reader use this section to test knowledge of dysrhythmias. Cover the interpretations in each legend, calculate intervals and irregularities as previously discussed, and determine the diagnosis. Consider also the significance of each dysrhythmia and what form of treatment would most likely be used. There may be disagreements in interpretation of rhythm strips, but the essential point is to make your diagnosis by using the analytic method described in this chapter. This approach offers a justification for your interpretation.

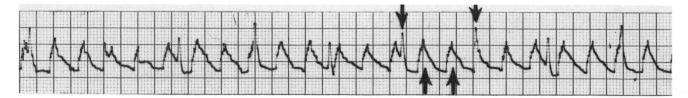

Fig. 5-93   Toothbrush tachycardia. This tracing was recorded from a patient brushing his teeth with an electric toothbrush at a rate of 188 brushes/min. Note the regularly occurring artifacts *(upright arrows)* that do not influence the QRS complexes *(inverted arrows)*.

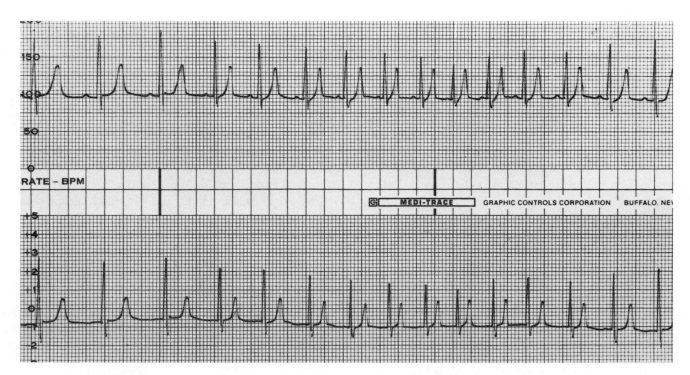

Fig. 5-94   Artifact simulating onset of supraventricular tachycardia. During playback of a tape-recorded ECG rhythm, the rate of revolutions per minute of the tape slowed and simulated the onset of a supraventricular tachycardia. The diagnosis of artifact is easily made, since in addition to shortening of the R-R interval, the PR, QRS, and QT intervals all decrease markedly. Both leads recorded simultaneously.

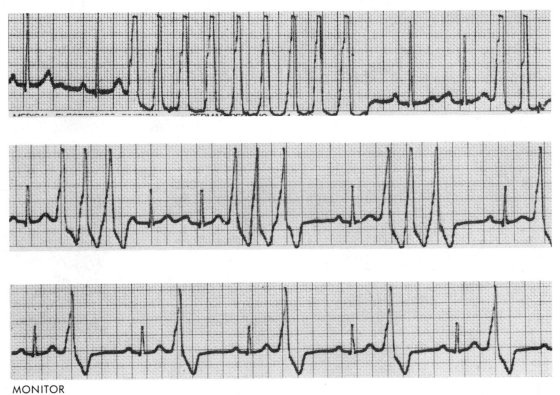

MONITOR

Fig. 5-95

Rate	Atrial, 60 to 75 beats/min; ventricular, 170 to 210 beats/min.
Rhythm	Atrial, slightly irregular; ventricular, irregular because of bursts of ventricular ectopy.
P waves	Normal for the sinus-initiated QRS complexes.
PR interval	Normal for the sinus-initiated QRS complexes, 0.16 second.
QRS complex	Normal for the sinus-initiated QRS complexes; wide, bizarre, prolonged (0.12 second) for ventricular ectopy.
Dysrhythmia	Paroxysmal ventricular tachycardia gradually decreasing in frequency to bigeminy and then complete disappearance. This result followed administration of lidocaine (50 mg intravenously) in a patient with an acute myocardial infarction.

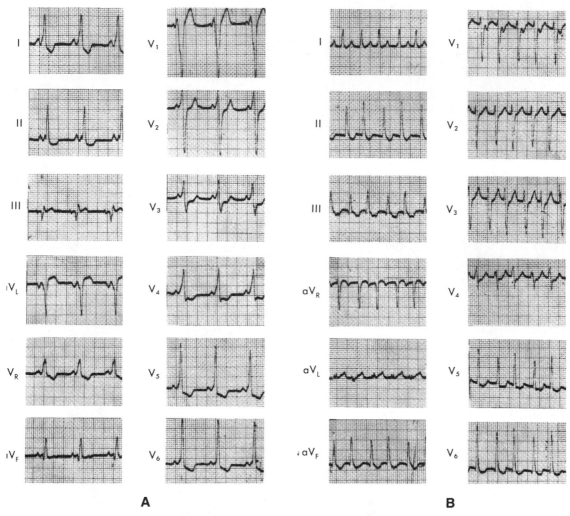

A

B

Fig. 5-96

Rate	**A,** 82 beats/min; **B,** varying between 150 and 180 beats/min.
Rhythm	**A,** Regular; **B,** slight variation in R-R intervals with long cycles alternating with short cycles.
P waves	**A,** Normal; **B,** retrograde; see lead V_1.
PR interval	**A,** 0.08 second; **B,** RP interval 0.12 second.
QRS complex	**A,** Prolonged, 0.12 second; **B,** normal, 0.08 second.
Dysrhythmia	**A,** Normal sinus rhythm during preexcitation syndrome; **B,** AVRT in the same patient.

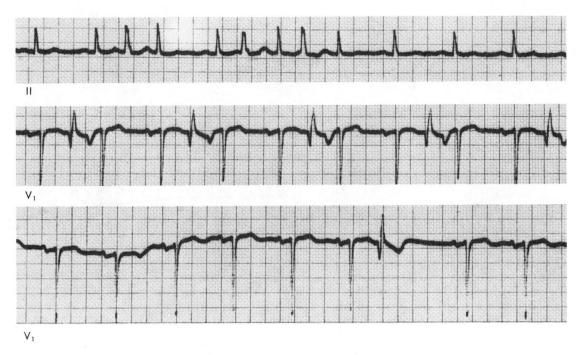

II

V₁

V₁

Fig. 5-97

Rate	75 beats/min, with premature complexes.
Rhythm	Irregular because of premature complexes.
P waves	Normal and precede each of the normal QRS complexes.
PR interval	Prolonged after the premature complexes.
QRS complex	Normal for sinus-initiated complexes; prolonged to almost 0.12 second for premature complexes.
Dysrhythmia	Interpolated premature ventricular complexes in the top and middle tracings. In the bottom tracing, premature ventricular complexes produce a compensatory pause and are therefore no longer interpolated.

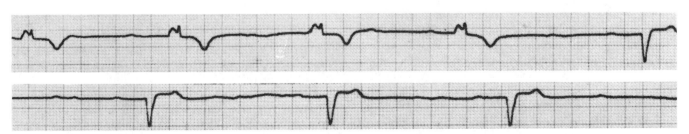

Continuous—MONITOR

Fig. 5-98

Rate	Atrial, 86 beats/min; ventricular, upright complexes at 38 beats/min and negative complexes at 28 beats/min.
Rhythm	Atrial, regular; ventricular, fairly regular.
P waves	Normal and have no relationship to the QRS complexes. Clear P waves cannot be seen throughout the entire tracing.
PR interval	Not measurable.
QRS complex	Abnormal; upright complexes at 0.14 second, negative complexes at 0.12 second.
Dysrhythmia	Complete AV block with a ventricular escape rhythm. The simultaneous change in ventricular contour and rate probably indicates a shift in the ventricular escape focus site.

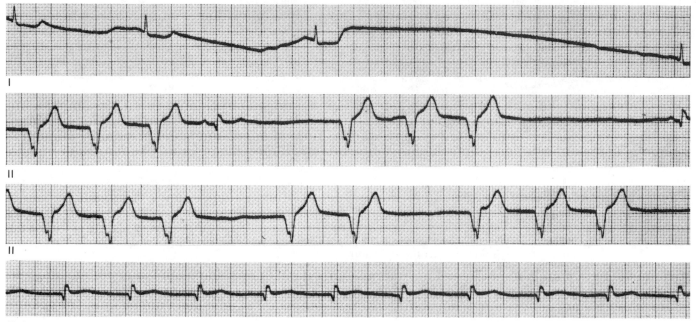

I

II

II

II Atropine, 0.75 mg IV

Fig. 5-99

Rate	Top tracing, slow with periods of asystole. Middle two tracings, 75 beats/min with periods of asystole. Bottom tracing, 65 beats/min.
Rhythm	Top three tracings, irregular; bottom tracing, regular.
P waves	Normal contour, preceding the sinus-initiated QRS complexes in lead II but hard to see in lead I.
PR interval	Normal for the sinus-initiated P waves, not present for the other QRS complexes. In the bottom tracing, no P wave or PR interval is apparent.
QRS complex	Normal for the sinus-initiated QRS complexes, prolonged (0.13 second) for the ventricular ectopic beats.
Dysrhythmia	Various dysrhythmias recorded in a patient with an acute inferior myocardial infarction. Top tracing, marked sinus bradycardia and periods of sinus arrest. Middle two tracings, an accelerated idioventricular rhythm, slightly irregular. The duration of the pauses in the third strip appears to be a multiple of the basic idioventricular cycle length, thus suggesting a possible intermittent exit block. Bottom tracing, a junctional rhythm after atropine administration suppresses the ventricular ectopy.

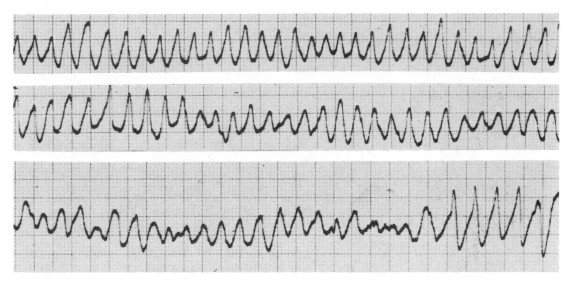

MONITOR

Fig. 5-100

Rate	300 to 500 beats/min.
Rhythm	Grossly irregular.
P waves	None seen.
PR interval	Not measurable.
QRS complex	Wide, bizarre, irregular.
Dysrhythmia	Ventricular flutter that becomes ventricular fibrillation in the bottom tracing. The ventricular fibrillation then seems to organize and merge into ventricular flutter or possibly ventricular tachycardia in the terminal portion of the tracing.

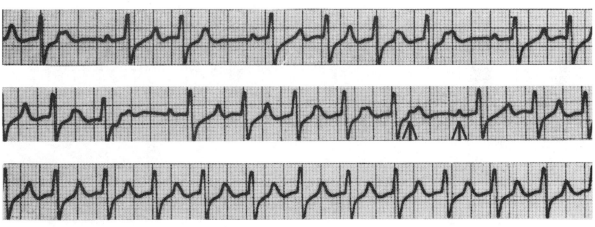

MONITOR

Fig. 5-101

Rate	Atrial, 115 beats/min; ventricular, varying, depending on the degree of block.
Rhythm	Atrial, regular; ventricular, irregular.
P waves	Precede each of the QRS complexes *(arrows)*.
PR intervals	Progressively lengthens until one P wave fails to conduct (type I second-degree AV block).
QRS complex	Normal (0.08 second).
Dysrhythmia	Atrial tachycardia with varying block. Note the varying T-wave contour as P waves fall during portions of the antecedent T wave. In the bottom tracing 1:1 AV conduction occurs.

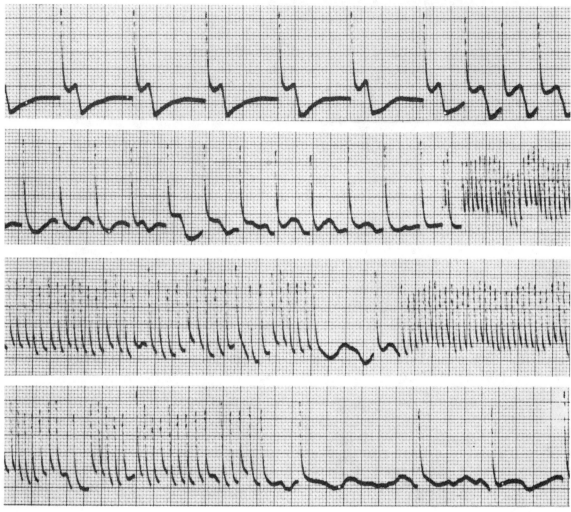

MONITOR

Fig. 5-102

Rate	Ventricular, 75 beats/min to very rapid rates.
Rhythm	Ventricular, periods of regularity replaced by gross irregularity.
P waves	None seen.
PR interval	Not measurable.
QRS complex	Wide, distorted, initiated by pacemaker spikes.
Dysrhythmia	Runaway pacemaker discharging at irregular and extremely rapid rates and finally initiating ventricular fibrillation. The pacemaker rate sped from 71 beats/min to approximately 145 beats/min and then greater than 1000 stimuli/min.

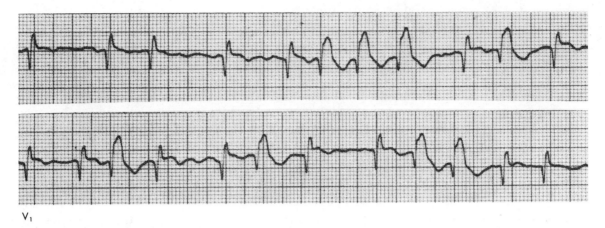

V_1

Fig. 5-103

Rate	Ventricular, 73 to 180 beats/min.
Rhythm	Ventricular, grossly irregular.
P waves	None seen.
PR interval	Not measurable.
QRS complex	Normal (0.08 second) and abnormal (0.12 second) with an RBBB contour.
Dysrhythmia	Atrial fibrillation with a rapid ventricular response. QRS complexes, which demonstrate an RBBB, terminate a short cycle or a series of short cycles that follow a long preceding cycle. The development of functional RBBB caused by cycle length changes in this fashion is called the *Ashman phenomenon*.

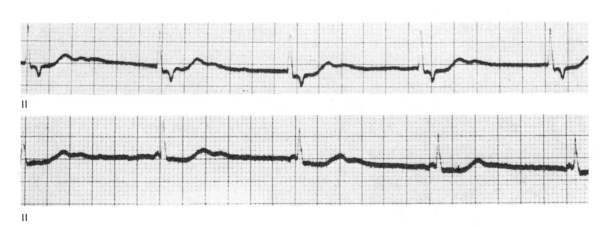

II

II

Fig. 5-104

Rate	*Top*, 52 beats/min.
Rhythm	Regular.
P waves	Retrograde.
PR interval	*Bottom*, 0.06 second.
RP interval	*Top*, 0.08 second.
QRS complex	Normal (0.06 second).
Dysrhythmia	AV junctional rhythm recorded on two occasions in the same patient. In the top tracing, retrograde P waves followed the QRS complex; in the bottom tracing, retrograde P waves preceded the QRS complex.

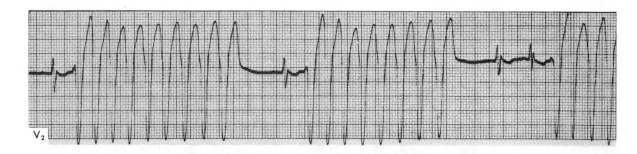

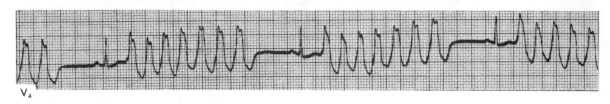

Fig. 5-105

Rate	Ventricular, 250 beats/min.
Rhythm	Ventricular, regular in a recurrent paroxysmal fashion.
P waves	Precede the normally conducted QRS complexes.
PR interval	Normal for the normally conducted QRS complexes.
QRS complex	Normal for the sinus-initiated QRS complexes, QRS complex prolonged for the ventricular ectopic systoles (0.14 second).
Dysrhythmia	Repetitive monomorphic ventricular tachycardia. Lack of fusion or capture beats and precise determination of atrial activity during tachycardia prevent an unequivocal diagnosis of ventricular tachycardia from this tracing, although the diagnosis is highly suggestive.

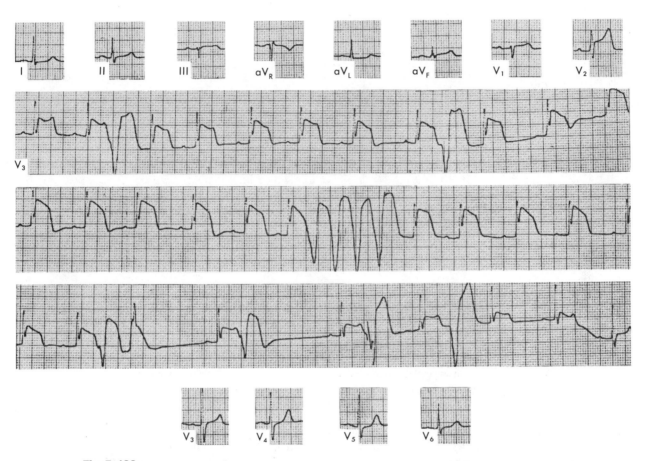

Fig. 5-106

Rate	During lead V_3, approximately 75 beats/min, interrupted by ventricular ectopy.
Rhythm	Fairly regular except when interrupted by ventricular ectopy.
P waves	Normal and precede each of the normally conducted QRS complexes.
PR interval	Normal (0.16 second) and constant.
QRS complex	Note abrupt ST-segment elevation between leads V_1 and V_2 and during lead V_3. Lead V_3 at the bottom shows a normal ST segment. Abnormal complexes have a QRS duration greater than 0.12 second.
Dysrhythmia	Atypical (Prinzmetal) angina pectoris characterized by ST-segment *elevation* probably is a result of coronary artery bypass. Premature ventricular complexes trigger a short run of ventricular tachycardia in the midportion of the tracing. ST segments return to the baseline as the chest pain abates and the ectopic ventricular activity ceases.

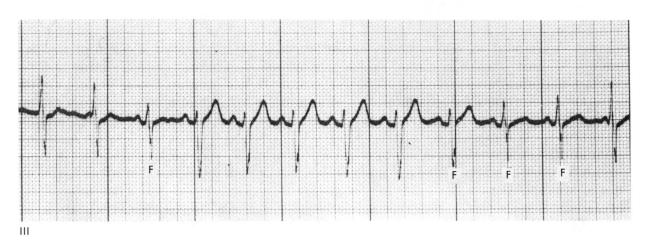

III

Fig. 5-107

Rate	107 beats/min.
Rhythm	Regular.
P waves	Normal and precede each of the QRS complexes in the midportion of the tracing.
PR interval	Constant (0.16 second) for the QRS complexes in the midportion of the tracing.
QRS complex	Normal duration (0.08 second) for both types of QRS complexes, *F,* Fusion QRS complexes.
Dysrhythmia	Ventricular tachycardia at beginning and end of tracing, which generates QRS complexes with a slightly different contour than during sinus tachycardia that occurs in the midportion of the tracing. The supraventricular origin of the tachycardia is suggested by the QRS duration (less than 0.12 second). However, recent data suggest that such a tachycardia may be ventricular, originating in the upper portions of the fascicular system and generating a QRS complex with a duration less than 0.12 second. The presence of fusion beats *(F)* supports this conclusion. In any event, during the tachycardia at the beginning and end of the ECG, QRS complexes are not related to atrial activity. Thus AV dissociation is present because of ventricular tachycardia. In the midportion of the tracing, slight acceleration of the sinus rate allows the sinus node to regain capture of the ventricles, suppress the tachycardia, and eliminate the periods of AV dissociation.

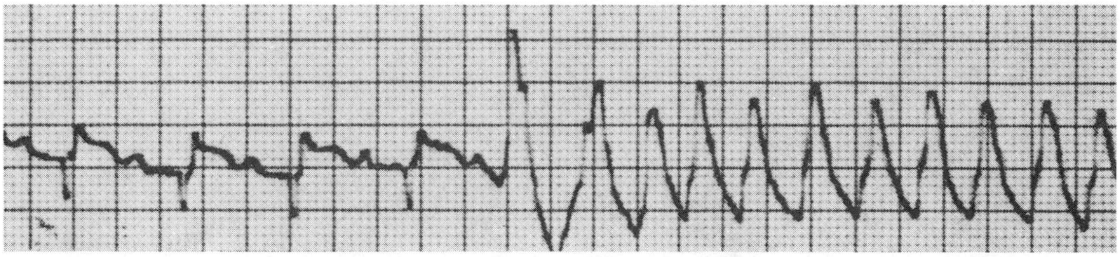

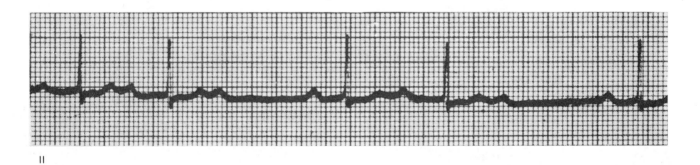

MONITOR

Fig. 5-108

Rate	Atrial, 110 beats/min; ventricular, 230 beats/min.
Rhythm	Regular.
P waves	Precede the normal QRS complexes but not seen during the tachycardia to the right.
PR interval	0.24 second, preceding the normal QRS complexes; not measurable during the tachycardia.
QRS complex	Normal (0.07 second) for the sinus-initiated QRS complexes; prolonged (0.14 second) during the tachycardia.
Dysrhythmia	Ventricular tachycardia that began in this patient who experienced an acute myocardial infarction without preexisting or precipitating ventricular complexes. Although it is possible that the P wave preceding the widened QRS complex initiates a supraventricular tachycardia with aberration, it is unlikely.

II

Fig. 5-109

Rate	Atrial, 75 beats/min; ventricular, 3:2 conduction, average 50 beats/min.
Rhythm	Atrial, regular; ventricular, irregular.
P waves	Normal and precede each QRS complex.
PR interval	Progressively lengthens before the nonconducted P wave.
QRS complex	Normal (0.06 second).
Dysrhythmia	Type I second-degree AV block.

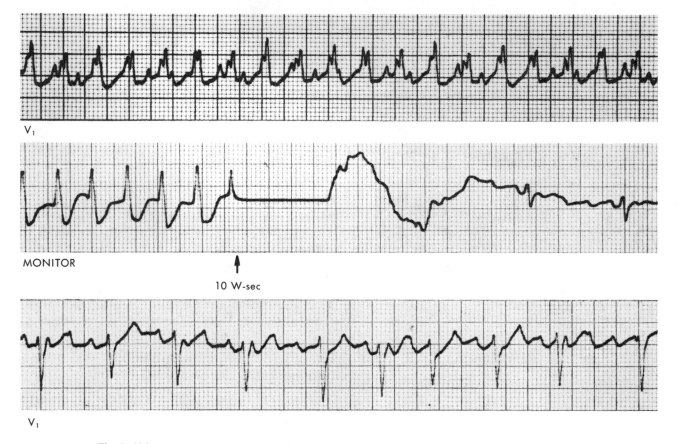

V₁

MONITOR

↑

10 W-sec

V₁

Fig. 5-110

Rate	Atrial, 300 beats/min *(top)*; ventricular, 200 beats/min *(top)*.
Rhythm	Atrial, regular; ventricular, regular.
P waves	Atrial flutter.
PR interval	Completely variable.
QRS complex	Wide, prolonged (0.12 second).
Dysrhythmia	Atrial flutter and ventricular tachycardia in top tracing (lead V₁). Thus complete AV dissociation is present. In the monitor recording (middle tracing) the left portion reflects the same activity seen in lead V₁. However, the particular monitor lead fails to reveal the atrial flutter waves. DC cardioversion *(arrow,* 10 joules) terminates the ventricular tachycardia but allows the atrial flutter to persist, seen more clearly in lead V₁ below. The atrial flutter at this point is not as precisely regular as it was before the cardioversion.

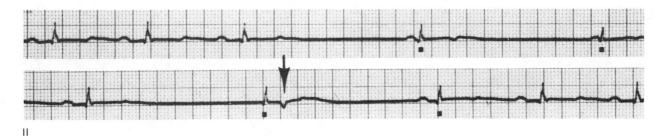

II

Fig. 5-111

Rate	30 to 50 beats/min.
Rhythm	Fairly irregular.
P waves	Precede and conduct to the QRS complexes that do not have dots beneath them. Those with dots beneath them are junctional escape beats.
PR interval	Prolonged (0.26 second) and constant for the QRS complexes that do not have a dot beneath them.
QRS complex	Normal duration and contour (0.08 second). Dots indicate AV junctional escape beats. The third AV junctional escape beat (lower tracing) retrogradely activates the atrium *(arrow)*.
Dysrhythmia	Sinus bradycardia with intermittent sinus arrest and AV junctional escape beats, the sick sinus syndrome.

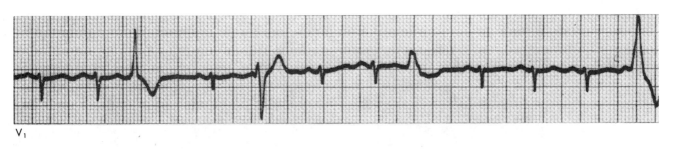

V₁

Fig. 5-112

Rate	98 beats/min.
Rhythm	Irregular because of premature ventricular systoles.
P waves	Normal and precede each sinus-initiated QRS complex.
PR interval	Normal for the sinus-initiated QRS complexes (0.14 second).
QRS complex	Normal for the sinus-initiated QRS complexes (0.08 second). Premature systoles are characterized by varied contour and a duration greater than 0.12 second.
Dysrhythmia	Multiform premature ventricular complexes with four different contours.

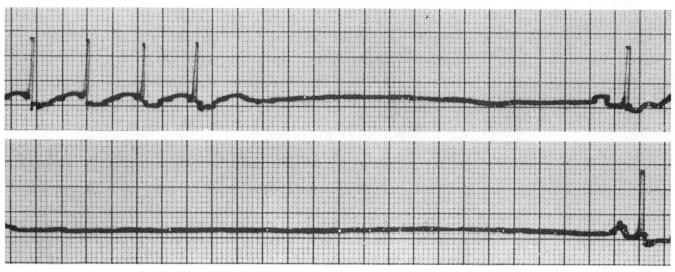

MONITOR

Fig. 5-113

Rate	140 beats/min, abruptly slowing after carotid sinus massage. Two periods of asystole are finally terminated by sinus rhythm.
Rhythm	Regular, followed by asystole, an atrial escape beat, and then sinus rhythm.
P waves	Can be seen when tachycardia terminates.
PR interval	Normal (0.18 second) in beats preceded by P waves.
QRS complex	Normal.
Dysrhythmia	Abrupt termination of paroxysmal supraventricular tachycardia by carotid sinus massage (at beginning of recording). A lengthy period of asystole results when the tachycardia stops, before sinus rhythm resumes.

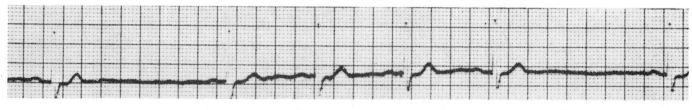

II

Fig. 5-114

Rate	33 to 66 beats/min.
Rhythm	Irregular.
P waves	Normal contour. Long P-P cycles are exactly twice the short P-P cycles.
PR interval	Normal (0.20 second).
QRS complex	Normal (0.08 second).
Dysrhythmia	2:1 sinus exit block.

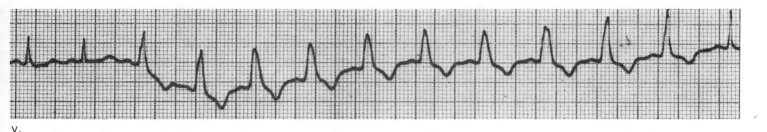

V₆

Fig. 5-115

Rate	Gradually accelerates from 105 to 115 beats/min.
Rhythm	Fairly regular.
P waves	Normal and precede each QRS complex.
PR interval	Normal (0.14 second) and constant.
QRS complex	Normal at the slower rates; LBBB (0.12 second) at the faster rates.
Dysrhythmia	Rate-dependent aberration with functional LBBB.

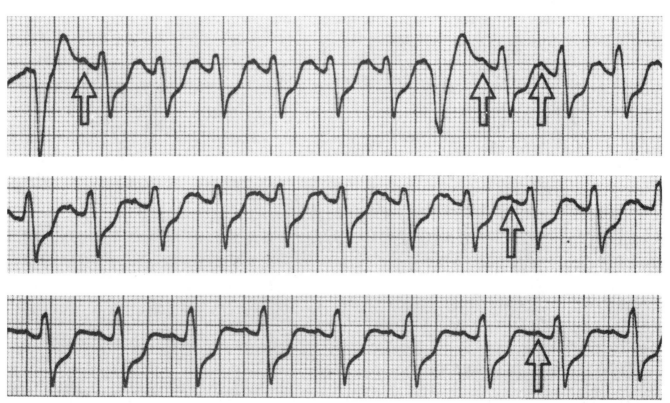

II—noncontinuous

Fig. 5-116

Rate	125 beats/min in top tracing; gradually slows to 100 beats/min in bottom tracing.
Rhythm	Regular.
P waves	Normal, but hidden by preceding T waves *(arrows).*
PR interval	0.16 second.
QRS complex	Abnormal, prolonged (0.14 second) because of the presence of a preexisting LBBB.
Dysrhythmia	Sinus tachycardia. Patient has a preexisting bundle branch block. Clear P waves *(arrows)* can be seen in the pause that follows the two premature ventricular complexes (top tracing). The heart rate gradually slowed after edrophonium (Tensilon) administration (middle and bottom tracings).

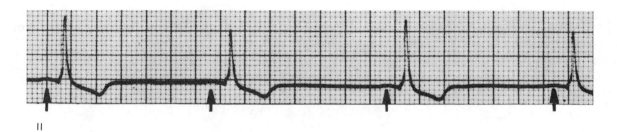

II

Fig. 5-117

Rate	41 beats/min.
Rhythm	Fairly regular.
P waves	Precede each QRS with a normal contour.
PR interval	0.16 second.
QRS complex	Borderline prolonged (0.11 second).
Dysrhythmia	Sinus bradycardia. Patient is receiving methyldopa for hypertension. Normal rate was restored after discontinuation of methyldopa therapy. Low-amplitude P waves indicated by arrows.

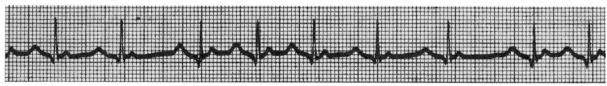

II

Fig. 5-118

Rate	Sinus rate increases with inspiration and decreases with expiration (70 to 110 beats/min).
Rhythm	Irregular with a repetitive phasic variation in cycle length according to respiratory cycles. Cycle lengths vary by more than 0.16 second. Breath-holding eliminates rate variations.
P waves	Precede each QRS with a normal, fairly constant contour.
PR interval	0.12 second.
QRS complex	Normal (0.08 second).
Dysrhythmia	Respiratory sinus dysrhythmia. The phasic variation corresponds to a respiratory rate of approximately 18 breaths/min.

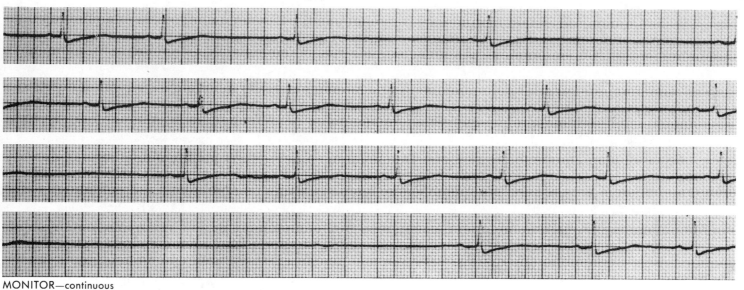

MONITOR—continuous

Fig. 5-119

Rate	Varying, slow (maximum rate of 5 beats/min).
Rhythm	Irregular; periods of asystole not a multiple of basic sinus cycle length.
P waves	Precede each QRS with a normal contour; may be altered by escape beats.
PR interval	Slightly prolonged (0.21 second).
QRS complex	Normal (0.09 second).
Dysrhythmia	Sinus arrest. Patient also has an acute inferior myocardial infarction. Asystolic intervals are not interrupted by escape beats.

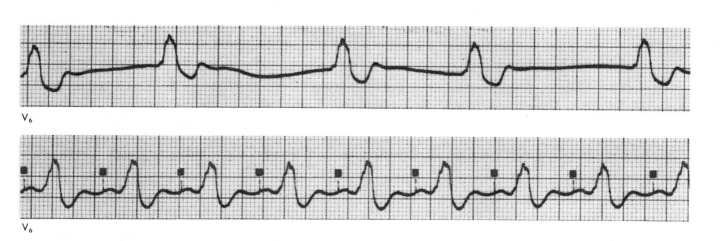

V_6

V_6

Fig. 5-120

Rate	Varying, slow (36 to 50 beats/min) *(top)*; normal (81 beats/min) *(bottom)*.
Rhythm	Irregular *(top)*; regular *(bottom)*.
P waves	Not seen *(top)*; follows pacemaker stimulus *(bottom)*.
PR interval	Not measurable *(top)*; 0.16 second *(bottom)*.
QRS complex	LBBB (0.20 second).
Dysrhythmia	Sinus arrest *(top)* and right atrial pacing *(bottom)*. Patient also has an LBBB. A supraventricular escape focus controls the rhythm in the top panel, but atrial activity is not apparent. Atrial pacing (stimuli indicated by filled squares, bottom tracing) results in atrial capture, producing a P wave and an unchanged QRS contour.

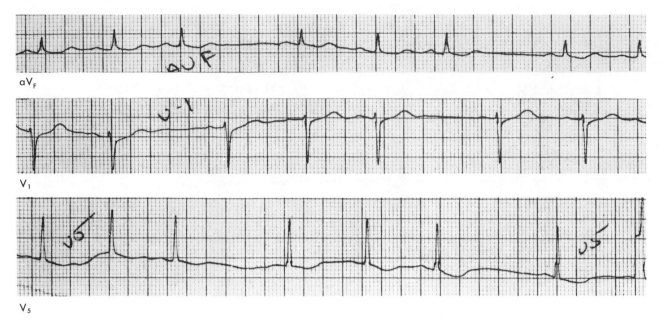

aV_F

V_1

V_5

Fig. 5-121

Rate	Varying, slow (50 to 88 beats/min).
Rhythm	A pause in atrial activity occurs. The P-P interval progressively shortens until the pause. The duration of the pause is less than twice the shortest P-P interval. The P-P interval after the pause exceeds the P-P interval preceding the pause.
P waves	Contour normal, precede each QRS complex; intermittent loss of P wave.
PR interval	Normal, constant (0.20 second).
QRS complex	Normal (0.08 second).
Dysrhythmia	Sinus exit block (type I). The four characteristic rhythm changes of this tracing allow the diagnosis of a type I exit block from the sinus node.

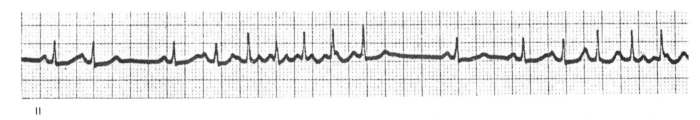

II

Fig. 5-122

Rate	Varying.
Rhythm	Irregular because of premature atrial complexes.
P waves	Premature atrial complexes have different contour; some are buried in preceding T wave.
PR interval (of atrial systole)	0.14 second.
QRS complex	Generally normal; may be aberrantly conducted (normal, 0.08 second).
Dysrhythmia	Single and multiple premature atrial complexes can be seen hidden with preceding T waves and appear to initiate short bursts of anatrial tachydysrhythmia, probably atrial flutter-fibrillation.

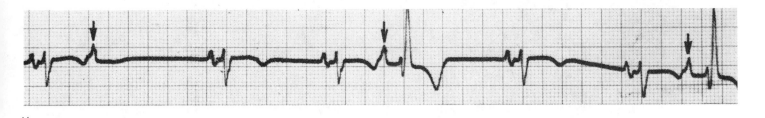

V₁

Fig. 5-123

Rate	Slow, because of nonconducted premature atrial complexes.
Rhythm	Irregular.
P waves	Premature atrial complexes have different contour and are buried in preceding T wave *(arrows)*.
PR interval (of premature atrial systoles)	First two premature atrial complexes are completely blocked; third and fourth premature atrial systoles conduct with a prolonged PR interval (0.21 second).
QRS complex	Third and fourth premature atrial complexes initiate aberrantly conducted QRS complex with an RBBB pattern.
Dysrhythmia	Nonconducted premature atrial complexes and premature atrial complexes initiating functional RBBB. Sinus-initiated P waves are abnormal and suggest left atrial enlargement. Premature atrial complexes *(arrows)* can be seen hidden in the preceding T waves. The first two premature atrial complexes are blocked and generate a pause in the ventricular rhythm. The second two premature atrial complexes conduct to the ventricle with a prolonged PR interval and initiate a functional RBBB.

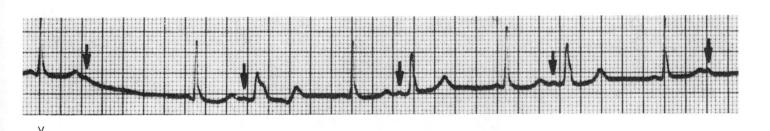

V₆

Fig. 5-124

Rate	Varying.
Rhythm	Irregular because of premature atrial complexes.
P waves	Premature atrial complexes have different contour and look like U waves *(arrows)*.
PR interval (of premature atrial complexes)	Later premature atrial complexes (second, third, and fourth) conduct, whereas early premature atrial complexes (first, fifth, and sixth) fail to reach the ventricles.
QRS complex	Second, third, and fourth premature atrial complexes produce varying degrees of LBBB.
Dysrhythmia	Nonconducted premature atrial complexes and premature atrial complexes that produce a functional LBBB. Premature atrial complexes can be seen in the terminal portion of the preceding T waves and look like the U wave *(arrows)*. Fairly early premature atrial complexes block, whereas slightly later premature atrial complexes conduct to the ventricles with an increase in PR interval and varying degrees of LBBB.

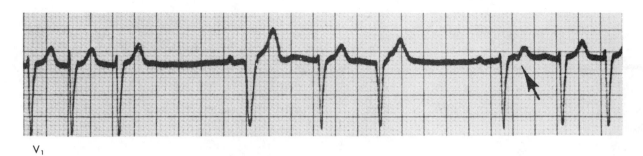

V₁

Fig. 5-125

Rate	150 beats/min.
Rhythm	Varying.
P waves	Not seen consistently.
PR interval	Cannot determine.
QRS complex	0.08 second.
Dysrhythmia	Paroxysmal supraventricular tachycardia. Paroxysmal supraventricular tachycardia suddenly terminates, begins briefly, stops, and then restarts again after a premature atrial complex *(arrow)* that conducts with a prolonged PR interval.

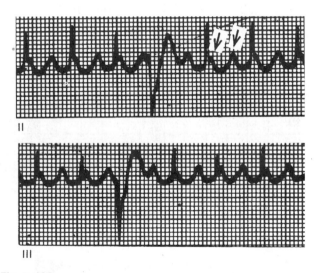

II

III

Fig. 5-126

Rate	Atrial, 280 beats/min; ventricular, 140 beats/min.
Rhythm	Atrial, regular; ventricular, 2:1.
P waves	Flutter waves with regular oscillations resembling a sawtooth pattern.
PR interval	Flutter-R interval is constant.
QRS complex	Normal (0.08 second).
Dysrhythmia	Uncommon form of atrial flutter. Flutter waves indicated by arrows. Single premature ventricular complex occurs in each lead. The conduction ratio is 2:1; that is, flutter waves are conducted alternately to the ventricle.

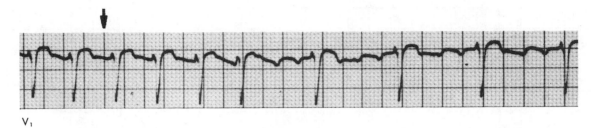

V₁

Fig. 5-127

Rate	Atrial, 300 beats/min; ventricular, 150 beats/min decreasing to 75 beats/min.
Rhythm	Atrial, regular; ventricular, regular.
P waves	Flutter waves clearly seen after carotid sinus massage *(arrows)* decreases the ventricular response.
PR interval	Flutter-R interval fairly constant.
QRS complex	Normal (0.08 second).
Dysrhythmia	Atrial flutter. Atrial flutter with a 2:1 ventricular response is present in the left portion of the tracing but cannot be clearly diagnosed from this lead. At the arrow, carotid sinus massage increases the degree of AV block to 4:1 and clearly exposes the atrial flutter waves.

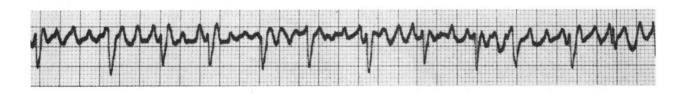

V₁

Fig. 5-128

Rate	Atrial, 300 to 500 beats/min; ventricular, 72 to 150 beats/min.
Rhythm	Atrial, irregular; ventricular, irregular.
P waves	Variability in the contour and spacing of the flutter-fibrillation waves.
PR interval	Nonmeasurable.
QRS complex	Normal (0.09 second).
Dysrhythmia	Impure atrial flutter (coarse atrial flutter or flutter-fibrillation). Impure atrial flutter is characterized by a faster atrial rate than pure atrial flutter, and more variability shows in the contour and spacing of the flutter waves.

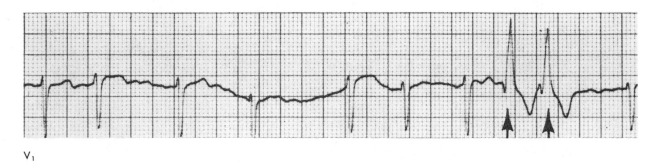

V₁

Fig. 5-129

Rate	Atrial, 350 to 600 beats/min; ventricular, 65 to 160 beats/min.
Rhythm	Atrial and ventricular, irregularly irregular.
P waves	Irregular rapid baseline undulations indicate fibrillatory atrial activity.
PR interval	Not measurable.
QRS complex	0.08 second; two complexes indicated by arrows are functional RBBB QRS complexes with a duration of 0.13 second.
Dysrhythmia	Atrial fibrillation. A long ventricular pause followed by a short ventricular pause precedes the QRS complex with an RBBB contour *(left arrow);* this QRS complex is followed after a short interval by a second QRS complex, also with RBBB *(right arrow).* The aberrant QRS pattern indicates functional RBBB (Ashman phenomenon).

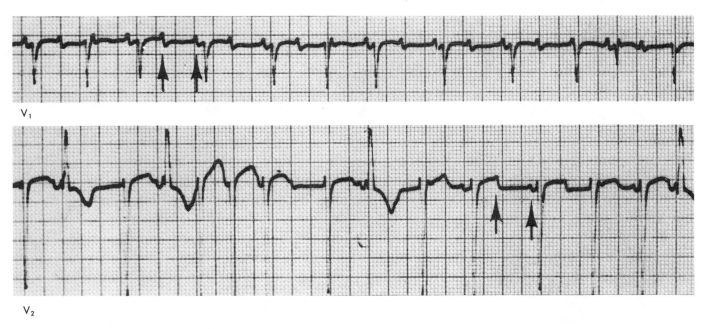

V₁

V₂

Fig. 5-130

Rate	Atrial, 167 beats/min; ventricular, varies according to the degree of AV block (83 to 120 beats/min).
Rhythm	Atrial, regular; ventricular, irregular (2:1, 3:2, and 4:3).
P waves	Contour differs from sinus-initiated P waves.
PR interval	Wenckebach cycles.
QRS complex	0.08 second; functional RBBB in lower tracing with a duration of 0.12 second.
Dysrhythmia	Atrial tachycardia with AV block. In the lower tracing, long-short QRS intervals, which follow longer intervals, set the stage for aberrant ventricular conduction that is manifest as a functional RBBB. Arrows indicate P waves.

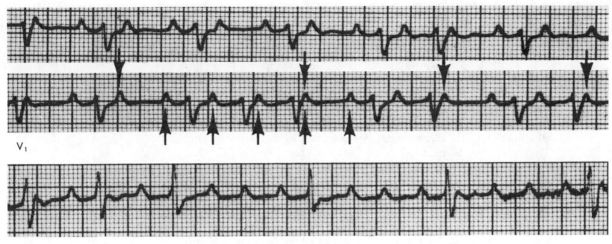

V₁

MONITOR

Fig. 5-131

Rate	Atrial, 157 beats/min, *top;* 193 beats/min, *bottom.* Ventricular, 83 to 125 beats/min, *top;* 50 to 94 beats/min, *bottom.*
Rhythm	Atrial, regular; ventricular, irregular (2:1, 3:1, 4:1, 4:3, etc.).
P waves	Contour differs from sinus-initiated P waves.
PR interval	Wenckebach cycles.
QRS complex	0.09 second.
Dysrhythmia	Atrial tachycardia with AV block caused by digitalis toxicity. Top two tracings recorded on admission. In the bottom tracing, continued digitalis administration increased the atrial rate to 193 beats/min and increased the degree of AV block. *Upright arrows,* P waves; *inverted arrows,* nonconducted P waves.

II

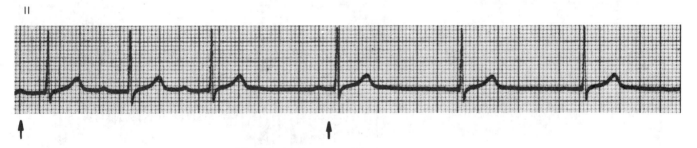

Fig. 5-132

Rate	Atrial, 75 beats/min initially, atrial activity not apparent during the junctional rhythm; ventricular, 48 to 50 beats/min during junctional rhythm.
Rhythm	Ventricular, generally regular.
P waves and PR interval	Relationship between P and QRS as explained under premature AV junctional complexes. (P waves not apparent). PR interval not determinable during junctional rhythm.
QRS complex	Normal (0.08 second); may be conducted with slight aberration.
Dysrhythmia	AV junctional rhythm. Carotid sinus massage (between arrows) produces significant sinus slowing to allow the escape of an AV junctional rhythm (fifth QRS). Note unchanged QRS complexes. Atrial activity to the right of the last arrow is not apparent and may be caused by the AV junctional rhythm with retrograde capture of the P wave, lost within the QRS complex.

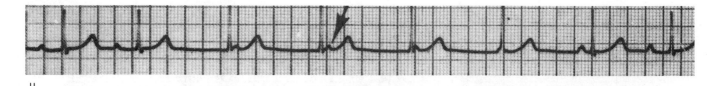

II

Fig. 5-133

Rate	Atrial, 45 to 70 beats/min; ventricular, 58 to 70 beats/min.
Rhythm	Atrial, slowing; ventricular, slowing but fairly regular.
P waves	Normal.
PR interval	See premature AV junctional complexes (AV dissociation in this tracing).
QRS complex	Normal (0.08 second).
Dysrhythmia	AV junctional rhythm. Transient, spontaneous sinus slowing allows the escape of an AV junctional rhythm. P waves occur just after the onset of the QRS complex *(arrow)* and represent normal sinus-initiated P waves. Gradual acceleration of the sinus rate reestablishes sinus control to the ventricular activity at the end of the tracing and thus terminates the period of AV dissociation in the midportion of the tracing. The PR interval is prolonged.

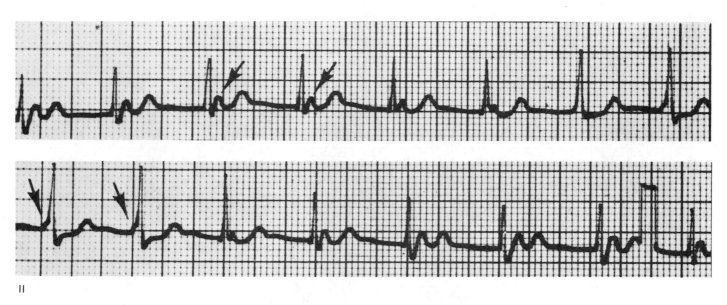

II

Fig. 5-134

Rate	Atrial and ventricular, 100 beats/min.
Rhythm	Atrial, regular; ventricular, fairly regular.
P waves	Normal.
PR interval	Varying.
QRS complex	0.08 second.
Dysrhythmia	NPJT. Atrial activity *(arrows)* follows, then slightly precedes, and then once again follows the inscription of the QRS complex. Therefore AV dissociation is present because of the accelerated AV junctional discharge. This type of AV dissociation is called *isorhythmic*.

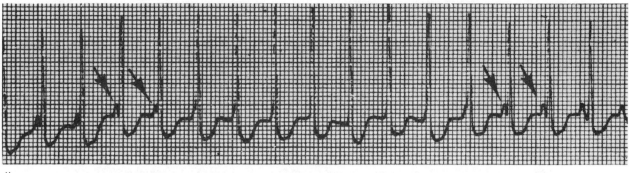

II

Fig. 5-135

Rate	Atrial and ventricular, 166 beats/min.
Rhythm	Atrial, regular; ventricular, regular.
P waves	Normal.
PR interval	Varying.
QRS complex	0.06 second.
Dysrhythmia	NPJT. Atrial activity *(arrows)* at a very similar rate and rhythm to the QRS complex can be seen to precede, then occur simultaneously with, and once again precede the onset of the QRS complex. This type of AV dissociation is called *isorhythmic*.

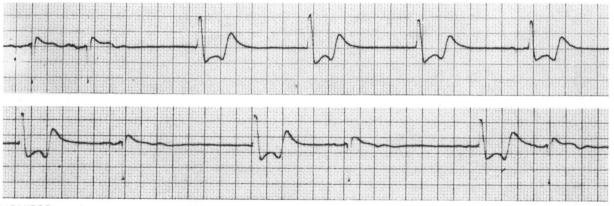

MONITOR—continuous

Fig. 5-136

Rate	Atrial, intermittent sinus arrest; ventricular, 43 beats/min.
Rhythm	Atrial, irregular; ventricular, regular.
P waves	Normal.
PR interval	Varying.
QRS complex of ventricular escape rhythm	0.13 second.
Dysrhythmia	Ventricular escape beats. Intermittent sinus arrest produced periods of asystole terminated by ventricular escape beats that are characterized by a prolonged, abnormal QRS complex. Intermittent return of sinus node activity establishes periods of supraventricular capture. The reason that AV junctional escape beats did not terminate the asystolic periods is not known.

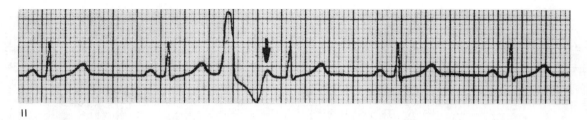

II

Fig. 5-137

Rate, rhythm, and P waves	Same as Fig. 5-55.
PR interval	Prolonged after the interpolated premature ventricular complex (0.20 second).
QRS complex	0.14 second.
Dysrhythmia	Interpolated premature ventricular complex. A sinus-initiated P wave *(arrow)* immediately after the premature ventricular complex conducts to the ventricles with a long PR interval. The PR interval after the premature ventricular complex is prolonged due to incomplete recovery of the AV node because of partial retrograde penetration by the interpolated ventricular complex.

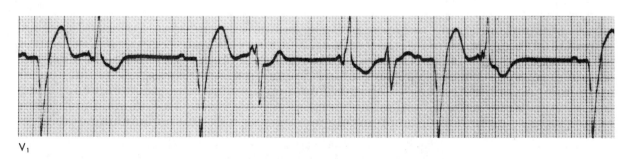

V₁

Fig. 5-138

Rate, rhythm, P waves, and PR interval	Same as Fig. 5-54.
QRS complex	Wide, bizarre, greater than 0.12 second with varying contours and coupling intervals.
Dysrhythmia	Multiform premature ventricular complexes. The normally conducted QRS complexes have an LBBB morphology. The PR interval is slightly prolonged (0.24 second). Premature QRS complexes with varying contours and coupling intervals are present and called *multiform ventricular complexes.*

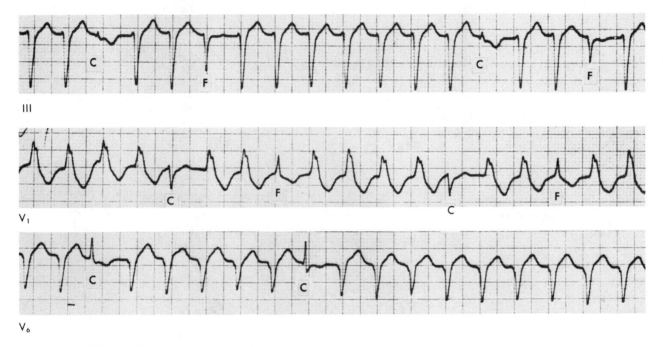

Fig. 5-139

Rate	Atrial, clear P waves not seen; ventricular, 150 beats/min.
Rhythm	Atrial and ventricular, regular.
P waves	Atrial activity is probably under independent control of sinus node.
PR interval	Not measurable.
QRS complex	0.14 second.
Dysrhythmia	Ventricular tachycardia. QRS complexes with a prolonged duration and an RBBB morphology occur at a regular interval and are occasionally interrupted by QRS complexes with an intermediate contour (*C*, capture) or QRS complexes with a normal contour. (*F,* fusion). Atrial activity cannot be seen; most likely, the atria are discharging independently to produce intermittent QRS captures and fusion beats. Therefore the most reasonable diagnosis is a ventricular tachycardia with AV dissociation.

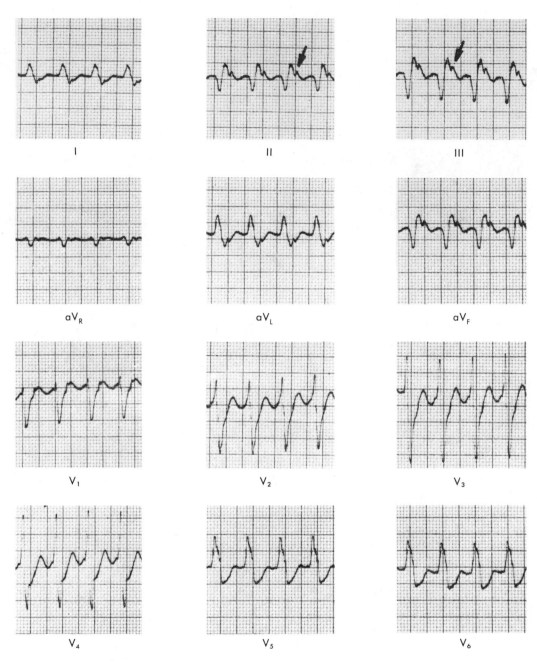

Fig. 5-140

Rate	Atrial, 150 beats/min; ventricular, 150 beats/min.
Rhythm	Atrial and ventricular, regular.
P waves	Retrograde P waves inverted in leads II and III *(arrows)* and aV$_F$.
RP interval	0.16 second.
QRS complex	0.12 second.
Dysrhythmia	Ventricular tachycardia with retrograde atrial capture. Ventricular tachycardia cannot be diagnosed with certainty from this surface ECG because all the features of this dysrhythmia can be mimicked by a supraventricular tachycardia with aberrant ventricular conduction of an LBBB type. Electrophysiologic study proved that this was a ventricular tachycardia, however. The importance of the illustration lies in demonstrating 1:1 retrograde conduction to the atrium. Retrograde atrial activity is indicated by arrows. Thus AV dissociation is not present during this ventricular tachycardia.

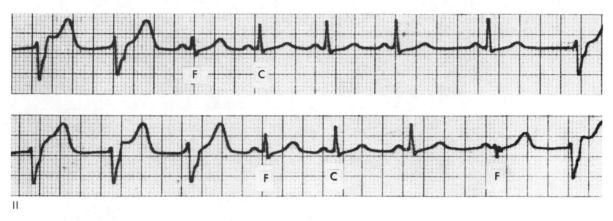

Fig. 5-141

Rate	Atrial, 70 to 90 beats/min; ventricular, 72 beats/min.
Rhythm	Atrial and ventricular, regular.
P waves	Independent.
PR interval	Not measurable during accelerated idioventricular rhythm.
QRS complex	0.14 second; fusion beats *(F)* and capture beats *(C)* often present.
Dysrhythmia	Accelerated idioventricular rhythm. An accelerated idioventricular rhythm is present at the beginning and termination of the top and bottom strips. In the midportion of each tracing, slight sinus node acceleration reestablishes sinus node control by capturing the ventricles and suppresses the accelerated idioventricular rhythm. When the sinus node shows, the accelerated idioventricular rhythm escapes. Fusion beats may occur in the beginning and end of such dysrhythmias because sinus and ventricular foci have similar rates.

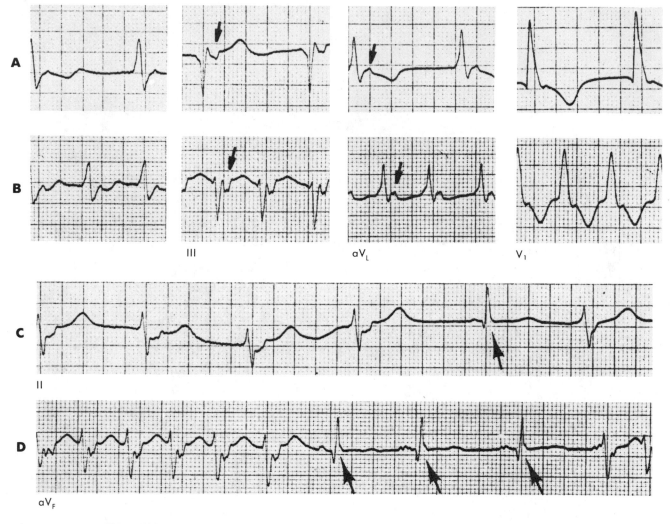

III   aV$_L$ V$_1$

II

D

aV$_F$

Fig. 5-142

Rate	Accelerated idioventricular rhythm (60 beats/min); ventricular tachycardia (varying slight, 150 beats/min).
Rhythm	Accelerated idioventricular rhythm (regular); ventricular tachycardia (regular).
P waves	Retrogradely captured.
PR interval	0.14 second.
QRS complex	0.14 second.
Dysrhythmia	Accelerated idioventricular rhythm and ventricular tachycardia. An accelerated idioventricular rhythm and a ventricular tachycardia occurred at different times in this patient. **A** illustrates leads I, II, aV$_L$, and V$_1$ during the accelerated ventricular rhythm, whereas **C** (lead II) illustrates the onset of the accelerated idioventricular rhythm. **B** illustrates the ventricular tachycardia in leads I, II, aV$_L$, and V$_1$, whereas **D** (aV$_F$) illustrates the onset and termination of the ventricular tachycardia. Retrograde atrial capture *(inverted arrows)* occurred during both tachycardias. Normally conducted QRS complexes present in **C** and **D** *(upright arrows)*. Note identical QRS contours for both tachycardias (leads aV$_L$, V$_1$, and V$_6$ in **A** were recorded at different standardization), indicating that they arose at same or similar areas of the ventricle.

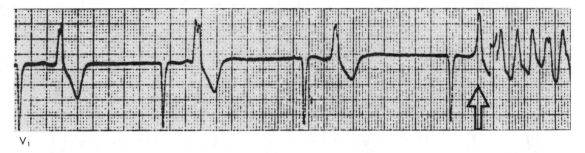

V₁

Fig. 5-143

Rate	Atrial, 60 to 100 beats/min; any independent atrial dysrhythmia may exist or the atria captures retrogradely. Ventricular, 400 to 600 beats/min.
Rhythm	Atrial, regular; may be irregular if the atria are retrogradely captured. Ventricular, grossly irregular.
P waves	Generally cannot be seen.
PR interval	Generally not measurable.
QRS complex	Baseline undulations without distinct QRS contours.
Dysrhythmia	Ventricular fibrillation. Premature ventricular complexes occurred in a bigeminal pattern with a decreasing coupling interval. The fourth premature ventricular complex discharged during the vulnerable period of the antecedent T wave and precipitated ventricular fibrillation *(arrow)*.

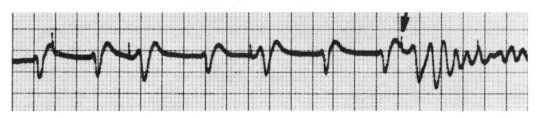

MONITOR

Fig. 5-144

Rate, rhythm, P waves, PR interval and QRS complex	Same as Fig. 5-143.
Dysrhythmia	Ventricular fibrillation. Pacemaker spikes *(arrow)* from a malfunctioning pacemaker fall randomly throughout the cardiac cycle at a slightly irregular interval. When the pacemaker spike discharged during the vulnerable period of the antecedent T wave *(arrow)*, it precipitated ventricular fibrillation. Ventricular rhythm preceding the onset of ventricular fibrillation is probably slightly irregular, accelerated idioventricular rhythm.

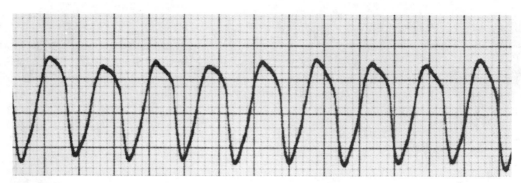

MONITOR

Fig. 5-145

Rate	Atrial, P waves not seen; ventricular, 195 beats/min.
Rhythm	Ventricular, regular.
P waves	Cannot be seen.
PR interval	Not measurable.
QRS complex	0.16 second.
Dysrhythmia	Ventricular flutter. Sine wave with regular large oscillations. The QRS complex cannot be definitely distinguished from the ST segment or T wave.

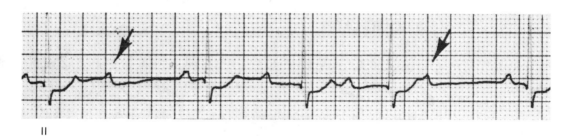

II

Fig. 5-146

Rate	Atrial, normal (83 beats/min); ventricular, depends on degree of AV block, which may vary between 2:1, 3:2, 4:3, 5:3, etc.
Rhythm	Atrial, regular; ventricular, varying, depending on the degree of AV block.
P waves	More numerous than QRS complexes but related to ventricular beats in a consistent, repetitive fashion.
PR interval	Progressive PR prolongation preceding the nonconducted P wave. Finally, one P wave is blocked, and the cycle then repeats.
QRS complex	Normal; R-R interval gradually shortens until the blocked P wave occurs; the cycle then repeats.
Dysrhythmia	Type I second-degree AV block. AV block is characterized by progressive PR prolongation preceding the nonconducted P wave. Type I AV block in the presence of a normal QRS complex is virtually always at the level of the AV node. Conduction ratios (that is, the number of P waves to the number of QRS complexes) 2:1, 4:3, and 3:2 in this tracing. Because the increment in conduction time is greatest in the second cycle of the Wenckebach group and then decreases progressively over succeeding cycles, the following characteristics are also present: the interval between successive R-R cycles before the nonconducted P wave progressively decreases; the duration of the pause produced by the nonconducted P wave is less than twice the shortest cycle, which is generally the cycle immediately preceding the pause; the duration of the R-R cycle after the pause exceeds the duration of the R-R cycle preceding the pause. These features can be seen in the middle 4:3 grouping. Blocked P waves indicated by arrows.

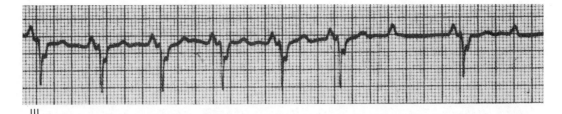

III

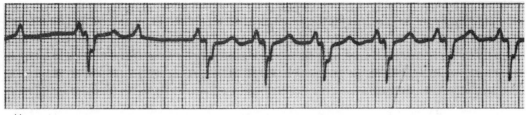

aV$_F$

Fig. 5-147

Rate	86 beats/min.
Rhythm	Atrial, regular; ventricular, varying, dependent on the degree of AV block.
P waves	Normal.
PR interval	Normal, constant (0.12 second) with sudden failure of conduction.
QRS complex	Prolonged; RBBB and left anterior hemiblock (0.12 second).
Dysrhythmia	Second-degree AV heart block, type II. RBBB (not readily apparent in leads III and aV$_F$) along with left anterior fascicular block is present in this patient. Sudden failure of AV conduction results without antecedent PR prolongation. The PR interval for the conducted beats is normal, as it often is during type II second-degree AV heart block.

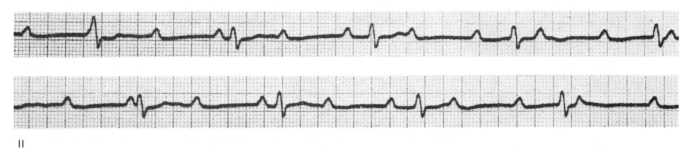

II

Fig. 5-148

Rate	Atrial, 85 beats/min; ventricular, 38 beats/min.
Rhythm	Atrial and ventricular, regular.
P waves	Normal.
PR interval	Completely variable.
QRS complex	Prolonged (0.12 second).
Dysrhythmia	Third-degree AV heart block. Complete AV dissociation is present resulting from complete heart block. The abnormal QRS complexes (prolonged duration) indicate a ventricular origin for the escape rhythm.

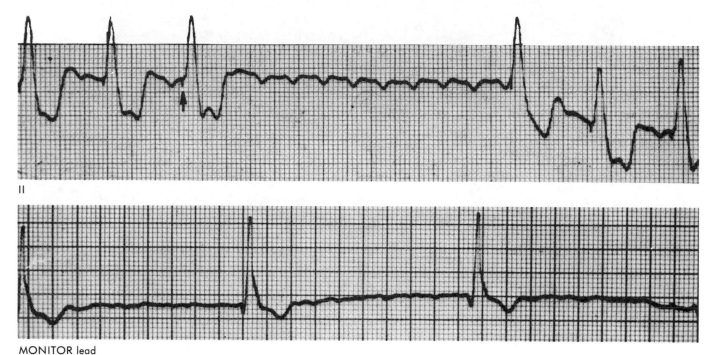

II

MONITOR lead

Fig. 5-149

Rate	Atrial, *top*, 250 beats/min; *bottom*, 400 to 600 beats/min. Ventricular, *top*, 100 beats/min; *bottom*, 32 beats/min.
Rhythm	Atrial, *top*, regular; *bottom*, irregular. Ventricular, *top*, regular; *bottom*, regular.
P waves	*Top*, atrial flutter; *bottom*, atrial fibrillation.
PR interval	Totally variable or nonmeasurable.
QRS complex	*Top*, ventricular paced beats (0.16 second); *bottom*, 0.14 second.
Dysrhythmia	Third-degree AV block during atrial flutter and atrial fibrillation. In the top tracing a ventricular pacemaker controls ventricular activity. (*Arrow*, pacemaker artifact.) In the midportion of the tracing the ventricular pacing was temporarily discontinued, and one can easily see the atrial flutter waves that fail to conduct to the ventricle. In the terminal portion of the tracing the ventricular pacemaker was turned on once again. In the bottom tracing the undulating baseline indicates the presence of atrial fibrillation. The regular ventricular rhythm establishes that none of the atrial fibrillatory impulses conduct to the ventricles; thus third-degree AV block is present during atrial fibrillation.

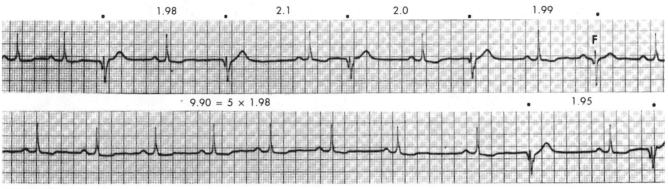

MONITOR—continuous

Fig. 5-150

Rate	Atrial, approximately 60 beats/min; ventricular parasystole, 30 beats/min.
Rhythm	Atrial, regular; ventricular parasystole, regular; interrupted by exit block or ventricular refractoriness.
P waves	Normal.
PR interval	During normally conducted beats, normal.
QRS complex (of ventricular parasystole)	Prolonged (0.13 second).
Dysrhythmia	Ventricular parasystole. The interval between ectopic ventricular systoles ranges between 1.98 and 2.1 seconds. This coupling interval varies between the sinus-initiated QRS complex and the parasystole complex. *F,* Ventricular fusion beat. Ventricular refractoriness prevents the emergence of the ventricular parasystole during the long interval in which it is absent. This interectopic interval equals 9.90 seconds and is 5 times the normal interectopic interval. The dark marks above the tracing indicate the parasystolic ventricular systoles.

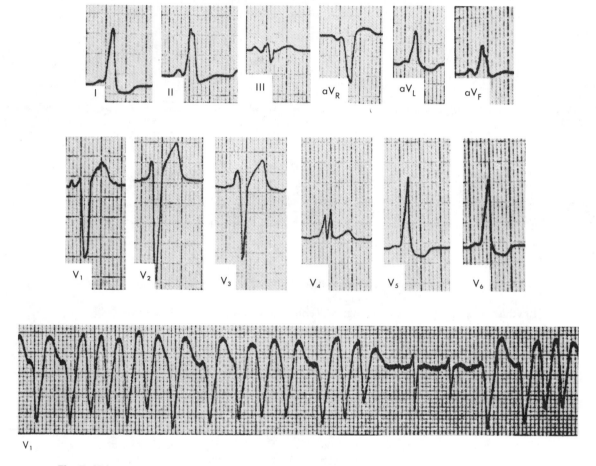

Fig. 5-151   Dysrhythmia: 12-lead ECG illustrating preexcitation syndrome with a right anterior or paraseptal pathway. The lower recording (lead V_1 half standard) demonstrates an extremely rapid ventricular rate during atrial fibrillation in the same patient. The grossly irregular ventricular rhythm, extremely rapid rate, and gradations in QRS contour from normal to prolonged (as conduction changes from the normal AV nodal pathway to the anomalous route) help distinguish this dysrhythmia from ventricular tachycardia. Bypass of the safety valve features provided by normal AV nodal delay accounts for the rapid ventricular rate that less commonly may cause the ventricles to fibrillate and result in sudden death.

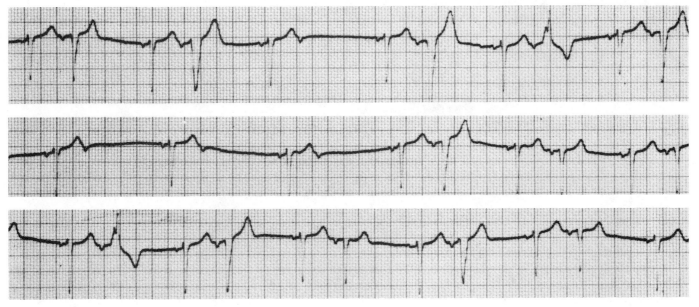

V₁—continuous

Fig. 5-152

Rate	Determined by the number of premature atrial complexes.
Rhythm	Irregular because of premature atrial complexes.
P waves	Both sinus-initiated and premature atrial P waves are abnormal.
PR interval	Normal (0.12 second) for the sinus-initiated P waves; prolonged after the premature atrial complexes. Some premature atrial complexes failed to conduct to the ventricle.
QRS complex	Normal after the sinus-initiated P waves; functional LBBB and functional RBBB after the premature atrial complexes.
Dysrhythmia	Functional RBBB and LBBB after atrial premature complexes. Premature atrial complexes occur at varying coupling intervals. When they occur with a very short PR interval, they fail to reach the ventricle and are therefore nonconducted atrial complexes. At slightly longer RP intervals, they conduct with both functional RBBB and functional LBBB. Differences in the duration of the preceding long cycle and in the duration of the short cycle account for whether functional RBBB or LBBB results.

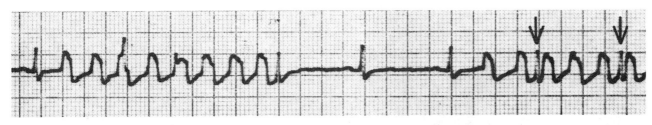

MONITOR

Fig. 5-153 Artifact. Regularly moving a loose electrode creates an artifact that mimics ventricular tachycardia. However, careful scrutiny uncovers the fairly regularly occurring normal QRS complexes *(arrows)*, each preceded by a P wave. The question of ventricular tachycardia may be eliminated, and the diagnosis of artifact is established by observing that the QRS complexes continue uninterrupted and unaffected by the apparent ventricular tachycardia.

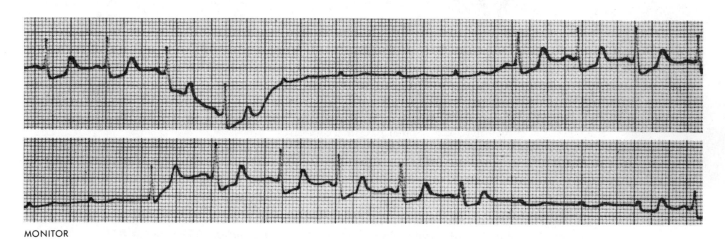

MONITOR

Fig. 5-154   Artifact simulating AV block. These tracings were recorded in a patient who presented with an acute anteroseptal myocardial infarction and 1 day later developed left anterior fascicular block. The monitored recording was interpreted as illustrating the development of advanced AV block with sequentially blocked P waves. Temporary transvenous pacemaker insertion was deemed immediately necessary. However, careful observation of the tracing reveals that the nonconducted P waves are artifactual in origin. In reality the "nonconducted P waves" are QRS complexes with a grossly diminished amplitude caused by intermittent poor ECG lead contact. The diagnosis is established by noting QRS complexes with intermediate amplitudes, by noting T waves that follow the diminutive QRS complexes, and by "matching out" the QRS complexes and finding that they occur at the same time as the apparent P waves.

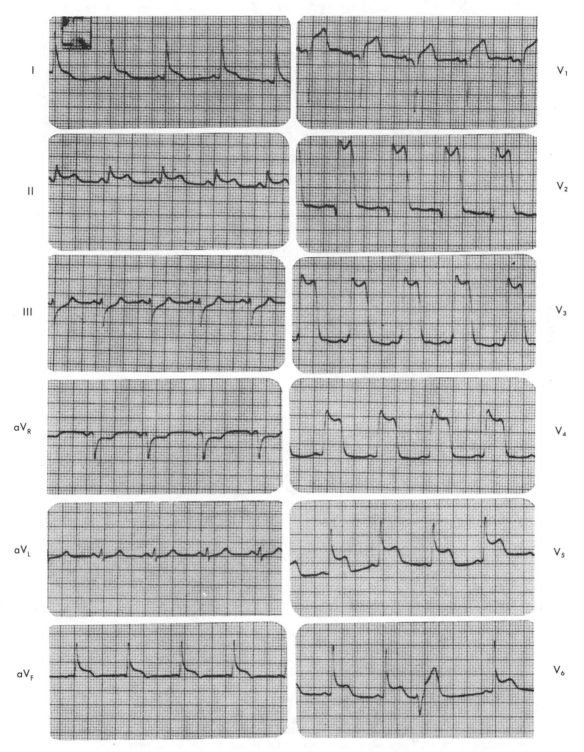

Fig. 5-155 Normal sinus rhythm, Q waves in leads V_1 and V_2. Marked ST-segment elevation in leads I, II, aV_F, and V_1 through V_6. T waves have not yet inverted. ECG reveals hyperacute anterolateral, possibly apical, myocardial infarction.

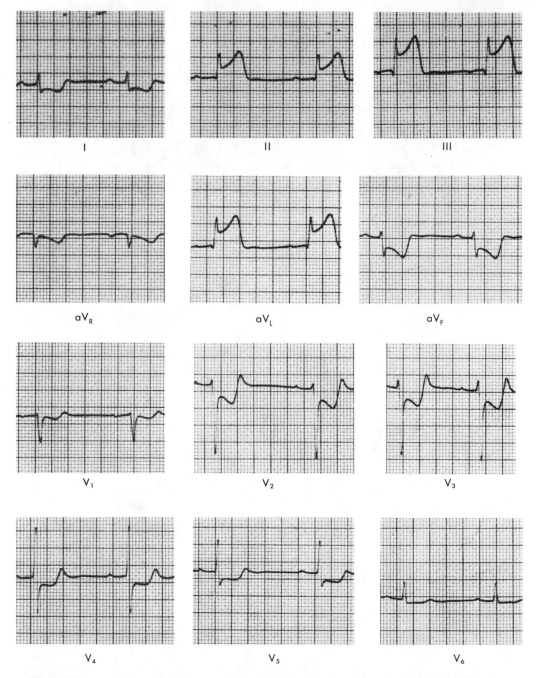

Fig. 5-156   Normal sinus rhythm. No pathologic Q waves have developed. Marked ST-segment elevation in leads II, III, and aV$_F$, with reciprocal depression in leads I, aV$_L$, and the anterior precordium. T waves are still upright. ECG reveals hyperacute inferior (diaphragmatic) myocardial infarction.

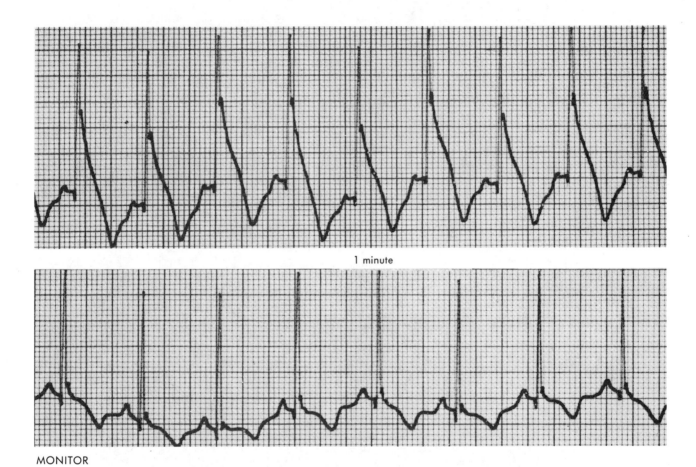

1 minute

MONITOR

Fig. 5-157 Top tracing demonstrates marked ST-segment elevation and T-wave inversion. One minute later (bottom tracing) the ST segments have returned to baseline. The T waves are still inverted. ECG reveals that the rapid ST-segment changes from elevation to normal are characteristic of atypical (Prinzmetal) angina pectoris.

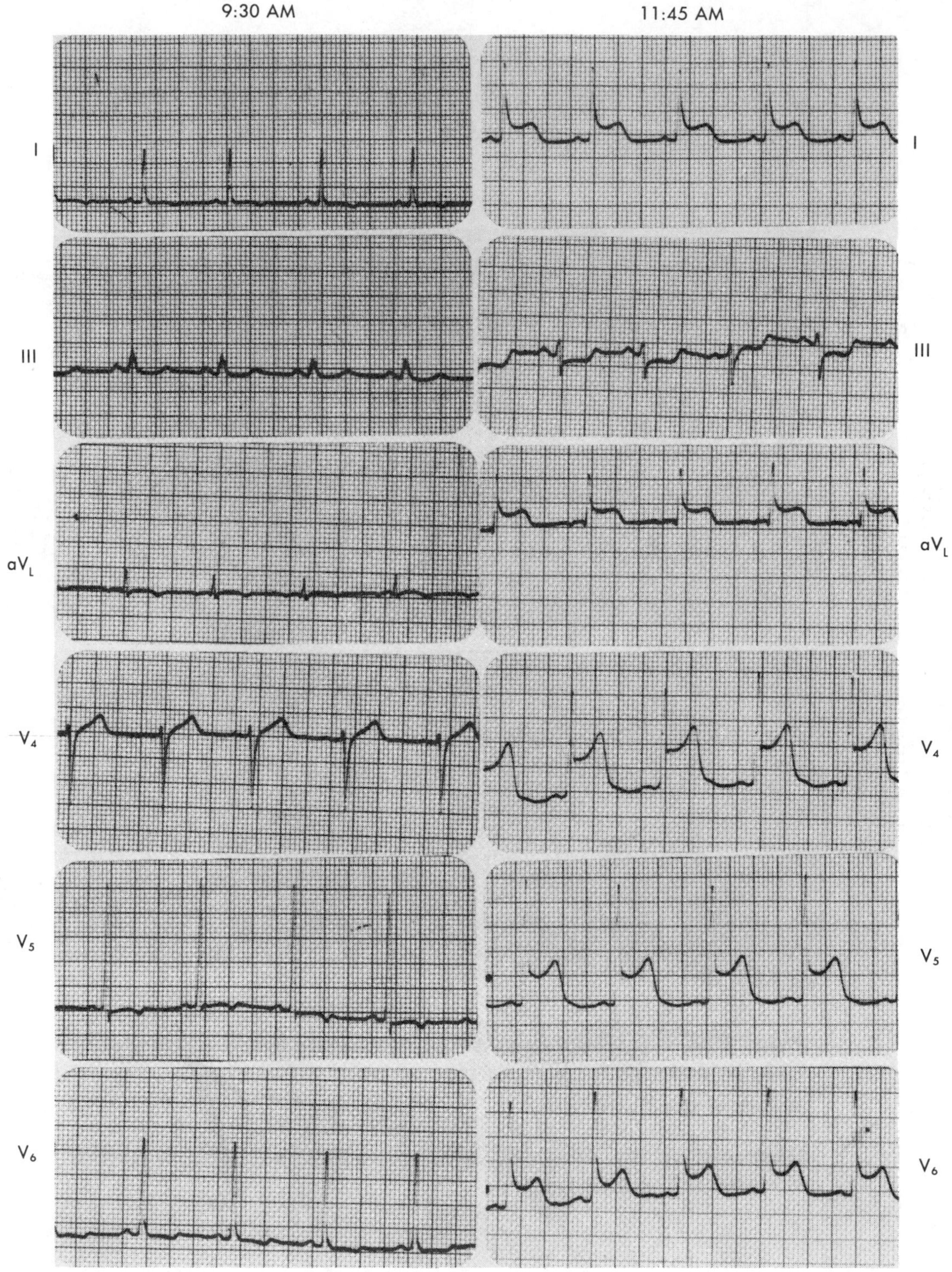

9:30 AM   11:45 AM

I

III

aV$_L$

V$_4$

V$_5$

V$_6$

Fig. 5-158 Normal sinus rhythm. Tracing at 11:45 AM (after the patient developed more chest pain) demonstrates ST-segment elevation in leads I, aV$_L$, and V$_4$ through V$_6$. The T waves are still upright, and no pathologic Q waves have developed. ECG reveals hyperacute lateral myocardial infarction.

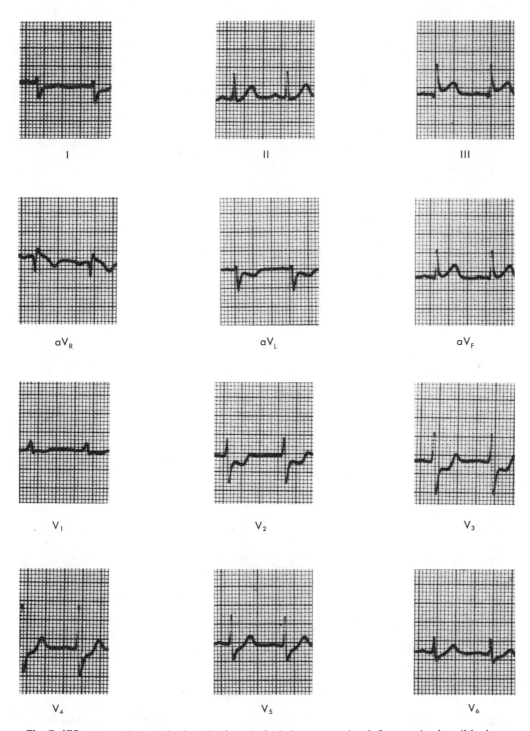

Fig. 5-159 Normal sinus rhythm. Right axis deviation suggesting left posterior hemiblock. ST-segment elevation in lead III, and slight ST-segment elevation in lead aV_F. Large R wave in lead V_1, with slight ST-segment depression in lead V_1, more marked in leads V_2 and V_3. T waves are still upright except for diphasic T waves in leads V_1 and V_2. ECG reveals acute posteroinferior myocardial infarction.

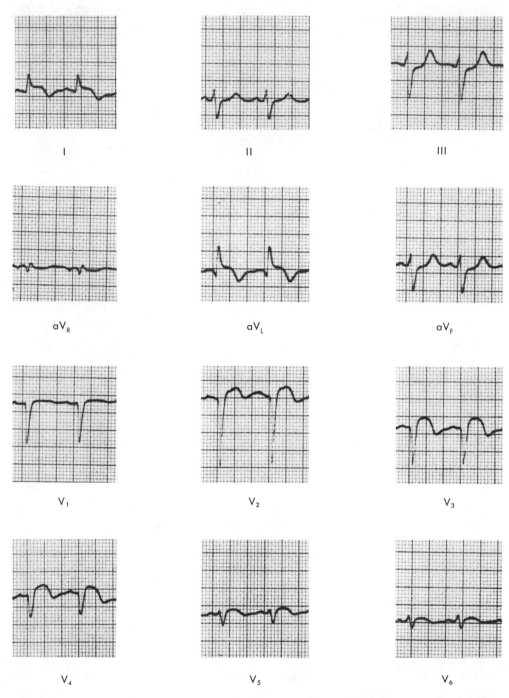

Fig. 5-160 Normal sinus rhythm. Left axis deviation characteristic of left anterior hemiblock. ST-segment elevation in leads I, aV_1 and V_2 through V_6. Abnormal Q wave in V_1 through V_4, with small R waves in V_5 and V_6. T wave inversion in leads l and aV_L and terminal T-wave inversion in V_2 through V_5. Impression is acute anterolateral myocardial infarction and left anterior hemiblock.

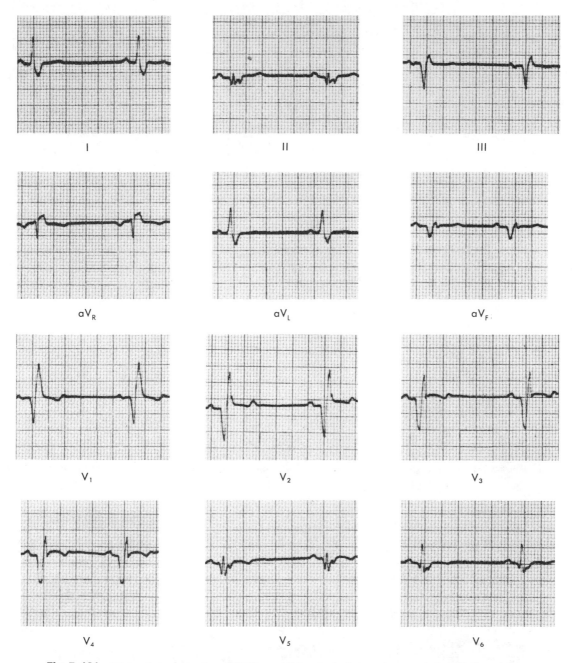

Fig. 5-161 Normal sinus rhythm, RBBB, and left axis deviation characteristic of left anterior hemiblock. ST segments are normal. There are nonspecific T-wave changes. A pathologic Q wave is present in leads II, III, aV$_F$ and V$_1$ through V$_4$ and makes the diagnosis of left anterior hemiblock difficult. ECG reveals RBBB, possible left anterior hemiblock, and anteroinferior myocardial infarction, probably old.

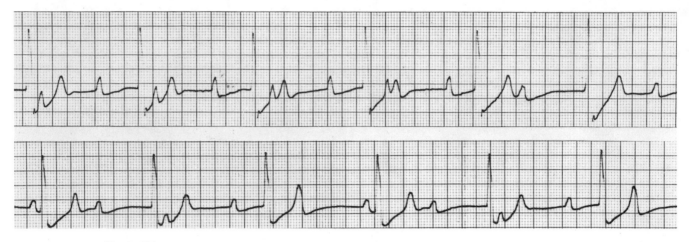

Fig. 5-162 Third-degree AV block. Complete AV dissociation is present caused by third-degree AV block. Atria and ventricles are under control of separate pacemakers, and the sinus node and an idioventricular escape rhythm, respectively. Monitor lead.

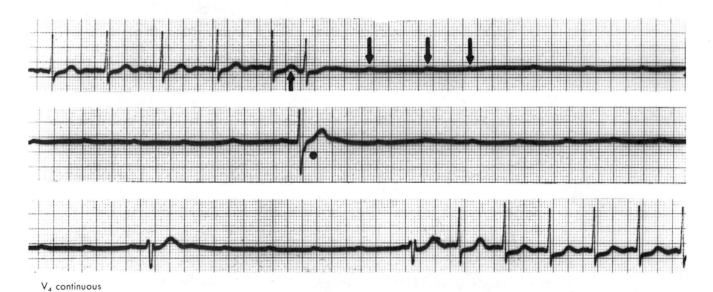

V₄ continuous

Fig. 5-163 Paroxysmal AV block. Periods of complete AV block interrupted only by an occasional escape beat occurred in this patient who had recurrent syncope. Each episode of AV block was always introduced by a premature atrial complex *(upright arrow)*, which then resulted in a series of successive nonconducted P waves *(inverted arrows)*. Finally, an escape beat occurred and restored conduction (bottom strip of this continuous recording of lead V₄). The electrophysiologic mechanism responsible for this form of paroxysmal AV block is not clear.

REFERENCES

1. Zipes DP: *Genesis of cardiac arrhythmias: electrophysiological considerations.* In Braunwald E, editor: *Heart disease: a textbook of cardiovascular medicine,* ed 4, Philadelphia, 1992, Saunders.

2. Rosenbaum MB: The hemiblocks: diagnostic criteria and clinical significance, *Mod Concepts Cardiovasc Dis* 39:141, 1970.

3. Jalife J, Moe GK: A biologic model of parasystole, *Am J Cardiol* 43:761, 1979.

4. Anzelovitch V and others: Characteristics of reflection as a mechanism of reentrant arrhythmias and its relationship to parasystole, *Circulation* 61:182, 1980.

5. Zipes DP: A consideration of antiarrhythmic therapy (editorial), *Circulation* 72:949, 1985.

6. Zipes DP and others: *The slow inward current and cardiac arrhythmias,* The Hague, 1980, Martinus Nijhoff.

7. Zipes DP: *Management of cardiac arrhythmias.* In Braunwald E, editor: *Heart disease: a textbook of cardiovascular medicine,* ed 4, Philadelphia, 1992, Saunders.

8. Zipes DP: *Specific arrhythmias: diagnosis and treatment.* In Braunwald E, editor: *Heart disease: a textbook of cardiovascular medicine,* ed 4, Philadelphia, 1992, Saunders.

9. Prystowsky EN, Zipes DP: *Treatment of tachycardia.* In Rakel RE, editor: *Conn's current therapy,* Philadelphia, 1984, Saunders.

10. Zipes DP, editor: Symposium on cardiac arrhythmias, *Cardiol Clin* vol 1, 1983.

11. Zipes DP, editor: Symposium on cardiac arrhythmias, *Med Clin North Am* 68:793, 1984.

12. Pick A, Langendorf R: *Interpretation of complex arrhythmias,* Philadelphia, 1979, Lea & Febiger.

13. Cummins RD, editor: *Textbook of advanced cardiac life support,* Dallas, 1994, American Heart Association.

14. Josephson ME: *Clinical cardiac electrophysiology,* ed 2, Philadelphia, 1993, Lea & Febiger.

15. Nattel S, Zipes DP: Clinical pharmacology of old and new antiarrhythmic drugs, *Cardiovasc Clin* 11:221, 1980.

16. Rinkenberger RL and others: Effects of intravenous and chronic oral verapamil administration in patients with supraventricular tachyarrhythmias, *Circulation* 62:996, 1980.

17. Arcebal A, Lemberg L: Mechanisms of supraventricular tachycardia, *Heart Lung* 13:205, 1984.

18. Prystowsky EN and others: Preexcitation syndromes: mechanisms and management, *Med Clin North Am* 68:831, 1984.

19. Huerta B, Lemberg L: Anticoagulation in atrial fibrillation, *Heart Lung* 14:521, 1985.

20. Zipes DP and others: Development of the implantable transvenous cardioverter, *Am J Cardiol* 54:670, 1984.

21. Kienzle M and others: Antiarrhythmic drug therapy for sustained ventricular tachycardia, *Heart Lung* 13:614, 1984.

22. Markmann P, Chellemi J: Surgical management of ventricular tachycardia, *Heart Lung* 13:622, 1984.

23. Rahimtoola S and others: Consensus statement of the conference on the state of the art of electrophysiological testing in the diagnosis and treatment of patients with cardiac arrhythmias, *Circulation* 75:11, 1987.

24. Zipes DP: Second-degree atrioventricular block, *Circulation* 60:465, 1979.

25. Hindman MC and others: The clinical significance of bundle branch block complicating acute myocardial infarction, *Circulation* 5X:689, 1978.

26. Chung EK: *Electrocardiography: practical applications with vectorial principles,* Norwalk, Conn, 1985, Appleton-Century-Crofts.

27. Miles WM and others: Evaluation of the patient with wide QRS tachycardia, *Med Clin North Am* 68:1015, 1984.

28. Wellens HJJ and others: The value of the electrocardiogram in the differential diagnosis of a tachycardia with a widened QRS complex, *Am J Med* 64:27, 1978.

29. Green M and others: Value of QRS alteration in determining the site of origin of narrow QRS supraventricular tachycardia, *Circulation* 68:368, 1983.

30. Shaw M and others: Esophageal electrocardiography in acute cardiac care: efficacy and diagnostic value of a new technique, *Am J Med* 82:689, 1987.

31. Bense DW: Transesophageal electrocardiography and cardiac pacing: state of the art, *Circulation* 75(111):86, 1987.

32. Gallager JJ and others: Esophageal pacing: a diagnostic and therapeutic tool, *Circulation* 65:336, 1982.

33. Commerford PJ, Lloyd EA: Arrhythmias in patients with drug toxicity, electrolyte and endocrine disturbances, *Med Clin North Am* 68:1051, 1984.

34. Vacek J and others: Cardiac electrophysiology: an overview, *Pract Cardiol* 10(13):83-97, 1984.

35. Akhtar M and others: NASPE Ad Hoc Committee 011 Guidelines for Cardiac Electrophysiological Studies, *PACE* 8:611, 1985.

SUGGESTED READINGS

Chung EK: *Electrocardiography: practical applications with vectorial principles,* Norwalk, Conn, 1985, Appleton-Century-Crofts.

Conover MB: *Pocket guide to electrocardiography,* ed 3, St Louis, 1994, Mosby.

Fenstenmachen: *Dysrhythmia recognition and management,* ed 2, Philadelphia, 1993, Saunders.

Huang PL: *Introduction to electrocardiography,* Philadelphia, 1993, Saunders.

Josephson ME, Wellens HJJ, editors: *Tachycardias: mechanisms and management,* Mt Kisco, NY, 1993, Futura.

Surawicz B: *Electrophysiologic basis of ECG and cardiac arrhythmias,* Baltimore, 1995, Williams & Wilkins.

Wagner GS, Marriott HJL: *Marriott's practical electrocardiography,* ed 9, Baltimore, 1994, Williams & Wilkins.

Zipes DP, editor: *Catheter ablation of arrhythmias,* Cermonk, NY, 1994, Futura.

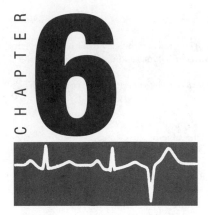

CHAPTER 6

Artificial Cardiac Pacemakers and Implantable Cardioverter Defibrillators

Nancy Stephenson
William J. Combs

Artificial cardiac pacemakers and implantable cardioverter defibrillators are electronic devices that each year maintain, sustain, and improve the lives of hundreds of thousands of men, women, and children throughout the world. These marvels of engineering excellence are now sufficiently complex that many are implanted minicomputers, storing and analyzing information and then responding as programmed to an astounding variety of cardiac conduction system abnormalities, including bradydysrhythmias and tachydysrhythmias. Their many functions include automatic rate variability in response to physiologic need, automatic mode switching to provide optimal functioning, various pacing protocols to induce and terminate specific cardiac rhythms, recognition of life-threatening dysrhythmias, and delivery of noninvasively programmable low- and high-energy shocks as needed to terminate potentially lethal dysrhythmias.

This chapter provides an overview of the functions and indications for artificial cardiac pacemakers and implantable cardioverter defibrillators, implant and follow-up procedures, and management of patients. However, since entire books now exist on these devices, readers are urged to consult the appropriate references for more detailed information and study.

ARTIFICIAL CARDIAC PACEMAKERS

The artificial cardiac pacemaker is an electronic stimulator used in place of the natural cardiac pacemaker, the sinoatrial (SA) node, and the specialized atrioventricular (AV) conducting system in the diseased, congenitally malformed, or iatrogenically damaged heart. The pacemaker system is composed of a power source, usually a battery; electronic circuitry for generating appropriately timed stimuli; and an electrode and wire system ("lead") used to complete the electrical connection between the circuitry and the myocardium. Pacemakers may be packaged for implantation totally within the body (permanent pacemakers), or they may be configured so that the electronics and power source remain outside the body (temporary pacemakers).

The first completely implantable devices were reported in the late 1950s.[1,2] There are an estimated 1 million patients worldwide who have implanted pacemakers. Advances in technology have been rapidly introduced into pacemaker systems, providing noninvasively programmable single- and dual-chamber pacemakers typically weighing 25 to 40 g and lasting an estimated 6 to 10 years. These highly reliable devices are dramatically different from the 250-g, asynchronous, 18-month devices of the early 1960s.

Indications
Permanent pacing

The most common indications for permanent pacing in the United States, as reported by the latest survey, are sinus node dysfunction and AV node and His-Purkinje conduction disorders.[3] These indications accounted for 93% of all implants. Sick sinus syndrome may be manifested as sinus arrest or block, severe sinus bradycardia, or alternating periods of bradycardia and supraventricular tachycardia (bradycardia-tachycardia syndrome). Further indications for permanent pacing include the following[4]:

1. Mobitz type II second-degree AV block distal to the bundle of His
2. Hypersensitive carotid sinus syndrome causing symptomatic severe slowing of the sinus rate, AV block, or both[5]
3. Chronic atrial fibrillation with a slow ventricular response that results in symptoms
4. Bifascicular block with prolonged His-ventricular intervals in patients who have syncope or presyncope and no other demonstrated cause of syncope (Bifasicular block with prolonged His-ventricular intervals in asymptomatic conditions is generally accepted as not being an indication for permanent pacing, although the issue is not entirely resolved.[4])
5. Termination or overdrive suppression of supraventricular tachycardia and less frequently ventricular tachycardia (VT) resistant to drug therapy and not amenable to surgical correction[6-8]

6. Periods of bradycardia or asystole after abrupt termination (overdrive suppression) of supraventricular tachycardia or VT resistant to drug therapy and not amenable to surgical correction

7. Prophylactic implantation in patients after myocardial infarction (MI) complicated by advanced AV block during the acute stages of infarction. (This indication also causes some controversy, and the issue is not completely settled.)

8. Prevention of tachydysrhythmias by providing rate maintenance with drugs or by control of AV conduction through the use of dual-chamber pacemakers

New indications for pacing under assessment include the following[9]:

1. Regularization of atrial rates during paroxysmal atrial fibrillation by the use of AAI or DDD mode pacing (see section on pacemaker modalities)

2. Dual-chamber pacing in patients with dilated cardiomyopathy for optimization of cardiac output

3. Dual-chamber pacing in patients with hypertrophic obstructive cardiomyopathy

Of these applications, pacing in patients with hypertrophic obstructive cardiomyopathy is the least controversial. The changes in septal and ventricular activation patterns for paced ventricular complexes reduce the left ventricular outflow gradient, reduce systolic anterior motion, and improve patient symptoms.[10]

Temporary pacing

Indications for temporary pacing include the following[4,6,7]:

1. Maintenance of an adequate heart rate and rhythm in patients during a variety of circumstances, such as after surgery, during catherizations or surgery, during administration of some drugs that might inappropriately slow the rate, and before implantation of a permanent pacemaker

2. Prophylaxis after open heart surgery

3. Acute (generally anterior) MI with type II second-degree or third-degree AV block

4. Acute (generally anterior) MI with concurrent onset of right bundle branch block with left axis deviation or concurrent onset of left bundle branch block

5. Acute inferior MI with third-degree AV block that is refractory to pharmacologic intervention and that produced ventricular dysrhythmias, hemodynamic compromise, or both

6. Termination of AV nodal reentry or reciprocating tachycardia associated with Wolff-Parkinson-White syndrome, atrial flutter, and VT

7. Suppression of ectopic activity (atrial or ventricular)

8. Electrophysiologic studies to evaluate diagnoses, mechanisms, and therapy in patients with a variety of bradydysrythmias and tachydysrythmias[11]

Modalities
NBG code

The North American Society for Pacing and Electrophysiology (NASPE) and the British Pacing and Electrophysiology Group (BPEG) code designed a shorthand notation to identify the many pacing modes (Table 6-1).[12]

The symbols of the notation indicate the following: the first two positions, the chambers in which the pacemaker functions; the third position, the mode of operation of the pacemaker; the fourth position, the pacemaker's programmability or rate-modulation characteristics; and the fifth position, the pacemaker's antitachycardia features. For example, if the pacing lead is inserted into the ventricle and the pulse generator is a ventricular demand type, the chamber paced is the ventricle, and the first letter in the five-position code is V. If the chamber sensed is the ventricle, the second letter is also V. If the mode of response of the pacemaker is to inhibit a pacing spike when spontaneous electrical activity is sensed, I is in the third position. If the mode of pacing is rate adaptive (responsive), R is in the fourth position. If the rate, output, or both of the pulse

---

TABLE 6-1   Five-Position Pacemaker Code (NBG)

Chamber Paced	Chamber Sensed	Mode of Response	Programmability/ Rate Modulation	Antitachydysrhythmia Functions
V = Ventricle	V = Ventricle	I = Inhibited	P = Simple programmable	P = Pacing
A = Atrium	A = Atrium	T = Triggered	M = Multiprogrammable	S = Shock
D = Atrium and ventricle	D = Atrium and ventricle	D = Atrial triggered and ventricular inhibited	C = Communicating	D = Pacing and shock
O = None	O = None	O = None	R = Rate modulation	O = None
			O = None	

From Bernstein A and others: The NASPE/BPEG pacemaker code, *PACE* 10(4):794, 1987.

generator can be programmed externally, *P* is in the fourth position. If the pacemaker is used to treat tachycardias, the tachydysrhythmic function is indicated in the fifth position.

Pulse generators that pace or sense in both the atrium and the ventricle are indicated by the designation *D*, meaning "dual." If the pacemaker does not have a function in one of the classifications, *O* is used. The different types of tachydysrhythmic functions are discussed in this chapter.

On the left in Figs. 6-1 through 6-5 are schematic diagrams of the heart; the right and left atria are represented by the top regions of the diagrams, and the right and left ventricles are represented by the bottom regions. The name of the pacemaker is placed beneath the hearts. The "output" circuit (part of the pacemaker that creates the electrical stimulus) is connected to the heart in the cardiac chamber marked with an asterisk and indicates the chamber *stimulated* by the pacemaker. The triangular element labeled *AMP* (portion of the pacemaker that has an electric amplifying circuit to enable sensing of cardiac activity) is connected to the heart in the cardiac chamber marked with a circle and indicates the cardiac chamber *sensed* by the pacemaker. Circled asterisks indicate that both sensing and stimulation can be accomplished at the location marked. NBG codes are given in the middle panel. The right panel shows ECG tracings of the pacemaker's function.

Atrial and ventricular asynchronous pacemakers

The first pacemakers simply stimulated the myocardium at a constant rate independent of the underlying cardiac rhythm; these pacemakers only paced and did not sense any spontaneous activity. If the pacemaker was connected to the atria, it was referred to as an *asynchronous atrial pacemaker (AOO)*, and if it was applied to the ventricles, it was referred to as a *ventricular asynchronous pacemaker (VOO)*. Asynchronous pacemakers are rarely used today, since it is relatively simple to provide noncompetitive pacemakers that avoid the potential risks of pacing during spontaneous rhythms.

Atrial and ventricular demand pacemakers

In the early 1970s, sensing circuits were added to pacemakers, so they would stimulate only when there was no appropriate underlying spontaneous rhythm. These pacemakers paced and sensed spontaneous activity. This prevented competitive pacing and the attendant risk of inducing fibrillation.

Demand pacemakers are supplied in two versions, inhibited and triggered. Inhibited devices withhold the stimulus and reset their timing when they sense spontaneous cardiac activity. Triggered devices are activated to deliver a stimulus just after spontaneous depolarization into the refractory tissue and reset their timing immediately when they sense spontaneous cardiac activity. Both types of pacemakers deliver a stimulus at the end of their timing cycle

(pacemaker escape interval) if no spontaneous cardiac activity is detected. The triggered mode was invented to address concerns that unipolar inhibited devices might allow a patient's heart to become asystolic if extracardiac signals (for example, pectoral muscle potentials, electrical signals from radio transmitters and power lines) were sensed, erroneously interpreted to be cardiac signals, and permitted to inhibit pacemaker output. Modern circuitry has reduced the likelihood of such occurrences, and the disadvantages of stimulating when not really necessary with a triggered mode (electrocardiogram [ECG] waveform distortion and high-power requirements for the pacemaker) have resulted in relatively little use of this form of pacing. However, it can be of value to achieve termination of some tachycardias (by externally triggering the pacemaker to deliver trains of stimuli) or to be certain diagnostically when or if the pacemaker has sensed a spontaneous event; it is therefore generally available in modern pacemakers as an option. Block diagrams and typical ECGs for the ventricular demand inhibited (VVI), ventricular demand triggered (VVT), atrial demand inhibited (AAI), and atrial demand triggered (AAT) devices are shown in Fig. 6-1.

Atrial synchronous ventricular pacemakers

To approximate normal cardiac function more closely, sophisticated dual-chamber (atrium and ventricle) "physiologic" pacemakers were developed. The atrial synchronous ventricular pacemaker (VAT) was designed for use in patients with normal sinus function and impaired AV conduction.[13] This device senses atrial activity by means of an electrode in the atrium and after a suitable delay, paces the ventricle, thereby providing an artificial AV node in lieu of the malfunctioning natural AV pathway. The VAT pacemaker does not pace the atrium. This method of atrial sensing and ventricular pacing preserves the atrial contribution to ventricular filling and maintains sinus control of ventricular rate. Rate limits are designed into the pacemaker so that during periods of atrial bradycardia at rates slower than the lower rate limit of the pacemaker, the unit paces as an asynchronous ventricular pacemaker at a predetermined backup rate. During atrial tachycardia the pacemaker paces no faster than its upper rate limit, yielding an AV response to sensed atrial activity similar to type I or type II AV block. The VAT device has been refined by the addition of circuitry that enables it to detect ventricular activity (ventricular sense amplifier). This modified pacemaker is called the *atrial synchronous ventricular inhibited pacemaker (ASVIP)*, described in the NBG code as VDD.[14] (The VDD pacemaker, like the VAT pacemaker, cannot pace in the atrium, but it does sense in both the atrium and the ventricle and paces in the ventricle.) Early VDD pacemakers required separate leads for atrial sensing and ventricular sensing and pacing. A resurgence of interest in VDD pacemakers occurred with the devel-

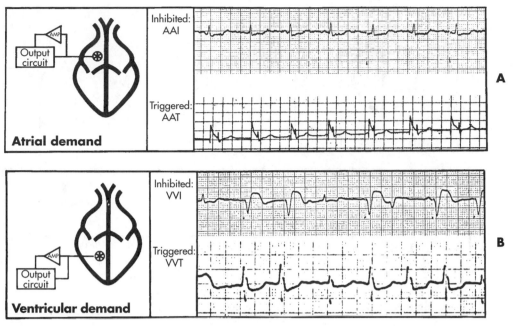

Fig. 6-1 Atrial and ventricular demand pacemakers (AAI, AAT, VVI, and VVT). **A,** In the left panel, a circled asterisk indicates that atrial demand pacemakers sense and pace in the atrium. In the top ECG of the right panel, the action of an atrial inhibited (AAI) pacemaker is illustrated. Note that the pacing spike is inhibited from discharging until the fifth and seventh complexes, when atrial rhythm slows slightly and allows escape of the atrial demand pacemaker. In the second ECG, each sensed P wave elicits a pacing spike delivered within the P wave (third, fourth, and fifth P waves). A pacing spike initiates the first, second, sixth, and seventh P waves. This is an example of AAT pacing. **B,** In the left panel, a circled asterisk indicates that ventricular demand pacemakers sense and pace in the ventricle. In the top ECG, the action of a ventricular demand pacemaker (VVI) is illustrated. Note that spontaneous ventricular activity inhibits pacemaker discharge, and pacing spikes are delivered only when the ventricular rate becomes slower than the escape interval of the pacemaker. In the bottom ECG, pacing spikes are delivered into each of the appropriately sensed QRS complexes; this is correct operation of the VVT pacemaker.

opment of single-pass leads with dedicated free-floating electrodes for atrial sensing and with standard ventricular electrodes on a common lead for ventricular sensing and pacing.[15,16] Block diagrams and ECGs for the VAT and VDD devices are shown in Fig. 6-2.

AV sequential pacemakers

In patients who have bradycardia and impaired AV conduction, the atrial contribution to ventricular filling can be preserved by using an AV sequential pacemaker (DVI).[15] This pacemaker senses only ventricular activity but can pace both the atrium and ventricle. After sensed or paced ventricular events, the DVI pacemaker monitors the ventricle for intrinsic electrical activity. If none is detected within a prescribed pacemaker escape interval, the pacemaker stimulates the atrium. It then waits long enough to allow pas-

sage of a normal AV interval and if no ventricular activity occurs, paces the ventricle.* Sensed ventricular activity inhibits the ventricular stimulus and resets all pacemaker timing. If the ventricular rate is sufficiently rapid, atrial stimuli are also inhibited. It is important to emphasize that the DVI pacemaker does not sense spontaneous atrial activity.

A variant of the DVI pacemaker, the DDI pacemaker, does sense atrial activity. This device inhibits the atrial stimulus to avoid competition between the pacemaker and an underlying atrial rhythm, but it does not provide atrial synchronous pacing. Fig. 6-3 contains the block diagram and representative ECG for the DVI pacemaker. DVI or DDI

---

*Some AV sequential pacemakers are of the committed type; that is, they do not wait for normal AV conduction to occur but instead always deliver a stimulus to the ventricle one AV interval after delivery of an atrial stimulus.

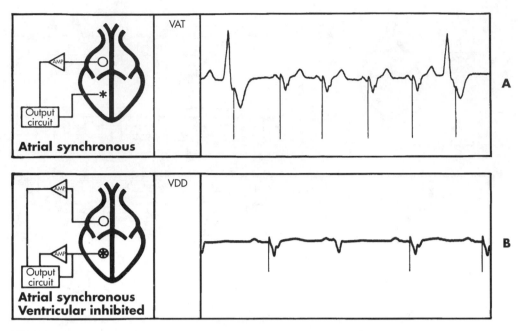

Fig. 6-2   Atrial synchronous pacemaker (VAT and VDD). For the VAT pacemaker **(A),** the circle in the atrium and the asterisk in the ventricle indicate that the pacemaker senses atrial activity and paces the ventricle. **B,** The circle in the atrium and the circled asterisk in the ventricle indicate that the pacemaker senses both atrial and ventricular activity and paces the ventricle (VDD). In the midportion of ECG in **A** the pacemaker delivers stimuli after each sensed P wave and produces a paced QRS complex. The first and last QRS complexes are spontaneous premature ventricular complexes (PVCs) that are *not* sensed by the pacemaker. The sinus P wave (hidden within the QRS complex) is sensed by the pacemaker and triggers it to deliver a pacing spike to the ventricle. Conceivably, such a response can deliver a stimulus into the T wave of the PVC. To avoid this problem, the VDD pacemaker has been equipped with a sensing circuit to sense spontaneous ventricular activity. Note in the ECG in **B** (VDD pacemaker) that the second P wave conducts to the ventricle with a PR interval shorter than the P-stimulus interval of the pacemaker. This conducted QRS complex is sensed by the pacemaker, and the pacing spike is inhibited, thus eliminating problems of pacemaker competition with spontaneous ventricular activity.

pacing is most often obtained by programming a DDD or DDDR pacemaker to the DVI or DDI mode.

Fully automatic or universal stimulation

In 1977 came the first clinical implants of the DDD pacemaker, a dual-chamber device that functions in the atrial synchronous mode during normal sinus activity and provides AV sequential pacing during periods of bradycardia.[16] Thus the DDD pacemaker senses and paces the atrium and the ventricle. This pacemaker operates in four modes, adapting automatically to the patient's underlying rhythm according to the schema in Table 6-2. Fig. 6-4 shows a block diagram and representative ECGs for the DDD pacemaker.

Rate-responsive devices

As the benefits of rate variability associated with atrial synchronous ventricular pacing became appreciated, it

was recognized that similar advantages might be available to patients with impaired atrial function.[17] However, an appropriate physiologic parameter independent of sinus nodal function is needed to set the pacemaker's rate. Clinical experience exists with single- and dual-chamber pacemaker designs that vary pacing rate in response to changes in the sensed mechanical activity of the body,[18] respiratory rate or minute ventilation,[19-21] QT interval,[22-24] central venous temperature,[25] right ventricular pressure,[26-27] oxygen saturation,[28] preejection index[29] and stroke volume,[30] ventricular depolarization gradient,[31] and pH.[32] Initial rate-responsive pacemakers were single chamber (AAIR and VVIR). They were soon followed by dual-chamber, rate-responsive pacemakers (DDDR) in which the sensor essentially modulates the pacemaker's lower rate, resulting in atrial pacing at a rate driven by the sensor or in atrial tracking if the intrinsic atrial rhythm is faster than the sensor or lower rate.[33] Fig. 6-5 shows a

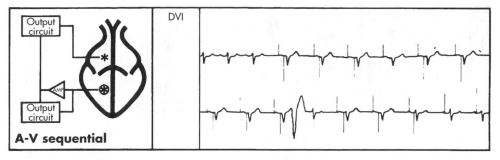

Fig. 6-3 AV sequential pacemaker (DVI)). The asterisk in the atrium and the circled asterisk in the ventricle indicate that the pacemaker paces the atrium and ventricle and senses spontaneous activity in the ventricle. The ECG demonstrates this operation. The first three sinus-initiated QRS complexes occur at a rate faster than the escape rate of the pacemaker, and the pacemaker is completely inhibited. At this point, the SA node discharge rate slows, and the pacemaker delivers a stimulus (upward spike) to the atrium. Because the paced P wave does not conduct to the ventricle within the escape interval of the pacemaker, the pacemaker then paces the ventricle (downward spikes). This occurs for three beats. Then the PR interval shortens slightly, inhibiting ventricular pacemaker discharge. The last two beats in the top strip and first three beats in the bottom strip indicate pacing in the atrium and ventricle. Then a PVC occurs and is sensed, and pacemaker activity is inhibited. The pacemaker then resumes delivery of spikes to the atrium and ventricle. In the terminal portion of this ECG the atrial rate speeds slightly. Since atrial activity is not sensed, pacemaker spikes "march" through the P wave, but ventricular spikes are inhibited.

TABLE 6-2	Operating Modes of DDD Pacemakers
Underlying Rhythm	**Pacemaker Function**
Normally conducted sinus rhythm	Totally inhibited
Normally conducted sinus bradycardia	Atrial pacing
Atrial bradycardia and prolonged or blocked AV conduction	AV sequential pacing
Normal sinus rhythm and prolonged or blocked AV conduction	Atrial synchronous ventricular pacing

block diagram and representative ECGs for the VVIR and DDDR pacemaker modes.

Body-motion-sensing pacemakers use one of two sensor types: activity crystal or accelerometer. Activity-sensing pacemakers use conventional lead systems for sensing and pacing and incorporate a microphone-like sensor that is inside the pacemaker and bonded to the inside of the titanium pacemaker can. This sensor responds to the mechanical vibrations of the body, producing electrical signals proportional to the patient's physical exercise. These "activity" signals are used to determine an appropriate pacing rate. This approach affords a rapid response to patient needs, uses a sensor that is hermetically sealed within the

pacemaker for reliable long-term service, and requires no change in implant technique. The disadvantages are an inability to respond to non-exercise-induced metabolic demands and the potential for minor rate increases in the presence of infrasonic environmental noises. Accelerometer-based, rate-responsive pacemakers use accelerometers mounted on the internal pacemaker hybrid or circuit board to measure the acceleration forces caused by exercise on the human body. Accelerometer signals in the frequency range of 1 to 4 Hz are correlated to metabolic equivalents during walking exercise.[34] Many of the advantages and disadvantages are common to activity- and accelerometer-based, rate-responsive pacemakers. Accelerometer-based pacemakers are less susceptible to inappropriate rate increases caused by pressure on the pacemaker.

Minute ventilation is better correlated and sensitive to metabolic demand than respiration rate. Consequently, minute ventilation is the primary respiratory parameter used in rate-responsive pacing systems. These systems require implantation of a bipolar lead in the atrium or ventricle for measurements of minute ventilation. Minute-ventilation-measuring pacemakers measure the transthoracic impedance variations caused by respiration by injecting current between the ring of a standard bipolar pacing lead and the pacemaker case. The resultant induced voltage is measured between the lead tip and the pacemaker case. Advantages of this system include a proportional pacemaker rate increase to varying workload and no special system lead requirements. Disadvantages include contraindication for use in patients with high breathing rates, rate

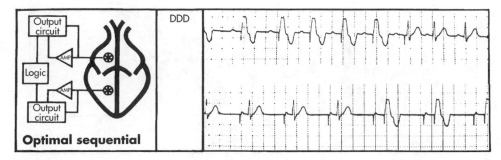

Fig. 6-4   Fully automatic sequential pacemaker (DDD). The circled asterisks indicate that the DDD pacemaker senses and paces in the atrium and ventricle. The top ECG on the right illustrates this feature. In the first five complete complexes, spontaneous atrial activity (P wave) is not followed by a spontaneous QRS complex within an appropriate PR interval. Therefore a pacemaker spike is delivered to the ventricle after each sensed P wave. The third QRS complex from the end occurs in time to be normally conducted from the P wave but not quite early enough to inhibit the pacemaker spike. The next QRS complexes follow a normal PR interval and thus inhibit pacemaker output. In the bottom strip, the development of sinus bradycardia triggers atrial pacemaker discharge, and pacemaker spikes precede the onset of P waves. Finally, in the bottom right portion, an atrial stimulus paces the atrium, and a ventricular stimulus paces the ventricle.

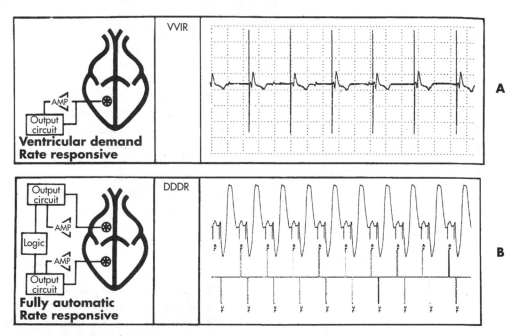

Fig. 6-5   Ventricular (VVIR) and fully automatic sequential (DDDR) rate-responsive pacemakers. **A,** For the VVIR pacemaker, the circled asterisk indicates sensing and pacing in the ventricle. The *R* in the fourth position of the NBG code indicates that the pacemaker escape interval is modulated by a sensor. **B,** The circled asterisks indicate that the DDDR pacemaker senses and paces in the atrium and ventricle. The *R* in the fourth position of the NBG code also indicates rate modulation by a sensor. The ECG illustrates rapid sensor-driven sequential pacing in the atrium and ventricle. Below the ECG is an example of a marker channel™, which in this case indicates both atrial and ventricular paced events when received by a pacemaker programmer.

increases caused by certain maneuvers such as arm waving, and rate changes caused by talking during exercise.

The QT-sensing pacemaker uses a conventional pacing lead to sense and pace, but it has circuitry designed to determine the interval between stimulation and the peak of the intracardiac T wave. Its operation is based on the physiologic concept that sympathetic tone increases in response to the body's need for an increased heart rate. Heightened sympathetic tone shortens the QT interval, and this shortening produces an increase in the pacemaker rate. Advantages of this pacemaker include the use of a standard pacing lead that requires no change in implant technique and device response to a parameter reflecting metabolic demand. Disadvantages include a relatively slow response time, changes in QT interval caused by drug interactions, and unreliable sensing of the T wave.

Temperature-sensing pacemakers measure the temperature in the right ventricle using a thermistor in a dedicated lead. The temperature in the right ventricle falls slightly at the beginning of exercise and gradually increases as exercise continues. Temperature sensing allows pacemaker rate changes to be proportional to workload. Disadvantages of this system include the use of a complicated dedicated lead, potentially blunted response of the system to short periods of low-level exercise, and rate responses resulting from temperature changes not initiated by exercise.

Additional but not extensive clinical experience exists with pacemakers that vary pacing rate in response to changes in the ventricular depolarization gradient. This gradient is derived from the evoked potential and varies with changes in circulating catecholamine levels. Clinical experience also exists with pacemakers that measure and vary pacing rate in response to the derivative of the right ventricular pulse-pressure waveform, which is measured with a dedicated pressure sensor on the lead, and to the preejection interval and stroke volume, which are derived from intracavitary impedance measurements. A limited number of pacemakers that measure right ventricular oxygen saturation using a dedicated lead with a built-in optical oxygen-saturation sensor have been implanted. Lead complexity, fibrotic growth over the sensor, and signal differences resulting from mechanical impingement of physical structures in the right ventricle are major obstacles to the general use of this technology for rate-responsive pacing.

To date, no single sensor ideally replaces the sinus node. The various sensors in use today typically contain one of the following shortcomings: slow response, nonproportionality for various workloads, nonproportionality for various types of exercise at equal workloads, and inappropriate sensor-driven rate increases.

Various combinations of sensors in which the sensors are complementary, which allows compensation for individual sensor shortcomings, have been proposed. Proposed sensor combinations have included respiration and stroke volume; respiration and activity; QT interval and stroke volume or activity; oxygen saturation and temperature; temperature and activity; and oxygen saturation, pressure, and stroke volume.[35] Many dual-sensor, single-chamber, rate-responsive pacemakers are being used clinically. These sensor combinations include QT interval and activity and minute ventilation and activity.[36,37] Both of these sensor combinations combine physiologic sensors: QT or minute ventilation with a fast-responding nonphysiologic activity sensor. The QT and activity pacemaker combines both sensors proportionally and requires confirmation by both sensors for a sustained rate increase.[38] The minute ventilation and activity pacemaker calculates an independent pacing rate for each sensor and compares the two. The fastest calculated sensor rate determines the pacemaker pacing rate and is limited by separate upper rates for both sensors. Programming separate upper rates allows limiting the contribution of the activity sensor to pacing rates between the lower rate and an intermediate rate, taking maximal advantage of the activity's fast response to the onset of exercise. Programming the minute ventilation rate to the maximum rate for sustained exercise allows the pacemaker to use the proportional response of minute ventilation to various types of sustained exercise.

The next generation of pacemakers will include multisensor DDDR pacemaker systems. The challenge for these systems will be to provide improved rate-responsive pacing therapy while simplifying the complexity of setting up or optimizing the therapy in individuals. These pacemakers will also include advanced timing features such as an automatic decrease in the pacemaker's lower rate at night and automatic mode switching from atrial tracking to nontracking modes when atrial dysrhythmias occur, which would drive the ventricular pacing rate inappropriately high.[39,40] The use of advanced techniques such as fuzzy logic controllers[41] and increased automatic operation may allow pacemakers to provide improved therapy to patients while reducing the time required for system initialization or follow-up.

Mode selection

Selection of the optimal pacemaker modality for a patient can be complex, requiring knowledge of the electrophysiologic performance of the SA node, AV conduction pathways, and hemodynamic status. A summary of each of the pacemaker modes described is presented in Table 6-3. A reasonable though less rigorous selection of modes can be made by considering the patient's atrial rhythm and AV conduction status, as indicated in Table 6-4.

Patients who have normal atrial rhythms do not require pacemakers if AV conduction is also normal. If AV function is interrupted, atrial synchronous ventricular pacing (VDD and DDD) provides a means for maintaining sinus control of the ventricular rate. If the patient also has sinus node chronotropic incompetence, a device that provides rate variability via another sensor (DDDR) adds a means

TABLE 6-3   Summary of Pacemaker Modalities

Pacemaker Type	NBG Code	Atrium	Ventricle
Atrial asynchronous	AOO	Pace	
Ventricular asynchronous	VOO		Pace
Atrial demand	AAI/AAT/AAIR	Pace/sense	
Ventricular demand	VVI/VVT/VVIR		Pace/sense
Atrial synchronous	VAT	Sense	Pace
Atrial synchronous, ventricular inhibited	VDD	Sense	Pace/sense
AV sequential	DVI/DVIR	Pace	Pace/sense
Fully automatic	DDD/DDDR	Pace/sense	Pace/sense

TABLE 6-4   Guide to Pacemaker Mode Selection*

| AV Conduction | Atrial Rhythm | | |
	Normal	Bradycardia	Brady/Tachy
Normal, no hypersensitive carotid sinus syndrome	None	AAIR	AAIR
Antegrade and retrograde block	VDD DDD	DDDR	DVIR/DDIR VVIR/DDDR (MS)
Antegrade block, prolonged retrograde conduction	DDIR/DVIR VVIR	DDIR/DVIR VVIR	DVIR/DDIR VVIR/DDDR (MS)

*By matching the patient's AV conduction and atrial rhythm to those in this table, an appropriate pacemaker mode can be determined. *R* after an NBG code indicates rate-responsive pacing.
MS, Mode switching.

of compensating for the slow sinus node. However, in patients who have prolonged retrograde conduction times, atrial activation after ventricular stimulation may trigger atrial synchronous devices, producing pacemaker-mediated tachycardia. If this cannot be prevented (for example, by use of a long atrial refractory period in the pacemaker), then DVI or DDI pacing may be used. DVI pacemakers are not triggered by atrial signals; hence they cannot induce pacemaker-mediated tachycardias. DDI pacemakers inhibit atrial pacing when an atrial signal is present but do not track atrial signals. However, rate-responsive VVIR, VVTR, DVIR, and DDIR pacemakers may be preferred to the DVI device because such pacemakers vary ventricular rate as the patient's needs change.

Atrial pacing (AAI and AAT) is appropriate in patients who have atrial bradycardia and normal AV conduction. In these patients, dual-chamber pacing (DDD and DVI) provides atrial pacing for benefits already cited and ventricular stimulation to compensate for the lack of AV conduction. Rate-responsive, dual-chamber pacing (DDDR, DVIR, and DDIR) may be preferred, since additional compensation during exercise is provided.

Finally, in patients who have atrial bradycardia and tachycardia (bradycardia-tachycardia syndrome), atrial synchronous devices without mode switching during atrial dysrhythmias are inappropriate because they accelerate ventricular rhythm during periods of atrial tachycardia. A mode-switching feature allows dual-chamber pacemakers to automatically switch from atrial synchronous (DDD and DDDR) modes to atrial nontracking (DDI, DDIR, and VVIR) on recognition of inappropriately fast atrial rates. Atrial synchronous operation is reestablished on return to a physiologic atrial rate. In all other respects mode-selection factors are comparable to those cited for patients who have only atrial bradydysrhythmias.

Ultimately, selection from among the several possible modes depends on additional factors, such as pacemaker size and patient physique, the availability and unique traits of specific devices, follow-up capabilities, patient age and hemodynamic needs, and economics (dual-chamber pacemaker and lead systems typically cost 35% more than comparably advanced single-chamber systems, which in turn may cost 60% more than nonprogrammable single-chamber devices).

Pacemaker Programmability[42-45]

The majority of permanent pacemaker implants use a programmable pacemaker. *Programmability* can be defined as noninvasive, reversible alteration of the electronically controlled performance of an implantable device such as a pacemaker. Use of a simple magnet to convert a demand pacemaker to its asynchronous mode generally is excluded from this definition, although it is in reality a simple form of programming. In the most advanced pacemakers, many performance characteristics are programmable; these include rate, stimulus output amplitude or duration, amplifier sensitivity, amplifier refractory period, hysteresis, pacing mode (for example, unipolar or bipolar system and VVIR/VVI/VVT/VOO), and operation of special information channels (telemetry of intracardiac electrograms, sensor output waveforms, programmed settings, and device-operation indicators such as "marker channel" battery™ status, lead impedance, and event counters). Furthermore, in dual-chamber pacemakers it is frequently possible to program AV intervals, atrial tracking and sensor upper rates, and the pacing mode (for example, DDD to DDDR).

Programmability is of benefit to the clinician and patient in that it allows optimization of pacemaker function for specific patient needs, minimizes the need for invasive procedures to correct malfunctions or to revise the system to meet changing patient needs, and facilitates troubleshooting procedures. Some pacemakers can tabulate past pacemaker operation in terms of the number of paced and sensed events (for example, rate). These types of data are commonly displayed in a histogram format. Analysis of event data provides documentation of pacemaker operation. This information may aid in troubleshooting and in optimizing pacemaker performance. Table 6-5 indicates applications for many of the commonly available programmable parameters. Programmability must be used with care, since it presents the risk of establishing inappropriate parameter settings (for example, insufficient output energy

to maintain capture and dangerously high or low rates) and imposes a greater need for maintaining accurate records to prevent erroneous decisions based on lack of knowledge about the rationale for the current status of the programmed settings in a patient. Thus it is essential to document the rationale for program changes at the time they are made.

Programming devices produce printed records of the parameter settings of the implanted pacemaker. Some printers are activated automatically when the programmers are turned on, although others require specific activation. When possible, it is advisable to include the printouts in the patient's records. It is also advisable to routinely determine and record all programmed parameters as a first step in each follow-up session and as a final step. This ensures that spontaneous reprogramming of the implanted device, a rare phenomenon, can be correctly identified.

Power Sources[46-48]

Nearly all pacemakers and defibrillators are battery powered. External devices, especially pacemakers, typically use standard alkaline or mercury batteries of the type found in common household appliances (such as transistor radios and flashlights), although an occasional external device uses a rechargeable or lithium battery.

Virtually all implantable devices are powered by lithium batteries. These batteries share certain characteristics that make them especially suitable for implantation; yet they are also significantly different. Each of the lithium systems offers high-energy density and a low self-discharge characteristic that ensures the delivery of maximal energy where it is needed and minimizes wasted energy. Most of the systems can be hermetically sealed to prevent ingress of body fluids and egress of tissue-damaging battery materials. Each system offers unique electrical characteristics and varying degrees of reliability. The most commonly used lithium batteries are the lithium iodide and lithium cupric sulfide batteries.

Reported performances of the major power sources clearly show the substantial progress made toward creating a pacemaker that will have sufficient longevity to curtail the need for replacement in the majority of patients. In 1994, survival probabilities were reported for large groups of pacemakers using lithium power sources.[48] A total of 15,749 lithium iodide–powered pacemakers showed a cumulative survival probability of 82.6% at 8 years; 3506 lithium cupric sulfide–powered pacemakers showed a survival probability of 77.5% at 8 years. These clinical results demonstrate the success of lithium power sources.

Electrode Systems (Leads)[49,50]

The pulse generator is electrically connected to the heart by a wire and electrode system referred to as a *lead*. The electrodes may be unipolar or bipolar. In bipolar lead systems the positive and negative electrodes are located within

TABLE 6-5   Applications of Programmable Pacemaker Parameters

Patient/Pacemaker Optimization	Diagnostic Applications	Correction of Malfunctions
RATE		
Improve cardiac output by allowing greater range of conducted sinus activity.	Suppress pacing to access underlying rhythm by ECG.	—
Minimize angina by keeping the rate below that which produces pain.	Test AV conduction with an atrial pacemaker by determining rates at which AV nodal Wenckebach behavior occurs.	
Suppress dysrhythmias.		
Adapt pulse generator to pediatric needs (faster rates).	Test sinus function with an atrial pacemaker by using bursts of rapid pacing to determine SA node recovery times.	
Terminate tachycardias with short, rapid bursts.		
Minimize "pacemaker syndrome" (caused by AV dissociation) by selecting low rate.	Confirm atrial capture by altering pacemaker rate and observing concomitant ventricular rate change.	
OUTPUT, AMPLITUDE, OR DURATION		
Maximize pulse generator longevity by selecting output energy that provides the minimum level of stimulation consistent with reliable maintenance of pacing.	Evaluate pacing threshold.	Regain capture after threshold increases caused by infarcts, electrolyte disturbances, and drugs.
Provide increased energy for high-threshold patients.		Eliminate diaphragmatic or pectoral muscle stimulation.
Avoid extracardiac stimulation (pectoral muscle, phrenic nerve).		
AMPLIFIER SENSITIVITY		
Establish appropriate sensitivity to detect intracardiac electrogram while avoiding sensing of extraneous signals (pectoral muscle potentials, electromagnetic interference).	Alter sensitivity to evaluate possible sources of oversensing or undersensing.	Compensate for changes in intracardiac electrogram amplitude.
Increase sensitivity for atrial sensing applications.		Resolve oversensing of T waves, muscle potentials, and electromagnetic interference.
REFRACTORY PERIOD*		
Extend duration for atrial applications to avoid sensing conducted R waves.	Alter duration to evaluate possible causes of oversensing or undersensing.	Lengthen duration to avoid T-wave sensing.
Shorten duration in ventricular applications to detect closely coupled ectopic events.		Shorten duration to eliminate failure to sense closely coupled ectopic events.
HYSTERESIS		
Minimize pacemaker syndrome by allowing sinus rhythm over widest possible rate range while establishing adequately high pacing rate when needed.	—	—

*Refractory period: that portion of a pacemaker's timing cycle during which intrinsic cardiac activity will not be allowed to reset the pacemaker's lower rate escape. Upper rate limits, noise reversion timing, and other pacemaker timing sequences may be reset during the refractory period, depending on the specific design.

TABLE 6-5   Applications of Programmable Pacemaker Parameters—cont'd

Patient/Pacemaker Optimization	Diagnostic Applications	Correction of Malfunctions
UNIPOLAR/BIPOLAR		
—	Evaluate lead fracture (bipolar changing to unipolar). Enhance stimulus artifact visibility on ECG (bipolar changing to unipolar). Evaluate oversensing (unipolar changing to bipolar).	Convert to unipolar operation to regain capture in case of lead fracture. Change mode to adapt to altered electrogram causing sensing failure. Convert to bipolar to eliminate sensing of myopotentials. Convert to bipolar to avoid extracardiac stimulation.
MODE		
Select optimum mode (for example, VDD for patients who have normal sinus function and impaired AV conduction). Alter mode if patient's needs change (for example, VDD changed to DVI if patient develops sinus bradycardia).	Establish triggered mode to enable external control of pacemaker from chest electrodes and external stimulator to perform noninvasive electrophysiologic studies of sinus function, AV conduction, and efficacy of antidysrhythmic agents. Confirm oversensing signal source by selecting triggered mode.	Change to backup mode (for example, VVIR) if atrial portion of dual-chamber system is nonfunctional (for example, lead displacement). Prevent oversensing by selecting asynchronous mode.
AV DELAY		
Maximize hemodynamic efficacy. Control or prevent tachydysrhythmias.	—	—
ATRIAL RATE-TRACKING LIMIT		
Maintain widest range of sinus rate control without incurring angina. Control ventricular response to atrial dysrhythmias. Prevent rapid synchronization to dissociated atrial activity during ventricular escape pacing in VDD mode. Prevent occurrence of retrograde atrial activity that would result from a long delay between the triggering event in the atrium and the resultant stimulus in the ventricle. (This retrograde activity can continuously trigger the pacemaker causing "pacemaker tachycardia.")	Select high rate limit for stress testing.	Reduce tracking rate limit if pectoral muscle activity triggers rapid pacing.
MODE SWITCHING		
Control ventricular response to atrial dysrhythmias.	—	Adjust mode switching parameter if adjustable to discriminate between atrial dysrhythmia and normal sinus response.

Continued.

TABLE 6-5	Applications of Programmable Pacemaker Parameters—cont'd	
Patient/Pacemaker Optimization	Diagnostic Applications	Correction of Malfunctions
TELEMETRY		
—	Compare programmed settings to actual device operation.	—
	Use marker channel indicators to determine which events pacemaker is causing and which events are being sensed.	
	Use electrogram to evaluate causes of undersensing or oversensing.	
	Use electrogram to evaluate drug effect on myocardium.	
	Use measurement of lead impedance to evaluate lead integrity.	
	Use event counters to evaluate undersensing or oversensing.	
	Use event counters to evaluate attainment of proper rates in rate-response modes.	

the cardiac chamber and are in contact with the endocardium. Unipolar systems place only the negative electrode in the heart and use a large-surface-area anode electrode, usually the metallic housing of the pulse generator, at a remote location. Either approach is clinically acceptable. Bipolar systems are less susceptible to extraneous electromagnetic interference (such as electrical signals generated by nearby power lines, automobile spark plugs, and radio transmitters), extracardiac myopotential interference, unwanted extracardiac stimulation, or threshold changes caused by defibrillatory currents. In unipolar systems, pacing spikes are usually more easily discernible on surface ECGs, which aids follow-up, and require a single electrical conductor that in certain instances increases reliability and allows construction of smaller-diameter lead bodies.

During the initial implantation of a pacemaker system and each replacement of a pacemaker or lead, electrical measurements must be made to ensure that the system functions correctly. The stimulation threshold is the minimal amount of energy necessary to capture the chamber of the heart to be paced; output of the pacing device must therefore be higher than this amount. Measurement of cardiac signal amplitudes (intracardiac electrogram) ensures that these signals are large enough to be sensed by the pacing device to enable it to respond appropriately to spontaneous cardiac electrical activity. These measurements are typically made using a pacing system analyzer.

Transvenous leads

Permanent pacing leads are designed for transvenous or epicardial placement. Transvenous leads are usually implanted within the right ventricular apex for ventricular pacing and in the right atrial appendage or coronary sinus for atrial applications. The leads are typically inserted via the cephalic, subclavian, or external jugular vein using fluoroscopy for visualization and stiff wires (stylets) inserted within the lumen of the leads for control during positioning. (The stylets must be removed after lead placement to avoid damaging the lead.) A rapid technique for lead placement in the subclavian vein with minimal trauma involves a simple venipuncture using a special percutaneous lead introducer.[51] A potential complication for this technique is subclavian lead crush. If the pacing lead passes between the first rib and clavicle before entering the vein, clamping between the first rib and clavicle can cause lead damage (insulation failure or conductor fracture).[52] This approach has gained favor and involves minimal risk in skilled hands, although there is a possibility of inadvertently entering the pleural cavity or arterial system. Urethane-insulated leads have reduced diameters and a decreased coefficient of friction, making it possible to pass an atrial and ventricular lead through a single vein and facilitating the use of dual-chamber pacemakers.[53,54] There are, however, insulation-failure mechanisms specific to polyurethanes: environmental stress cracking and metal ion oxidation. Changes in lead design and material composition will address these issues in newer polyurethane lead designs.[55]

Transvenous leads come in a variety of designs, each purporting to ensure stable permanent positioning of the electrodes. Fig. 6-6 includes examples of ventricular and atrial leads with a variety of fixation mechanisms. Many atrial leads also incorporate a J shape to aid in proper positioning within the atrial appendage. The transvenous approach is associated with very low morbidity and with current lead designs, a very low rate of displacement.[56-58]

New designs in transvenous leads offer improvements in electrical efficiency. Electrodes with titanium nitride and iridium coatings and carbon and platinized platinum surfaces result in improved sensing and stimulation thresholds. Available for clinical use are atrial and ventricular leads that incorporate a steroid-containing pellet behind a porous electrode, permitting minute amounts of the steroid to be dissolved by body fluids and deposited into the tissues immediately around the electrode. This design decreases stimulation thresholds and increases short- and long-term cardiac signal amplitudes.[59-62] This approach may offer significant benefits, particularly to patients in whom high stimulation thresholds and low cardiac signal amplitudes have resulted in repeated clinical problems with their pacemaker systems, often necessitating the use of short-lived, high-output pulse generators. Examples of advanced leads in clinical trials include combining low-threshold steroid leads with small-surface-area electrodes,[63] yielding highly efficient low-threshold lead systems[63] and combining steroid leads with active fixation lead mechanisms.[64]

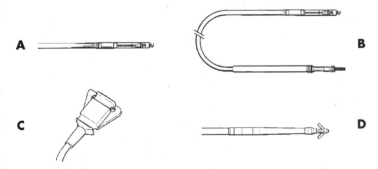

Fig. 6-6 Example of atrial and ventricular pacemaker electrodes. **A,** Bipolar endocardial urethane lead with screw-in tip electrode for active fixation to ventricular endocardial surface (Medtronic model 4068). **B,** Bipolar endocardial urethane lead with J shape and screw-in tip electrode for active fixation to the atrial endocardial surface (Medtronic model 4568). **C,** Bipolar epicardial electrode attached by suturing into the myocardium (Medtronic model 4965). **D,** Bipolar ventricular endocardial silicone lead with passive lead fixation by lodging within the trabecular structure of the ventricle (Medtronic model 5034).   (Courtesy Medtronic, Inc, Minneapolis.)

Epicardial leads

Epicardial leads are used far less frequently than transvenous systems, but they are of particular benefit in patients who have smooth, dilated right ventricles and in patients who have truncated right atrial appendages. The placement approach depends on the type of epicardial electrode used.

Temporary leads

Temporary pacing leads include transvenous catheter electrodes, wire electrodes, and in extreme circumstances, precordial surface electrodes. Electrodes for a temporary transvenous catheter can be placed in a fashion similar to that used for permanent leads. Placement is facilitated by designing the catheters to be stiffer than would be acceptable for permanent use and by sometimes incorporating additional aids such as inflatable balloons or cuffs that "float" the catheter in the bloodstream to the right ventricle. In the absence of fluoroscopy, ECG recordings from the catheter enable the user to determine the location of the electrodes (Fig. 6-7).

Heart wires are frequently placed in the atria and ventricles of patients during open heart surgery. These stainless steel wires are used during the surgical procedure and the postoperative recovery phase. In emergencies, wire electrodes can be inserted percutaneously into the heart by a pericardiocentesis (or similar) needle.

Similarly, during emergencies, surface skin electrodes placed on the chest wall can be stimulated with very high voltages to achieve cardiac pacing transthoracically. Such an approach should be used only until a transvenous catheter electrode can be positioned. One technique for noninvasive pacing has been reported to be of minimal discomfort and is suitable for prolonged use. Special, large-surface-area electrodes and external pulse generators with very wide (about 40 msec) stimulus pulse widths are required.[65]

For temporary and permanent pacing it is important to place the electrodes in a position that provides acceptably low stimulation thresholds and sufficiently large intracardiac signals to be sensed by the pulse generator. Generally this implies acute thresholds of less than 2 milliamperes (mA) and 1.25 V, with ventricular electrograms greater than 4 mV or atrial electrograms in excess of 2 mV. These values are lower with steroid-eluting permanent transvenous leads. Thresholds generally rise after short-term positioning, reaching a peak of 2 to 4 times the acute values within the first 2 to 6 weeks and falling to intermediate values.[66] The electrogram typically decreases in amplitude by 15%; its rate of rise with respect to time (slew rate) decreases as much as 50% with maturation of the implant.[67] These factors must be considered when evaluating the appropriateness of a given lead position. Again, these changes may not be observed when steroid-eluting permanent transvenous leads are used.

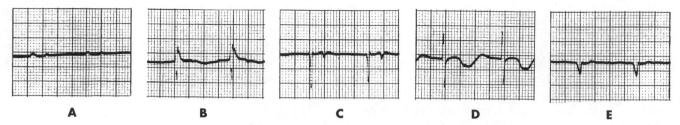

Fig. 6-7 Electrograms obtained when bipolar electrode is located in high superior vena cava (**A**), superior vena cava and right atrium (**B**), right atrium (**C**), right ventricle (**D**), and pulmonary artery (**E**). All tracings were calibrated at 1 mV/cm except **D**, which was recorded at half standard.

Follow-Up

Despite the reliability demonstrated by current pacemakers, it is important to regularly monitor the patient and the pacemaker system after implantation. Such monitoring has five major goals: evaluation of the electrical function of the pacing system to detect malfunctions or imminent power-source depletion; evaluation of the proper rate-adaptive function if applicable; evaluation of the implant site for possible mechanical difficulties such as erosion or infection; detection of progression of the patient's cardiac problems, which may necessitate reprogramming or revision of the pacing system or accompanying drug regimen; and reassurance of patients that concern and attention is being given their progress and offering of opportunities to discuss concerns.

The follow-up schedule should be arranged to provide close monitoring during the immediate postimplantation period, moderately frequent observation during the routine service life of the system, and increased surveillance as the system nears completion of its service life. A suggested schedule is 6 weeks after implantation, annually beginning 6 months after implantation, and monthly once initial signs of power-source depletion are observed (in almost all pacemakers this appears as a rate decrease with a magnet over the pulse generator). Given the longevity of modern systems, it may be counter-productive to attempt to stretch out the last few months of service by frequent monitoring, since this probably adds only 5% to 10% to the total service life while increasing monitoring costs by 30% to 40%.

Follow-up visits should be scheduled in the physician's office or in a special pacemaker clinic where the patient can be seen in person. (Telephone monitoring of the patient's ECG, pacing rate, and pulse generator stimulus duration can be of value as a supplement between personal evaluations but should not replace office visits.) Each visit should include a recording of a 12-lead ECG with a rhythm strip showing that the pacemaker appropriately captures and senses; a measurement of pacemaker parameters, including rate and pulse width; and a general physical examination, including careful scrutiny of the pacemaker pocket. If a

problem is evident or if the patient reports symptoms, an x-ray film may be obtained to evaluate the lead and its position, blood tests may help reveal threshold problems related to electrolyte imbalances, and long-term ambulatory monitoring may be indicated if intermittent failures are suspected. The results of the follow-up procedure should be carefully recorded,[68] since much of the required analysis depends on changes in operation rather than on absolute values of measured parameters. This record is especially important for patients who have programmable pacemakers and for whom intentional changes may be totally innocuous (such as a rate change programmed to improve cardiac output) or for whom the changes may signify device-performance problems (such as a rate decrease caused by battery depletion).

Care should be exercised in selecting follow-up equipment, and data must be analyzed with full understanding and knowledge of the idiosyncrasies of the equipment used. For example, digital monitoring and recording systems frequently do not reliably and reproducibly register the pacemaker stimulus artifact because of its extremely short duration. As a result, the pacemaker artifact may not always be recorded even if it is present, or its polarity and amplitude may vary markedly throughout the recording. On the other hand, such systems may substitute a standardized artifact for the real signal, eliminating diagnostic information in the process. As another example, some follow-up clinics perform waveform analysis using an oscilloscope or special ECG machine to display the waveshape of the pacemaker stimulus. The clinician must be fully aware of the correct waveshape for each pacemaker. Modern pacemakers frequently produce more complex stimulus pulse shapes than the traditional "square wave," and it is not unusual for such waveforms to be misread as signs of malfunction.

An often underestimated benefit of follow-up is reduction of patient anxiety. A clear answer to a simple question can be extremely important to a patient's well-being. In fact, some clinics have formed pacemaker clubs that allow patients to meet periodically to compare notes and provide mutual support.

Troubleshooting [69-72]

Complex systems involving electrical, mechanical, and physiologic interactions inevitably develop malfunctions, and pacemakers are no exception. Fortunately, the detection and correction of such problems are relatively straightforward for the knowledgeable user if appropriate equipment is available.

Equipment

The most useful troubleshooting tool is a 12-lead analog ECG machine. This permits evaluation of pacemaker sensing, capture, and approximate rate; evaluation of electrode positioning by vector analysis of ventricular activity; and confirmation of appropriate function for the mode of pacing used. Multiple ECG leads are necessary for vector analysis of lead positioning and frequently help in increasing the visibility of small artifacts produced by bipolar systems or in evaluating atrial activity when dealing with dual-chamber or atrial demand pacemakers.

A digital counter is useful in obtaining accurate rate and pulse width information. These counters may be supplied as specialized monitors, may be built into pacemaker programmers, or may be purchased alone. Such devices are necessary when evaluating pacing rate and pulse width changes caused by battery depletion, component failure, or reprogramming.

A magnet should always be available for troubleshooting sessions. Nearly all pacemakers can be converted to asynchronous operation by the placement of a magnet over the generator site. This enables evaluation of capture when the patient's intrinsic rhythm inhibits the pacemaker and can be useful in diagnosing oversensing by disabling all sensing function. Magnet application should be used with care, since some pacemakers can be programmed by application of a suitable magnet and there is always a definite but slight risk of inducing tachydysrhythmias when pacing asynchronously.

Carotid sinus massage or the Valsalva maneuver may slow a patient's intrinsic rhythm and induce pacing. Such a procedure may be used to evaluate capture if a pacemaker fails to respond to magnet application because of a component failure or a unique design having no asynchronous magnet mode.

Exercise may be used to speed the patient's spontaneous rate in the evaluation of sensing capability or in the evaluation of a pacemaker rate increase in response to exercise in rate-adaptive modes.

Chest wall stimulation with an external stimulator connected to precordial surface electrodes can be used to test sensing function and to determine rate tracking limits for atrial tracking pacemakers (VAT, VDD, DDD, and DDDR).

Manipulation of the pulse generator in its pocket can sometimes elicit ECG signs of a loose connection or damaged lead close to the generator site.

X-ray examination or fluoroscopy of the chest and pacemaker system in multiple views helps determine lead position, gross lead fracture, and disconnections at the generator. A baseline x-ray film should be obtained before the patient is discharged after implantation of the system.

An oscilloscope or special ECG recorder designed to display the waveshape of the pacemaker stimulus is used by some centers to evaluate lead problems or unusual component failures.

A pacemaker programmer is an extremely useful troubleshooting tool in dealing with a programmable pacemaker; it allows the user to vary stimulus strength, amplifier sensitivity, rates, refractory periods, and pacing modes. This permits noninvasive threshold evaluation and in many systems permits the user to obtain noninvasive intracardiac electrograms to evaluate sensing operation. Many systems include digital telemetry of the programmed settings of the pacemakers; some systems provide a marker channel™, a noninvasively telemetered signal indicating pacemaker sensing and pacing, which with a surface ECG, clearly identifies pacemaker operation (Fig. 6-8). Most modern systems allow measurement of lead impedance, a helpful parameter for lead troubleshooting. Other systems provide telemetered event counter data that display the number of paced and sensed events for various rate ranges (Fig. 6-9). Programmers may also be used to determine the pacemaker model number and serial number for some pacing systems when patient information is lacking.

Invasive procedures are necessary if noninvasive approaches fail. A pacing system analyzer is the primary tool for invasive troubleshooting. This instrument typically can analyze the implantable pulse generator function (sensitivities, refractory periods, rates, pulse widths, and amplitudes), evaluate lead integrity and positioning, and provide electrophysiologic patient data (stimulation thresholds, electrogram amplitudes, AV conduction, and sinus function).

In addition to the troubleshooting hardware, it is important to have detailed patient records, including prior ECGs and x-ray films, and information on the characteristics of the implanted system. Unfortunately, it is common for a normally functioning pacemaker to be diagnosed as malfunctioning simply because of inadequate understanding of proper device operation. Systems with hysteresis,* mode switching,† special antitachycardia pacemakers, and

---

*Pacemakers with hysteresis are designed to work as follows: The escape interval (before pacing) after the last sensed spontaneous activity exceeds the interval between subsequent consecutive pacing artifacts. This allows maintenance of normal sinus rhythm over a wide range of rates (pacemaker inhibited) while ensuring an adequate pacing rate when needed. This type of operation is diagrammed in Fig. 6-10.

†*Mode switching* refers to a pacemaker system feature in which during atrial tracking modes (DDD and DDDR) the pacemaker distinguishes between high atrial rates related to exercise or atrial tachycardias. In the presence of inappropriate high atrial rates, the pacemaker switches to an atrial nontracking mode (VVIR and DDIR). On return to appropriate atrial rates, the pacemaker again returns to atrial synchronous operation. Detection of atrial tachycardias can use atrial rate criteria and sensor rates to differentiate between atrial tachycardia and appropriate high atrial rates.

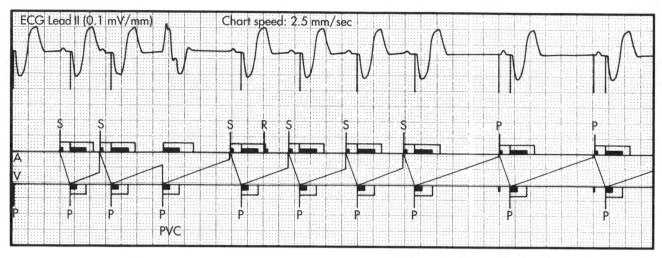

Fig. 6-8 Marker channel™–generated diagnostic ladder diagram for a DDD pacemaker. The ladder diagram clarifies pacemaker response to a short run of atrial tachycardia seen in the surface ECG. In the diagram, *S* represents sensing; *P*, pacing; *R*, refractory sensing; *white rectangular area*, pacemaker refractory periods; *solid rectangular area*, absolute refractory periods (blanking). Sloping lines between the horizontal parallel lines indicate timing of AV and ventriculoatrial escape intervals. Atrial sensing, pacing, and refractory periods are marked above the top horizontal line, and ventricular events are marked beneath the lower line. The marker channel indicates atrial synchronous ventricular pacing followed by a premature ventricular contraction and atrial synchronous ventricular pacing with a refractory atrial sensed event followed by atrial and ventricular sequential pacing.

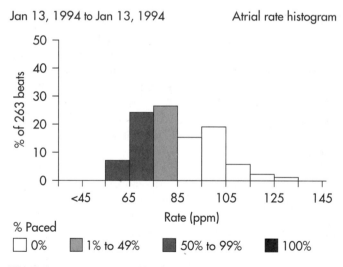

Fig. 6-9 Pacemaker event counter data. The number of sensed and paced intervals are stored as events in rate ranges and presented in a graph. The percentage of paced beats in each bin (rate change) are presented as 0%, between 1 and 49%, between 50 and 99%, and 100%.

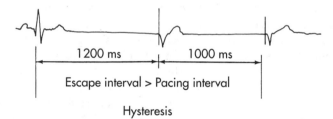

Fig. 6-10 Diagrammatic representation of operation of a VVI pacemaker incorporating hysteresis. The last beat of the sinus rhythm is the first complex on the left. Spontaneous sinus bradycardia results, and the pacemaker "escapes" at an interval of 1200 msec. The subsequent pacing interval is 1000 msec, however; thus the escape interval of the pacemaker exceeds the pacing interval (in other words, the initial escape rate of pacemaker discharge is slower than the subsequent rate of pacing) to allow the patient's heart to remain in a normally conducted rhythm for as much of the time as possible.

Failure to pace

Failure to pace implies nondelivery of a stimulus or loss of capture (delivery of an ineffective stimulus that fails to depolarize the myocardium).

Failure to deliver a stimulus can result from various factors, including improper connection of the lead to the generator (as when set screws are not tightened); broken lead wires with no insulation defect; "crosstalk" between atrial and ventricular portions of dual-chamber pacemakers so

synchronous pacemakers are especially vulnerable to misdiagnosis.

Pacemaker-related problems fall into four broad categories: failure to pace, loss of sensing or oversensing, pacing at an altered rate, and undesirable patient-pacemaker interactions.

that the atrial stimulus is sensed by the ventricular amplifier, thus inhibiting the ventricular stimulus (caused by improper electrode placement or incorrect electrode types); pulse generator component failure; and power source depletion. Occasionally, a misdiagnosis of failure to pace is made when a normally functioning pacemaker is merely inhibited by the patient's intrinsic rhythm. This is especially common with programmable pacemakers set at relatively low rates. (Inappropriate nondelivery of a stimulus also may be caused by oversensing, which is discussed later.)

Loss of capture may be caused by lead dislodgment (the most common cause); myocardial perforation with lead migration to an extracardiac position; failure of lead insulation or wire fracture; increased stimulation threshold caused by infarction, drug effects, electrolyte imbalances, and fibrosis at the electrode site; and inappropriate programming of pacemaker stimulus strength. Lack of capture when a stimulus is delivered during the myocardial refractory period is a frequent source of misdiagnosis.

Loss of sensing or oversensing

A pacemaker may fail to sense intracardiac signals, resulting in competitive pacing or in the case of atrial synchronous units, loss of AV synchrony. This may be caused by lead dislodgment (the most common cause); inadequate amplitude or waveshape of the intracardiac electrogram caused by inappropriate lead placement, fibrosis, infarct, drugs, or electrolyte disturbances; inappropriate programming of amplifier sensitivity or polarity, refractory periods, or mode (for example, AOO and VOO); wire fracture or insulation defect; connector defect; and component failure (such as a stuck magnetic reed switch).

Occasionally, a misdiagnosis of sensing failure is made when spontaneous activity occurs with delivery of the pacemaker stimulus and results in fusion beats. This occurs because electrical activity may occur within the myocardium and be visible on the surface ECG record before it reaches the pacemaker electrode site. Concurrently, the pacemaker escape interval may elapse, with resultant stimulation just before arrival of the spontaneous depolarization. This apparent failure to sense is, in fact, perfectly normal operation. Another case of apparent sensing failure is reversion to asynchronous operation in the presence of electromagnetic interference—also a normal mode of operation for many pacemakers. Finally, closely coupled intracardiac signals may occur when a lead with a hairline fracture or loose connection makes intermittent contact or when two endocardial leads come into contact. Electromagnetic interference from power lines, radio or television transmitters, and other electrical noise sources may occasionally be sensed, especially by unipolar pacemakers. Sometimes this may result in inhibition or triggering, but it more commonly produces reversion to the asynchronous mode that provides continued pacing support. Very rarely, a pacemaker may sense the afterpotentials remaining on a lead after delivery

of a stimulus. This is most commonly the result of using very wide pulse widths, excessively short refractory periods, and short cross-channel blanking periods (blanking of the ventricular sense amplifier for a short period during delivery of an atrial channel pacing stimulus).

In all cases of suspected oversensing, placing the pacemaker in an asynchronous mode (applying a magnet if it is a permanent pacemaker or turning off the sensitivity if it is an external pacemaker) abolishes the symptoms caused by the pacemaker malfunction and confirms the diagnosis.

Pacing at an altered rate

A fairly common cause for concern is apparent operation of a pacemaker at an unexpected rate. This can be an indication of a real problem with the pacemaker system but more frequently reflects a diagnostic error.

The possible true causes of unexpected pacing at an altered rate include the following: oversensing that induces rate slowing caused by inhibition or rate acceleration caused by triggering or rate-responsive sensor malfunction, rate slowdown built into most pacemakers to indicate approaching power-source depletion, and component failure (usually causing a stimulus output or a rapid stimulation rate typically limited to less than 150 beats/min by "runaway" protection circuits).

Frequent causes of pacing at an altered rate when there is no system failure include the presence of a rate hysteresis that produces a long escape interval after sensed activity; reprogramming of a programmable pacemaker without proper recording of the change in patient records; tracking of spontaneous intrinsic cardiac accelerations with VVT, AAT, VAT, VDD, DDD, and DDDR pacemakers; sensor-driven rate increases in rate-adaptive pacing modes; failure of the reader to note a nearly isoelectric atrial or ventricular complex in a single-lead ECG tracing so that the pacemaker appears to have a prolonged stimulus-to-stimulus interval; misinterpretation of nonpacemaker artifacts such as rapid spike potentials generated by muscle fasciculation or electrical noise in the ECG recording system; and lack of familiarity with device operation (such as a DDDR pacemaker with mode-switching operating asynchronous to atrial electrical activity in the presence of inappropriately high atrial rates).

Undesirable patient-pacemaker interactions

Occasionally, undesirable patient-pacemaker interactions develop. The pacemaker pocket may become infected or develop hematomas, or the generator may erode through the pocket site. These problems occur less frequently with small, lightweight generators. Some patients exhibit "twiddler's syndrome," playing with their pulse generators and rotating them in their pockets, causing retraction of the lead and total system failure.

Extracardiac stimulation of the pectoralis muscles or diaphragm may be observed. These problems are generally restricted to unipolar pacemakers; are less likely with the newer low-threshold, high-impedance leads; and have been reported, in rare instances, with bipolar systems. Decreasing the pulse width, voltage, or current of the stimulus can be useful in eliminating or reducing such extracardiac stimulation.

Incorrect pacing mode selection for a given patient or changes in a patient's postimplantation status can have serious consequences. For example, atrial tracking pacemakers (VAT, VDD, DDD, and DDDR) may detect slowly conducted retrograde atrial activity (long RP interval) after ventricular stimulation, inducing pacemaker-mediated tachycardia with a pacing interval equal to the programmed AV interval plus the retrograde conduction time (RP interval). Patients may respond poorly to other specific pacing modes, depending on their underlying hemodynamic and electrophysiologic conditions. In many such cases, the use of multiprogrammable pacemakers allows the clinician to alter the pacing system characteristics without resorting to invasive procedures.

Table 6-6 summarizes various pacemaker problems and their likely causes.

Example of troubleshooting

The following hypothetical example demonstrates how a clinician troubleshoots a pacemaker malfunction, in this case intermittent loss of capture and failure to sense spontaneous ventricular activity (Fig. 6-11). The patient has a ventricular demand pacemaker implanted 1 year before.

The first step in troubleshooting is to list the likely causes of the symptoms. Since there are two malfunctions in this example, it is highly probable, although not absolutely certain, that there is a common cause. The most likely causes follow:

Lack of capture	Lack of sensing
Lead dislodgment or perforation	Lead dislodgment or perforation
Lead wire fracture	Lead wire fracture
Lead insulation failure	Lead insulation failure
Pulse generator failure	Pulse generator failure
Inappropriate programming of output energy	Inappropriate programming of amplifier sensitivity or refractory period
High threshold	Inadequate electrogram amplitude caused by infarct, electrolyte disturbance, and myocardial disease
Misread ECG ("loss of capture" seen only when stimulus occurs during cardiac refractory period)	Electromagnetic interference–induced reversion to asynchronous mode
	Stuck reed switch
	Misread ECG (fusion beats)

Analysis should begin by comparing a current 12-lead ECG with a baseline tracing predating the occurrence of the problem. The current tracing should be carefully reviewed to prevent misinterpretation of fusion beats as sensing failure or pacing artifacts during the cardiac re-

fractory period as lack of capture. Electromagnetic interference–induced reversion to the asynchronous mode can usually be eliminated as a cause if the problem of nonsensing persists in a 12-lead ECG that shows no signs of electrical interference. Comparison of the current and baseline ECGs establishes the presence or absence of lead position changes, including perforation as evidenced by shifts in the pace QRS vector and pacing artifact vector.* An x-ray examination provides confirmation of significant dislodgements. Insulation defects in the lead result in vector changes in the pacing artifact but usually not in the paced QRS complex.

Application of a magnet should result in pacing without sensing. In most pacemakers, magnet application alters the pacing rate (sometimes by only a few milliseconds), confirming that the reed switch is functioning and allowing elimination of the possibility of nonsensing caused by a stuck reed switch.

If inappropriate programming is thought to be the problem, it is a simple matter to reprogram the amplifier sensitivity and refractory period to restore sensing and increase the stimulus intensity to restore capture. If such reprogramming fails to resolve the problem or if the parameter settings required are not within normally accepted bounds, inappropriate programming can be excluded.

Wire fracture can produce nonsensing and lack of capture, but it is generally accompanied by random resetting of the escape interval as the broken wire ends intermittently touch. An x-ray examination can sometimes help confirm wire fracture, but not all fractures are visible on the x-ray film. In this example the regularity of the escape intervals probably eliminates wire fracture as the cause of the problem.

Noninvasive procedures have been explored to evaluate the majority of potential causes for the reported malfunctions. Threshold elevation, inadequate electrogram characteristics, and pulse generator failure require invasive evaluation, although some noninvasive determinations can be obtained if the patient has a sophisticated multiprogrammable pulse generator. Some of these devices can telemeter the intracardiac electrogram, facilitating evaluation of sensing problems. In addition, some devices allow noninvasive measurement of lead impedance. They also allow the user to obtain noninvasive threshold measurements. Nevertheless, correction of sensing and pacing failure caused by any of these factors requires invasive procedures.

In the example, ECG evidence (Fig. 6-12) indicates a lead dislodgement. There is an axis shift in the pacemaker stimulus artifact and in the paced QRS complexes. Lead placement is the most common cause of sensing and capture failures.

---

*Digital ECG systems with low sampling rates cannot be used to determine the reliability of the vector of the pacemaker artifact.

TABLE 6-6   Pacemaker System Problems and Causes*

Problem	Nonpacing Noncapture	Nonsensing	Oversensing	Altered Rate	Undesirable Patient/IPG Interactions
ACTUAL MALFUNCTIONS					
Lead dislodged or perforated myocardium (possibly caused by twiddler's syndrome)	NC	X	X	X	X
Lead insulation failure	NC	X	X	X	X
Lead fracture with fluid in lumen	NC	X	X	X	
Skeletal muscle potentials, electromagnetic interference, hairline lead fracturees	NP	X	X	X	
Pulse generator failure	NP, NC	X	X	X	
Poor lead/IPG connection	NP	X	X	X	
Power source depletion	NC, NP	X	X		
Lead fracture with dry lumen	NP	X			
Electric interference resulting in asynchronous pacing		X		X	
Cross-talk between atrial and ventricular channels			X	X	
Sensitivity too high			X	X	
Refractory period too short			X	X	
High threshold: fibrosis, infarct, drugs, electrolyte imbalance, lead position	NC				
Low-output energy setting	NC				
Poor electrogram: fibrosis, infarct, drugs, electrolyte imbalance, lead position		X			
Sensitivity too low		X			
Refractory period too long		X			
Asynchronous mode: magnet or programmed		X			
End-of-service-life indicator activated				X	
High-output energy setting: extracardiac stimulation					X
Infection, hematoma, erosion					X
Sensor malfunction				X	
POTENTIAL MISDIAGNOSES					
Recording system masks ECG signal (for example, lead switching)	NP, NC		X	X	
Recorder malfunction (for example, paper speed error)		X	X	X	
Hysteresis mode			X	X	X
Fusion of activity from pacemaker and cardiac source	NC	X			
Artifacts from source other than IPG (for example, muscle fasciculation)	NC			X	

*The column headings are symptoms of a malfunctioning pacemaker system. The left column includes entries that are mechanisms that can produce the symptoms marked with an X, NC (noncapture or ineffective stimulus), or NP (nonpacing or no stimulus artifact). After determining the type and number of symptoms exhibited by a system, one can find a match to entries in this table, thereby determining the most probable cause of the malfunction. The lower half of the table links apparent symptoms with mechanisms that do not result from pacemaker malfunction.

Continued.

TABLE 6-6   Pacemaker System Problems and Causes—cont'd

Problem	Nonpacing Noncapture	Nonsensing	Oversensing	Altered Rate	Undesirable Patient/IPG Interactions
POTENTIAL MISDIAGNOSES—cont'd					
Stimulus falls in tissue refractory period	NC				
Atrial stimulus misread as ventricular without capture or vice versa	NC				
Cardiac activity is within IPG refractory period (for example, QRS within AV interval of committed DVI pacemaker)		X			
Rate-responsive pacemaker changing rate in response to parameter not reflected in ECG record (for example, activity)				X	

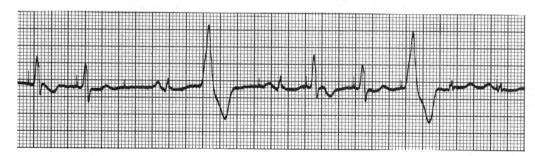

Fig. 6-11 Failure of a VVI pacemaker. Note that pacing stimuli occasionally fail to elicit a paced QRS complex and also occasionally fail to sense spontaneous electric activity. Lead II.

Conclusions

Artificial cardiac pacemakers of today are very different from their predecessors of the early 1960s; today, pacemakers offer a variety of sophisticated modes and programmable features. Advancements will further optimize function while increasing automatic operation, providing enhanced therapy for patients and reducing the time demands of the health care provider.

IMPLANTABLE CARDIOVERTER DEFIBRILLATORS

The implantable cardioverter defibrillator (ICD) is an electronic device used primarily to detect and terminate potentially lethal ventricular dysrhythmias through the delivery of low- or high-energy shocks. Antitachycardia and bradycardia pacing therapies are also available in most de-

vices. The ICD system consists of a power source, electronic circuitry for generating appropriately timed shocks and pacing stimuli, and an electrode and wire system (lead) to complete the electrical connection between the circuitry and the heart. The first ICD was implanted in a human in February 1980.[73,74] It is estimated that there are over 75,000 patients worldwide who have implanted ICDs, and today's devices are vastly different from the early versions,[75] which weighed 250 to 300 g, delivered only 25 to 30 joule shocks, required open chest procedures for implantation, and lasted 18 to 24 months.[76,77] Current models weigh 150 to 200 g or less, provide pacing therapies and low- or high-energy shocks that are noninvasively programmable, can be implanted without open chest procedures, have memory storage for recording episode history, and may last 5 to 6 years.[78]

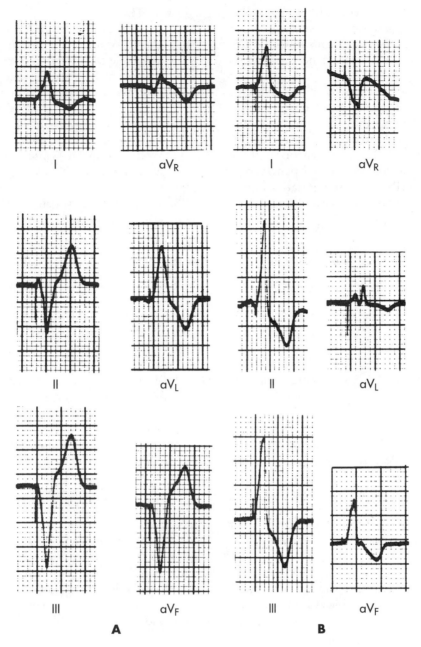

I aV_R I aV_R

II aV_L II aV_L

III aV_F III aV_F

A **B**

Fig. 6-12 ECG leads I, II, III, aV_R, aV_L, and aV_F were recorded before **(A)** and after **(B)** pacemaker malfunction. The VVI pacemaker developed sensing and capture problems. Note that the vector and amplitude of the spikes are different in the two 12-lead ECGs and that the generated QRS complexes are also different. This ECG example is most consistent with migration of the pacing electrode from its initial appropriate location in the right ventricular apex to a different position in the ventricle. This was the case, and the lead was repositioned.

Indications

During the 1980s, commercially available ICDs provided shock therapy only and had no programmability. Therefore their use was extremely limited during the early clinical studies under Food and Drug Administration regulations and when they became commercially available in 1985. Patients had to have survived at least one episode of cardiac arrest not associated with an MI and believed to result from hemodynamically unstable VT or ventricular fibrillation (VF). Patients with recurrent VTs who had not had an arrest could also be considered for an ICD if VT or VF was inducible in the electrophysiology (EP) laboratory while the patient was on what was believed to be optimal antidysrhythmic drug therapy.[79]

Almost from the beginning, however, it became apparent that the ICD was highly effective in preventing sudden cardiac death. Thus consideration of patients for ICD therapy began to expand beyond the rather narrow criteria originally used.[80-85]

As a result of these seemingly expanding indications for the use of the ICD, panels representing three main professional organizations issued summaries of indications for the use of these devices in 1991. One panel consisted of representatives from the American Heart Association and the American College of Cardiology. The other panel representatives were from NASPE. Recommendations from both panels were similar and divided their indications into the following categories:

Class I	ICD Therapy is indicated by general consensus.
Class II	ICD therapy is a recognized option, but there is no general consensus.
Class III	ICD therapy is generally not justified.

The following are the panels' recommendations by class:[86,87]

Class I

1. Patients with spontaneous sustained VT or VF in whom EP testing or Holter monitoring cannot be used to accurately predict the efficacy of other therapies; includes patients whose VT or VF is not inducible at EP testing
2. Patients with recurrent VT or VF despite antidysrhythmic therapy guided by EP testing or Holter monitoring; includes patients in whom drugs predicted to be effective at initial EP testing fail
3. Patients with VT or VF whose VT or VF remains persistently inducible at EP testing despite the best drug therapy, surgical therapy, or catheter ablation

Class II

1. Patients with syncope of undetermined origin who have sustained VT or VF inducible at EP testing and in whom antidysrhythmic drug therapy is limited by inefficacy, intolerance, or noncompliance

Class III

1. Patients with sustained VT or VF related to acute ischemia or infarction or toxic or metabolic etiologies amenable to correction or reversibility
2. Patients with recurrent syncope of undetermined origin whose syncopy is not inducible at EP testing into sustained ventricular tachydysrhythmias
3. Patients with incessant VT or VF
4. Patients with VF secondary to atrial fibrillation in Wolff-Parkinson-White syndrome whose bypass tracts are amenable to surgical or catheter ablation therapy
5. Patients with surgical, medical, or psychiatric contraindications

Modalities
NBD code

NASPE and BPEG, based on the success and use of the generic code developed to identify the various pacing modes (see Table 6-1), have also developed a defibrillation code to identify the functions of ICDs. This new code (Table 6-7) was patterned after the pacemaker (NBG) code and is compatible with it.[88]

Table 6-7 provides a shorthand description of implantable defibrillator operation. The first position indicates the chambers in which cardioversion and defibrillation shocks are delivered, and the second position specifies the locations of antitachycardia pacing. In the third position, the method by which tachycardias are detected is specified, and the fourth position identifies the chambers in which antibradycardia pacing is provided. For example, currently available devices shock only in the ventricle, so the first letter in the four-position code is *V*. The first devices available for human implants had no antitachycardia pacing functions, so the second letter in the code for these devices is *O*. They detect VF using changes in the electrogram, and therefore *E* is in the third position; since they also have no antibradycardia pacing available, the fourth and final position is designated *O*. The complete code is therefore *VOEO*.

TABLE 6-7   NASPE/BPEG Defibrillator (NBD) Code

Shock Chamber	Antitachycardia Pacing Chamber	Tachycardia Detection	Antibradycardia Pacing Chamber
O = None	O = None	E = Electrogram	O = None
A = Atrium	A = Atrium	H = Hemodynamic	A = Atrium
V = Ventricle	V = Ventricle		V = Ventricle
D = Dual (A+V)	D = Dual (A+V)		D = Dual (A+V)

From Bernstein A and others: The NASPE/BPEG defibrillator code, *PACE* 16:1776, 1993.

Devices available today are considerably more complex than the early devices. Therefore a "short form" code was also developed to quickly identify devices limited to only cardioversion defibrillation and those that also incorporate antitachycardia and antibradycardia pacing. This code is shown in the box.

Devices with only shock capability

ICDs that provided shock-only therapy were, as previously indicated, the only devices commercially available during the 1980s.[76,77] Since they typically lasted 18 to 24 months, with later models lasting approximately 3 years, most of these devices have now been explanted from surviving patients and replaced with newer models. Currently, only a few devices with shock-only capability are being implanted. They are considered "first-generation" devices.[89]

Devices with shock capability and antibradycardia pacing

ICDs with shock capability and antibradycardia pacing are currently being implanted, but there are differences of opinion among physicians regarding whether they are needed and which patients should receive them. These devices are considered "second-generation" devices.

Devices with antitachycardia and antibradycardia pacing and shock capabilities

ICDs with antitachycardia pacing for termination of VT as well as shock therapy and antibradycardia pacing were approved for commercial use in 1993 but had been undergoing clinical trials for several years before then.[90] Most of the devices now being implanted are of this type. They are considered "third-generation" or "tiered-therapy" devices.[89]

Next-generation devices

Next-generation ICDs will continue to improve on the technologic advances made during the past few years, primarily in the areas of simplified implantation procedures and improved detection algorithms for tachydysrhythmias appropriate for intervention by the implanted device. Systems referred to as "fourth-generation ICD systems" are now undergoing clinical trials in the United States and are commercially available elsewhere.[91-92] These systems differ from third-generation systems in that they are unipolar, single-shocking electrode, transvenous, tiered-therapy systems usually implanted in the subcutaneous or submuscu-

---

**NASPE/BPEG DEFIBRILLATOR (NBD) CODE,
SHORT FORM**

ICD-S = ICD with shock capability only
ICD-B = ICD with bradycardia pacing as well as shock
ICD-T = ICD with tachycardia (and bradycardia) pacing as well as shock

From Bernstein A and others: The NASPE/BPEG defibrillator code, *PACE* 16:1776, 1993.

---

lar pectoral area. The ICD can is "active" and becomes the second-shocking electrode. Early experience suggests that these systems may limit the time and cost of the surgical procedure, decrease the morbidity rate and length of stay in the hospital, minimize the expertise required for successful use, and function as effectively as epicardially placed systems or systems with multiple leads and electrodes. If so, they will make more widespread use of ICDs both practical and likely, assuming appropriate and satisfactory resolution of continuing controversies.

Improved detection algorithms will also be highly beneficial. Current systems use various methods for discriminating VTs from sinus tachycardias and atrial fibrillation, but these methods are not completely perfected, resulting in inappropriate detections and therefore inappropriate shocks.[93-94] Early experience with new algorithms incorporating interval stability (designed to distinguish VTs from atrial fibrillation) and onset criteria (designed to distinguish VTs from sinus tachycardias) have shown promise in reducing the number of inappropriate detections while maintaining or increasing the number of appropriate detections of VTs.[95] Such algorithms will continue to be improved as experiences with them increase.

Mode selection

Selection of the optimal ICD modality for the individual can be a challenging task requiring detailed knowledge of specific dysrhythmias that have been documented and the patient's hemodynamic response to them. An additional challenge exists if a patient has experienced significant hemodynamic compromise or collapse without documentation of the dysrhythmia or dysrhythmias that preceded it. Clearly, VF must be detected by the ICD 100% of the time. To achieve this high degree of *sensitivity* may require somewhat less *specificity,* the result of which can be the unnecessary delivery of high-energy shocks.[96]

It has been repeatedly demonstrated that antitachycardia pacing of various types is highly effective in terminating sustained VT in patients with ICDs, with reported success rates ranging from 91% to 99%.[97-102] It has also been demonstrated that low-energy cardioversion is effective in terminating some ventricular dysrhythmias that do not respond to antitachycardia pacing.[90,100,102,103]

Therefore most current ICD recipients receive tiered-therapy devices programmed to deliver progressively aggressive and separate treatment for VT and VF, using the full capabilities of the devices. This full function mode (VVEV) promotes patient comfort without compromising patient safety by eliminating many unnecessary high-energy shocks.

Programmability[104-107]

The first ICDs of the early 1980s were not programmable; the rate at which a ventricular dysrhythmia was deemed to be VT or VF, prompting delivery of a shock, was set by the manufacturer. The shock energy level was also preset.

It quickly became apparent, however, that patients' VT rates could change and that atrial or supraventricular tachydysrhythmias could develop at rates equal to or above the VT rate, prompting unnecessary shocks. Research also began to indicate that the hearts of conscious patients with slower ventricular tachydysrhythmias could be effectively cardioverted with shocks of much lower energy levels that were more comfortable for the patients. Therefore the first programmable features of ICDs were dysrhythmic detection rates and shock energy levels.

Today all ICDs are programmable, the extent depending on their number of features. Third- and fourth-generation systems, which are the most widely used, have extensive programmability of all features. These include but are not limited to standard bradycardia sensing and pacing features (rate, stimulus output amplitude and duration, amplifier sensitivity, and amplifier refractory period); VT and VF detection criteria (rate, onset, duration, stability, and morphology); antitachycardia pacing therapies to treat VT (type of therapy, pulse intervals, number of sequences in the therapy, and number of therapy attempts); and cardioversion/defibrillation therapies (shock energy level, waveforms, current pathways, pulse width, and number of attempts).

The programmability of ICDs is of immense benefit to clinicians and patients because it permits these highly sophisticated devices to be tailored to changing patient conditions. Programmability also minimizes the need for invasive procedures to correct malfunctions and greatly enhances troubleshooting procedures. It further allows the noninvasive induction of VT, VF, or both to ensure that the device correctly terminates the dysrhythmia if it occurs spontaneously, which is absolutely essential. Table 6-8 indicates applications of some of the most common ICD programmable parameters, and Fig. 6-13 illustrates device therapeutic operations and evaluation and testing capabilities.

Programming needs to be done with extreme caution and performed only by thoroughly trained personnel who have extensive knowledge of each patient's cardiac and dysrhythmic history, since incorrect programming could cause failure to detect a potentially lethal dysrhythmia and result in death. It is also extremely important to note that magnet application, which is, as previously mentioned, a simple form of programming, is entirely different when applied to ICDs than it is when applied to permanent pacemakers. In addition, unlike pacemakers, in which magnet application results in the same basic change for all manufacturers' devices (conversion to an asynchronous pacing mode), the results of magnet application to ICDs differ from manu-

---

TABLE 6-8   Applications of Programmable ICD Parameters

Parameter(s)	Patient/ICD Optimization	Diagnostic Applications	Correction of Malfunctions
Brady pacing support (see Table 6-5)	Ensure that heart rate does not drop below a specified value; ensure that heart function resumes after application of a shock.	Suppress pacing to assess underlying rhythm by ECG; evaluate the heart's ability to resume functioning after a shock.	Adjust rate, output sensitivity, and refractory period.
VT and VF detection criteria	Help differentiate between sinus tachycardia and VT and VF; ensure that nonsustained VT and VF are appropriately treated.	Induce VT and VF to evaluate appropriateness and timeliness of programmed detection criteria.	Adjust rate, onset, duration, stability, and morphology.
Antitachycardia pacing therapies	Permit VT termination with painless pacing therapies as much as is possible and safe.	Induce VT to ensure that selected pacing therapies are working promptly and appropriately.	Adjust therapy type, number of intervals, number of sequences, and number of attempts.
Cardioversion/defibrillation therapies	Ensure cardioversion/defibrillation as rapidly as possible; permit cardioversion/defibrillation at lowest effective energies to optimize patient safety and device longevity.	Induce VT and VF to evaluate promptness and effectiveness of cardioversion/defibrillation; permit therapy at lowest effective thresholds; assess stability of thresholds to ensure patient safety.	Adjust shock energy level, waveforms, current pathways, pulse width, and number of attempts.

THERAPEUTIC OPERATIONS

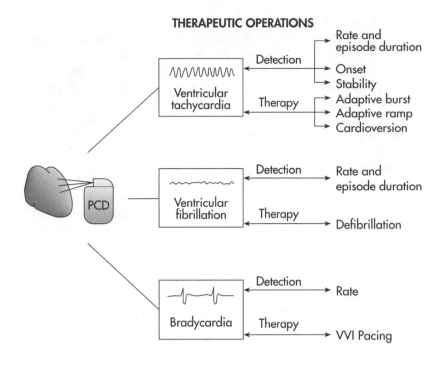

EVALUATION AND TESTING OPERATIONS

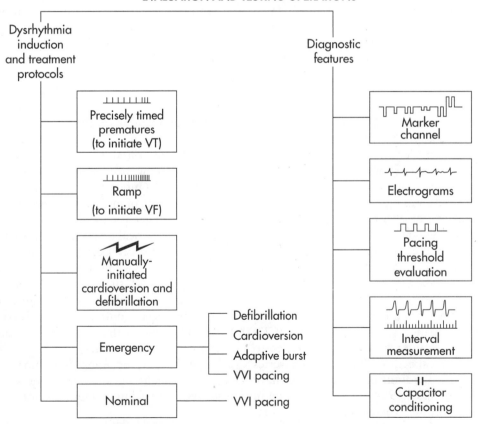

Fig. 6-13   Therapeutic operations and evaluation/testing capabilities of a third-generation ICD (Medtronic PCD model 7217).   (Courtesy Medtronic, Inc, Minneapolis.)

facturer to manufacturer. A magnet placed over an ICD prevents the device from sensing VT, VF, or both, but whether this is only while the magnet is in place or whether it results in automatic reprogramming requiring reactivation of sensing through another programming sequence differs from one manufacturer to another. Devices that are automatically reprogrammed by application of a magnet can also have their sensing circuits deactivated through inadvertent exposure by the patient to strong magnetic fields. Therefore it is essential that patients know the magnet response of their particular device. Patients with devices that are automatically reprogrammed by magnet application must be taught to avoid areas with high magnetic fields and to have their devices rechecked at the follow-up clinic if they have any concerns about possible inadvertent exposure to such areas.

Currently, ICD programming devices produce printed records of all programmed parameters, including the VT and VF detection and therapy settings. They also produce specific data regarding which therapies were used and whether these therapies were successful in terminating the VT or VF. Fig. 6-14 is an example of such a printout. These data are very useful in optimizing device function. A printout of all current programmed parameters should be evaluated and included in the patient's record every time the patient is seen for follow-up examination. This ensures that inadvertent reprogramming is accurately identified and corrected.

Power Sources[108-110]

Power sources (batteries) for ICDs have posed unique challenges to designers from the very beginning. Like batteries for implantable pacemakers, batteries for ICDs must be able to provide maximal energy when needed, minimize wasted energy, and be hermetically sealed into a can to prevent ingress of body fluids and egress of tissue-damaging battery materials. Unlike pacemaker batteries, however, defibrillator batteries must also be capable of charging high-voltage capacitors very rapidly (up to 750 V in less than 10 sec). There must also be a constant low-level background current to power the monitoring and bradycardia pacing circuits of the ICD.

The lithium iodide and lithium cupric sulfide batteries used in implantable pacemakers are not suitable for ICDs because they cannot deliver energy as rapidly as needed to charge the high-voltage capacitors. Therefore batteries based on lithium–silver vanadium oxide chemistry have been under development since 1984 and are now used in virtually all ICDs. An additional characteristic of these batteries is a gradual voltage decline, which is useful and necessary for predicting when device replacement is required.

The reported performance of newer models of ICDs shows the progress that has been made toward increasing the overall longevity of these devices. The 1994 survival probabilities for newer devices reported that two models

of ICDs from two different manufacturers, comprising 473 units, showed a cumulative survival probability of 100% at approximately 40 months. This contrasts with two of the earliest models of ICDs, comprising 558 units, which showed a cumulative survival probability of significantly less than 50% at approximately 40 months. These data reflect clinical results and clearly demonstrate the progress that has been made with lithium–silver vanadium oxide chemistry for ICD batteries.[48]

Electrode Systems (Leads)[111-122]

ICDs, like permanent pacemakers, are electrically connected to the heart by means of wires and electrode systems referred to as *leads*. These systems are needed for pacing, sensing, and delivery of cardioversion/defibrillation shocks. The newest fourth-generation systems available from one manufacturer are unipolar defibrillation systems, with the shocking coil lead located within the cardiac chamber (and adjacent vessels if necessary, depending on the defibrillation waveforms needed for obtaining adequate defibrillation thresholds). The metallic housing of the ICD serves as the other electrode for defibrillation. The polarity of this lead system (designation of the negative/cathodal and positive/anodal electrodes) is programmable. Pacing and sensing is standard bipolar, however, and these electrodes are located on the same lead as the main shocking coil. Older systems use bipolar, tripolar, and quadripolar electrode lead systems for defibrillation (the ICD housing is not an electrode), again depending on the waveforms needed for obtaining adequate defibrillation thresholds. Pacing and sensing for these older systems may be standard bipolar, using ring (anodal) and tip (cathodal) electrodes on the lead containing the main shocking coil, or integrated bipolar, using the shocking coil itself as the pacing/sensing (anodal) electrode.

At the time of initial implantation of an ICD system and when the generator and any leads are replaced or modified, the same electrical measurements needed when implanting a permanent pacemaker (stimulation threshold and cardiac signal amplitudes) must be made. In addition, the defibrillation threshold (the minimum amount of energy required to successfully terminate VF) must be determined and compared to the output of the ICD to ensure that the difference between the two is high enough to ensure adequate defibrillation safety margins. Other testing may also be performed, including determination of the cardioversion threshold and the effectiveness of one or more antitachycardia pacing therapies for the termination of VT.

Transvenous leads

Permanent ICD leads are designed for transvenous, epicardial, and subcutaneous chest placement. Transvenous leads, commonly referred to as *nonthoracotomy leads*, can be placed in a variety of positions to minimize the amount of energy needed for defibrillation. Positions for the shock-

```
PACING AND SENSING                            VT THERAPY #4:                                VF onset counter                    14
  Pacing mode             VVI                   Therapy type      CARDIOVERSION
  Pacing rate             65    PPM              VT therapy enable     ON                  VT EPISODE AND THERAPY DATA:
  Pacing pulse width      1.59  MS               CV pulse width        3.9     MS            Episode count                      6
  Pacing amplitude        5.4   V                CV energy (joules)    34.0    J             VT therapy #1 success count        3
  Sensitivity             0.3   MV               CV current pathway    SEQ                   VT therapy #2 success count        2
  Refractory after pace   320   MS                                                          VT therapy #3 success count        1
                                              VF DETECTION AND THERAPIES:                    VT therapy #4 success count        0
VT DETECTION AND THERAPIES                      VF detect:                                   # of VT's PCD ineffective          0
VT Detect:                                        VF detection enable     ON                 PCD efficacious on last VT        YES
  VT detection enable     ON                      VF detection interval   320     MS         Last therapy used                 #3
  # intervals to detect   16                      # intervals to detect   18                 # Seq in last pace therapy         5
  VT detection interval   400   MS                                                          R-R avg for last pace therapy     370   MS
  Interval stability      OFF   MS            VF DEFIBRILLATION THERAPY #1:
  Onset criteria enable   OFF                   VF therapy enable       ON                 VF EPISODE AND THERAPY DATA:
  Onset value (R-R%)      81    %               Defib pulse width       3.9     MS           Episode count                      5
  Onset counter enable    ON                    Defib energy (joules)   34.0    J            VF therapy #1 success count        3
                                                Defib current pathway   SEQ                  VF therapy #2 success count        2
VT THERAPY #1:                                                                               VF therapy #3 success count        0
  Therapy type            RAMP%              VF DEFIBRILLATION THERAPY #2:                    VF therapy #4 success count        0
  VT therapy enable       ON                   VF therapy enable       ON                    # of VF's PCD ineffective          0
  Initial # of S pulses   5                    Defib pulse width       3.9     MS            PCD efficacious on last VF        YES
  First R-S interval      97    %              Defib energy (joules)   34.0    J             Last therapy used                 #2
  Per pulse decrement     10    MS             Defib current pathway   SEQ
  # of sequences          8                                                               LAST EPISODE DETECTION SEQUENCE:
  Minimum interval        200   MS           VF DEFIBRILLATION THERAPY #3:                    −19. R-R interval-920 MS
                                                VF therapy enable       ON                    −18. R-R interval-910 MS
VT THERAPY #2:                                   Defib pulse width       3.9     MS            −17. R-R interval-230 MS
  Therapy type            BURST%                Defib energy (joules)   34.0    J             −16. R-R interval-210 MS
  VT therapy enable       ON                    Defib current pathway   SEQ                        :
  # of S1 pulses          6
  S1-S1 interval          84    %            VF DEFIBRILLATION THERAPY #4:                     −0. R-R interval-210 MS
  Per sequence decrement  10    MS             VF therapy enable       ON                      −0. VF detected
  # of sequences          5                    Defib pulse width       3.9     MS
  Minimum interval        200   MS             Defib energy (joules)   34.0    J           EVENTS AFTER LAST THERAPY:
                                                Defib current pathway   SEQ                    +0. VF therapy #2 delivered
VT THERAPY #3:                                                                                +1. R-R interval-650 MS
  Therapy type            CARDIOVERSION     DATA                                              +2. R-R interval-920 MS
  VT therapy enable       ON                 PCD Status:                                      +3. R-R interval-920 MS
  CV pulse width          6.3   MS             Memory retention      OK                            :
  CV energy (joules)      3.0   J              Charge circuit        OK                       +10. R-R interval-920 MS
  CV current pathway      SNGL                 Last charge time      3.12    SEC             +10. Therapy was successful
                                               Battery voltage       6.19    V
```

Fig. 6-14 Sample printout from a third-generation ICD (Medtronic PCD model 7217). (Courtesy Medtronic, Inc, Minneapolis.)

ing coil leads include the right ventricular apex, coronary sinus, and high or low superior vena cava. Pacing and sensing electrodes are usually positioned in the right ventricular apex, but this will change as ICDs with dual-chamber pacing and sensing are developed. Patches for subcutaneous chest placement, functioning as additional shocking electrodes, can be positioned in the apical, infraclavicular, or subscapular regions. Fig. 6-15 illustrates a variety of placements for nonthoracotomy lead systems.

Like permanent pacemaker leads, transvenous ICD leads are usually inserted via the cephalic or subclavian veins, with positioning stylets in place and under fluoroscopic control. Insertion using lead introducers is increasingly performed but is not as common as with pacemaker leads, since ICD leads are usually larger in diameter. This will change, however, as advances in lead technology permit overall reduction in the size of the leads.

Epicardial leads

Epicardial leads, the only systems available for ICD implantation in the early 1980s, have largely been abandoned for initial device implants. Even patients who are undergoing open heart surgery for other reasons and who need ICDs usually have transvenous systems implanted as separate procedures. Some patients may have previously implanted epicardial lead systems, which may be connected to their current ICDs. These systems may continue to be used, provided that they are still functioning appropriately and remain in the proper position on the heart. If new leads are required when generator replacement is needed,

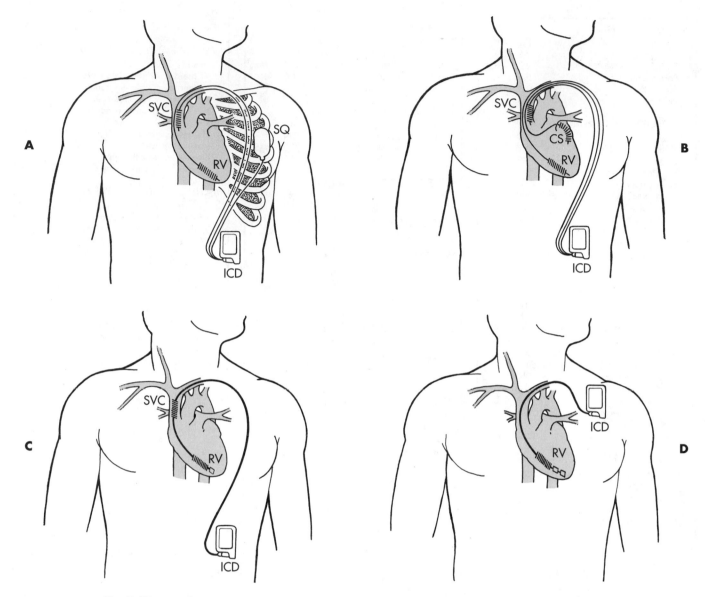

Fig. 6-15 Examples of various placements for nonthoracotomy lead systems. **A,** A three-lead system with shocks delivered from the right ventricular *(RV)* electrode to the superior vena cava *(SVC)* electrode and also to the subcutaneous patch *(SQ)* electrode. **B,** A three-lead system with shocks delivered from the RV to SVC electrodes and also to the coronary sinus *(CS)* electrode. **C,** A single-lead system with shocks delivered form the RV to SVC electrodes. **D,** A single-lead system with shocks delivered form the RV electrode to the pulse generator can.

epicardial leads are usually abandoned in situ. Epicardial leads may occasionally be used for an initial implant if adequate defibrillation thresholds cannot be obtained using endocardial systems, an increasingly rare event.

Waveforms and Current Pathways[123-127]

In addition to lead positioning and the number of leads used, defibrillation waveforms may affect the effectiveness of defibrillation shocks in terminating VF. A number of words are used to describe defibrillation waveforms. These include *shape, duration,* and *tilt* (the percentage that the pulse amplitude decreases from the beginning to the end of the pulse output). Electrical characteristics of defibrillation waveforms include factors such as the leading edge voltage or current of the pulse and total delivered energy.

Current ICD systems use primarily monophasic or biphasic waveforms. Monophasic waveforms are single pulses that decay from the beginning to the end of the pulse through control of the tilt. The total amount of voltage or current delivered to the heart depends on the capacitor used in the ICD and the resistance of the total circuit. Biphasic waveforms are dual pulses of opposite polarity. If delivered by a single capacitor, they are really one pulse with both negative and positive phases. This results in current flows in both directions over the same pathway, first from positive/anodal to negative/cathodal and then in the opposite direction. The total amount of voltage or current delivered again depends on the capacitor or capacitors used in the device and the resistance of the total circuit. Fig. 6-16 illustrates a biphasic waveform.

Some studies have suggested that the use of biphasic waveforms reduces the total amount of energy needed for defibrillation in some patients. However, since waveforms are only one of the many factors influencing defibrillation thresholds, personnel involved with implantation and follow-up of ICDs must be thoroughly familiar with the many ways to optimize defibrillation thresholds at the time of initial device implant and for long-term therapy.

Current may be delivered over a single pathway between two electrodes or over two or more pathways between three or more electrodes. When multiple pathways are used, the defibrillation pulses can be delivered simultaneously or sequentially.

Follow-Up[128-132]

Follow-up of patients with ICDs is best done in an organized and systematic manner at regular intervals and using specific procedures. The frequency of follow-up may be influenced by the type of device implanted, the length of time it has been in place, shocks received, the patient's general overall mental and physical state, and many other considerations. However, consistent evaluation helps ensure that the device performs appropriately when needed.

Therefore many patients are followed at intervals of approximately 3 months.

The following general steps are usually performed at each follow-up session:

1. Assessment of the patient's overall clinical status: This includes obtaining from the patient a description of all device-related experiences since the patient's last visit and information about whether any shocks have occurred.

2. Analysis of the device: By use of the programmer and programming head as specified by the manufacturer, the current parameters of the implanted device and all other data stored in the device's memory are obtained and printed; this is usually accomplished with a single programming sequence.

3. Evaluation of battery status: The battery information contained on the printout of device parameters is checked, and manufacturer recommendations for specific voltages are followed; this may include increasing the frequency of follow-up, scheduling the patient for elective or urgent replacement of the device, or maintaining regularly scheduled follow-up evaluations.

4. Evaluation of the condition of the high-voltage capacitors: This is done by evaluating the charge time and ensuring that it is at or below manufacturer specifications; a charge time that is too long may delay the delivery of a shock or may result in the shock being delivered at less than maximal voltage, possibly compromising defibrillation efficacy.

5. Evaluation of spontaneous episode and therapy data: The clinician should compare the current printout with the final printout for the previous follow-up

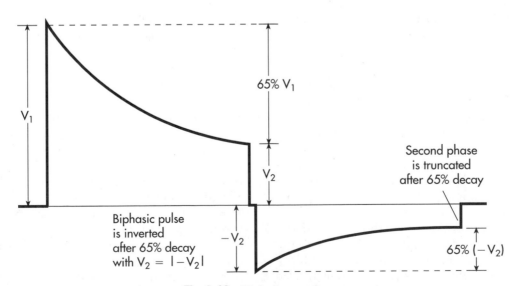

Fig. 6-16   Biphasic waveform.

visit, noting the number of VT and VF episodes reported and the specific therapies effective in terminating them; should make any needed parameter adjustments based on this information; and should determine whether device-reported episodes are consistent with patient-reported experiences and address inconsistencies as needed.

6. Determination of the pacing threshold: This is done in the same manner as with permanent pacemakers and ensures the ability of the ICD to capture during pacing and the integrity of the pacing leads.

7. Tests for oversensing: The clinician adjusts output and sensitivity to determine whether P waves, T waves, or postpacing polarizations are inappropriately sensed, which could result in VF not being detected appropriately or failure to pace when needed.

Additional tests may be appropriate and necessary at some or all follow-up sessions. These include induction and termination of the clinical dysrhythmia, stress testing, an ambulatory ECG, x-ray studies (posteroanterior and lateral), and several others.

At the conclusion of each follow-up visit, a printout of all device parameters should be obtained and placed in the patient's chart, and the episode event counters may be cleared if desired. This documents any programming changes that may have been made and permits the device to "start over" in tracking VT and VF episodes; it also documents the therapies used to terminate these episodes.

Troubleshooting

ICDs are among the most complex of systems involving electrical, mechanical, and physiologic interactions, and it is therefore inevitable that malfunction or inappropriate function of these systems occur. Whether the detection and correction of these improper functions is prompt and relatively straightforward or whether it is difficult depends largely on two things: the availability of appropriate equipment and the availability of thoroughly trained and knowledgeable medical and nursing personnel.

Equipment

Much of the same equipment used to evaluate implantable pacemaker systems is also useful in evaluating the performance of ICD systems. This includes a 12-lead ECG, magnet, x-ray examination or fluoroscopy, oscilloscope, and of course, programmer. Most current ICD programmers provide some kind of a diagnostic channel to assist in ECG interpretation and telemetered event counters that summarize dysrhythmic events and whether they were successfully treated.

Equally as important as the troubleshooting hardware are detailed patient records, including documentation of prior programmed parameters, ECGs, and x-ray films. Normally functioning ICD systems may be misinterpreted as malfunctioning by personnel who are not thoroughly fa-

miliar with system operation or do not have the patient's records. Therefore it is imperative that consistent follow-up be performed by highly trained and knowledgeable medical and nursing personnel.

NURSING CARE OF PATIENTS WITH PERMANENT CARDIAC PACEMAKERS AND ICDs[133-142]

Nursing care of patients with permanent cardiac pacemakers and ICDs presents unique challenges because of the need for implantation of a device within the body. Cultural differences in beliefs concerning such practices may greatly influence patient and family acceptance, and health care professionals should be sensitive to these issues during interactions. When possible, family members should be included in as many aspects of the patient's care as possible, since they may influence adherence to follow-up procedures and specific instructions and affect other aspects of overall management.

Because of what patients have seen or heard in the broadcast or print media or from their friends, patient knowledge may range from knowing nothing to having a reasonably accurate understanding of pacemakers and ICDs. Whatever the level of knowledge, thorough and accurate information presented in a clear and logical manner will help reassure patients and families and stimulate acceptance of the need for an implanted device while providing an understanding of what life after the procedure will be like.

Before the implant, the use of charts, drawings, or models helps patients understand the parts of the implanted system and the locations where they will be placed. Such visual aids also help patients and families understand the ways in which the heart functions, the specific abnormality in function that the patient has, and the reasons that the system chosen is necessary. Showing patients a model of the device and leads may also be helpful, since patients may have vague ideas regarding the size of the devices. These models, as well as the visual aids, are often available from the manufacturers, sometimes at a nominal charge. Additional teaching aids such as videos, slide series, and materials written specifically for children are also usually available.

A patient booklet is usually packaged with each device. Since these are not available until the time of the procedure, when the package containing the device is opened, extra copies can be ordered from the manufacturer so that patients can review them in advance. Patients should be encouraged to read the booklet, share it with their families, and ask questions.

An additional source of stress for patients and families may arise if preauthorization or approval for implant is required or if financial coverage for the recommended device is unavailable or in question. During this waiting period, support and reassurance will be necessary. If an alternative form of therapy is required for financial reasons, explanations regarding why the alternative approach is also appropriate and beneficial will be required.

Implantation of a pacemaker or an ICD may take place in a cardiac catheterization laboratory, an EP laboratory, or an operating room. It may be done as an outpatient procedure, as an inpatient procedure during a hospitalization, and in some cases, in a surgical center not directly connected with a hospital. Wherever it is performed, all device-implant procedures must be performed under sterile conditions to the greatest extent possible, and all personnel associated with the implant should wear clothing and other protective coverings appropriate to this kind of environment. These precautions minimize the risk of an infection at the generator and/or lead sites, which is potentially disastrous for the patient.

Many device-implant procedures are performed with patients only partially sedated. Under these conditions, all personnel should exercise caution during conversations, since their words can be heard and misinterpreted by conscious patients who may be listening. Patients should be told in advance if there are specific things they will be asked to do during the procedure, such as coughing or deep breathing to help ensure that the lead has been securely stabilized. The absence of general anesthesia also means that patients should be told that they will be covered with surgical drapes, that their arms and legs will be secured, and that they should not move unless asked to do so. They should be told to indicate if they are in pain, such as when the device pocket is being created, so that additional local anesthesia can be given if necessary. In general, patients should be prepared for what they will see, feel, and hear, and medical and nursing personnel should be constantly attentive to minimize anxiety, to answer questions, and to reassure patients regarding the progress of the procedure.

Patients undergoing ICD placement need special attention and support because the implant procedure may be somewhat longer and because more than one incision site may be required. In all cases, it is necessary to induce VT, VF, or both to ensure that the implanted device appropriately detects and terminates these rhythms, which can be extremely stressful for patients if they are not fully anesthetized. Patients will therefore require extensive reassurance that these procedures are safe and necessary and that highly skilled people and equipment are available to restore the normal heart function.

Postimplant nursing care is specific to the type of implant, the device system involved, the area where the patient is cared for, and the policies and procedures of the institution. Continuous ECG monitoring for a period helps ensure that the newly implanted device is functioning appropriately. In addition, a postoperative chest x-ray study may be requested to confirm proper positioning of the leads. The implant sites should also be checked to ensure that sutures are intact and drainage is not excessive. In some institutions, restrictions are placed on body movement during the first several hours or days after implantation of a new lead system, and practices concerning length of hospitalization differ. If patients are discharged within 24 to 48 hours, as is becoming increasingly common, instructions regarding when they are to return for follow-up should be emphasized. It is also important to ensure that before discharge, documentation of all programmed parameters is placed in the patient's chart and that a temporary identification card for the device is given to the patient. Assuming that the implant is appropriately registered with the device manufacturer, which should always be done, a permanent identification card will be mailed to the patient from the manufacturer within a few weeks.

Resumption of normal activities after device implantation varies from patient to patient and chiefly depends on the patient's state of health before the implant and the reasons that a device was felt to be necessary. Patients should be encouraged to resume normal daily activities and recreational pursuits, gradually increasing the levels as their state of health permits.

Lifestyle adaptation, the most important aspect of which is regular follow-up care, should also be emphasized. Patients should know the reasons that they now need to have regular follow-up, and the type of follow-up chosen for them (clinic visits, transtelephonic monitoring, or both) should be fully explained to them. This is also the time to discuss the safe use of common electric devices such as microwave ovens, razors, electric toothbrushes, and hair dryers (all properly functioning household electric devices are generally considered safe to use); symptoms they might experience with strong continuous electrical interference (commonly a return of their preimplant symptoms or an unexpected discharge of an implantable defibrillator); and steps to take if this occurs (move away from or stop using the device in question and then telephone their medical contact person). Patients who have been using or working with complex electric devices on the job or for leisure activities may need special information. Such devices might include welding equipment, automobile engines, or power tools. If a patient must continue using such equipment, the manufacturer of the device can be asked to assess the situation and determine whether continued use of the equipment in question is safe or if the equipment can be modified to ensure safety. In general, the use of electric devices by patients with implanted pacemakers or cardioverter defibrillators does not present problems unless the electrical signals generated are interpreted by the device's sensing circuits as being generated by the heart. Depending on the type of device implanted, this could result in appropriate inhibition of the implanted device or inappropriate triggering, especially in antitachycardia pacemakers and implantable defibrillators. Since devices differ from one manufacturer to another and since various electric devices generate different signals, individual assessment of specific situations is essential, and it is important not to assume that patients with implanted pacemakers or defibrillators are automatically restricted in their use of certain electric devices.

Some patients may enjoy participating in support groups for pacemaker or ICD recipients or receiving newsletters and magazines designed for them. Medical and nursing personnel involved in caring for patients with these devices should therefore become familiar with available support measures. Information can be obtained from local heart associations and from device manufacturers. Patients should also be encouraged to carry with them at all times the identification card issued by the manufacturer of their devices and other medical identification information if appropriate. This is particularly important when traveling, since implanted devices can sometimes trigger airport security systems. In addition, if adjustment of device parameters becomes necessary, the device identification card will enable medical and nursing personnel to accurately identify the implanted device and quickly locate the equipment needed to reprogram it. If external defibrillation is required, it is essential that defibrillation paddles not be placed directly over an implanted device and that assessment of the device be made as soon as possible after external defibrillation. This includes verification of the device's programmed parameters as well as verification of appropriate pacing and sensing, which in most cases should not be affected by the external defibrillation.

SUMMARY

The implantable pacemakers of the mid-1990s are highly reliable and sophisticated devices that have been modified and perfected in over 3 decades of use. They now offer most patients the opportunity for completely normal lifestyles, with minimal requirements for follow-up by medical and nursing personnel. Over 1 million people worldwide now benefit from such devices.

The ICDs of the mid-1990s have been in clinical use for 1 decade and have undergone rapid technologic advancement. They are now relatively easy to implant, although their extensive programmability and many therapeutic options require thorough knowledge and training of medical and nursing personnel. These devices may prolong patients' lives. However, whether this has been achieved remains to be established, as does the issue of the cost effectiveness of this therapy. As these and other therapies for overall cardiac care continue to be developed and improved, answers to these and other issues will become more clear, and new directions for the application of these therapies will begin to emerge.

REFERENCES

1. Elmquist R, Senning A: *An implantable pacemaker for the heart*, *Proceedings of the Second International Conference of Medical-Electric Engineers*, London, 1959, Iliffe & Sons.
2. Zoll P, Linenthal A: Long-term electrical pacemakers for Stokes-Adams disease, *Circulation* 22:341, 1960.
3. Parsonnet V and others: Cardiac pacing practices in the United States in 1985, *Am J Cardiol* 62(1):71, 1988.
4. Zipes DP, Duffin E: *Cardiac pacemakers.* In Braunwald E, editor: *Heart disease: a textbook of cardiovascular medicine*, ed 3, Philadelphia, 1988, Saunders.
5. Sutton R and others: Physiological cardiac pacing, *PACE* 3(2):207, 1980.
6. Osborn MJ, Holmes DR: Antitachycardia pacing, *Clin Prog Electrophysiol Pacing* 3(4):239, 1985.
7. Duffin E, Zipes DP: *Chronic electric control of tachydysrhythmia.* In Mandel WJ, editor: *Cardiac arrhythmias, their mechanisms, diagnosis and management*, Philadelphia, 1987, Lippincott.
8. Zipes DP: Electrical therapy of cardiac arrhythmias (editorial), *N Engl J Med* 309:1179, 1983.
9. Furman S and others: *A practice of cardiac pacing*, ed 3, Mount Kisco, 1993, Futura.
10. Fananapazir L and others: Impact of dual-chamber permanent pacing in patients with obstructive hypertrophic cardiomyopathy with symptoms refractory to verapamil and beta adrenergic blocker therapy, *Circulation* 85:2149, 1992.
11. Akhtar M and others: NASPE ad hoc committee on guidelines for cardiac electrophysiological studies, *PACE* 8(4):611, 1985.
12. Bernstein A and others: The NASPE/BPEG generic pacemaker code for antibradyarrhythmia and adaptive-rate pacing and antitachyarrhythmia devices, *PACE* 10(4):794, 1987.
13. Nathan D and others: An implantable synchronous pacemaker for long-term correction of complete heart block, *Am J Cardiol* 11:362, 1963.
14. Kruse I and others: Clinical evaluation of atrial synchronous ventricular inhibited pacemakers, *PACE* 3(6):641, 1980.
15. Berkovits B and others: Bifocal demand pacing, *Circulation* 39:44, 1969.
16. Funke HD: Three years experience in optimized sequential cardiac pacing, *Stimucoeur* 9(1):26, 1981.
17. Fananapazir L and others: Atrial synchronized ventricular pacing: contribution of the chronotropic response to improved exercise performance, *PACE* 6(3):601, 1983.
18. Humen D and others: Activity-sensing, rate-responsive pacing: improvements in myocardial performance with exercise, *PACE* 8(1):52, 1985.
19. Rossi P and others: Physiological sensitivity of respiratory dependent cardiac pacing: 4-year follow up, *PACE* 11(9)1267, 1988.
20. Lau CP and others: Rate responsive pacing with a pacemaker that detects respiratory rate (biorate), *Clin Cardiol* 11:318, 1988.
21. Lau CP and others: Initial clinical experience with a minute ventilation sensing rate modulated pacemaker: improvements in exercise capacity and symptomatology, *PACE* 11(11):1815, 1988.
22. Rickards AF, Norman J: Relation between QT interval and heart rate: new design of physiological adaptive cardiac pacemaker, *Br Heart J* 45:56, 1981.
23. Fananapazir L and others: Reliability of the evoked response in determining the paced ventricular rate and performance of the QT or rate responsive (TX) pacemaker, *PACE* 8(5):701, 1985.
24. Goicolea de Ore A and others: Rate responsive pacing: clinical experience, *PACE* 8(3):322, 1985.
25. Fearnot NE and others: Increasing cardiac rate by measurement of right ventricular temperature, *PACE* 7(6):1240, 1984.
26. Sharma AD and others: Physiological pacing based on beat to beat of right ventricular dp/dt initial feasibility studies in man (abstract), *J Am Coll Cardiol* 7:3A, 1986.
27. Sutton R and others: Ventricular rate responsive pacing using the first derivative of right ventricular pressure on a sensor (abstract), *J Am Coll Cardiol* 11:167, 1988.
28. Wirtzfeld A and others: Regulation of pacing rate by variations of mixed venous oxygen saturation, *PACE* 7(6):1257, 1984.
29. Chirife R: Physiological principles of a new method for rate responsive pacing using the preejection interval, *PACE* 11(11):1545, 1988.

30. Salo RW and others: Continuous ventricular volume assessment for diagnosis and pacemaker control, *PACE* 7(7):1267, 1984.

31. Paul V and others: Closed loop control of rate adaptive pacing: clinical assessment of a system analyzing the ventricular depolarization gradient, *PACE* 12(12):1896, 1989.

32. Cannilli L and others: Preliminary experience with the pH-triggered pacemaker, *PACE* 1(4):448, 1978.

33. Kappenberger LJ, Herpers L: Rate responsive dual chamber pacing, *PACE* 9(6):987, 1986.

34. Alt E and others: The basis for activity controlled rate variable cardiac pacemakers: an analysis of mechanical forces on the human body induced by exercise and environment, *PACE* 12(10):1667, 1989.

35. Stangl K, Laule M: *Combinations of parameters.* In Alt E and others, editors: *Rate adaptive cardiac pacing,* Berlin, 1993, Springer Verlag.

36. Connelly D and others: Initial experience with a new single chamber dual sensor rate responsive pacemaker, *PACE* 16(9):1833, 1993.

37. Slade A and others: Clinical experience with a new dual sensor rate responsive pacemaker generator (abstract) *PACE* 16(4):894, 1993.

38. Cowell R and others: Are we being driven to two sensors? Clinical benefits of sensor cross-checking, *PACE* 16(7):1441, 1993.

39. Lee M, Baker R: Circadian rate variation in rate-adaptive pacing systems, *PACE* 13(12):1797, 1990.

40. Mond H, Barold S: Dual chamber, rate adaptive pacing in patients with paroxysmal supraventricular tachyarrhythmias: protective measures for rate control, *PACE* 16(11):2168, 1993.

41. Suguira T and others: A fuzzy approach to the rate control in an artificial cardiac pacemaker regulated by respiratory rate and temperature: a preliminary report, *J Med Eng Tech* 15(3):107, 1991.

42. Parsonnet V, Rodgers T: The present status of programmable pacemakers, *Prog Cardiovasc Dis* 23(6):401, 1981.

43. Furman S, Pannizzo F: Output programmability and reduction of secondary intervention after pacemaker implantation, *J Thorac Cardiovasc Surg* 81(5):713, 1981.

44. Hayes DL and others: Initial and early follow-up assessment of the clinical efficacy of a multiparameter-programmable pulse generator, *PACE* 4(4)417, 1981.

45. Billhardt RA and others: Successful management of pacing system malfunctions without surgery: the role of programmable pulse generators, *PACE* 5(5):675, 1982.

46. Parsonnet V: Cardiac pacing and pacemakers, VVI, power sources for implantable pacemakers. I. *Am Heart J* 94(4):517, 1977.

47. Brennen KR and others: A capacity rating system for cardiac pacemaker batteries, *J Power Sources* 5:25, 1980.

48. Song SL and others: Performance of implantable cardiac rhythm management devices, *PACE* 17(4):692, 1994.

49. Greatbatch W: Metal electrodes in bioengineering, *CRC Crit Rev Bioeng* 5(1):1, 1981.

50. Smyth NPD: Techniques of implantation: atrial and ventricular, thoracotomy and transvenous, *Prog Cardiovasc Dis* 23(6):435, 1981.

51. Littleford P and others: Method for the rapid and atraumatic insertion of permanent endocardial pacemaker electrodes through the subclavian vein, *Am J Cardiol* 43:980, 1979.

52. Stokes K and others: A possible new complication of subclavian stick: conductor fracture (abstract), *PACE* 10(3):748, 1987.

53. Parsonnet V and others: Transvenous insertion of double sets of permanent electrodes *JAMA* 243(1)62, 1980.

54. Parsonnet V: Routine implantation of permanent transvenous pacemaker electrodes in both chambers: a technique whose time has come, *PACE* 4(1):109, 1981.

55. Stokes K: *Pacing leads for rate-adaptive pacing.* In Benditt DG: *Rate-adaptive pacing,* Boston, 1993, Blackwell.

56. Furman S and others: Comparison of active and passive adhering leads for endocardial pacing. I. *PACE* 2(4):417, 1979.

57. Furman S and others: Comparison of active and passive adhering leads for endocardial pacing. II. *PACE* 4(1):78, 1981.

58. Kertes P and others: Comparison of lead complications with polyurethane tines, silicone rubber tined and wedge tip leads: clinical experience with 822 ventricular endocardial leads, *PACE* 6(5):957, 1983.

59. Timmis GC and others: *A new steroid-eluting low threshold pacemaker lead.* In Steinbeck K, editor: *Proceedings of the Seventh World Symposium on Cardiac Pacing,* Vienna, 1983.

60. Kruse IM, Terpstra B: Acute and long-term atrial and ventricular stimulation thresholds with a steroid-eluting electrode, *PACE* 8:45, 1985.

61. Timmis GC and others: Late effects of a steroid-eluting porous titanium pacemaker lead electrode in man (abstract), *PACE* 7:479, 1984.

62. King KH and others: A steroid-eluting endocardial pacing lead for treatment of exit block, *Am Heart J* 106:1438, 1983.

63. Stokes K, Bird T: A new efficient nanoTip lead, *PACE* 13(12):1901, 1990.

64. Schwaab B and others: A new bipolar steroid eluting screw-in lead (abstract), *PACE* 16(4):945, 1993.

65. Zoll P and others: External noninvasive electric stimulation of the heart, *Crit Care Med* 9(5):393, 1981.

66. Furman S and others: Cardiac pacing and pacemakers. IV. Threshold of cardiac stimulation, *Am Heart J* 94(1): 115, 1977.

67. Furman S and others: Cardiac pacing and pacemakers. III. Sensing the cardiac electrogram, *Am Heart J* 93(6):794, 1977.

68. MacGregor D and others: Computer assisted reporting system for the follow-up of patients with cardiac pacemakers, *PACE* 3(5):568, 1980.

69. Furman S: Cardiac pacing and pacemakers. VI. Analysis of pacemaker malfunction, *Am Heart J* 94(3):378, 1977.

70. Barold S: *Modern cardiac pacing,* Mt Kisco, NY, 1985, Futura.

71. Mond HG: *The cardiac pacemaker: function and malfunction,* New York, 1983, Grune & Stratton.

72. Adler S and others: Advances in single-chamber pacemaker diagnostic data, *PACE* 9:1141, 1986.

73. Mirowski M and others: Termination of malignant ventricular arrhythmias with an implanted automatic defibrillator in human beings, *N Engl J Med* 303:322, 1980.

74. Mirowski M: The automatic implantable cardioverter-defibrillator: an overview, *J Am Coll Cardiol* 6:461, 1985.

75. Sneed N and others: The impact of device recall on patients and familiy members of patients with automatic implantable cardioverter defibrillators, *Heart Lung* 23(4):317, 1994.

76. Kolenik S and others: Engineering considerations in the development of the automatic implantable cardioverter defibrillator, *Prog Cardiovasc Dis* 36(2):115, 1993.

77. Mower M, Hauser R: Developmental history, early use, and implementation of the automatic implantable cardioverter defibrillator, *Prog Cardiovasc Dis* 36(2):89, 1993.

78. Callans D, Josephson M: Future developments in implantable cardioverter defibrillators: the optimal device, *Prog Cardiovasc Dis* 36(3):227, 1993.

79. US Food and Drug Administration, 50 *Fed Reg* 47276, 1985.

80. Reid P and others: *The automatic implantable cardioverter-defibrillator: five-year clinical results.* In Breithardt G and others, editors: *Nonpharmacological therapy of tachyarrhythmias,* Mount Kisco, 1987, Futura.

81. Kelly P and others: The automatic implantable cardioverter-defibrillator: efficacy, complications and survival in patients with malignant ventricular arrhythmias, *J Am Coll Cardiol* 11:1278, 1988.

82. Tchou P and others: Automatic implantable cardioverter defibrillators and survival of patients with left ventricular dysfunction and malignant ventricular arrhythmias, *Ann Intern Med* 109:529, 1988.

83. Winkle R and others: Long-term outcome with the automatic implantable cardioverter defibrillator, *J Am Coll Cardiol* 13:1353, 1989.

84. Manolis A and others: Clinical experience in seventy-seven patients with the automatic implantable cardioverter defibrillator, *Am Heart J* 118:445, 1989.

85. Winkle R and others: Ten year experience with implantable defibrillators, *Circulation* 84(suppl 2):II-426, 1991.

86. Dreifus Y and others: Guidelines for implantation of cardiac pacemakers and antiarrhythmia devices: a report of the American College of Cardiology/American Heart Association Task Force on Assessment of Diagnostic and Therapeutic Cardiovascular Procedures (Committee on Pacemaker Implantation), *J Am Coll Cardiol* 18:1, 1991.

87. Lehman M, Saksena S (for the NASPE Policy Conference Committee): Implantable cardioverter defibrillators in cardiovascular practice: report of the Policy Conference of the North American Society of Pacing and Electrophysiology, *PACE* 14:969, 1991.

88. Bernstein A and others: The NASPE/BPEG defibrillator code, *PACE* 16:1776, 1993.

89. Cannom D: *Current indications and contraindications for ICD implantation*. In Naccarelli G, Veltri E, editors: *Implantable cardioverter defibrillators*, Boston, 1993, Blackwell.

90. U.S. Food and Drug Administration, 58 *Fed Reg* 17594, 1993.

91. Vergara G and others: New implanting procedure and clinical results with 4th generation ICD: Proceedings of the 11th International Congress, *New Frontiers of Arrhythmias* 9(2):99, 1994.

92. Bardy G and others: A simplified, single-lead unipolar transvenous cardioversion-defibrillation system, *Circulation* 88(2):543, 1993.

93. Schmitt C and others: Significance of supraventricular tachyarrhythmias in patients with implanted pacing cardioverter defibrillators. I. *PACE* 17(3):295, 1994.

94. Hamer M and others: Evaluation of outpatients experiencing implantable cardioverter defibrillator shocks associated with minimal symptoms. I. *PACE* 17(5):938, 1994.

95. Swerdlow C and others: Discrimination of ventricular tachycardia from sinus tachycardia and atrial fibrillation in a tiered-therapy cardioverter-defibrillator, *J Am Coll Cardiol* 23(6):1342, 1994.

96. Jones G, Bardy G: Considerations for ventricular fibrillation detection by implantable cardioverter defibrillators. II. *Am Heart J* 127(4):1107, 1994.

97. Almendral J and others: The importance of antitachycardia pacing for patients presenting with ventricular tachycardia, *PACE* 16(2):535, 1993.

98. Wietholt A and others: Clinical experience with antitachycardia pacing and improved detection algorithms in a new implantable cardioverter-defibrillator, *J Am Coll Cardiol* 21:885, 1993.

99. Fromer M and others: Efficacy of automatic multimodal device therapy for ventricular tachyarrhythmias as delivered by a new implantable pacer cardioverter-defibrillator: results of a European multicenter study incorporating 102 implants, *Circulation* 86:374, 1992.

100. Leitch J and others: Reduction in defibrillation shocks with a device combining antitachycardia pacing, cardioversion and defibrillation (abstract), *J Am Coll Cardiol* 17:128A, 1991.

101. Block M and others: Pacer-cardioverter-defibrillator (PCD): utilization, efficacy and complications of antitachycardia pacing (abstract), *J Am Coll Cardiol* 17:54A, 1991.

102. Trappe H-J and others: Role of antitachycardia pacing in patients with third generation cardioverter defibrillators. II. *PACE* 17(3):506, 1994.

103. Nathan A: The role of cardioversion therapy in patients with implanted cardioverter defibrillators. II. *Am Heart J* 127(4):1046, 1994.

104. Winkle W: *The implantable defibrillator: progression from first- to third-generation devices*. In Zipes D, Jalife J, editors: *Cardiac electrophysiology from cell to bedside*, Philadelphia, 1990, Saunders.

105. Zipes D and others: Clinical transvenous cardioversion of recurrent life-threatening ventricular tachyarrhythmias: low-energy synchronized cardioversion of ventricular tachycardia and termination of ventricular fibrillation in patients using a catheter electrode, *Am Heart J* 103:789, 1982.

106. Miles W and others: The implantable transvenous cardioverter: long-term efficacy and reproducible induction of ventricular tachycardia, *Circulation* 74:518, 1986.

107. Thakur R and others: *Clinical use of implantable cardioverter-defibrillators*. In Tacker W Jr, editor: *Defibrillation of the heart: ICDs, AEDs, and manual*, St Louis, 1994, Mosby.

108. Takeuchi E, Quattrini P: Batteries for implantable defibrillators, *Med Electron* 10:114, 1989.

109. Visvisky M, Holmes C: Long-term testing of defibrillator batteries, *PACE* 14:341, 1991.

110. Tacker W: *Design of implantable cardioverter defibrillators (ICDs)*. In Tacker W Jr, editor: *Defibrillation of the heart: ICDs, AEDs, and manual*, St Louis, 1994, Mosby.

111. Timmis G: The development of implantable cardioversion defibrillation systems: the clinical chronicle of defibrillation leads. II. *Am Heart J* 127(4):1003, 1994.

112. Saksena S and others: Innovations in pulse generators and lead systems: Balancing complexity with clinical benefit and long-term results, *Am Heart J* 127(4, part 2):1010, 1994.

113. Manolis A: Transvenous endocardial cardioverter defibrillator systems: Is the future here? *Arch Intern Med* 154(6):617, 1994.

114. Marchlinski F: Nonthoracotomy defibrillator lead systems: a welcomed addition but still a lot to learn, *Circulation* 87(4):1410, 1993.

115. Bardy G and others: Implantable transvenous cardioverter-defibrillators, *Circulation* 87(4):1152, 1993.

116. Bardy G and others: A simplified, single-lead unipolar transvenous cardioversion-defibrillation system, *Circulation* 88(2):543, 1993.

117. Vergara G and others: New implanting procedure and clinical results with 4th generation ICD, *New Trends Arrhythmias* 9(2):99, 1993.

118. Bardy G and others: Prospective, randomized comparison in humans of a unipolar defibrillation system with that using an additional superior vena cava electrode, *Circulation* 89(3):1090, 1994.

119. Stanton M and others: Consistent subcutaneous prepectoral implantation of a new implantable cardioverter defibrillator, *Mayo Clin Proc* 69:309, 1994.

120. Kudenchuk P and others: Efficacy of a single-lead unipolar transvenous defibrillator compared with a system employing an additional coronary sinus electrode: a prospective, randomized study, *Circulation* 89(6):2641, 1994.

121. Raitt M, Bardy G: Advances in implantable cardioverter-defibrillator therapy, *Curr Opin Cardiol* 9:23, 1994.

122. The PCD Investigator Group: Clinical outcome of patients with malignant ventricular tachyarrhythmias and a multiprogrammable implantable cardioverter-defibrillator implanted with or without thoracotomy: an international multicenter study, *J Am Coll Cardiol* 23(7):1521, 1994.

123. Hayes D, Bardy G: *Various pulses and lead systems to lower defibrillation thresholds*. In Naccarelli G, Veltri E, editors: *Implantable cardioverter-defibrillators*, Boston, 1993, Blackwell.

124. Bardy G and others: Electrode system influence on biphasic waveform defibrillation efficacy in humans, *Circulation* 84(2):665, 1991.

125. Davidson T and others: Implantable cardioverter defibrillators: a guide for clinicians, *Heart Lung* 23(3):205, 1994.

126. Jung W and others: Clinical efficacy of shock waveforms and lead configurations for defibrillation. II. *Am Heart J* 127(4):985, 1994.

127. Blanchard S and others: *Defibrillation waveforms*. In Singer I, editor: *Implantable cardioverter defibrillator*, Armonk, 1994, Futura.

128. Singer I and others: *Post operative care and follow-up of implantable cardioverter-defibrillator patients*. In Singer I, editor: *Implantable cardioverter defibrillator*, Armonk, 1994, Futura.

129. Biblo Y and others: *Follow-up of patients with implantable cardioverter-defibrillator devices.* In Estes III N and others, editors: *Implantable cardioverter-defibrillators: a comprehensive textbook,* New York, 1994, Marcel Dekker.

130. *PCD system reference guide,* Minneapolis, 1993, Medtronic.

131. Thomas A, Moser S: *Nursing aspects of ICD patient care: patient education and perioperative and long-term care.* In Naccarelli G and others, editors: *Implantable cardioverter defibrillators,* Boston, 1993, Blackwell.

132. Luceri R: *Implantable defibrillators: physician's role after hospital discharge.* In Naccarelli G and others, editors: *Implantable cardioverter defibrillators,* Boston, 1993, Blackwell.

133. Collins M: When your patient has an implantable cardioverter defibrillator, *Am J Nurs* 94(3):34, 1994.

134. Schaefer Y and others: Caring for a patient with an A.I.C.D., *Nursing 92* 22(12):48, 1992.

135. Dougherty C: Longitudinal recovery following sudden cardiac arrest and internal cardioverter defibrillator implantation: survivors and their families, *Am J Crit Care* 3(2):145, 1994.

136. Dunbar S and others: Internal cardioverter defibrillator device discharge: experiences of patients and family members, *Heart Lung* 22(6):494, 1993.

137. Lüderitz B and others: Patient acceptance of implantable cardioverter defibrillator devices: changing attitudes. II. *Am Heart J* 127(4):1179, 1994.

138. Molchany C, Peterson K: The psychosocial effects of support group intervention on AICD recipients and their significant others, *Prog Cardiovasc Nurs* 9(2):23, 1994.

139. Frame R: Implantable cardioverter defibrillators: past, present, and future, *Crit Care Choices* 94:34, 1994.

140. Boley T and others: The patient with an automatic implantable cardioverter defibrillator, *J Am Acad Nurse Pract* 5(5):205, 1993.

141. Porterfield L and others: The cutting edge in arrhythmias, *Crit Care Nurse* 131(suppl)3:8, 1993.

142. Witherell C: Cardiac rhythm control devices, *Crit Care Nurs Clin North Am* 6(1):85, 1994.

7

Coronary Artery Disease

Elizabeth Van Beek Carlson
Lynne T. Braun
Marcia Pencak Murphy

INCIDENCE, PREVALENCE, MORBIDITY, AND MORTALITY

Despite the recent decline in age-adjusted death rates, cardiovascular disease remains the leading cause of death in the United States. The American Heart Association (AHA) estimates that 6.23 million Americans have a history of coronary heart disease. Among the more than 70 million Americans with some form of heart disease, coronary artery disease (CAD) ranked second to hypertensive heart disease in prevalence. Of all acute myocardial infarctions (AMIs), 5% occur in people under the age of 40, and 45% occur in people under the age of 65. CAD caused 489,340 deaths in the United States in 1990. Sudden cardiac death occurs in 250,000 adults in the United States each year. Among the approximately 500,000 Americans who die annually from AMI, 20% are under the age of 65. Furthermore, two thirds of the deaths from AMI occur outside the hospital, and half of victims wait more than 2 hours before seeking help.[1]

Pathogenesis

Atherosclerosis is a degenerative arterial disease often clinically expressed as myocardial and cerebral infarction, ischemic cardiomyopathy, and ischemia of the lower extremities. It develops as atheromatous plaque formation as a fundamental injury, which combines changes within the arterial lumen and the outer layers. Atherosclerosis results from an interaction among the structural and metabolic properties of the arterial vessels, blood components, and hemodynamic parameters.[2]

Atherosclerotic lesions vary according to the anatomic site; the age and genetic and physiologic status of the affected individual; and the risk factors to which the individual has been exposed. Modern techniques of cell and molecular biology reveal that each lesion contains elements of three cellular categories: smooth muscle proliferation; formation of connective tissue matrix, including collagen, elastic fibers, and proteoglycans; and accumulation of intracellular and extracellular lipids. Atherosclerotic lesions occur primarily within the intimal layer of the arterial wall.

The process includes three stages: the fatty streak, the fibrous plaque, and the advanced or complicated lesion.[3]

Fatty streaks begin in childhood and consist of lipids, macrophages, and T lymphocytes. As the lesions expand, they contain smooth muscle cells that have also migrated into the intima. Fatty streaks can be found in the aorta shortly after birth; however, their number increases between the ages of 8 and 18 years. Fatty streaks appear in the coronary arteries at about age 15 and increase in frequency throughout the third decade of life. Fatty streaks are yellowish in appearance and cause little or no obstruction of the affected artery.[3]

Fibrous plaques begin to develop around age 25 in populations prone to atherosclerosis and its clinical sequelae. The fibrous plaque is white in appearance and becomes elevated; therefore if this lesion progresses, it can occlude the arterial lumen and interfere with the myocardial blood supply. During this stage of lesion formation, smooth muscle cells proliferate, forming a fibrous cap that includes a connective tissue matrix, macrophages, T lymphocytes, and intracellular and extracellular lipids. This fibrous cap covers a deeper deposit of lipid and cellular debris. The presence of T lymphocytes in the lesions suggests that an immune response may be important in lesion genesis or progression.[3]

Advanced lesions of atherosclerosis occur as age increases. The fibrous plaque becomes vascularized from the luminal and medial aspects, resulting in hemorrhage. The lipid-rich core increases in size and often becomes calcified. The intimal surface may develop fissures (cracks), disintegrate, and ulcerate, which attracts the cellular components of clot formation. Thrombi organize and increase plaque size, which further reduces the size of the arterial lumen.[3]

Over the years a number of theories regarding the pathogenesis of atherosclerosis have been proposed, but only three are discussed here. The *response-to-injury theory* states that some form of injury to the endothelium results in structural changes, functional changes, or both in the endothelial cells. Various factors may modify the permeability of endothelial cells, including hypercholesterolemia; altered shear stress from blood flow over branch points or bifurcations in arteries, which occurs in hypertension; and dysfunction induced by toxins. Injury to the endothelium and enhanced permeability allow blood constituents (that is, lipoproteins, platelets, macrophages) to access the arterial wall, which leads to proliferation of arterial smooth muscle cells.[3]

The *lipid theory* describes the attraction, deposition, and proliferation of lipid substances within the intima of arteries. Elevated levels of low-density lipoprotein (LDL) lead to cholesterol internalization and esterification within smooth muscle cells. The lipid may accumulate in monocytes within the cell wall; the monocytes are subsequently converted to macrophages. Although the exact mechanism of lipid accumulation and proliferation within the arterial intima is unknown, studies suggest that oxidation of LDL within the vascular wall stimulates further accumulation of lipid components within the macrophage.[4,5]

The *monoclonal hypothesis* suggests that each atherosclerotic lesion is derived from a single smooth muscle cell, which stimulates cell proliferation within the lesion. Cell transformation may occur by various agents, such as viruses or chemicals.[3]

Historically, clinicians regarded blood vessels as inert tubes that carried blood and that had little to do with the life-sustaining processes occurring within them. Today we recognize that the cells of the vessel wall and their chemical messengers are responsible for the maintenance of normal homeostasis and the genesis and progression of atherosclerosis. Several potent biologic mediators are derived from and convey signals among endothelial and smooth muscle cells.[6] The vascular cell adhesion molecule lines the surface of endothelium over atherosclerotic lesions, which increases the adherence of leukocytes (monocytes and T lymphocytes) to the endothelial cells at particular sites in the artery wall.[3] Studies have demonstrated a diminished release of endothelium-derived relaxing factor identified as nitric oxide, which normally inhibits smooth muscle contraction and cellular proliferation.[7] Growth factors, such as platelet-derived growth factor (PDGF) and interleukin-1 (IL-1), mediate smooth muscle cell growth.[4] In addition, IL-1 transforms the normal blood-compatible surface of the endothelial cell into one that promotes coagulation and thrombosis and inhibits fibrinolysis.[6]

In summary, atherogenesis is a complex process that involves endothelial cells, smooth muscle cells, and platelets. It represents an inflammatory response to injury caused by well-recognized risk factors. The function of cells is modified because of their interaction with chemical mediators and lipoprotein particles. Therapeutic investigations are directed at inhibiting lesion progression by interfering with subcellular triggering mechanisms. For example, antioxidant agents such as probucol may retard the lipid core of plaque formation. Angiotensin-converting enzyme in-

hibitors and calcium channel blockers can inhibit smooth muscle cell proliferation.

Natural History and Prognosis

Considering the natural history of CAD, it is important to distinguish factors that affect the underlying atherosclerosis from those that influence the occurrence of clinical manifestations such as angina pectoris, MI, or sudden death.

Some degree of CAD is present in most individuals older than 30 in Western industrialized nations. However, such disease is almost always clinically silent until it occludes greater than 50% of the diameter (75% by cross-sectional area) of a major coronary vessel.[8] Even at this degree of obstruction, blood flow to the region of the myocardium supplied by the occluded vessel is usually acceptable at rest, and it becomes inadequate only when the oxygen demands of the myocardium are high (for example, during strenuous exercise). This is called *stable angina pectoris* and is identified by chest pain that shows a consistent pattern in terms of threshold, duration, and setting.

When the arterial lumen is almost completely obstructed, blood flow is insufficient to maintain a normal oxygen supply to the myocardium in the resting state. Unstable angina pectoris is diagnosed when there is a lower exercise threshold for inducing pain, which may last longer than usual. The pain may occur at rest. Unstable angina pectoris frequently leads to *myocardial infarction*, which denotes injury to the myocardium. A common pathologic feature of unstable angina pectoris and MI is the presence of a mural thrombus, which significantly or totally occludes the arterial lumen.[9]

Even when stenoses are severe, myocardium once served by diseased arteries may receive blood through alternative channels, termed *collaterals*, which may delay the onset of symptoms. The degree to which a patient's heart forms such collaterals is unpredictable[10]; therefore the relationship between the severity of the stenosis and the severity of symptoms is also unpredictable. Furthermore, some individuals may have serious limitations to myocardial blood flow, even developing MI without chest pain, an occurrence that complicates the clinical assessment of patients with CAD.

The coronary arteries are muscular structures capable of rapid variations in diameter and are under the influence of autonomic nerves and vasoactive substances released by the vascular endothelium and platelets. The degree to which an atherosclerotic plaque within a coronary artery limits blood flow depends on the severity of the plaque itself and on the muscular tone of the vessel around the plaque. Thus an insignificant 25% stenosis may rapidly become a critical 99% stenosis under the influence of a vasoconstrictive stimulus. This occurrence is termed *vasospasm* and may be suspected clinically with observation of transient ST-segment elevation on the electrocardiogram (ECG). Although some degree of vasospasm is present in virtually all patients with CAD, it occasionally occurs in the absence of clinically demonstrable atherosclerosis. This is called *variant angina*.[11]

In addition to the marked variability in the rate of progression of the underlying atherosclerosis, these pathophysiologic considerations account for the unpredictability of prognoses for an individual with CAD. These considerations also explain part of the difficulty in detecting CAD in the early stages. However, it is possible to use anatomic and physiologic data to estimate prognoses. An important variable is the number of major coronary vessels with significant obstructions. CAD occurs most frequently in the left anterior descending artery, less frequently in the right coronary artery, and still less frequently (although not rarely) in the circumflex artery. Narrowing tends to be most severe in the proximal 2 to 3 cm of each artery, but distal involvement is also common. The site of vessel obstruction is clinically important, since proximal lesions are more amenable to therapy by angioplasty, atherectomy, or bypass grafting.

In summary, coronary atherosclerosis may have no symptoms for many years until the disease progresses to produce an obstruction that interferes with the arterial blood supply to the myocardium. If the obstruction progresses gradually over years, intercoronary collateral circulation may develop, and clinical evidence of disease may be deferred or may never occur. Despite marked obstructive disease, the myocardial cells may receive adequate oxygen regardless of demands. On the other hand, when an artery is partially obstructed and sufficient collateral circulation has not yet developed, the obstruction may impair blood flow during conditions of increased demand, producing symptoms of intermittent vascular insufficiency.

RISK FACTORS

Large-scale epidemiologic studies have identified cardiovascular risk factors associated with a higher incidence of CAD.[13] The 25% decline in the mortality rate from cardiovascular disease in the last decade is partially attributable to increased public awareness of risk factors and subsequent lifestyle changes. Well-established major risk factors include hypertension, hypercholesterolemia, smoking, and diabetes mellitus. Other factors that may affect the risk for CAD are obesity, a sedentary lifestyle, and an aggressive response to stress. In this context, risk is viewed as the probability of developing CAD, and that probability is determined by the number of risk factors in any individual, by the level of each factor (that is, the level of blood pressure or cholesterol), and by age. It is important to consider the cumulative nature of risk factors in the clinical evaluation of the patient. For example, a person who smokes and is hypertensive has approximately twice the risk as one who smokes and is normotensive. Although the disease is more common when multiple risk factors are present, it can occur in the absence of any identifiable risk factors. Clearly, genetic or environmental variables can act independently of established risk factors and influence the clinical outcome. Nonetheless, identification and elimination of risk factors remain a priority to further lower the incidence of CAD.

Age, Gender, and Race

Atherosclerosis is more prevalent in older people. In 1990, 930,477 deaths were caused by diseases of the heart, with 489,340 or 52.6% attributed to CAD. In addition, the death rate for persons with CAD rose steeply with age among older adults. The death rate of men with CAD was higher than that of women in age groups 65 to 80. However, after 81 years of age, women had higher death rates (55%) than men (45%).[12] Men have a greater risk of cardiovascular disease than women,[1] but cardiovascular disease remains the leading cause of death among women in the United States. The Framingham study[13] reported that after age 55 women's risk of CAD increases tenfold and approaches but does not reach the risk of men.

Black men have slightly lower CAD death rates (3.5%) compared with white men. Black women have higher CAD death rates (approximately twice the rate) than white women until age 74.[1] Gender-related changes in the prevalence of risk factors occur as people age. The Stanford Five-City Project found that smoking, hypertension, and hypercholesterolemia were more prevalent among men than among women aged 25 to 49 years. This dominance of risk factors in men was not present in men aged 50 to 74 years. Women's risk profiles became more similar to men's as they aged, and by ages 65 to 74, women's risk profiles were worse than men's with respect to smoking and hypercholesterolemia. Hypertension risk remained approximately the same in men and women by ages 65 to 74.[14]

Hypertension

Hypertension is the most common form of cardiovascular disease and is a primary risk factor for CAD. Approximately 50 million Americans have elevated blood pressure, which is a systolic blood pressure (SBP) greater than or equal to 140 mm Hg, a diastolic blood pressure (DBP) greater than or equal to 90 mm Hg, or both.[15] *Essential hypertension* refers to the 90% to 95% of cases in which the cause is unknown.

The Fifth Report of the Joint National Committee on Detection, Evaluation, and Treatment of High Blood Pressure (JNC V) contains a new classification scheme for adult blood pressure (Table 7-1).[15] Hypertension is divided into stages 1 through 4 based on blood pressure level, which reflects the increasing risk for cardiovascular disease and other complications.

The risk for heart disease associated with hypertension is directly proportional to the level of elevated blood pressure, and either the SBP or the DBP may be used to predict risk. Diastolic hypertension is related to an increase in

TABLE 7-1   Classification of Blood Pressure for Adults Age 18 Years and Older*

Category	Systolic (mm Hg)	Diastolic (mm Hg)
Normal†	<130	<85
High normal	130-139	85-89
Hypertension‡		
Stage 1 (mild)	140-159	90-99
Stage 2 (moderate)	160-179	100-109
Stage 3 (severe)	180-209	110-119
Stage 4 (very severe)	≥210	≥120

*Not taking antihypertensive drugs and not acutely ill. When SBP and DBP fall into different categories, the higher category should be selected to classify blood pressure status. For instance, 160/92 mm Hg should be classified as stage 2, and 180/120 mm Hg should be classified as stage 4. Isolated systolic hypertension (ISH) is an SBP ≥140 mm Hg and DBP <90 mm Hg and staged appropriately (for example, 170/85 mm Hg is defined as stage 2 ISH).

†Optimum blood pressure with respect to cardiovascular risk is SBP <120 mm Hg and DBP <80 mm Hg. However, unusually low readings should be evaluated for clinical significance.

‡Based on the average of two or more readings taken at each of two or more visits after initial screening.

NOTE: In addition to classifying stages of hypertension based on average blood pressure levels, the clinician should specify the presence or absence of target-organ disease and additional risk factors. For example, a patient with diabetes and a blood pressure of 142/94 mm Hg plus left ventricular hypertrophy should be classified as "Stage 1 hypertension with target-organ disease (left ventricular hypertrophy) and with another major risk factor (diabetes)." This specificity is important for risk classification and management.[15]

From National Heart, Lung, and Blood Institute; National Institutes of Health: *The Fifth Report of the Joint National Committee on Detection, Evaluation, and Treatment of High Blood Pressure* (JNC V). Oct 30, 1992, The Institutes.

total peripheral resistance (arteriolar), and systolic hypertension reflects an elevated cardiac output, large vessel (arterial) stiffness, or both. A young hypertensive person may have an elevated SBP as a result of an increased cardiac output related to sympathetic nervous system overactivity. In middle-aged and older adults, systolic hypertension is usually due to atherosclerosis of the aorta and its major branches.[16] Systolic and diastolic hypertension may exist together, however.

Data from the Framingham study[17,18] revealed that hypertensive persons (blood pressure greater than 160/95 mm Hg) have more than twice the risk for CAD compared with normotensive persons (blood pressure less than 140/90 mm Hg). Individuals with borderline hypertension have a 50% increase in risk. SBP exerts an even greater influence than DBP on rates of morbidity and mortality for coronary heart disease.[19,20] Elevated blood pressure is best thought of as one facet of the cardiovascular risk profile, since the existence of concomitant risk factors markedly increases risk.

Among patients 60 years and older, systolic hypertension is a strong predictor of cardiovascular morbidity and mortality.[21] The prevalence of isolated systolic hypertension (defined as an SBP of 140 mm Hg or greater with a DBP of less than 90 mm Hg) increases after age 60. Hypertension is present in approximately 60% of non-Hispanic whites, 71% of non-Hispanic blacks, and 61% of Mexican Americans aged 60 years or older.[15] The Systolic Hypertension in the Elderly Program demonstrated a 27% reduction in the incidence of coronary heart disease, a 36% reduction in the incidence of strokes, and a 32% reduction in the incidence of all major cardiovascular events after drug treatment.[22]

A major focus of nursing is identifying risk factors specific for hypertension and assisting patients in reducing them. Congenital and environmental risk factors, including heredity, age, race (black), obesity, salt intake, use of alcohol or caffeine, smoking, use of oral contraceptives, socioeconomic factors, and stress, have been identified. Public education has raised the detection and treatment rates of hypertension among Americans. Practices in reducing the risk factors have contributed to the 50% decline in CAD mortality rates and 57% decline in stroke mortality rates over the last 2 decades.[15]

The goal of hypertension treatment is to prevent the morbidity and mortality associated with elevated blood pressure and to control blood pressure by the least possible intrusive means. Blood pressure reduction should occur with control of other cardiovascular risk factors; therefore lifestyle modifications, including weight reduction, moderation of dietary sodium and alcohol intake, avoidance of tobacco, and increased physical activity, are used alone or with drug therapy for hypertension.[15]

A strong association exists between obesity and elevated blood pressure.[15] The mechanism by which obesity leads to hypertension appears to be related to an increase in blood volume, stroke volume, and cardiac output.[23] Weight reduction reduces blood pressure in hypertensive individuals who are more than 10% above ideal body weight.[24]

The American diet contains sodium much beyond the body's physiologic needs. Excess dietary sodium may be a mechanism of essential hypertension in some individuals. An analysis of published reports of 24 different communities ($n = 47,000$) showed that an average lower sodium intake of 100 mmol/day was associated with an average lower SBP of 5 to 10 mm Hg. Older individuals with ISH may respond to sodium restriction because their hypertension usually is volume dependent.[26] Dietary counseling encourages refraining from adding salt to foods, avoiding processed foods, and reading labels of purchased food items for sodium content.

Alcohol, caffeine, and tobacco are related to hypertension in some studies. The prevalence of hypertension increases with the consumption of more than 1 to 2 ounces of ethanol per day, which produces an acute pressor response. Caffeine ingestion and smoking may cause an acute rise in blood pressure; however, some studies have not shown a higher incidence of hypertension with chronic use.[27] Smoking should be discouraged, however, since its combination with hypertension greatly potentiates the risk of CAD.

Regular aerobic physical activity may be beneficial in the prevention and treatment of hypertension.[15] Normotensive individuals with low levels of physical fitness have a 52% greater risk of developing hypertension compared with highly fit persons.[28] Furthermore, regular aerobic exercise lowers SBP and DBP by approximately 10 mm Hg in individuals with essential hypertension.[29] Blood pressure is most effectively lowered by exercise of moderate intensity (40% to 60% of maximal oxygen consumption), which translates into 30 to 45 minutes of brisk walking 3 to 5 times per week for most sedentary individuals.[15] However, the reduction in blood pressure elicited by exercise training may not normalize blood pressure. In this case, it should be used as an adjunct to drug therapy.

Studies on behavioral approaches to hypertension management have shown that various relaxation and biofeedback methods produce little to modest long-term reduction in blood pressure in selected groups.[30,31] The combination of biofeedback and relaxation techniques produces greater effects than either approach alone.[32] These approaches are primarily recommended for mild hypertension and may be used to reduce medication requirements. For evaluation of long-term effectiveness, blood pressure should be closely monitored at rest and during daily activities.

Numerous studies have shown that reduction of blood pressure with medications clearly decreases cardiovascular morbidity and mortality rates.[15,33-37] Protection has been shown for stroke, coronary heart disease events, congestive heart failure, progression to more severe levels of hypertension, and all-cause mortality.

The JNC recommends drug therapy if blood pressure remains at or above 140/90 mm Hg over 3 to 6 months despite attempts to modify lifestyle.[15] Drug therapy is particularly important for individuals with target-organ damage or other cardiovascular risk factors. Initial therapy should begin with a single drug for stages 1 and 2 hypertension. Since diuretics and β blockers reduce cardiovascular morbidity and mortality rates in clinical trials, they are the preferred drug classes for initial therapy. However, other drug classes may be selected—calcium channel blockers, angiotensin-converting enzyme inhibitors, α blockers, and α-β blockers—which are also effective in lowering blood pressure. Drug selection must take into account individual characteristics (race, age), concomitant diseases that may be beneficially or adversely affected by the drug chosen, use of other drugs that may lead to drug interactions, quality of life (untoward side effects), physiologic

and biochemical measurements (resting heart rate, plasma renin activity, body weight), and lifestyle and economic considerations.

If blood pressure is not adequately controlled after 1 to 3 months, the clinician may increase the dose of the first drug, substitute an agent from another class, or add a second drug from another class. Patients with stage 3 or 4 hypertension may require the addition of a second or third agent after a short interval.

Hypercholesterolemia

Cholesterol is a lipid that is a primary component of cell membranes and a precursor of bile acids and steroid hormones. It is transported through the circulation by lipoproteins, which are particles containing apolipoproteins and several lipids (including triglycerides, cholesterol, cholesteryl esters, and phospholipids). The apolipoproteins assist in maintaining the structural integrity and functional specificity of plasma lipoproteins. Generally, the apolipoprotein B concentration in plasma is positively associated with CAD, and apolipoprotein A is negatively associated with CAD. Knowledge about lipoproteins and apolipoproteins has increased dramatically in the last decade, providing the framework for understanding lipid metabolism in normal individuals and in those with lipid disorders. Lipoprotein metabolism is complex and beyond the scope of this chapter, but the reader is referred to current literature for more information.[38]

Three major classes of plasma lipoproteins can be measured in a fasting individual: very low-density lipoproteins (VLDLs), low-density lipoproteins (LDLs), and high-density lipoproteins (HDLs). VLDLs contain mostly triglycerides and 10% to 15% of the total serum cholesterol. Derived from the metabolism of VLDL, LDLs contain 60% to 70% of the total serum cholesterol. The HDLs are mostly protein and contain about 20% to 30% of the total cholesterol. Studies have demonstrated that HDL levels are inversely correlated and LDL levels are directly correlated with the risk of CAD.[39]

Comparisons of world populations demonstrate the direct association between serum cholesterol levels and the incidence of CAD.[40] People who move to a country with higher average serum cholesterol levels eventually acquire the dietary habits, serum cholesterol levels, and CAD rate of their new country. Prospective epidemiologic studies have demonstrated that serum cholesterol levels predict future CAD morbidity and mortality, with risk increasing steadily as cholesterol levels rise above 200 mg/dl.[41]

In addition to the data that support the causal relationship between elevated serum cholesterol levels and CAD, several clinical trials have demonstrated that lowering LDLs by dietary or drug interventions can reduce the incidence of CAD. In the Lipid Research Clinics Coronary Primary Prevention Trial,[42] investigators compared the cholesterol-lowering drug cholestyramine with a placebo and found that a 12.5% decrease in LDLs was associated with a 19% decrease in the incidence of AMI and death in the cholestyramine treatment group.[42]

In the Helsinki Heart Study,[43,44] drug treatment associated with an 11% decrease in LDL levels and an 11% increase in HDL levels was also associated with a 34% decrease in the CAD endpoints of definite heart attack or death. In both studies the benefits of therapy were not evident until after 24 months. Data from the Coronary Drug Project[45] also evidenced a significant decrease in overall mortality in a 15-year follow-up in men after AMI who were treated with nicotinic acid, a cholesterol-lowering agent.

The pooled analysis of clinical findings therefore suggest that intervention is as effective in preventing recurrent MI and death in patients who have had an MI as it is in the primary prevention of CAD. The evidence is strongest in middle-aged men with initial high cholesterol levels. Evidence suggests, however, that decreasing total cholesterol and LDL cholesterol levels also is likely to reduce CAD incidence in adults and in individuals with more moderate elevations of cholesterol.[46]

A recent review of the nine prospective studies that have examined the correlation between total cholesterol levels and CAD in women revealed that elevated total cholesterol and possibly LDL levels are risk factors for CAD in women.[47] A high triglyceride level is an independent risk factor for women, and an increased HDL level is negatively associated with subsequent CAD.[48] Data indicate that women have much lower rates of CAD than men with similar cholesterol values.[47] Nevertheless, a recent study confirms the need for screening women for the risk of CAD because lifestyle changes can reduce the incidence of CAD morbidity and mortality.[49]

The Bogalusa Heart Study,[50] which included a 15-year span, established that cardiovascular risk can be predicted early in life and that the interrelationships of risk factors in children are similar to those observed in adults. Approximately 5% of 5- to 18-year-old American children have total plasma cholesterol levels exceeding 200 mg/dl.[51] In a recent study of 786 fourth-grade schoolchildren, 10% had blood cholesterol levels of 200 mg/dl or more, and only 33% had a family history of early CAD.[52]

The National Cholesterol Education Program (NCEP), which was established by the Heart, Lung and Blood Institute to reduce the prevalence of elevated blood cholesterol levels in the United States, recently published recommendations on testing and managing cholesterol levels in children and adults.[53,54] The NCEP recommends a strategy incorporating population and individualized approaches.[55] The population approach aims to lower the average levels of blood cholesterol among all children and adolescents through population-wide changes in eating patterns. The NCEP recommends a diet that includes a saturated fat intake of less than 10% of total calories, of 30% or

less of calories from total fat, and of less than 300 mg of cholesterol a day for all healthy children over 2 years of age.[55] Educating the public through the media, schools, health care professionals, and government agencies will play a key role in the success of this approach.

The individualized approach is aimed at identifying and treating children and adolescents at the greatest risk for high blood cholesterol levels as adults. Although the NCEP did not recommend universal screening, it did recommend that selective screening was appropriate for a certain subset of children. The NCEP recommended screening of children whose (1) parents or grandparents, at 55 years of age or less, underwent procedures such as balloon angioplasty or bypass surgery; (2) parents or grandparents, at 55 years of age or less, had a documented MI, angina, peripheral vascular disease, or sudden cardiac death; or (3) parents' or grandparents' history is unobtainable, particularly those with other risk factors.[55]

The NCEP recommends dietary therapy as the primary approach to treating children and adolescents with elevated blood cholesterol levels. The NCEP recommends consideration of drug therapy in children 10 years of age and older if the LDL cholesterol level remains above 190 mg/dl after an adequate trial of diet therapy, if the LDL cholesterol level is 160 mg/dl with a positive family history, or if two or more risk factors are present after vigorous attempts to control them.[55]

Rates of CAD are much higher in older adults than in younger people. In fact, studies show that even advanced CAD responds to cholesterol-lowering therapy. Therefore older adults may benefit by using a cholesterol-lowering diet. Many older individuals may not be suitable candidates because of advanced age or other severe competing illnesses.[54]

Mean serum total cholesterol levels in American adults aged 20 through 74 years have consistently declined from 1960 through 1991.[55] More than half the decline occurred from 1976 to 1991. Many changes in nutritional, lifestyle, and medical therapeutic factors may have influenced the declines in blood cholesterol levels. In addition, it appears that public health efforts to reduce cholesterol levels are proving effective.

As part of its activities, the NCEP established the Expert Panel on Selection, Evaluation, and Treatment of High Blood Cholesterol in Adults, which has recently published its second report regarding cholesterol management. The Panel recommends that total serum cholesterol levels as well as HDL cholesterol levels should be measured in all adults at least every 5 years.[54] For people without CAD, total cholesterol levels are categorized as desirable (less than 200 mg/dl), borderline high-risk (200 to 239 mg/dl), or high-risk (greater than 240 mg/dl). In addition to measuring the total and HDL cholesterol levels, the Panel recommends an individual assessment of other risk factors. It describes the following positive risk factors for

CAD: age (men 45 and women older than 55 or who have had premature menopause without estrogen replacement), family history of early CAD, smoking, hypertension, HDL cholesterol level of less than 35 mg/dl, and diabetes. An HDL cholesterol level of 60 mg/dl or more is considered a negative risk factor.[54]

For individuals without CAD and desirable blood cholesterol levels, the HDL level dictates further follow-up. Those with HDL cholesterol levels of 35 mg/dl or above are given information regarding diet and exercise and have another HDL analysis in 5 years. Those with an HDL cholesterol level of less than 35 mg/dl should have further lipoprotein analyses. For individuals with borderline high-risk total cholesterol levels, the level of HDL cholesterol and presence of multiple other risk factors determine follow-up. Those with an HDL level of 35 mg/dl or greater and fewer than two other risk factors are given information on diet and exercise and require follow-up in 2 years. Those with a borderline total cholesterol level and an HDL level of less than 35 mg/dl or at least two risk factors should have lipoprotein analysis.[54]

The LDL cholesterol level is calculated from the lipoprotein analysis. Subsequent decisions for management of individuals without CAD who require further lipoprotein analysis are based on the LDL cholesterol level. Individuals with a desirable LDL level (less than 130 to 159 mg/dl) do not need further evaluation. Those with borderline LDL cholesterol levels (less than 130 to 159 mg/dl) who have fewer than two other risk factors are given instruction or diet and exercise and require 1 year follow-up. Those with borderline high-risk LDL levels and at least two other risk factors and those with high-risk LDL levels (greater than 160 mg/dl) require clinical evaluation and cholesterol-lowering diet therapy.[54]

The Panel recommends that all individuals with CAD have lipoprotein analysis, with follow-up being based on the LDL cholesterol level. For these individuals, the optimum LDL cholesterol level is 100 mg/dl or less. With an optimum LDL cholesterol level, individuals with CAD are given instructions on diet and exercise and require annual lipoprotein analysis. With an LDL cholesterol level greater than 100 mg/dl, individuals require clinical evaluation, and cholesterol-lowering therapy should be initiated.[54]

Dietary therapy and physical activity are the first therapies used to reduce elevated serum cholesterol levels. Dietary therapy occurs in two steps. The step-one diet involves an intake of saturated fat of 8% to 10% of total calories, of 30% or less of calories from total fat, and of less than 300 mg of cholesterol per day. Foods high in saturated fat include whole milk, cream, butter, cheeses, animal fats, organ meat, and palm and coconut oils. Reduction in cholesterol intake is best achieved by decreasing the intake of egg yolks and fats of animal origin. If goals are not met with the step-one diet, the individual proceeds to the step-two diet. This diet includes a further decrease in saturated fat to less than 7% of total calories and in cholesterol to less than 200 mg/dl.[54]

The Panel recommends that dietary measures be undertaken for at least 6 months in primary prevention before initiating drug therapy. Medications can be considered earlier in patients with severe elevations of LDL cholesterol of 220 mg/dl or greater.[54] The ATP recommends that for primary prevention, drug therapy should be considered for an individual who despite dietary therapy has an LDL cholesterol level of 190 mg/dl or greater without two other risk factors or of 160 mg/dl or greater with two other risk factors. For individuals with CAD, drug therapy is recommended if LDL cholesterol levels are 130 mg/dl or greater after maximal dietary therapy.

The primary classes of lipid-lowering drugs include those that (1) stimulate the removal of LDL through receptor-mediated mechanisms (bile acid sequestrants); (2) decrease the rate of synthesis of VLDL, the precursor of LDL (nicotinic acid); (3) hasten the clearance of VLDL (fibric acid derivatives); (4) lower LDL cholesterol levels (statins); and (5) stimulate the clearance of LDL via nonreceptor mechanisms (probucol). Because of their long-standing efficacy, nicotinic acid and bile acid sequestrants are the drugs of choice for lowering LDL cholesterol levels.[56]

Smoking

Cigarette smoking has been identified as a major health problem, and it is the single most preventable cause of death in the United States.[57] During the last several decades, significant public health effort has been focused on decreasing the prevalence of smoking. Although these efforts have had a positive impact in reducing overall smoking prevalence, the rate of decline has been variable among population subgroups such as women, blacks, adolescents, and individuals with lower educational levels and socioeconomic status.

According to the current estimates, 27.9% of white men and 23.5% of white women smoke.[1] Studies show that in the United States, smoking has declined by more than 32% since 1965.[1]

There is a variation in smoking prevalence among racial subgroups. For example, a higher proportion of black men smoke than white men. Data reveal that 32.6% of black men and 21.2% of black women smoke. In addition, 30.9% of Hispanic men and 16.3% of Hispanic women smoke.

Years of education and socioeconomic status are also factors that influence smoking prevalence. Smoking prevalence is several times higher among those with fewer than 12 years of education compared with those with at least 16 years of education. Furthermore, 20% to 35% of women in wealthy nations smoke compared with 2% to 10% of those in the Third World.[1]

Smoking continues to be a problem in the adolescent age group. An estimated 2.4 million teenagers aged 12 through 17 are smokers. The Centers for Disease Control and Prevention estimate that every day approximately 3000 American young people become smokers. This is a serious problem, since the majority of adults, approximately 75%, started smoking before age 18.[1]

There has been a great deal of effort to reduce smoking in the worksite, in public, and in the home. A significant trend is the negative attitude toward cigarette smoking reflected in numerous regulations separating smokers and nonsmokers in schools, restaurants, worksites, airplanes, and other public places. Nonsmokers have become outspoken in their demand for clean indoor air. By 1991, 43 states and the District of Columbia had restricted public smoking. The range was from simple laws, such as no smoking in school buses in operation, to comprehensive clean indoor air laws.[57]

Smoking is a major risk factor for coronary and peripheral vascular disease. It has been associated with a two-to-fourfold increased risk of CAD, a greater risk of death from CAD, and an elevated risk of sudden death.[58] In fact, for each 10 cigarettes smoked there is an incremental increase in cardiovascular mortality in men (18%) and in women (31%).[59]

Available data suggest that smoking cessation markedly decreases future CAD risk. In a recent study, the coronary heart disease mortality rate in 5 years decreased among men who had quit smoking to almost the level of a lifelong nonsmoker.[60] Even in older adults aged 65 to 74 years, smoking cessation is associated with decreased cardiovascular risk, indicating that it is worthwhile to encourage patients of all ages to stop smoking.[61]

Smoking a cigarette causes an infusion of nicotine, which stimulates the sympathetic nervous system. In healthy people, this results in an increased heart rate, blood pressure, stroke volume, cardiac output, and coronary blood flow. The peripheral vascular changes include cutaneous vasoconstriction associated with decreased skin temperature, systemic vasoconstriction, and increased muscle blood flow.[62]

The specific mechanism whereby cigarette smoking accelerates the development of CAD or precipitates its manifestations is yet to be defined. In patients with CAD, nicotine may contribute to the magnitude and frequency of reversible myocardial ischemia. There is increased oxygen consumption with the increased heart rate and blood pressure. The carbon monoxide inhaled also decreases the oxygen-carrying capacity of the blood. Carbon monoxide may also produce direct damage to the arterial endothelium. When a healthy person smokes a cigarette, blood flow increases to meet the increased demand. In the presence of CAD, however, coronary blood flow cannot increase sufficiently to meet the increased demand because of a decreased coronary artery lumen size, which may cause angina pectoris or myocardial dysfunction. Cigarette smoking also causes constriction of epicardial arteries and a further decrease in coronary blood flow in patients with CAD, despite an increase in myocardial oxygen demand.[63]

Smoking may contribute to CAD through its effects on hemostasis and the development of thrombosis, which is a factor in the atherogenic process and AMI. Blood coagulates more easily in smokers than nonsmokers, fibrinogen levels are higher, platelets are reported in some studies to be more reactive,[64] and platelet survival is shortened in smokers compared with nonsmokers. Smokers also tend to have a relatively unfavorable lipoprotein pattern, with a lower polyunsaturated to saturated fat rate that may contribute to the increased LDL cholesterol concentrations found in smokers.[65] In addition, smoking appears to be a major risk factor for vasospastic angina.[66]

The majority of smokers who quit do so without the help of structured groups or prescription medications. Successful smoking cessation usually follows repeated attempts to quit. Several personal characteristics are positively correlated with successful efforts to quit, including a high expectation of success, high number and long duration of past smoking-cessation attempts, fewer cigarettes smoked per day, low stress, and a sense of personal control and security. Barriers to successful cessation include lack of understanding about the health consequences of smoking and fear of failure, nicotine withdrawal, and weight gain.[67]

Several methods exist to assist with smoking cessation. A review of smoking-cessation programs conducted by the U.S. Department of Health and Human Services identified the following factors that improved success: (1) use of multiple cessation methods, which can address the behavioral and pharmacologic components of addictions; (2) payment, as in commercial programs, which increases commitment; (3) the presence of illness or risk factors that improve motivation to quit; and (4) good maintenance procedures, which provide ongoing support to the ex-smoker.[68]

Among medical patients, the rate of spontaneous quitting is 1% per year, but this rate can be increased several-fold with minimal intervention by the health care provider, including simple instructions to stop smoking. Further treatment may require pharmacologic or behavioral therapy or both.[69]

Behavioral therapy is often critical to successful smoking cessation. These methods are categorized into four types: (1) self-help methods, self-help aids, and mass media approaches; (2) health professional–directed minimal interventions, such as brief counseling, hypnosis, or single-session acupuncture; (3) comprehensive smoking-cessation programs; and (4) either the second or third method combined with a pharmacologic aid such as Nicorette gum or clonidine.

Self-help methods, including books, cassettes, or tapes, are readily available to smokers. The use and efficacy of these approaches have not been thoroughly studied.[70]

Nasopuncture and auriculopuncture are the two primary methods of acupuncture used for smoking cessation. There are few published studies on the efficacy of acupuncture, and most of these are methodologically flawed. In a review of these studies, Godenick[70] concluded that there is no substantive evidence that acupuncture relieves withdrawal symptoms or promotes smoking cessation.

Studies on the effectiveness of hypnosis as a treatment for smoking are also difficult to evaluate because of poor study design and limited follow-up. However, in a review of smoking-cessation methods, Schwartz[68] concluded that the skill and experience of the therapist and multiple sessions appear to improve cessation rates.

Behavioral methods for smoking cessation include aversive methods and self-management techniques. Aversive methods include rapid smoking and mild electric shock. Self-management methods include nicotine fading, gradual reduction of the number of cigarettes smoked over time, and relaxation techniques. A recent review of these methods concluded that the best successful rates have been achieved by a combination of aversive and self-management methods. Data indicate that aversion therapy is effective in initiating smoking cessation, whereas abstinence is better helped by self-management strategies.[70]

Pharmacologic therapies to assist smoking cessation include receptor antagonists (such as clonidine), and nicotine-substitution therapy. Mecamylamine decreases the satisfaction and other effects of smoking. Clonidine decreases the severity of the craving for nicotine and that of nicotine-withdrawal symptoms, probably by acting on the α-adrenergic receptors of the central nervous system. In a recent clinical trial, clonidine therapy for 6 weeks was found to be more effective than a placebo in assisting smoking cessation, although the benefit was observed only in women.[71]

The most effective pharmacologic approach for smoking cessation has been nicotine-substitution therapy. In some studies, nicotine gum has been useful in helping subjects to quit smoking. The gum is most effective when used as a component of a comprehensive program that includes behavioral therapy. Side effects from the gum such as hiccups and nausea may be controlled by lowering the dose of nicotine and by slow, paced chewing.[72]

A number of methods or a combination of them can help smokers to achieve abstinence. Programs with an effective maintenance component have the best long-term success. Social support, training in coping strategies, and use of substitutes such as exercise may enhance long-term maintenance.[68]

Physical Inactivity

The Centers for Disease Control and Prevention has recently identified physical inactivity as a strong and independent risk factor for coronary heart disease. Physically inactive individuals have almost a twofold increase in the risk for coronary heart disease (relative risk is 1.9), which is comparable to the relative risks associated with elevated SBP (2.1), cigarette smoking (2.5), and elevated serum cholesterol levels (2.4).[73] In addition, physical activity favorably influences other risk factors, such as reducing blood pressure, assisting in weight loss, and increasing HDL cholesterol levels.

Investigators have studied the effects of occupational or leisure time physical activity or both on coronary heart disease morbidity and mortality rates. Over 40 years ago, Morris and others[74] reported that physically active London transit workers and postal carriers had lower coronary heart disease events than bus drivers and sedentary postal clerks. Follow-up work showed that the conductors had half the coronary heart disease mortality rate of the drivers.[75] These differences may not appear very large; however, they are significant when considering the mild form of exercise involved in collecting tickets or delivering mail. It was later determined, however, that the bus drivers weighed more than the conductors, which may have contributed to the difference in heart disease rates.[76]

Among the most well-controlled occupational studies was an investigation of Israeli workers living on farm settlements.[77] Many extraneous variables were eliminated because all subjects were of the same ethnic origin, lived in the same environment, ate the same diet in communal dining halls, and received similar medical care. There were no statistically significant differences in body weight and cholesterol levels within the sample. In the 15-year retrospective survey of more than 10,000 men and women who were 40 to 64 years of age, there was a 2.5 and 3.1 greater incidence of coronary heart disease respectively for men and women engaged in sedentary work compared with those engaged in physical work.

A prospective study of 6351 longshoremen[78,79] demonstrated a strong inverse relationship between energy expenditure at work and coronary heart disease morbidity and mortality rates. The death rate for heart disease among the men who expended 8500 kcal/week or more (cargo handlers who loaded and unloaded ships) was about half that of those who were less physically active (foremen and clerks). This difference remained significant when cigarette smoking, SBP, and body weight were excluded.

The Framingham study[80] used a subjective measure of physical activity based on recall of daily activities. The index used in this study was the product of hours spent at each physical activity level and a weight based on oxygen consumption of that activity. Men with the highest scores on this index (that is, men who were more active) had fewer deaths related to heart disease than men who were less active, even when other risk factors were excluded. The significant relationship diminished for women when adjustment was made for age.

The largest body of evidence regarding the relationship between exercise and reduced cardiovascular risk originates from studies of several thousand Harvard alumni by Paffenbarger and others.[81-84] The age-adjusted incidence of coronary heart disease was inversely related to energy expenditure. Men who expended less than 2000 kcal/week had a 64% greater risk than men who had a higher energy expenditure. In addition, alumni who had been college athletes and did not continue exercising had a higher risk for coronary heart disease compared with alumni who were physically active and had not been athletes in college. The implication of this study was that current physical activity is the relevant factor in determining the influence of exercise on the risk of coronary heart disease. Continual follow-up of these alumni has demonstrated that exercise is inversely related to mortality, especially death from cardiovascular diseases.

One of the proposed mechanisms for the reduced incidence of coronary heart disease in those who regularly exercise is an increase in the HDL level. Wood and others[85,86] studied 81 healthy, sedentary men aged 30 to 55 for 1 year; these men were randomly assigned to participate in a running program or to remain sedentary. At the end of 1 year, the runners had a significantly higher fitness level as measured by maximal oxygen consumption and less body fat than the sedentary controls. In addition, total cholesterol, LDL, and triglyceride levels were reduced, and the HDL level was increased in the runners. Opposite changes were observed in sedentary subjects. These changes in lipid measurements, however, were not significant. Data from the group who averaged running at least 8 miles/week revealed an increase in the HDL level that was significant. Thus beneficial lipoprotein changes may be related to the quantity and quality of exercise. A significant increase in HDL level and reductions in the LDL and triglyceride levels were also found in 237 patients enrolled in phase 2 cardiac rehabilitation programs.[87] In this study, patients with the worse lipid profiles showed the most improvement in lipid values after exercise rehabilitation.

Exercise produces other effects that reduce cardiovascular risk. Resting and submaximum exercise heart rates decrease as a result of exercise training, and blood pressure may be reduced in normotensive and hypertensive individuals,[88,89] producing an increase in myocardial oxygen supply and a reduction in myocardial oxygen consumption. Additional cardiovascular benefits of exercise training include increases in stroke volume, cardiac output, and arteriovenous oxygen difference. Along with the direct benefits of exercise, individuals who exercise regularly are more likely to engage in other healthy behaviors that contribute to a lower risk, such as eating moderately, coping more effectively with stress, and avoiding smoking.

Significant cross-sectional associations between physical activity level and cardiovascular risk have been observed in community-based investigations. The sample of the Stanford Five-City Project included 380 men and 427 women (ages 18 to 74) who were followed from 1979 to 1985. For men, an improvement in the total physical activity score significantly correlated with an increase in the HDL level and a decrease in body mass index. For women, an improvement in the physical activity score was associated with an increase in the HDL level and a decrease in the resting heart rate.[90]

Parents and educators should emphasize to children the importance of regular physical activity. Children must be encouraged to participate in school-related and community physical education programs that address the health benefits of exercise. This early exposure to exercise will help to form life-long physical activity habits.

When adults decide to initiate an exercise program for the prevention of CAD, they should be encouraged to first obtain physical examinations. Ideally these examinations include graded maximal exercise tests to determine aerobic capacity and evaluate cardiovascular status.

An exercise prescription based on an individual's functional capacity may be provided. An exercise prescription should address the type, intensity, duration, and frequency of physical activity. The type of exercise includes any activity that uses large muscle groups and is aerobic in nature, such as running, jogging, walking, swimming, bicycling, rowing, cross-country skiing, skating, or jumping rope. The intensity of training should begin at 65% of one's age-related maximal heart rate ($220 - age$). Intensity may be increased as conditioning effects, such as a lower resting heart rate, are observed. However, cardiovascular benefits are achieved with low- to moderate-intensity exercise, and patients with known coronary heart disease should seek consultation from health care professionals before exercising at high intensities. The duration of exercise is 15 to 60 minutes of continual or intermittent aerobic activity, and frequency is 3 to 5 days per week.[91,92]

Exercise scientists have recently proposed "lifestyle exercise" as an approach to increasing physical activity.[92] Lifestyle exercise involves the integration of multiple short bouts of physical activity into one's daily life. Experts speculate that if the total daily energy expenditure is the same as that with traditional training regimens, similar health benefits should accrue.

Glucose Intolerance

Coronary heart disease is more prevalent in patients with adult-onset diabetes mellitus, although the precise mechanisms are unclear. Patients with diabetes have more connective tissue degeneration, which expedites atheroma formation. A 14-year study of the gender-specific effect of non-insulin-dependent diabetes mellitus (NIDDM) on the risk of fatal ischemic heart disease showed that the age-adjusted relative hazard in diabetic vs. nondiabetic persons was 1.8 in men and 3.3 in women. The relative hazard remained greater in women (3.3) than in men (1.9) when adjusted for other risk factors (age, plasma cholesterol level, SBP, and smoking).[93] Another study by Liao and others[94] showed similar results. Age-adjusted relative risk for cardiac death in diabetics was 1.0 in men and 1.96 in women.

Personality Factors

For many years, CAD has been thought to be more prominent among individuals with personality type A. The characteristics of type-A behavior pattern as described by Friedman and Rosenman[95] include aggressiveness, ambition, competitive drive, and a chronic sense of urgency. Two characteristics, easily aroused anger and hostility, have been added to the original definition.[96] Recent studies have raised doubts concerning the relationship between type-A behaviors and CAD. An analysis of multiple risk-factor intervention trial (MRFIT) data for 3110 men revealed that the type-A behavior pattern was not significantly associated with the risk of first major coronary events (coronary death and definite nonfatal MI) after a mean follow-up of 7.1 years. The same study analyzed the Jenkins Activity type-A score for 12,772 men and found no significant association with the risk of first major coronary event.[97] Subsequently, 257 men with CAD in the Western Collaborative Group Study were evaluated to determine whether behavior type was related to subsequent CAD mortality. The researchers found that behavior type was not related to mortality in patients who died within 24 hours of the coronary event. Unexpectedly, patients who survived for 24 hours showed a lower mortality rate for type-A patients (12.7 years/1000 person-years) than type-B patients (19.1 years/1000 person-years).[98]

Maruta and others[99] evaluated hostility as measured by the 50-item Minnesota Multiphasic Personality Inventory (MMPI) Hostility Scale and the development of CAD, CAD-related mortality, and total mortality. When only the hostility score was considered, it was a significant factor for predicting the development of CAD, CAD-related mortality, and total mortality. However, when age and gender were also considered, the hostility score was no longer a significant predictive factor.

Other factors that appear related to type-A behavior patterns include age and sympathetic nervous system function. One study reported that a type-A behavior pattern was associated with a consistent elevation of sympathetic nervous system function among healthy middle-aged men. Williams and others[100] suggest that maladaptive changes in sympathetic function may occur during the transition from late adolescence to middle age in type-A men. A 9-year cohort study found evidence that individuals with type-A behavior patterns are more likely to experience a steeper increase in blood pressure and rate of cigarette smoking during their third decade of life than their type-B counterparts. The investigators offered the possibility that type-A behaviors and these two risk factors may become less strongly associated during middle age as life situations become more predictable and manageable.[101]

Stress

The question of the relationship of stress to the development of cardiovascular disease remains unsettled, although several authors have made a strong case for the link among cardiovascular reactivity, stress, and cardiovascular disease.[102] Weiner[103] stated that stressful experiences are probably only one factor among many other factors that predispose individuals to CAD.

Eliot[104] has associated the glucocorticoid excess of long-term stress (perceived as a persistent loss of control) and the catecholamine excess of short-term stress (repeated episodic events occurring about 20 to 30 times/day) with a number of risk factors for cardiovascular disease. Glucocorticoid excess has been related to potential weight gain resulting from the conversion of protein to carbohydrates and fat, an alteration in cholesterol levels (decreased HDL and increased total cholesterol levels), and a lowering of the stimulation threshold in the brain.

Vasoconstriction from catecholamine excess related to short-term stress is increased because the arterioles have been sensitized by long-term stress resulting in endothelial damage. Glucocorticoid excess results in an increase in angiotensin II, predisposing the individual to hypertension. Increased retention of sodium and fluid results from the stimulation of the adrenal cortex, thus adding to the potential for hypertension. Depletion of potassium and magnesium levels related to adrenal cortex stimulation increases the risk of dysrhythmias, whereas a catecholamine excess lowers the dysrhythmia threshold.[104]

Long- and short-term stress affect platelets by increasing their number, adhesiveness, and aggregation. Catecholamine excess also increases myocardial oxygen demand, mobilizes free fatty acids, and decreases insulin secretion. These alterations are associated with the development of atherosclerosis.[104]

Other work in this area lends strength to Eliot's conclusions. In a study done in Great Britain, a strong association was found between job stress score and plasma fibrinogen concentration.[105] Italian researchers demonstrated the existence of a direct link between emotional stress and platelet function. Mental stress induced significant increases in heart rate, SBP and DBP, cardiac output, platelet aggregation, the formation of circulating platelet aggregates, and thromboxane B_2 levels in plasma and serum.[106] Similar results were found in patients after infarction and in control subjects, although they were less evident in the control subjects. Although it is not definitive, it appears that stress is a risk factor that interacts with other risk factors in the development or progression of CAD.

Stress management refers to the identification and analysis of problems related to stress and the use of a variety of therapeutic interventions to alter the source or experience of stress. The goal of stress management is not to minimize or eliminate stress but to achieve a balance between an individual's resistance to stress and the amount of stress in the environment.[107]

In general, there are six types of interventions used in stress management. Problem-focused physiologic strategies focus on the stressor itself and altering that stressor. These strategies are most often used when the stressor is physiologic such as a chronic disease involving a lifestyle change that would affect the course of the disease. Problem-focused behavioral strategies such as assertiveness training, time management, or the acquisition of new skills work to alter the nature of the stressor.[107]

Cognitive strategies are used to alter the perception of stress. Problem-solving techniques, thought stopping of ruminative or obsessive thoughts, and cognitive hypothesis testing are examples of problem-focused cognitive strategies.[107]

Techniques that enable the individual to deal more effectively with the physiologic arousal accompanying stress are termed *emotion-focused physiologic strategies*. Some examples of this approach include relaxation therapies and particular lifestyle interventions. These techniques do not alter the stressor but help the individual change the physiologic response. Emotion-focused cognitive strategies alter the emotional, affective, or cognitive response to stress. Individuals use techniques such as cognitive hypothesis testing, challenges to negative thoughts, or cognitive reinterpretation to deal with the cognitive sequelae of stress.[107]

Finally, emotion-focused behavioral strategies address the behavioral response to stress. These strategies include learning new behaviors to counter maladaptive response and using recreation and leisure time activities to offset the effects of stress.[107]

Obesity

It is estimated that 47 million American adults are 20% or more over their desirable weight. Overweight individuals account for 24.4% of white men, 25.7% of black men, 25.1% of white women, and 43.8% of black women.[1] Although this remains a controversial issue, most epidemiologic studies show a positive relationship between obesity (any weight greater than 30% over ideal weight) and morbidity and mortality from CAD.[108,109] The risk of CAD increased in men and women as their mean weights increased, with this association being most pronounced in those younger than 50 years of age.[108] A 26-year follow-up study of participants in the Framingham Heart Study showed that weight is a relatively potent risk factor for total cardiovascular disease in women (0.199) versus men (0.143).

The distribution of body fat as opposed to overall obesity has been investigated. Researchers in Sweden found the relation between the ratio of waist-hip circumference and cardiovascular disease and death to be stronger than any other anthropometric variable studied in 1462 women aged 38 to 60.[110] Subsequent work investigated the relationship between body fat distribution and death in women aged 55 to 69 years. This 5-year follow-up study had 1504 deaths occur among the accumulated 198,000 person-years. Overall obesity was measured using body mass index, and a J-shaped association with mortality was found. Death rates were highest in the leanest as well as the most obese women. Use of the waist-hip circumference ratio revealed a strong, positive association with mortality in a monotonic dose-response fashion. An increase of 0.15 units in the waist-hip circumference ratio (for example, a 6-inch increase in waist measurement in a woman with 40-inch hips) was associated with a 60% greater relative risk of death after adjusting for age, body mass index, smoking, education level, marital status, and estrogen and alcohol use. These data support the idea that the distribution of body fat may be more indicative of cardiovascular risk in women than overall obesity.[111,112]

Caffeine and Alcohol Intake

Although there is a substantial amount of literature describing the deleterious effects of caffeine, the association between caffeine use and cardiovascular risk has not been established.[113-116] The influence of alcohol on cardiovascular risk continues to be debated. Several epidemiologic studies have shown that drinking alcohol in moderation reduces the risk of CAD.[117,118]

This controversy has been fueled by recent evidence on the effect of alcohol on lipoprotein subfractions. It is known that the regular use of alcohol can reduce HDL levels. A British study of 1048 women found that moderate alcohol consumption (1 to 2 drinks/day) is associated with lower plasma concentrations of triglycerides, cholesterol, and insulin and a lower body mass index. Moderate alcohol consumption was also associated with higher plasma concentrations of HDL, HDL_2 cholesterol, and HDL_3 cholesterol. All of these were independent of body mass index, smoking habits, and oral contraceptive use.[119] Continued investigation concerning moderate alcohol use and its "protective" effect is warranted.

Other Risk Factors

Additional signs associated with increased risk of coronary heart disease are hyperuricemia and ECG abnormalities at rest and in response to exercise. Some major risk factors may be determined by familial or genetic factors. The tendency toward development of hypertension, diabetes, and hyperlipidemia may be inherited. Also, certain habits and lifestyles such as smoking, overeating, and lack of exercise may be passed down in a family. There may also be other inherited traits, currently unmeasurable, that affect risk. It is vitally important to recognize that risk is multifactorial, that the influence of two or more factors may be synergistic, and that risk is influenced by any given factor's degree of abnormality, not just its presence or absence. The emphasis for the future is on primary prevention, which includes risk factor education, basic research support, and acceptance by the public or responsibility for health maintenance. Secondary risk factors, including MI and dysrhythmias, will be discussed in subsequent chapters.

Summary

The most important primary prevention strategies for coronary artery disease are better nutrition, increased physical activity, cessation of smoking, weight reduction, effective stress management, moderate alcohol consumption (a limit of 50 g or 2 to 3 average drinks per day), and control of hypertension. The best strategy is one that includes each of these goals, a comprehensive "lifestyle change" strategy.

PREVENTION IN THE COMMUNITY

Primary preventive strategies can be implemented singularly or in combination in a number of settings and through community and national health information programs. In general, health education programs aimed at providing information and altering the behavior of large groups of individuals are the most cost effective.

Home

The importance of beginning preventive strategies in childhood cannot be overemphasized. Although many heart, lung, and blood diseases are not manifest until middle age or later, their development begins during childhood and adolescence.[120] The fatty streaks and fibrous plaques that apparently result in end-stage cardiovascular disease have frequently been observed in children and youth.[121] Individuals with higher-than-average blood pressures as teenagers are also more likely to have elevated blood pressures as adults.

The majority of unhealthy behaviors seen in adults are learned during childhood and have their origins in the home. Eating habits, exercise patterns, smoking, use of alcohol, attitudes that relate to self-confidence and to society, management of stress, involvement with others, and decision-making abilities are all first learned in the home. Obesity, like other coronary risk factors, is more difficult to correct in adults than in children. Children of parents who set examples conducive to health are more likely to assume a healthy lifestyle than if the opposite were true. Primary prevention programs in the home must therefore involve children and adults.

School

Based on the results of pediatric epidemiologic studies, it is clear that the foundation for adult heart diseases is established in childhood.[122,123] Therefore screening for cardiovascular risk factors and specific health programs must be introduced into the educational system.

Numerous school-site programs have been implemented. A major focus is smoking prevention, since smoking is often initiated among adolescents. An assessment of school-based smoking-prevention programs in the United States showed that these programs are consistently effective in delaying the onset of smoking; however, they have not often demonstrated the long-term effects of preventing smoking. A panel of the National Cancer Institute proposed minimum components for smoking-prevention programs, which include instruction about social consequences, short-term physiologic effects of tobacco use, and social influences on tobacco use (peer, parent, and media influences) and training in refusal skills. The minimum length for these programs should be two, five-session blocks provided in separate school years between the sixth and ninth grades. Programs should include peer and parental involvement and teacher training.[124]

In 1983 the "Tobacco-Free Schools" project was initiated jointly by the American Lung Association of Minnesota and the Minnesota Department of Education. The project, which encourages local school districts to adopt tobacco-free policies, establishes nonsmoking as the norm in schools for adults and students. It assumes that prevention education is more effective when programs, school policies, and adult models provide a consistent message that tobacco use is unhealthy and unacceptable.[125]

In addition, the American Cancer Society, the American Lung Association, and the AHA began a 12-year collaborative program in 1988 aimed at including at least one third of the country's 3 million first-graders in the Smoke-Free Class of the year 2000. Specific lesson plans have been developed for participating schools.[126]

As a result of the data accumulated from the Bogulusa Heart Study on cardiovascular risk factors in children,[127] a program called "Heart Smart" was initiated to provide cardiovascular risk assessment and education for elementary schoolchildren. The long-term goal of the program is to reduce cardiovascular risk factors in children through adoption of healthy lifestyles. The program includes risk-factor screening (fasting lipid levels, anthropometrics, blood pressure); a strong physical education program, "Superkids—Superfit," which teaches aerobic activities and encourages children to adopt exercise as a lifelong habit; a school lunch program that includes menu items low in sodium, fat, and sugar; staff education; and a parent outreach program. The Heart Smart program was initiated in four elementary schools, wherein two schools were randomly assigned to intervention or control conditions. The total sample size was 556 fourth- and fifth-graders. Results showed that school lunch choices were successfully altered, and children whose lunch choices were heart healthy had the greatest reduction in total cholesterol levels. Improvements in run-walk performance were related to improvements in the overall cardiovascular risk profile. Increases in HDL levels were observed at intervention schools. Observations in this population of children indicate that behavior change is related to physiologic changes that reduce cardiovascular risk.[128]

The Class of 1989 Study, a component of the Minnesota Heart Health Program, was designed to reduce cardiovascular disease in three communities in the North Central United States.[129] This program included two physical activity interventions implemented for eighth- and tenth-grade students. Beginning in the sixth grade, self-report questionnaires that contained measures for physical activity were administered. Physical activity scores were significantly higher for girls in the intervention group throughout the 7-year follow-up period; boys showed a trend toward increasing physical activity scores. Therefore comprehensive behavioral school programs can produce lasting improvement in adolescent physical activity.

Worksite

Industry has taken an increasing interest and played a growing role in health promotion and disease prevention among employees. The first National Survey of Worksite Health Promotion Activities conducted in 1988 surveyed a random sample of all private-sector worksites with 50 or more employees.[130] Of the 1358 responding worksites, 65.5% had one or more areas of health-promotion activity. Overall prevalence by type of activity included health-risk assessment (29.5%), smoking cessation (35.6%), blood pressure control and treatment (16.5%), exercise and fitness (22.1%), back problem prevention and care (28.5%), and off-the-job accident prevention. Health-promotion activities increased with worksite size and varied considerably by types of industry.[130]

With 100 million adult Americans at work every day, the worksite is an ideal setting for offering preventive health services and health-education programs aimed at the prevention of CAD. The development of secondary prevention strategies is also important.

Prevention and promotion programs at the worksite are numerous and diverse. The Heart at Work program developed by the AHA is one example of a comprehensive program.[131] Over 3000 companies nationwide have implemented this program. Heart at Work is a multifaceted educational program designed to teach employees how to prevent or reverse the effects of cardiovascular disease. The program includes high blood pressure screenings and counseling, cholesterol screening and counseling, smoking-cessation classes, cardiopulmonary resuscitation training, and exercise and nutrition education.[131]

Worksite health promotion programs have had varying degrees of success. Tenneco, Inc., found that health care costs were lower among exercisers than nonexercisers.[132] A recent study, however, found that participation in a health-promotion program was not associated with reduced health care costs.[133] A large, diversified industrial company found that program participants experienced a 14.0% decline in disability days.[134] Also, a year-long smoking-cessation program in nine worksites employing approximately 700 smokers produced high participation rates (29%) and moderate cessation rates (20%).[135]

A primary motivation for the development of worksite health-promotion programs is the potential financial benefit to employers. Employers now pay approximately half of the nation's health care bill. There is strong evidence that poor employee health behaviors are associated with increased health care costs. Additional business costs adversely affected by preventable illness in workers include life insurance, absenteeism, disability insurance, workman's compensation, decreased productivity, and turnover. In general, the claims of programs' profitability are based on anecdotal evidence or analyses that included methodologic flaws. The authors recommend the development of a new research-based body of knowledge to clearly document the economic merits of health-promotion programs.

Community

During the past 25 years a number of community-wide health-promotion programs have been undertaken, both in the United States and in other industrial nations. The Stanford Health Disease Prevention Program[136] was originally a 2-year experimental program in three California communities whose major objective was to determine whether intensive educational efforts could reduce cigarette smoking, blood cholesterol levels, and high blood pressure. Two communities were exposed to a mass media campaign designed to influence adults to change their living habits in ways that could reduce the risk of heart attack and stroke. In one of these towns the media campaign was supplemented with intensive face-to-face instruction for people identified as being at high risk. A third community, which was relatively isolated from the media shared by the two communities, served as a control. After 2 years the overall risk of cardiovascular disease in the control community increased about 7%, while in the other two towns there was a substantial (15% to 20%) decrease in risk. In the community that had the media campaign plus personal instruction, the initial improvement was greater than in the other experimental town, and health education was more successful in reducing cigarette smoking. At the end of the second year the decrease in risk was roughly the same in both experimental communities. The program concluded that intensive face-to-face instruction and counseling seem important for changing behaviors such as smoking and inadequate diet; however, where resources are limited, mass media education campaigns are an effective influence in reducing the risk of cardiovascular disease.

The Five-City Project, a major outgrowth of the original Stanford Heart Disease Project, is designed to stimulate and maintain lifestyle changes that would result in reduction of cardiovascular disease risk in the community. The project recognized the need to reach persons who do not speak English, and it developed health-promotion messages for Spanish radio stations. Field trials were undertaken to determine the impact of educational programs in the community on changes in cardiovascular risk factors and morbidity and mortality rates.[136]

Analysis of various aspects of the Stanford Five-City Study reveals that community-based intervention studies can affect the health of the population and therefore serve as a model for other communities. One report[137] indicates that an increase in physical activity over 5 years is favorably associated with changes in risk factors for men and women. For men, an increase in physical activity significantly correlated with an increase in HDL levels and a decrease in body mass index and the 10-year coronary heart disease risk score. For women, increased physical activity was associated with changes in HDL levels and resting pulse rate.

Using the Stanford Five-City data, Winkleby and others[138] looked at risk-factor reduction by educational levels. Over 8 years, men and women aged 25 to 74 from each educational group in the treatment cities showed significant declines in smoking prevalence and levels of blood pressure and cholesterol (with the exception of women and cholesterol levels). These authors concluded that broad-based education efforts in the United States are succeeding across educational levels.

Smoking cessation education as part of the Stanford Five-City Project showed positive results from intervention. Smoking prevalence decreased over 8 years in the control and treatment cities, but the decrease tended to be greater in the treatment rather than the control cities, with the difference being consistent over time. Smoking decreased in the control cities as well, but this decrease was not linear, and rates varied within cities between times. Smokers were more likely to quit in the treatment versus control cities.[139]

However, researchers learned that it was necessary to target the groups for which a response was desired by an analysis of adolescent and young adult smokers from the Five-City Project. Smoking cessation was targeted to the adults, so researchers asked about the diffusion of information to other groups. Smoking prevalence decreased by 50% among young adults but increased among adolescents, so the diffusion effect was determined to be limited or nonexistent.[140]

Analysis of data from the Stanford Five-City Project concerning weight gain showed that subjects in the treatment cities gained significantly less weight than subjects in control cities. Although this study provided some evidence that community health-education programs may help reduce weight gain over time, the authors felt that different effective measures must be developed to alter this risk factor in a broad population.[141]

The North Karelia Project in Finland, begun in 1972, was the first major community-based cardiovascular disease–prevention program. The program activities were primarily educational, aiming to teach the community how to adopt healthy lifestyles and reduce cardiovascular risk. Other strategies included development of a hypertension screening process and environmental changes such as smoking restrictions and introduction of low-fat food products. Follow-up surveys have indicated that health behaviors and risk factors changed over a 5-year period, with a decreased risk of 17% for cardiovascular disease in men and 12% in women. In addition, approximately 17,000 hypertensives were recruited to the hypertension register as a result.[142]

Subsequent follow-up of North Karelia for the years 1971 to 1987 showed mortality from ischemic heart disease and the rate of AMI declining steeply in men and women. This decline was accompanied by a decline in total mortality rates. Comparisons were made to the population of Kaunas, Lithuania, and the mortality and AMI rates increased in men but remained unchanged in women.[143]

Other community-based intervention trials have included the Interuniversity Study on Nutrition and Health in Belgium, the Pawtucket Heart Health Project (Rhode Island), and the Minnesota Heart Health Program.[144,145] Some results from the latter are discussed in the section on school risk-factor preventions.

Recently, many communities have passed local initiatives requiring all public places to restrict smoking to designated areas. Research will demonstrate the comparative effect of community-wide behavioral restrictions versus educational efforts alone.

Based on the results of these demonstration programs, community-wide programs have been implemented. Program initiatives arise from organizational and individual efforts. Many programs are jointly sponsored and publicized by voluntary organizations working in the community.

Prevention of cardiac disease through nutritional intervention is widely seen. Within many communities, restaurants provide heart-healthy meals that follow the AHA dietary guidelines. Participating restaurants work with volunteer dieticians to modify the food served and the manner of preparation to meet heart-healthy guidelines. Guides to restaurants offering heart-healthy menus are distributed by local organizations and are advertised as having heart-healthy menu selections. Food Festivals,[146] such as the week-long event in September sponsored by the Chicago Heart Association, are held to focus public attention on AHA dietary guidelines and their impact on cardiovascular health. Stores allow volunteers to work at information displays promoting proper nutrition and to give cooking demonstrations and tours when appropriate. Corporate and nonprofit institutional cafeterias use heart-healthy menus for the week and provide nutritional information to their employees. An annual heart-healthy recipe contest has encouraged development of recipes using the nutritional guidelines. These recipes are then distributed through the area. The AHA has recently developed a program called *Culinary Hearts Kitchen*. The program is a demonstration course on cooking meals low in calories, cholesterol, fat, and sodium.[147]

Video messages of 45 to 60 seconds on the selection and use of lean meats and poultry are being developed. These videos are being tested in grocery stores to target consumers who may not read nutritional information. They are intended to inform the consumer at the point of purchase with the goal of increasing purchases of lean protein sources.[147]

Cookbooks directed at adults and children are available with heart-healthy recipes. Some cookbooks combine nutritional information from the cardiovascular, diabetic, and cancer literature.

The prevention and detection of risk factors is a community-based activity. The Northeast Oklahoma City Cholesterol Education program, a church-based cholesterol-intervention program, found hypertension, elevated cholesterol levels, and obesity to be prevalent among the members. Because churches are central institutions in most African-American communities and because of the high prevalence of modifiable risk factors among their members, the authors concluded that churches serve as appropriate sites for the implementation of community-based risk-factor–control programs.[148]

One such project is the Heart, Body, and Soul program in East Baltimore, which focuses on smoking cessation.[149] The essential components in this project were building trust and acceptance and providing the technical support to encourage smoking-cessation strategies.

In addition, church-based hypertension screening and counseling programs have targeted medically underserved areas.[149] Church members are trained to conduct blood pressure screening and present education concerning risk factors. Appropriate referrals are then made as necessary.[149]

These are but a few examples of the programs designed to have community impact on cardiovascular health. Information concerning programs of this nature can be obtained from local voluntary associations.

NATIONAL PRIORITIES

In 1987, the Public Health Service and the Institute of Medicine of the National Academy of Sciences convened a national consortium to help guide the development of health-promotion and disease-prevention objectives for the year 2000. Various organizations and professionals across the United States contributed to the objectives by gathering information, providing testimony, and commenting on drafts. The resultant document, known as *Healthy People 2000,* sets three broad goals that challenge the nation to (1) increase the span of health life for Americans, (2) reduce health disparities among Americans, and (3) achieve access to preventive services for all Americans. *Healthy People 2000* identifies 300 discrete objectives among 22 priority areas. It is from these areas that research needs can be identified. Health-promotion strategies, health protection, and preventive services are the bulk of the areas identified. Health-promotion strategies are pertinent to the cardiovascular population, since they involve personal choices related to lifestyle and the resultant influence on health prospects.

Aspects of many of the 22 priority areas are pertinent to cardiovascular disease prevention and health promotion, but certain areas can be highlighted. Although progress has been made in the control of high blood pressure and the reduction of blood cholesterol levels, this continues to be a priority. The goals for these two priority areas are to increase the number of hypertensive individuals whose blood pressures are under control and the number of individuals whose blood cholesterol levels have been reduced below 200 mg/dl. Nutritional objectives include the reduction of the prevalence of overweight individuals by 23% and reduction of dietary fat intake by 17%. Specific objectives related to smoking include a 48% reduction in the prevalence of smoking and a focus on children and adolescents to reduce the initiation of smoking by 50%. Physical activity, as it relates to various risk factors, is emphasized in relation to a healthy lifestyle. To enable these objectives to be accomplished. *Healthy People 2000* cites the importance of beginning health education at the primary school level and continuing this emphasis into the worksite.[150,151]

Similarly, the National High Blood Pressure Education Program Working Group emphasizes the primary prevention of hypertension in target populations: African-Americans, persons with high-to-normal blood pressure, those with a family history of hypertension, and individuals with lifestyle factors that contribute to age-related increases in blood pressure. Interventions for primary prevention include weight control, reduced sodium and calorie intake, increased physical activity, reduced alcohol consumption, and stress management.[152]

In addition, the current health care reform plan incorporates primary prevention strategies to improve the health of our nation and reduce health care costs. Opportunities will exist for nurses to assume leadership roles in the provision of primary care.

RESEARCH NEEDS IN HEALTH PROMOTION

A comprehensive approach to health promotion has been described as an essential part of a primary prevention program directed against the premature onset of CAD. Given the acceptance of disease prevention and health promotion by the American people, the scientific evidence on which these concepts are based must be strengthened: program evaluation techniques must be refined, ways must be found to allocate resources fairly, the needs of special populations must be accommodated, and new organizational structures must be developed. These and other issues must be carefully and intelligently considered for all levels of society.

Preventive strategies must be tested through longitudinal, multidisciplinary, invasive studies of the intersection of high-risk groups and high-risk situations against control groups. Research is also needed to identify the developmental determinants of unhealthful behavior during childhood and adolescence. Genetic research is already making inroads in this regard, adding to the knowledge base about the genes involved in heart disease, especially those responsible for lipid metabolism and transport. More studies on the impact of risk-factor reduction on women, older adults, and ethnic groups are also necessary.

Many ramifications of health education are still unknown. For example, what kinds of national education models will work most effectively on the heterogeneous U.S. population? Will benefits accrue rapidly or slowly? Will they be temporary or permanent? Will they occur in the general population or only in high-risk groups? Unfortunately, there are major weaknesses in much of the evaluation of patient education: oversimplification of the behavior and causes of behavior that must be influenced by patient education, failure to make explicit the theoretic or assumed connection between educational interventions and behavioral or health results, and limited analyses of data, which leave many questions unanswered. These issues are further complicated by the lack of reimbursement for patient education in the health care delivery system.

Clearly, successful health education programs offer great promise; consumers will assume more responsibility for adopting health practices that protect health and prevent illness or complications, and they will make more timely and appropriate use of health resources. Already we have seen fewer hospital admissions, and shorter hospital stays as a result of past research in this area. Further research is necessary to determine the effects on patient satisfaction and quality of life.

REFERENCES

1. American Heart Association: *1993 heart and stroke facts and statistics,* Dallas, 1992, The Association.
2. Pamplona R and others: Mechanisms of glycation in atherosclerosis, *Med Hypotheses* 40:174, 1993.
3. Ross R: *Factors influencing atherogenesis.* In Schlant RC, Alexander RW, editors: *The heart, arteries and veins,* New York, 1994, McGraw-Hill.
4. Chobanian AV: Pathophysiology of atherosclerosis, *Am J Cardiol* 70:3G, 1992.
5. Kottle BA: Current understanding of the mechanisms of atherogenesis, *Am J Cardiol* 72:48C, 1993.
6. Libby P: Do vascular wall cytokines promote atherogenesis? *Hosp Pract* 27:51, 1992.
7. Flavahan NA: Atherosclerosis or lipoprotein-induced endothelial dysfunction, *Circulation* 85:1927, 1992.
8. Hangartner JRW and others: Morphological characteristics of clinically significant coronary artery stenosis in stable angina, *Br Heart J* 56:501, 1986.
9. Alexander RW: *The coronary ischemic syndromes: relationship to the biology of atherosclerosis.* In Schlant RC, Alexander RW, editors: *The heart, arteries and veins,* New York, 1994, McGraw-Hill.
10. Piek JJ, Becker AE: Collateral blood supply to the myocardium at risk in human myocardial infarction: a quantitative postmortem assessment, *J Am Coll Cardiol* 11:1290, 1988.
11. Prinzmetal M and others: Angina pectoris. I. A variant form of angina pectoris: preliminary report, *Am J Med* 27:375, 1959.
12. Roberts WC and others: Ages at death and sex distribution in age decade in fatal coronary artery disease, *Am J Cardiol* 66:1379, 1990.
13. Castelli WP: Cardiovascular disease and multifactorial risk: challenge of the 1980's, *Am Heart J* 109:1191, 1983.
14. Williams EL and others: Changes in coronary heart disease risk factors in the 1980s: evidence of a male-female crossover effect with age, *Am J Epidemiol* 137:1056, 1993.
15. National Heart, Lung, and Blood Institute; National Institutes of Health: *The Fifth Report of the Joint National Committee on Detection, Evaluation, and Treatment of High Blood Pressure* (JNC V). Oct 30, 1992, The Institutes.
16. Brest AN: Antihypertensive therapy in perspective. I. *Mod Conc Cardiov Dis* 57:65, 1988.
17. Kannel WB: Role of blood pressure in cardiovascular morbidity and mortality, *Prog Cardiov Dis* 17:5, 1974.
18. Castelli WP: Cardiovascular disease and multifactorial risk: challenge of the 1980s, *Am Heart J* 106:1191, 1983.
19. Kannel WB and others: Perspectives on systolic hypertension: the Framingham study, *Circulation* 61:1179, 1980.
20. Neaton JD, Wentworth D: Serum cholesterol, blood pressure, cigarette smoking, and death from coronary heart disease, *Arch Intern Med* 152:56, 1992.
21. Mann SJ: Systolic hypertension in the elderly: pathophysiology and management, *Arch Intern Med* 152:1977, 1992.
22. The Systolic Hypertension in the Elderly Program Cooperative Research Group: Implications of the Systolic Hypertension in Elderly Program, *Hypertension* 21:335, 1993.
23. Raison J and others: Extracellular and interstitial fluid volume in obesity with and without associated systemic hypertension, *Am J Cardiol* 57:223, 1986.
24. Langford HG and others: Effect of drug and diet treatment of mild hypertension on diastolic blood pressure, *Hypertension* 17:210, 1991.
25. Law MR and others: By how much does dietary salt reduction lower blood pressure? I. Analysis of observational data among populations, *Br Med J* 302:811, 1991.
26. Niarchos AP and others: Comparison of the effects of diuretic therapy and low sodium intake in isolated systolic hypertension, *Am J Med* 77:1061, 1984.
27. Kaplan NM: *Clinical hypertension,* Baltimore, 1990, Williams & Wilkins.
28. Blair SN and others: Physical fitness and incidence of hypertension in healthy normotensive men and women, *JAMA* 252:487, 1984.
29. Hagberg JM: *Exercise, fitness, and hypertension.* In Bouchard C and others, editors: *Exercise, fitness and health,* Champaign, Ill, 1990, Human Kinetics.
30. Health and Public Policy Committee, American College of Physicians: Biofeedback for hypertension, *Ann Intern Med* 102:709, 1985.
31. Patel C and others: Trials of relaxation in reducing coronary risk: four-year follow-up, *Br Med J Clin Res* 290:1103, 1985.

32. Fahrion SL: Hypertension and biofeedback, *Primary Care* 18:663, 1991.

33. Collins R and others: Blood pressure, stroke, and coronary heart disease. II. Short term reductions in blood pressure: overview of randomized drug trials in their epidemiological context, *Lancet* 335:827, 1990.

34. MacMahon S and others: Blood pressure, stroke, and coronary heart disease. I. Prolonged differences in blood pressure: prospective observational studies corrected for the regression dilution bias, *Lancet* 335:765, 1990.

35. SHEP Cooperative Research Group: Prevention of stroke by antihypertensive drug treatment in older persons with isolated systolic hypertension, *JAMA* 265:3255, 1991.

36. Dahlof B and others: Morbidity and mortality in the Swedish trial in old patients with hypertension (STOP-hypertension), *Lancet* 338:1281, 1991.

37. MRC Working Party: Medical research council trial of treatment of hypertension in older adults: principal results, *Br Med J* 304:405, 1992.

38. Schaefer E and others: Genetics and metabolism of lipoproteins, *Clin Chem* 34:89, 1988.

39. Mannihen V and others: Lipid alterations and decline in the incidence of coronary heart disease in the Helsinki Heart Study, *JAMA* 260:641, 1988.

40. Martin MJ and others: Serum cholesterol, blood pressure, and mortality: implications from a cohort of 361,662 men, *Lancet* 2:933, 1986.

41. Stamler J and others: Is the relationship between serum cholesterol and risk of death from CHD continuous and graded? *JAMA* 356:2823, 1988.

42. Lipid Research Clinics Program: The Lipid Research Clinics Coronary Primary Prevention Trial results. I. Reduction in the incidence of coronary heart disease, *JAMA* 251:351, 1984.

43. Frick MH and others: Helsinki Heart Study: primary-prevention trial with gemfibrozil in middle-aged men with dyslipidemia, *N Engl J Med* 317:1237, 1987.

44. Mannimen V and others: Lipid alterations and decline in coronary heart disease in the Helsinki Heart Study, *JAMA* 260:641, 1988.

45. Canover PL and others: Fifteen years mortality in Coronary Drug Project patients: long term benefits with niacin, *Am Cardiol* 8:1245, 1986.

46. Goodman D and others: Expert Panel on Detection, Evaluation, and Treatment of High Blood Cholesterol in Adults, NIH publication No 88-2925, 1988.

47. Bush T and others: Cholesterol, lipoproteins, coronary heart disease in women, *Clin Chem* 34:B60, 1988.

48. Castelli W: Cardiovascular disease in women, *Am J Obstet Gynecol* 1553, 1988.

49. Perlman J and others: Cardiovascular risk factors, premature heart disease, and all cause mortality in a cohort of northern California women, *Am J Obstet Gynecol* 1658, 1988.

50. Newman WP and others: Relation of serum lipoprotein levels and systolic blood pressure to early atherosclerosis: the Bogalusa Heart Study, *N Engl J Med* 314:138, 1986.

51. Weidman W and others: Diagnosis and treatment of primary hyperlipidemia in childhood, *Circulation* 74:1181A, 1986.

52. Davidson D and others: School-based blood cholesterol screening, *J Pediatr Health Care* 3:3, 1989.

53. McCabe E: Monitoring the fat and cholesterol intake of children and adolescents, *J Pediatr Health Care* 7:61, 1993.

54. Expert Panel on Detection, Evaluation, and Treatment of High Blood Cholesterol in Adults: Summary of the second report of the National Cholesterol Education Panel (NCEP) expert panel on detection, evaluation, and treatment of high blood cholesterol in adults (adult treatment panel), *JAMA* 269:3009, 1993.

55. Sempos CT and others: Prevalence of high blood cholesterol among US adults: an update based on guidelines from the second report of the National Cholesterol Education Program Adult Treatment Panel, *JAMA* 269:3009, 1993.

56. Blum C, Levy R: Current therapy for hypercholesterolemia, *JAMA* 261:3582, 1989.

57. Ehrich B, Emmons KM: Addressing the needs of smokers in the 1990s, *Behav Therapist* 17(6):119, 1994.

58. Lakierm JR: Smoking and cardiovascular disease, *Am J Med* 93:88, 1992.

59. Kannel WB, Higgins M: Smoking and hypertension as predictors of cardiovascular risk in population studies, *J Hypertens* 8(suppl):93, 1990.

60. Tverdal A and others: Mortality in relation to smoking history: 13 year follow up of 68,000 Norwegian men and women 35-49 years, *J Clin Epidemiol* 46:475, 1993.

61. LaCroix AZ, Omenn GS: Older adults and smoking, *Clin Geriatr Med* 8:69, 1992.

62. Benowitz N: Pharmacologic aspects of cigarette smoking and nicotine addiction, *N Engl J Med* 319:1328, 1988.

63. Quillen JE and others: Acute effect of cigarette smoking on the coronary circulation: constriction of epicardial and resistance vessels, *J Am Coll Cardiol* 22:642, 1993.

64. Felts JD and others: Effects of cigarette smoking and nicotine on platelets and experimental coronary artery thrombosis, *Adv Exp Med Biol* 273:339, 1990.

65. Thompson R and others: Cigarette smoking, polyunsaturated fats, and coronary heart disease, *Ann N Y Acad Sci* 686:130, 1993.

66. Sugiishi M, Takatsu F: Cigarette smoking is a major risk factor for coronary spasm, *Circulation* 87:76, 1993.

67. Joseph A, Byrd JR: Smoking cessation in practice, *Primary Care* 16:83, 1989.

68. Schwartz J: Review and evaluation of smoking cessation methods: the US and Canada, 1978-1985. US Department of Health and Human Services. Public Health Service, National Institute of Health, NIH Publication No 87-2940, April 1987.

69. Godenick M: A review of available smoking cessation methods, 1989. I. *Maryland Med J* 38:277, 1989.

70. Godenick M: A review of available smoking cessation methods, 1989. II. *Maryland Med J* 38:377, 1989.

71. Glassman AH and others: Heavy smokers, smoking cessation, and clonidine: results of a double blind randomized trial, *JAMA* 259:2863, 1988.

72. Buchkremer G and others: Combination of behavioral smoking cessation with transdermal nicotine substitution, *Addict Behav* 14:229, 1989.

73. CDC: Public health focus: physical activity and the prevention of coronary heart disease, *MMWR* 43:669, 1993.

74. Morris JN and others: Coronary heart disease and physical activity of work, *Lancet* 2:1053, 1953.

75. Morris JN and others: Incidence and prediction of ischaemic heart disease in London busmen, *Lancet* 2:552, 1966.

76. Morris JN: *Uses of epidemiology*, New York, 1975, Churchill Livingstone.

77. Brunner D and others: Physical activity at work and the incidence of myocardial infarction, angina pectoris and death due to ischemic heart disease: an epidemiological study in Israeli collective statements (kibbutzim), *J Chronic Dis* 27:217, 1974.

78. Paffenbarger RS, Hale WF: Work-activity and coronary heart disease mortality, *N Engl J Med* 292:545, 1975.

79. Paffenbarger RS and others: Work-energy level, personal characteristics, and fatal heart attack: a birth cohort effect, *Am J Epidemiol* 105:200, 1977.

80. Kannel WB, Sorlie P: Some health benefits of physical activity: the Framingham study, *Arch Intern Med* 139:857, 1979.

81. Paffenbarger R and others: Physical activity as an index of heart attack risk in college alumni, *Am J Epidemiol* 108:161, 1978.
82. Paffenbarger RS and others: A natural history of athleticism and cardiovascular health, *JAMA* 252:491, 1984.
83. Paffenbarger RS and others: Physical activity, all-cause mortality, and longevity of college alumni, *N Engl J Med* 314:605, 1986.
84. Paffenbarger RS and others: The association of changes in physical-activity level and other lifestyle characteristics with mortality among men, *N Engl J Med* 328:538, 1993.
85. Wood PD and others: Increased exercise level and plasma lipoprotein concentrations: a one-year, randomized, controlled study in sedentary, middle-aged men, *Metabolism* 32:31, 1983.
86. Wood PD: Impact of experimental manipulation of energy intake and expenditure on body composition, *Crit Rev Food Sci Nutr* 33:369, 1993.
87. Lavie CJ and Milani RV: Factors predicting improvements in lipid values following cardiac rehabilitation and exercise training, *Arch Intern Med* 153:982, 1993.
88. McArdle WD and others: *Exercise physiology*, Philadelphia, 1991, Lea & Febiger.
89. Tipton CM: Exercise, training, and hypertension: an update, *Exercise Sport Sci Rev* 19:447, 1991.
90. Young DR and others: Associations between changes in physical activity and risk factors for coronary heart disease in a community-based sample of men and women: the Stanford Five-City Project, *Am J Epidemiol* 138:205, 1993.
91. American College of Sports Medicine: Guidelines for exercise-testing and prescription, Philadelphia, 1991, Lea & Febiger.
92. Gordon NF and others: Life style exercise: a new strategy to promote physical activity for adults, *J Cardiopulmonary Rehabil* 13:161, 1993.
93. Barrett-Connor EL and others: Why is diabetes mellitus a stronger risk factor for fatal ischemic heart disease in women than in men? The Rancho Bernardo study, *JAMA* 265:627, 1991.
94. Liao Y and others: Sex differences in the impact of coexistent diabetes on survival in patients with coronary heart disease, *Diabetes Care* 16:708, 1993.
95. Friedman M and Rosenman RH: Association of specific overt behavior pattern with blood and cardiovascular findings, *JAMA* 169:1286, 1959.
96. Williams B and others: Type A behavior, hostility, and coronary atherosclerosis, *Psychomatic Med* 42:539, 1980.
97. Shekelle RB and others: The MRFIT behavior pattern study. II. Type A behavior and incidence of coronary heart disease, *Am J Epidemiol* 122:559, 1985.
98. Ragland DR, Brand RJ: Type A behavior and mortality from coronary heart disease, *N Engl J Med* 318:65, 1988.
99. Maruta T and others: Keeping hostility in perspective: coronary heart disease and the hostility scale on the Minnesota Multiphasic Personality Inventory, *Mayo Clin Proc* 68:109, 1993.
100. Williams RB and others: Biobehavioral bases of coronary prone behavior in middle-aged men. I. Evidence for chronic SNS activation in Type As, *Psychosomatic Med* 53:517, 1991.
101. Garrity TF and others: The association between Type A behavior and change in coronary risk factors among young adults, *Am J Public Health* 80:1354, 1990.
102. Blascovitch J, Katkin ES, editors: *Cardiovascular reactivity to psychological stress and disease,* Washington, DC, 1993, American Psychological Association.
103. Weiner H: Stressful experience and cardiorespiratory disorders, *Circulation* II:2, 1991.
104. Eliot RS: Stress and the heart, *Postgrad Med* 92:237, 1992.
105. Markowe HLJ and others: Fibrinogen: a possible link between social class and coronary heart disease, *Br Med J* 291:1312, 1985.
106. Grignani G and others: Platelet activation by emotional stress in patients with coronary artery disease, *Circulation* 83:II-128, 1991.
107. Cotton DHG: Stress management: an integrated approach to therapy, New York, 1990, Brunner/Mazel.
108. Hubert HB and others: Obesity as an independent risk factor for cardiovascular disease: a 26-year follow-up of participants in the Framingham Heart Study, *Circulation* 67:968, 1983.
109. Manson JE and others: A prospective study of obesity and risk of coronary heart disease in women, *N Engl J Med* 322:882, 1990.
110. Lapidus L and others: Distribution of adipose tissue and risk of cardiovascular disease and death: a 12 year follow up of participants in the population study of women in Gothenburg, Sweden, *Br Med J* 289:1257, 1984.
111. Folsom AR and others: Body fat distribution and 5-year risk of death in older women, *JAMA* 269:483, 1993.
112. Kris-Etherton PM, Krummel D: Role of nutrition in the prevention and treatment of coronary heart disease in women, *J Am Diet Assoc* 93:987, 1993.
113. Puccio EM and others: Clustering to atherogenic behaviors in coffee drinkers, *Am J Public Health* 80:1310, 1990.
114. Grobbee DE and others: Coffee, caffeine, and cardiovascular disease in men, *N Engl J Med* 323:1026, 1990.
115. Klatsky AL and others: Coffee use prior to myocardial infarction restudied: heavier intake may increase the risk, *Am J Epidemiol* 132:479, 1990.
116. Tverdal A and others: Coffee consumption and death from coronary heart disease in middle aged Norwegian men and women, *Br Med J* 300:566, 1990.
117. Klatsky AL and others: Alcohol and mortality, *Ann Intern Med* 117:646, 1992.
118. Jackson R and others: Alcohol consumption and risk of coronary heart disease, *Br Med J* 303:211, 1991.
119. Razay G and others: Alcohol consumption and its relationship to cardiovascular risk factors in British women, *Br Med J* 304:80, 1992.
120. Little JA: Coronary prevention and regression: studies updated, *Can J Cardiol* 4(A):11A, 1988.
121. Mannimen V and others: Lipid alterations and decline of coronary heart disease in the Helsinki Heart Study, *JAMA* 260:641, 1988.
122. Boreham C and others: Coronary risk factors in schoolchildren, *Arch Dis Child* 68:182, 1993.
123. Berenson GS and others: Cardiovascular risk factors in children and early prevention of heart disease, *Clin Chem* 34:B115, 1988.
124. Glynn TJ: Essential elements of school-based smoking prevention programs, *J Sch Health* 59:181, 1989.
125. Griffin GA and others: Tobacco-free schools in Minnesota, *J Sch Health* 58:236, 1988.
126. Turn-of-century high school class may turn tide against tobacco use, *JAMA* 260:13, 1988.
127. Newman WP and others: Relation of serum lipoprotein levels and systolic blood pressure to early atherosclerosis: the Bogalusa Heart Study, *N Engl J Med* 314:138, 1986.
128. Arbeit ML and others: The heart smart cardiovascular school health promotion: behavior correlates of risk factor change, *Prev Med* 21:18, 1992.
129. Kelder SH and others: Community-wide youth exercise promotion: long-term outcomes of the Minnesota heart health program and the class of 1989 study, *J Sch Health* 63:218, 1993.
130. Fielding JE, Piserchia PV: Frequency of worksite promotion activities, *Am J Public Health* 79:16, 1989.
131. American Heart Association of Metropolitan Chicago: *Heart at work,* Chicago, 1993, The Association.
132. Baun S and others: Health promotion for educators: impact on absenteeism, *Prev Med* 15:166, 1986.

133. Sciacca J and others: The impact of participation in health promotion on medical costs: a reconsideration of the Blue Cross and Blue Shield of Indiana study, *Am J Health Promotion* 7:374, 1993.

134. Bertera RL: The effects of workplace health promotion on absenteeism and employment costs in a large industrial population, *Am J Public Health* 80:1101, 1990.

135. Glasgow RE and others: Implementing a year long, work-site based incentive program for smoking cessation, *Am J Health Promotion* 5:192, 1991.

136. Farquhar JW and others: *The Stanford Five-City Project: an overview*. In Matarazzo JD and others, editors: *Behavioral health: a handbook of health enhancement and disease prevention*, New York, 1984, Wiley & Sons.

137. Young DR and others: Associations between changes in physical activity and risk factors for coronary heart disease in a community-based sample of men and women: the Stanford Five City Project, *Am J Epidemiol* 138:205, 1993.

138. Winkleby MA and others: Trends in cardiovascular disease risk factors by educational level: the Stanford Five City Project, *Prev Med* 21:592, 1992.

139. Fortmann SP and others: Changes in adult cigarette smoking prevalence after 5 years of community health education: the Stanford Five City Project, *Am J Epidemiol* 137:82, 1993.

140. Winkleby MA and others: Cigarette smoking trends in adolescents and young adults: the Stanford Five City Project, *Prev Med* 22:325, 1993.

141. Taylor CB and others: Effect of long-term community health education on body mass index: the Stanford Five City Project, *Am J Epidemiol* 134:235, 1991.

142. Puska P: *Community-breed prevention of cardiovascular disease: the North Karelia Project*. In Matarazzo JD and others, editors: *Behavioral health: a handbook of health enhancement and disease prevention*, New York, 1984, Wiley & Sons.

143. Rastenyte D and others: Comparisons of trends in ischaemic heart disease between North Karelia, Finland, and Kaunas, Lithuania, from 1971 to 1987, *Br Heart J* 68:516, 1992.

144. Kittel F: *The interuniversity study on nutrition and health*. In Matarazzo JD and others, editors: *Behavioral health: a handbook of health enhancement and disease prevention*, New York, 1984, Wiley & Sons.

145. Lasater T and others: *Lay volunteer delivery of a community-based cardiovascular risk factor change program: the Pawtucker Experiment*. In Matarazzo JD and others, editors: *Behavioral health: a handbook of health enhancement and disease prevention*, New York, 1984, Wiley & Sons.

146. American Heart Association of Metropolitan Chicago: Chicago, Ill, 1989, The Association.

147. American Heart Association National Center: Dallas, 1989, The Association.

148. Flack JM, Wiist WH: Cardiovascular risk factor prevalence in African-American adult screenees for a church-based cholesterol education program: the Northeast Oklahoma City Cholesterol Education Program, *Ethn Dis* 1:78, 1991.

149. Stillman FA and others: Heart, body, and soul: a church-based smoking-cessation program for Urban African Americans, *Prev Med* 22:335, 1993.

150. McGinnis JM and others: Health progress in the United States: results of the 1990 objectives for the nation, *JAMA* 268:2545, 1992.

151. US Department of Health and Human Services: *Healthy people 2000*, US Public Health Service Pub No 91-50212, Washington DC, 1992, US Government Printing Office.

152. National High Blood Pressure Education Working Group: National high blood pressure education program working group report on primary prevention of hypertension, *Arch Intern Med* 153:186, 1993.

153. Jorde LB, Carey JC, White R: *Medical genetics*, St Louis, 1995, Mosby.

CHAPTER 8

Care of the Cardiac Patient

Linda Baas

Coronary care units (CCUs) were established in the 1960s as a direct result of the practice of grouping patients who were more ill than other patients in a defined area and the availability of two pieces of equipment: continuous electrocardiographic (ECG) monitoring devices and external defibrillators.[1] This led to the training of nurses to perform both tasks.[2] The result has been the proliferation of CCUs to the point that almost every hospital in the United States has such a patient care unit. Shortly after the advent of CCUs, other forms of specialized intensive care units (ICUs) were established. CCUs and ICUs became havens of high technology, since they were areas that had specially educated nurses and had more nurses per patient than other areas of the hospital. Over time, the percentage of CCU and ICU hospital beds has increased, whereas the overall number of inpatient beds continues to decline. A national study reported that 8.09% of all hospital beds in 1991 were designated as critical care, increased from 6.5% in 1981.[3] In general, critical care is the most expensive area of inpatient costs, consuming 15% to 20% of the hospital budget and 1% of the gross national product.[3]

CCUs were credited with a major contribution to reduced mortality associated with myocardial infarction (MI) and its complications.[2,4] The two activities most likely to positively influence mortality are the prevention and successful management of ventricular fibrillation.[5] The patients who benefit most from treatment in a CCU are those who have angina at rest (preinfarction angina), MIs in progress, extensions of MIs, life-threatening dysrhythmias, severe heart failure, or cardiogenic shock.[6]

At a time when modern technology and scientific research are expanding the ability of health professionals to diagnose and treat patients with acute MI (AMI), some investigators are questioning the necessity of admitting all patients with chest pain to the CCU when only 15% to 30% actually have diagnosed AMIs.[7-9] Clearly the CCU is generally accepted as the most appropriate place for the care of the person experiencing an AMI, but the need for more precise and prompt diagnostic criteria is evident.[10] As

CCU costs rise, an acceptable method of triage for persons with chest pain may reduce unwarranted CCU admissions and ultimately reduce health care costs. An innovative approach to this concern is the development of the "heart emergency room," a special holding area for the person with chest pain who is not demonstrating obvious ECG and clinical signs of an AMI.[11] This area of the emergency department can provide continuous ECG and ST-segment monitoring of the person in a quiet area. Cardiac enzyme levels can be ascertained at 6- to 8-hour intervals to determine whether there are changes consistent with AMI. At the end of 24 hours, if there is no sign of AMI, the person may undergo a treadmill test and/or echocardiogram. Depending on the results of these diagnostic studies, it is possible that the person may be discharged from the emergency room and have appropriate follow-up. This approach is cost effective because a CCU admission is avoided and appropriate treatment is provided in a more expeditious manner.

A second concern about the treatment of the person with an AMI is related to early intervention to reduce the amount of myocardial damage and preserve more cardiac function. This approach has led to the coordination of the services offered by many areas of the hospital as well as public education and prehospital care. Many large institutions have developed interventional cardiology programs to ensure early recognition and treatment of AMI. This begins with prehospital care protocols that may include sending cellular transtelephonic 12-lead ECGs to the emergency department or cardiologist at the receiving hospital.[12-13] The prehospital care team can obtain initial information that would enable the receiving team to expedite thrombolytic or emergent percutaneous transluminal coronary angioplasty (PTCA) treatment. Success of either treatment requires early recognition and prompt action to salvage more area of the myocardium. It is essential that the patient be promptly evaluated in the emergency department. If the patient is a candidate for thrombolysis, the drug of choice should be started while the patient is in the emergency department. An additional hour of monitoring in the emergency department may be warranted to evaluate the effectiveness of the thrombolytic agent. The patient can be transferred to the CCU if there is evidence of reperfusion of the myocardium as demonstrated by the return of ST segments to baseline, relief of pain, and reperfusion dysrhythmias. If there is no evidence of reperfusion, the patient can be transferred to the cardiac catheterization laboratory for emergent salvage PTCA. After the procedure, the patient is then admitted to the CCU. Thus efforts to improve the time to treatment must focus on public awareness of symptoms, prehospital treatment, emergency department efforts to speed diagnosis and initiate therapy, and improved coordination of hospital services.[14-15]

Scientific and technologic advances have created an increasingly complex environment for the care of the cardiac patient. In an effort to improve patient care services, new or more specialized health practitioners have been introduced into the milieu of coronary care. The use of unlicensed personnel working under the direction of the nurse is increasing, even in the CCU.[16] Many units now employ monitor and cardiovascular technicians whose primary responsibility is maintenance of the equipment used in patient care. Many of these technicians are also responsible for monitoring cardiac rhythms and initiating appropriate therapy; others often assist in holding pressure over arterial puncture sites. A variety of respiratory, physical, and occupational therapists are also involved. Dieticians and pharmacists are often employed solely for the hospital's cardiac patient population. Cardiovascular nurse clinicians and cardiovascular clinical nurse specialists are commonplace in many CCUs and have varying responsibilities related to patient care and staff development. These new responsibilities include case management and primary care as an advanced critical care nurse practitioner.[17-20] Physicians seek consultation from specialists who have advanced knowledge and skill in cardiovascular nuclear radiology, ECGs, echocardiography, electrophysiology, and arteriography. Associated with these specialists are a variety of other technicians who interact with the patient.

The proliferation of health practitioners in coronary care introduces the potential for fragmentation of patient care and loss of focus on the patient as a whole being. This concern led the NIH Consensus Conference on Critical Care to conclude that "nurses are the key element in critical care."[21] To prevent fragmentation and to promote effective, efficient, and holistic care for the cardiac patient, collaboration and cooperation are essential among all care providers. The primary physician and nurse have the responsibility to seek advice and assistance as appropriate from other health practitioners, the patient, and the family and to use these contributions as they make decisions concerning patient care. The physician and nurse together need to develop a comprehensive plan that encompasses the goals and activities of all who interact with the patient.[22-23] Furthermore, the nurse and physician can foster patient- and family-focused care, resulting in improved outcomes and patient satisfaction.[24-26]

MI is one manifestation of coronary artery disease; other manifestations include heart failure, pulmonary edema, cardiogenic shock, dysrhythmias, and sudden cardiac death. This chapter presents a comprehensive approach to planning and implementing the care of the patient exhibiting the complications of coronary artery disease; this care is based on individual needs from admission to discharge. Such an approach is important because patients are likely to be moved from one hospital area to another as their condition improves. Needs change as the patient and family adjust to the suddenness of admission to a CCU and as they plan for discharge and resumption of normal activities. Of course, recovery is not always uneventful, and the patient and family must address crises as they occur.

PRIORITIES IN ADMISSION TO THE CCU

Patients are admitted to a CCU for rapid management of existing problems, surveillance for and early management of dysrhythmias, and initial rehabilitation. At the time of admission it is important to collect baseline data for initiating therapy and for comparison at later stages of the patient's condition (Fig. 8-1).

Immediate Monitoring of Cardiac Rate and Rhythm

It is essential that electrodes be applied to the patient immediately on admission so that abnormal cardiac rhythms, which may be life-threatening, can be detected; ST segments must also be monitored. A brief explanation of the purpose of the electrodes should be given to the patient. As the patient's condition becomes stabilized, the monitoring equipment can be discussed with the patient more thoroughly. Heart rate alarms should *always* be set to alert the staff to tachydysrhythmias or bradydysrhythmias.

Establishment of Intravenous Access

At least one but preferably two intravenous catheters are inserted and secured in place as a means of administering fluids, pain medication, and emergency drugs, if they are required. A saline-flushed intravenous cannula that is capped is particularly advantageous because it minimizes the amount of fluid necessary for maintaining intravenous access; in patients with heart failure, it is important to limit fluid intake.

Relief of Pain and Anxiety

The effects of pain and anxiety may be synergistic and result in an increased myocardial oxygen demand by an already compromised heart. Therefore it is vital that pain and anxiety be promptly alleviated. The physician usually prescribes analgesics and nitrates for relief of pain, and these should be administered as needed.

*Stamp here with
patient's plate*

_____

ADMISSION NOTE

Admission status: Clinic_____ ER_____ Date _____ Time_____
Married_____ Single_____ Widowed_____ Divorced_____
Race and nationality_____ Religion _____ Age_____

Patient history

Chest pain _____ Onset_____ Duration_____ Location _____
  Radiation_____ Subjective description _____
Associated acute events:
  Loss of consciousness _____ Duration _____ Cardiac arrest _____
  Palpitations _____ GI _____ Perspiration _____ Anxiety _____
  Shortness of breath _____ Dizziness _____ Dyspnea_____
Medications taken or administered and time _____
Medical history and risk factors (check those appropriate):
  Myocardial infarction_____ Angina _____ Obesity_____
  Pacemaker_____ Heart failure _____
  Weight loss _____ Cerebrovascular accident_____ Alcohol_____
  Respiratory _____ Hypertension _____ Glaucoma _____ Diabetes _____
  Smoking _____ Prostatic hypertrophy _____ Blood transfusion _____
  Gout _____ Surgery_____ Reaction to anesthesia_____
Postcardiopulmonary resuscitation _____ Contraindications to anticoagulation _____
  Other_____

Personal information

  Height _____ Weight _____ Dentures _____ Glasses _____ Contacts _____
  Sleeping habits_____ Usual diet_____
  Food, medication, environmental allergies (especially to streptokinase) _____
  Prostheses_____ Family history_____
  Usual activity level _____ Living arrangements_____

Physical examination   Admission weight _____ Reported height _____

  General appearance _____ Mental status_____
  Vital signs: Temperature _____ Pulse _____ Respiration _____
  Blood pressure: Right _____ Left_____
  Lungs: Respiratory pattern _____ Wheezes _____ Crackles _____
  Cardiovascular: Heart sounds_____ Quality _____ Rhythm _____
    Lifts_____ Heaves_____ Thrills_____ Murmur _____ Rub _____
    Gallop_____
  Pulses (all extremities) _____ Neck Veins _____ Abdomen_____
  Skin: Color _____ Temperature _____ Cyanosis _____ Edema _____
  Clubbing _____ Ecchymosis lesions _____ Other _____

                              Signature _____

Insert ECG strip here.

Fig. 8-1   Sample form for admission note to the CCU.

Morphine sulfate is often used to alleviate pain and anxiety but may be contraindicated if second-degree atrioventricular (AV) block or sinus bradycardia is present. If morphine sulfate is given and the degree of AV block or sinus bradycardia worsens, atropine may be administered to counteract its effects. After morphine is given, blood pressure, heart rate, and respiratory rate must be carefully monitored for adverse effects. Brief explanations about activities and equipment may assist in relieving patient anxiety. A mild sedative such as diazepam may be prescribed to reduce anxiety and stress. Opiates and sedatives, however, should be given cautiously, if at all, to confused and restless patients suffering from shock or heart failure. Family visits may mitigate against stress and anxiety. However, visits may increase the patient's stress level, which increases myocardial oxygen demand. Visits should be carefully monitored for these effects. A booklet about the CCU that is tailored to the individual is helpful to families in understanding what is being done and why (Fig. 8-2).

Supplemental Oxygen

Even in patients with uncomplicated MI, hypoxemia may be present and necessitate the use of oxygen. Most often a binasal cannula administering 1 to 2 L/min is sufficient. Application of a lubricant or emollient to the nares helps prevent irritation and maintain skin integrity. Oxygen saturation monitoring is often sufficient to assess for hypoxemia if the condition warrants; a measurement of arterial blood gas levels 30 minutes after initiating oxygen therapy provides a baseline for arterial oxygenation.[27] Arterial blood gas levels are measured as necessary to guide oxygen administration and maintain acid-base balance. Caution should be taken when performing an arterial stick on a patient receiving thrombolytic or anticoagulant agents. An arterial cannula should be inserted if frequent measurements of blood gas levels are needed.

Decrease in Myocardial Oxygen Consumption

Myocardial oxygen consumption is determined by heart rate, preload, afterload, and contractility. An increase in any one of these factors will increase myocardial oxygen demand. Although it is difficult to precisely determine myocardial oxygen demand, it can easily be estimated by calculating the rate-pressure product (RPP). The following formula is used for the following calculation:[28]

$$RPP = \frac{HR \times SBP}{100}$$

where *HR* is heart rate and *SBP* is systolic blood pressure. Any nursing action of medical treatment that decreases heart rate or systolic blood pressure will reduce the RPP, which reflects the reduction in myocardial oxygen demand.

Recovery of the myocardium after an ischemic episode requires that the workload and subsequent oxygen demand of the heart be reduced. This is accomplished generally through bedrest, assistance with activities of daily living, and stress reduction. Although complete bedrest for several weeks was once thought to be necessary for the healing of the MI, current regimens are less restrictive. The concept of metabolic equivalents (METs) is frequently used to determine appropriate activity after MI. A MET is a unit of measurement for oxygen uptake, with 1 MET representing an oxygen uptake of 3.5 ml/kg of body weight per minute. Sitting quietly in a chair requires 1 MET, whereas slow walking requires 3 METs. In the CCU, activities that require 1.5 to 2 METs are generally permitted. Other protocols for increasing activity may include gradually increasing exercise to a level that raises the heart rate 20 beats per minute or less above resting heart rate. The systolic blood pressure also increases with exercise, and activity should be adjusted so that the systolic blood pressure does not increase by more than 30 mm Hg above resting pressure. Finally, the nurse plays a key role in reducing the patient's stress and anxiety. Identifying the patient's needs and focusing on providing personalized care is at great importance in reducing myocardial oxygen consumption.

Completion of Database

As soon as possible after admission, information necessary to complete the database should be obtained. The patient history and physical examination should be completed (see Chapter 2), paying particular attention to the following:

A. Patient history
B. Physical examination
  1. Inspection of skin for color, diaphoresis, and other abnormalities.
  2. Palpation of chest area for unusual movements, excursion, cardiac enlargement, apical impulse, and other signs.
  3. Percussion of chest for areas of dullness and of liver for edge and size. Cardiac borders are seldom defined by percussion.
  4. Auscultation of blood pressure, carotid arteries (bruit), apical heart rate, heart sounds, pericardial friction rub, gallops, and murmurs. The murmur of papillary muscle dysfunction may occur in the acute phase of MI as a result of ischemia, infarction of the papillary muscle, or both. The murmur of mitral regurgitation results when the injured papillary muscle fails to contract properly, allowing blood to regurgitate into the left atrium during systole. The murmur is often transient but may be permanent if the papillary muscle does not heal completely. A ventricular septal defect murmur may also occur during the first 10 days after infarction and is a very loud, grade 4 or 5 systolic murmur. There is usually an accompanying systolic thrill, and the murmur is best heard along the lower left sternal border. The ap-

CORONARY CARE UNIT INFORMATION

While you, a family member, or friend are in the CCU, you may hear terms such as *coronary, electrocardiogram (ECG)*, or *congestive heart failure* and be uncertain as to what they mean about the patient's condition. This may be a time when you have a lot of questions and anxieties.

The CCU staff understands this and has prepared this information sheet to help you understand what goes on in a CCU. If you want to know more about heart disease, there is literature available in our unit on request. Also we will be glad to try to answer any questions you may have.

Patient care

A CCU is for the "intensive" care of cardiac patients. This CCU has 16 beds and is attended 24 hours a day by registered nurses who are specially trained to read ECGs and recognize any early signs of complications. From the time a patient arrives in the unit until he or she is transferred to a room, there is a nurse near the bedside to render the care needed.

Because of the serious nature of heart disease, a patient is placed in the CCU during the critical phase of the heart's condition and remains there until this critical phase is over, usually 1 to 5 days. Progress is followed continuously with special monitoring equipment at each bedside and at the nurses' station to record the patient's ECGs, which indicate the heart rhythms.

While in the CCU, patients need only their necessary personal belongings. Shaving equipment (razor with nurse's approval), cosmetics, toilet articles, eyeglasses, and small change may be kept in the bedside drawer. Male patients may wear pajama bottoms. Female patients do not need their night gowns, since it is preferred that a hospital gown be worn. Reading materials and a few personal items are allowed. A television and radio are provided in each room. Large floral arrangements and suitcases are not allowed due to limited space.

When the physician approves transfer out of the CCU, the patient is usually taken to a room on another floor. Transferring patients is usually done during the day, but if an emergency situation arises and a bed is needed in the unit during the night, a patient may have to be moved then.

Visiting is permitted from 10 AM to 8 PM for members of the patient's immediate family or significant others. Because of the nature of the patient's illness, no more than two visitors should be in the patient's room at one time.

If emergency situations exist, visitation may be refused.

Phone

There is a pay phone available in the lobby. Direct calls to the unit are permitted so that you can get an update on your loved one's condition. Families may leave their phone numbers at the desk in the CCU. A phone is available so patients can make calls. If you want to telephone your loved one you may call the unit at (xxx-xxxx) and we will transfer your call unless the patient is resting.

Chaplain

This service is available on request at any time by contacting a CCU nurse or the chaplain's office.

Waiting rooms

The waiting room is open only until 8:30 PM. Those who wish to stay during the night must use the waiting room in the emergency department or arrange for a room in the family visitor wing.

If you have questions, please contact a CCU nurse.

The CCU Staff

Fig. 8-2 Sample fact sheet given to families of patients in the CCU.

pearance of this murmur is an ominous event prognostically, sudden in onset, and frequently accompanied by profound cardiogenic shock. It is also important to auscultate the lungs for crackles, rhonchi, wheezes, and increased or decreased breath sounds. Note the rate, character, and depth of respirations. These data are necessary to evaluate the presence or absence of congestive heart failure and are useful for comparison if this is a consideration at a later date.

C. Supportive data

1. Serum cardiac isoenzyme levels should be measured initially and then every 4 to 8 hours for 24 hours to document an abnormal increase in serum levels. If the patient has a sudden exacerbation of pain with associated ECG changes, cardiac enzyme level measurements may be indicated to assist in determining whether the previous infarction has continued.

2. Arterial blood gas levels may be measured initially and then as needed (depending on the patient's condition) to determine the adequacy of oxygenation and acid-base balance. Pulse oximetry may provide adequate monitoring for the patient without pulmonary disease.

3. Fluid and electrolyte balance should be monitored. It is imperative that fluid intake and output be accurately measured. Equally important is that an accurate daily weight of the patient be taken at admission and at the same time each day on the same scale. Many ICU beds now have built-in scales for patient comfort. Weight measurement can help determine the minimum weight gain that occurs in the early stages of heart failure or when other indicators, such as the chest x-ray film, are still normal. Personnel must be reminded to measure rather than to estimate intake, just as all output is measured. It should also be remembered that fluids, such as tube feedings, fluids used to flush the Swan-Ganz catheter and arterial lines, and fluids from any other sources, must be included in the total fluid intake measurement. Output should include bleeding and drainage from any site, as well as urine and stool. The patient's state of hydration may also be evaluated by the skin tone.

4. Edema may be a late sign of congestive failure and should be added to the database already gathered on the fluid balance of the patient. The extent of peripheral edema should be measured by palpation once it appears, and comparative evaluations should be performed frequently to determine changes in edema noted in the periphery. Edema in a cardiac patient on bedrest is frequently noted in dependent areas such as the sacrum or genitalia.

5. The dietary regimen, if different from the patient's usual diet, should be explained to the patient and family. Cardiac patients are usually placed on a low-sodium, low-fat, low-cholesterol diet. In some cardiac patients, sodium restriction may be unnecessary or impractical; these patients are given food with the usual sodium content. A soft diet may be prescribed with frequent, small feedings, although some physicians prefer liquids on the first day. Because metabolic demands increase after ingestion of food, the quantity of food at each serving should be kept small. Studies show that hot and cold liquids are not detrimental, so their exclusion from diets is unnecessary. Decaffeinated coffee and tea are permitted. The relationship between caffeine intake and heart problems has not been clearly established. There is no relationship between caffeine intake and MI, but there is a relationship between caffeine intake and dysrhythmias in the ischemic heart.

6. A 12-lead ECG (see Chapter 4) should be performed initially in the emergency room or in the CCU. A copy should be maintained on the patient's chart for comparison with later tracings, which are often performed daily for 3 days and with every exacerbation of chest pain and/or developing dysrhythmias. Personnel in the CCU should be adept at obtaining and interpreting the 12-lead ECG in a patient with MI.

Medical and nursing diagnoses are derived from the compiled data and serve as the basis for planning medical and nursing therapies.

EQUIPMENT
Monitoring System

In the CCU the first equipment with which the patient is likely to come in contact is the monitoring system. For a patient who has suffered an MI or who has had a pacemaker implanted, careful monitoring of cardiac performance is essential. The cardiac monitor simplifies such care by continuously displaying the cardiac rhythm, oxygen percent saturation, invasive and noninvasive blood pressure, and other parameters not readily followed by other means. Because most dysrhythmias occur during the first 48 to 72 hours after infarction and 80% to 90% of patients who have MIs experience dysrhythmias, constant surveillance is vital.

Components

The cardiac monitor is an instrument that displays electrical activity during the cardiac cycle as a wave pattern across a screen. An example of the basic components of cardiac monitors is shown in Fig. 8-3.

Oscilloscope

The screen on which the patient's ECG pattern appears is an oscilloscope.

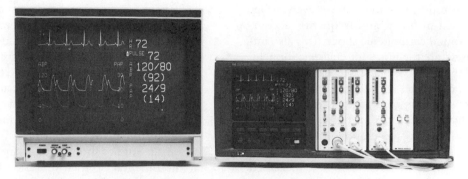

Fig. 8-3 Monitoring system shows oscilloscope, digital and numerical display, and wave forms. (Reprinted with permission of Hewlett-Packard Co, Palo Alto, Calif.)

Digital display

An electronic mechanism averages the number of ventricular complexes per minute, and this rate is shown on the rate scale indicator. Also, each QRS complex is indicated by an audible beep and flashing light. If the pulse rate can be relayed to a console at the nursing station, the bedside monitor beep should be silenced so that the patient does not hear it.

Rate display and alarm limits

Integrated with the alarm system is the rate display, which signals if the heart rate goes above or below predetermined limits. The limits vary according to the routine of a particular unit, based on the sensitivity of the electrodes and monitoring system. For example, the alarm may be triggered to sound at 25 beats above or below an individual's average heart rate, or it may be set to sound automatically at the high-low values of 150 beats/min and 50 beats/min.

Alarm control system

When the heart rate falls below or rises above the preset levels, audio and visual alarms alert the staff. Each time an alarm is triggered, the staff must observe the patient and make a prompt decision regarding the cardiac rhythm.

When the CCU personnel depend on an alarm system for warning, the rate limit indicators and alarm system must be checked regularly—not only for accuracy but also to be sure that the system is operative. In some situations, the limit settings are temporarily turned off in the patient's room. At these times, personnel must depend on visual observation of the oscilloscope and the related clinical picture. For instance, the limit settings are turned off to prevent false alarms from electric interference resulting from the use of a high-power machine (for example, a direct write-out ECG machine or a portable x-ray machine). False alarms may also be triggered by manipulation of the chest electrodes when repositioning them to other sites on the chest or when bathing the patient. The patient's welfare is endangered if the alarm limit settings remain off; therefore it is essential to check these settings periodically. Many monitoring systems now have an alarm suspension option that turns the alarm off for 3 minutes and then reinstates the same alarm parameters. When available, this option should be used. When such an alarm system is not available, personnel must develop another means of being alerted to changes in rhythm on the monitor oscilloscope. Only through an adequate method of observation can significant changes be identified and further rhythm disturbances prevented.

Most monitoring systems now have different levels of alarms based on a program that recognizes some dysrhythmias. The most serious alarm level alerts staff to rate limit changes, asystole, ventricular fibrillation, or tachycardia. The second level of alarm recognizes a change in rhythm such as heart block and frequent ectopy or atrial fibrillation. The lowest level of alarm advises the staff at occasional ectopy. These systems allow staff to modify the alarm system based on the patient's usual rhythm. Also, the computer learns the appearance of the patient's usual rhythm and subsequently sounds an alarm when the pattern deviates from the initial ECG tracing.

Sweep speed

The rate at which the electronic beam sweeps across the screen can be controlled, and the sweep can be set at trace speeds of 25 mm/sec (the beam sweeps across a standard screen in 6 seconds) or 50 mm/sec (the 3-second sweep position). The 6-second position is generally used for routine monitoring. The 3-second position often provides for better interpretation of the rhythm or the pressure waveform by spreading the complexes.

Filter

The filter reduces extraneous muscular artifacts. However, when a 12-lead ECG is recorded from the monitor, the filter must be switched off, since it may distort the ST segment.

Central console

Individual bedside monitors in a CCU are connected to a central console at the nursing station to permit continuous observation of the ECG patterns from all the monitors.

Additional components

Complementary parts can be added as necessary to the basic monitoring system. For example, a direct write-out ECG machine can be located in the central station; this is triggered to record the cardiac rhythm automatically during alarm situations or on demand. Such recordings may be used to demonstrate the patient's response to antidysrhythmic therapy.

Some monitor systems have memory tapes that store a predetermined duration of the patient's ECG, which can then be recalled at will. This allows a printout of the cardiac rhythm recorded over the previous 60 seconds. At the time of alarm, some monitors print out memory storage and then the current rhythm from the time of trigger. Memory mechanisms, however, erase after a period of time; therefore at the moment of an alarm, personnel must decide whether to record the stored memory information or the current rhythm. Use of 24-hour tape monitoring simplifies this problem. The monitoring system may also include multichannel recorders to monitor central venous and pulmonary artery (PA) pressures, pulse oximetry, temperature, respirations, invasive and noninvasive arterial pressures, and other physiologic parameters. In some centers, this information can be stored in and retrieved from a computer. Trends at these parameters can be plotted and displayed so that gradual or abrupt changes can be analyzed. Many new monitoring systems use computer analysis for dysrhythmia interpretation, pacemaker recognition, and ST-segment monitoring. Also, the monitor may contain a calculator programmed to compute parameters such as pulmonary and systemic vascular resistance and calculate drip rates for intravenous infusions.

Electrodes

Topical electrode patches are commonly used for patient monitoring. The following steps are involved in preparing the skin and in applying the electrodes:

1. At the sites chosen for electrode placement, clean the skin thoroughly with alcohol to remove all residues. If necessary, shave the hair at these sites.
2. The skin of some patients may require abrasion at the electrode sites to obtain an adequate ECG signal. If this is the situation, abrade each site by rubbing the area with a gauze pad.
3. Apply adhesive electrode pads and press them against the skin at the prepared sites. For extra adhesion, apply a strip of nonallergenic tape over electrodes.

Placement of electrodes

The most commonly used leads for cardiac monitoring are II, V_1, or MCL_1 (modified chest lead). The lead that best displays the QRS complexes and P waves (and pacing stimuli if pacing is used) is used for monitoring.

A positive electrode, a negative electrode, and a ground electrode are required to record one bipolar lead. The location for these electrodes determines the lead recorded by the monitor. For example, a modification of lead V_1 (MCL_1) is recorded by placing the negative electrode just under the outer quarter of the left shoulder and the ground electrode beneath the right clavicle, with the positive electrode being placed at the fourth right intercostal space at the right sternal border (the usual V_1 position).

Many of the computerized monitoring systems use lead II for interpretation. The negative electrode is placed just under the outer quarter of the right shoulder, and the ground electrode is positioned in the left lower abdominal area (left leg position).

To prevent interference with the physical examination, the chest electrodes should be placed away from the area near the apex of the heart. Placement of the electrodes on the chest reduces motion and muscle artifacts and allows the patient more freedom of movement than limb-lead monitoring. Electrodes should be repositioned daily to prevent local skin irritation caused by prolonged contact of the hypertonic electrode paste with one point of the skin surface.

The modified V_1 chest lead has the added advantage over the other chest leads (often haphazardly positioned on the chest) of giving a maximal amount of information about rhythm disturbances and conduction. The MCL_1 provides an easily recognized recording of the sequence of ventricular activation and therefore furnishes maximum information to discriminate between right and left bundle branch block and between premature ventricular contractions and aberrant supraventricular complexes (see Chapter 4). Because many monitors display two or more leads on the oscilloscope, the nurse can select the two best leads to provide information based on knowledge of the patient's condition and previous ECGs.

The electrode wires from the patient are attached to a connector unit pinned to the patient's gown. From this unit a cable leads to the monitor where the electrode wires are connected to their respective terminals: positive wire to positive terminal, negative wire to negative terminal, and ground wire to ground terminal. In certain machines the electrode terminals are specifically labeled. In other machines, it is necessary to be familiar with the terminal connections. Incorrect matching of electrodes and terminals will change the lead that is to be monitored.

Interference with Monitoring

External voltage and patient movements generally are responsible for interference in a properly operating monitoring system. External voltage interference (alternating 60-cycle current) appears on the screen as a smooth thickening of the baseline resulting from the 60 tiny peaks/sec (Fig. 8-4, *A*). Inadequate grounding of the monitor and other equipment or improper electrode placement and connection may produce this type of interference.

Because the cardiac monitor registers muscle potential, sudden voluntary or involuntary movement by the patient can cause interference. For example, coughing or turning over in bed may precipitate a wandering baseline and erratic or irregular fluctuations on the oscilloscope (Fig. 8-4, *B*). Placing the electrodes in areas of limited muscular activity reduces this problem.

In the tense, nervous, or cold patient, the monitor may display a harsh, jagged, uneven oscillation about the baseline. Another patient activity that can simulate ventricular fibrillation is brushing the teeth. Personnel must be careful not to interpret these baseline undulations as signifying fibrillatory waves.

Electric Hazards

The electric equipment used in a CCU increases the potential of electric shock hazard for the patient and equipment operator. Therefore it is important that CCU personnel have a basic understanding of the principles of current flow, current source, and grounding.

When ground connections of equipment are not at the same potential (zero volts or a few millivolts above zero), leakage current may flow between the source and its ground. Current flows through patients if they serve as links in this circuit. Skin offers resistance to current flow and therefore protects the heart from electric shock. If the voltage is high enough or skin resistance has been lowered or eliminated, ventricular fibrillation may result. On some equipment, built-in isolation circuits isolate patients from the ground and the power line, thus preventing conductive pathways. However, an intracardiac catheter or fluid column bypasses the skin and the protection from current flow that it affords, making the patient highly vulnerable to electric shock. Alternating current power-line levels of only millionths of amperes, undetectable when applied to the skin, can induce ventricular fibrillation if contact with the myocardium is made.

Any alternating current power-line–operated device from which some of the current flows through the metal frame, case, or another exposed part may serve as a current source. It may be an electric bed with a broken or missing ground connection or a device with two-wire power cords (two-pronged plugs) such as TV sets, bed lamps, or electric fans. Patients may lie in the path of the current source and ground directly by touching the electric device, or patients may ground indirectly by making physical contact with other people who touch the defectively grounded instrument. Either situation causes patients to become conductive pathways and allows current to flow through them to the ground.

Equipment operators should be cautious when using electronic equipment near water, steam pipes, radiators, or plumbing fixtures. Such pipes and fittings are excellent

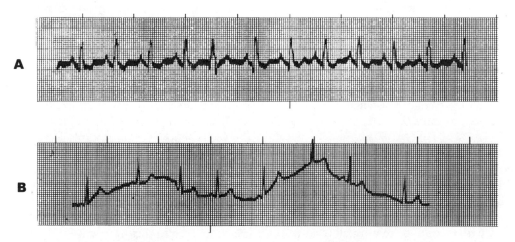

Fig. 8-4 **A,** ECG tracing that shows external voltage interference (alternating 60-cycle current) appearing as a smooth thickening of the baseline as a result of the 60 tiny peaks/sec. **B,** ECG tracing in which patient interference (for example, coughing and turning) is shown by a wandering baseline.

electric grounds. Consequently any electric device near them, including power cords, plugs, and wall receptacles, that exposes the user to live current can be extremely hazardous if the operator simultaneously contacts both the device and a grounded pipe or faucet. The operator then becomes the link between the current source and the ground that the current seeks. The resultant shock may not be fatal, but serious injury can result from the violent muscular reaction in "letting go" (Table 8-1).

Personnel may detect tingling sensations when touching or brushing against a piece of electronic equipment. The voltage necessary to produce this sensation is only one thousandth of an ampere. Under ordinary circumstances this is harmless; however, this voltage is nearly 50 times the amount necessary to produce ventricular fibrillation if current flows directly to the patient's heart.

Clearly, many considerations are necessary to ensure electric safety. Awareness of potential hazards, prompt correction of faulty equipment, and regular safety inspection checks are all needed. In 1993, the revised electrical safety standards for electromedical equipment was relaxed, raising the allowable current by 2.5 to 5 times the previously allowed current.[29] This change warrants increased caution in clinical settings. Personnel should be thoroughly briefed in the following rules for electric safety in the CCU:

A. All equipment should be grounded. This means that a pathway of least resistance is available for the currents within the machine to flow to ground.
  1. All equipment must have three-pronged plugs that connect the hospital ground to the equipment chassis.
  2. Adaptors fitting a three-prong plug into a two-slot electric outlet should not be used.
  3. Extension cords should not be used to connect electronic equipment. If extensions are necessary, only three-pronged grounding-type cords should be used.

B. Wet surfaces conduct current. Therefore hazards such as wet sheets and wet floors should be eliminated.
C. Safety inspection checks should be routine. A qualified electric technician should check all equipment for faulty or missing ground connections and hazardous voltages. (Equipment can still operate with defective ground connections.)
D. When two instruments are in use near a patient, they should be connected to the same power receptacle.
E. No one should ever plug or unplug equipment or turn on a light while any part of the body or the patient's body is in contact with water, steam pipes, radiators, or plumbing fixtures.
F. Equipment cords should not be allowed to kink, drape on pipes and plumbing, or lie on wet surfaces.
G. Tingling sensations emitted from objects such as a bed frame or an instrument case should be reported. Equipment not necessary to support the life of the patient is unplugged; this condition must be corrected immediately in equipment necessary for life support.
H. When an intracavitary lead is used, the electrode catheter is connected to the V lead of the ECG machine, since this circuit has a high electric resistance in relation to ground. Anyone or anything electrically grounded must not touch the V-lead electrode terminals.
I. Additional precautions should be taken for patients with temporary cardiac pacemakers.
  1. The electrodes at the end of the pacemaker should be well insulated. On older models a rubber glove is used to cover the exposed terminals at the junction with the external power source. Most newer models are adequately insulated.
  2. When possible, use external battery pacemakers that are isolated from the power-line sources.
  3. Personnel should wear rubber gloves when connecting or disconnecting the battery pacemaker and when adjusting electrodes at the end of the catheter.

TABLE 8-1 Effects of Electric Current

60-Cycle Current (1-Second Duration) Delivered Through Skin		60-Cycle Current (1-Second Duration) Leading to Heart	
Milliamperes	Effects	Microamperes	Effects
1	Threshold of perception; tingling	20 to 50	Ventricular fibrillation
16	"Let-go" current; muscle contraction		
50	Pain; possible fainting; mechanical injury		
100-3000	Ventricular fibrillation		
6000 or greater	Sustained myocardial depolarization followed by normal rhythm; temporary respiratory paralysis; burns		

4. Patients should use battery-operated razors rather than razors that require electricity.

The State Medical Device Act of 1990 requires health care facilities to investigate, document, and report serious events related to all medical devices, equipment, and supplies.[30]

COMPLICATIONS OF CORONARY ARTERY DISEASE

The most common complications of coronary artery disease are angina and MI. The clinical syndromes of heart failure, pulmonary edema, cardiogenic shock, dysrhythmias, and sudden cardiac death usually occur as a complication of myocardial ischemia or MI. In addition, psychologic alterations may be noted at any point during the illness.

Angina Pectoris

Angina pectoris is a syndrome characterized by chest discomfort that occurs as a result of transient myocardial ischemia. This myocardial ischemia is a result of an imbalance of myocardial oxygen supply and demand: a decreased supply, an increased demand, or both. An inadequate supply of oxygen can be caused by coronary artery obstruction, usually because of atherosclerosis. However, coronary artery spasm or coronary artery thrombosis may also cause or contribute to the obstruction. Severe anemia and hypoxia also can cause a decrease in myocardial oxygen supply. Many clinical conditions can cause an increased demand for myocardial oxygen, including tachycardia, hypertension, valvular stenosis, left ventricular hypertrophy, and hyperthyroidism, as well as pharmacologic effects.[31,32]

Various types of anginal pain occur. Exertional, or stable, angina is initiated by exertion, is predictable at a certain level of activity or the same RPP, and is associated with a fixed coronary obstruction. Variant angina produces symptoms similar to stable angina but is caused by coronary artery spasm.[31] Some patients with coronary artery spasm have normal coronary arteries;[33] however, many patients with spasm also have some degree of stenosis. Variant angina usually occurs at rest, often during the night or early morning, frequently happening at the same time each day. On ECG, ST segments are elevated during the attack and return to normal with pain relief. Variant angina may be stable, as in Prinzmetal angina, but more often it is unstable.[34]

Unstable angina, also called *crescendo angina, preinfarction angina,* or *progressive angina,* is any new onset of angina, acceleration of previously stable angina, or severe, prolonged ischemic pain at rest. Unstable angina is thought to be caused by acute changes, such as fissuring of the intracoronary plaque, thrombus formation, or spasm. These events cause transient myocardial ischemia. Unstable angina also is called *unstable myocardial ischemia,* and AMI is an extreme form of unstable ischemia.[34,35]

Although the term *angina pectoris* literally means chest pain, perhaps it should be referred to as *discomfort* because many patients may deny experiencing chest pain. Rather, they often refer to vague sensations, feelings, or aches. These unpleasant feelings have been described in a variety of ways, including a sense of pressure or burning, squeezing, heaviness, smothering, and very frequently as "indigestion." Since the discomfort of angina is usually located in the retrosternal region, patients often illustrate the nature and location of their symptoms by placing a clenched fist against their sternum. Often angina pectoris is not confined to the chest but may radiate to the neck, jaw, epigastrium, shoulders, or arms. Most often it radiates to the left shoulder and left arm. Occasionally, angina may produce discomfort in an area of radiation without affecting the retrosternal region.

Attacks of exertional angina are typically preceded by an elevation of the RPP as evidenced by changes in the blood pressure, heart rate, or both. During the attack, pulse rate and blood pressure usually increase further, presumably as a consequence of anxiety and as a physiologic response to pain. In some instances, however, blood pressure and pulse may fall dramatically as a result of vagally mediated reflexes. More important than the location is the duration of the pain and the circumstances under which it occurs. Angina pectoris lasts usually only a few minutes if the precipitating factor is relieved. Attacks are often induced by effort and occur *during* rather than after exertion. Exertion during cold weather or after meals is particularly likely to produce pain. Anxiety, smoking, stressful situations, worry, anger, hurry, and excitement are common precipitating factors. Patients have described the following situations as producing chest pain: running to catch a bus, driving in heavy traffic, having nightmares, experiencing painful stimuli, having sexual intercourse, and straining at stool.

Angina typically lasts from 1 to several minutes and usually no more than 3 to 5 minutes. It is relieved by rest, nitroglycerin, or any influence that drops arterial pressure or heart rate (RPP) and equalizes the supply of blood and nutrients with the demand.

Diagnosis

The diagnosis of angina pectoris is usually made from a characteristic history because frequently there are few abnormalities found through physical examination and the ECG may be normal at rest. It is best to allow patients to describe symptoms without using suggestive terms. Time and patience are necessary to explore the patient's lifestyle, habits, and emotions to obtain a clear picture of the pain and the extent of incapacitation.

On physical examination, the patient's blood pressure and pulse should be measured, because hypertension, tachycardia, or both can be precipitating factors. Also, signs of congestive heart failure such as rales, a third heart sound gallop, peripheral edema, and neck vein distention may be present. During episodes of angina, the patient may be di-aphoretic and restless. Heart rate, blood pressure, and res-piratory rate may be elevated but may return to normal with pain relief.[31,34]

A 12-lead ECG may show ST-segment or T-wave changes in the affected leads. These changes may be caused by transmural ischemia, such as in an AMI or coronary artery spasm. Return of the ST segment and T wave to baseline after relief of the angina indicates that coronary artery spasm was the precipitating factor.[36]

Also useful in the diagnosis of angina are stress testing, radionuclide studies, and Holter monitoring. In addition, cardiac catheterization is indicated to accurately determine the extent of coronary artery disease in patients with se-vere unstable angina. For documentation of coronary artery spasm, ergonovine maleate can be injected into the coronary artery during cardiac catheterization to induce spasm.[34,37]

Treatment

The first principle in treating angina pectoris is to min-imize the discrepancy between the demand of the heart muscle for oxygen and the ability of the coronary circula-tion to meet this demand. Accordingly, patients must learn to pace themselves so that physical activity is kept below the threshold of discomfort. Moderate exercise performed below the angina threshold should be encouraged. Tread-mill testing can determine a target heart rate for exercise that is below the ischemic threshold.[28]

Additional measures include adopting a diet designed to achieve the individual's ideal weight and the cessation of smoking. Hypertension, if present, should be treated. Smokers should be strongly encouraged to stop, using a planned strategy that includes behavioral change and ac-knowledges nicotine withdrawal symptoms[38]

Pharmacologic treatment is directed at two objectives: relief from symptoms when they occur and prevention of angina.[39-40] For the first objective, nitroglycerin taken sub-lingually is the treatment of choice. For prevention, β-adrenergic blocking agents are prescribed to slow the heart rate and attenuate the contractile response to phys-ical or emotional activity. Longer-acting nitrates such as isosorbide dinitrate (Isordil) or nitroglycerin paste (Nitrol) exert an action for 2 to 4 hours and are very effective. Re-ichek and others[41] have found that transdermal nitrogly-cerin patches did not offer 24 hours of stable antianginal protection. During sustained transdermal treatment, pa-tients develop tolerance to nitroglycerin, so antianginal ef-ficacy is diminished. An intermittent dosage schedule is recommended to avoid nitrate tolerance.

Recent reports indicate that vasodilators acting princi-pally on the arterial system (for example, hydralazine or prazosin) may attenuate the hypertensive response to exer-tion and aid in preventing angina. Calcium blocking agents (for example, nifedipine, verapamil, diltiazem) are another group of potent vasodilators for coronary and peripheral arteries that also have the ability to decrease afterload and myocardial contractility. The combination of nitrate ther-apy and calcium blockers has been extremely effective.[41] Other investigators have demonstrated improved left ven-tricular function, improved exercise tolerance, and delayed onset of chest pain with therapy consisting of nitrates, β-adrenoreceptor blockers and calcium antagonists.[40]

Other general measures for the management of angina include sedation, relief of anxiety, and supervised exercise programs designed to enhance physical condition and thereby reduce the blood pressure and heart rate response to exercise.[40,42,43]

In addition to nitrates, β blockers and calcium channel blockers, heparin and thrombolytic therapy may be con-sidered for patients with unstable angina. Angioplasty and coronary artery bypass grafting (CABG) provide relief of symptoms and prolong life in selected subgroups of pa-tients. A recent publication from the U.S. Agency for Health Care Policy and Research details clinical practice guidelines for the diagnosis and management of unstable angina endorsed by the American Heart Association, American College of Cardiology, and other professional groups.[40]

Although many persons experience angina during isch-emia, it is important to remember that myocardial ischemia can occur without symptoms. It is estimated that 3 to 4 million Americans with coronary artery disease and 50% of persons with AMIs have silent ischemia. This increases the need for continuous ST-segment monitoring after MI, af-ter an invasive intracoronary procedure, or with evidence of ischemia after an ECG.

AMI

An MI is an ischemic event that occurs over several hours and can induce ischemic injury and necrosis (cell death) in myocardial tissue (Fig. 8-5). Tissue damage oc-curs in a wavelike fashion; the center of the infarct is the area of necrosis, and this is surrounded by an area of in-jured myocardium, which in turn is surrounded by an area of ischemic tissue. The most common cause of MI is coro-nary arterial thrombosis, which is often superimposed on an already atherosclerotic vessel; another cause of MI is prolonged coronary artery spasm. The initial goals of treat-ment are to confirm the diagnosis and to preserve ischemic myocardium.

Chest pain is the presenting symptom in most patients with AMI. The pain is frequently severe, but there may be minimal or, on occasion, no discomfort. The discomfort is usually substernal and may radiate to the epigastric region, jaw, shoulders, elbows, or forearms. The pain is usually de-scribed as a heaviness, tightness, or constriction but occa-sionally as indigestion or a burning sensation. It usually persists for 30 minutes or longer, often until potent anal-gesics have been administered. In its classic presentation

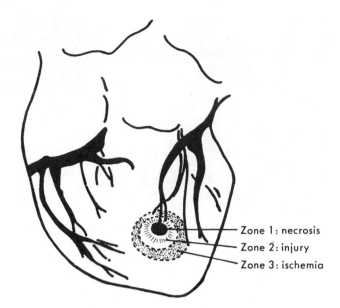

Zone 1: necrosis
Zone 2: injury
Zone 3: ischemia

Fig. 8-5   Tissue damage after myocardial infarction. *Zone 1,* Necrotic tissue; *zone 2,* injured tissue; *zone 3,* ischemic tissue.

the symptoms of MI are more severe than typical angina. On the other hand, the symptoms of infarction may be subtle, and very often, severity and duration of pain do not distinguish among prolonged angina, coronary insufficiency (prolonged ischemia), and MI.[44]

In addition to chest pain, patients with MI may experience shortness of breath, sweating, weakness or extreme fatigue, nausea, vomiting, and severe anxiety. On physical examination, they may show evidence of overactivity of the sympathetic nervous system, including tachycardia, sweating, and hypertension. Alternatively, evidence of vagal hyperactivity may predominate with bradycardia and hypotension. Many patients look surprisingly normal. Hypotension with tachycardia and peripheral cyanosis suggests a markedly reduced cardiac output and shock. In some patients, normal blood pressure is maintained, but a third heart sound gallop and pulmonary rales indicate acute left ventricular failure. Murmurs related to mitral insufficiency or a ruptured interventricular septum may develop, and a pericardial friction rub may be heard. Heart sounds are usually diminished in intensity, and particularly with anterior infarction, a paradoxical parasternal systolic lift can be felt inside the apex region.

The diagnosis of MI is initially made on the basis of the patient's history and ECG tracings and is finally confirmed with cardiac enzyme measurements. Ancillary but nonspecific findings of infarction include low-grade fever, elevation of the white blood cell count, and elevation of the erythrocyte sedimentation rate. The ECG may show typical findings of infarction or nonspecific changes of the ST segment or T wave. Rarely, if ever, are serial ECGs normal in a patient with documented infarction.

With necrosis of the heart muscle, enzymes normally confined within the myocardial cell leak out and appear in peripheral blood; serum glutamic-oxaloacetic transaminase (SGOT), lactate dehydrogenase (LDH), and creatine kinase (CK) are the enzymes measured most frequently. LDH and CK appear in more than one form and are referred to as *isoenzymes.* The isoenzymes of LDH and CK are distributed differently in different tissues so that elevations of the "heart" isoenzymes are more specific evidence of heart muscle necrosis than elevation of either the total CK or LDH level. Elevations of CK-MB and of LDH-1 (the predominant heart isoenzymes) are typically observed in MI.

Radionuclide imaging techniques used to confirm the diagnosis of MI have received considerable attention. These imaging methods include thallium-201 scintigraphy and technetium-99 pyrophosphate imaging.[45] Myocardial uptake of thallium-201 depends on blood flow; with decreased flow, an area of diminished activity is visualized. Because a single study cannot differentiate between ischemic and necrotic myocardium, serial studies are necessary, and the first thallium-201 study should be done within 6 hours after the onset of symptoms. In conjunction with other findings noted above, serial thallium-201 images can be used to diagnose an MI and to estimate the location and extent of decreased coronary perfusion and resulting necrosis. It is also used with angina to determine the extent of the ischemic area. The isotope is injected at peak exercise to look for ischemia. After the patient rests 1 to 3 hours, the heart is again imaged to look for reversal of perfusion defects that represent the area of reversible ischemia.

Thallium-201 scintigraphy with dipyridamole has been useful in identifying patients at high risk for cardiac events after MIs. Dipyridamole is a potent coronary vasodilator. When used with thallium-201, it simulates an exercise thallium-201 test.[45] This test is a useful predictor of events after MI and has high levels of sensitivity and specificity.

The radionuclide imaging test using technetium-99 pyrophosphate is regarded as a fairly sensitive technique for confirming myocardial damage. The isotope is taken up by necrotic cells 12 to 18 hours after the onset of infarction; uptake persists for 4 to 5 days and then typically decays. Even small areas of infarction can be identified by appropriate scanning equipment from the "hot spot" produced on the scintigram. For optimal results the test should be done 48 to 72 hours after the onset of infarction. The ideal candidate for this test is the person who has a history of several days of pain, since cardiac enzyme tests done at admission may have returned to normal levels.[45-46]

Because wall-motion abnormalities and wall thinning correlate with ischemia and infarction, two-dimensional echocardiography may be used to assess the ischemic heart. Systolic wall thickening is normally seen as part of the remodeling process. Systolic wall thinning is seen when the infarct involves more than 20% of the transmural thickness. Although echocardiographic wall-motion abnormalities seem to consistently overestimate infarct size, echocardiography can give a reasonable estimate of overall left ventricular function. It is also useful in determining acute and chronic mechanical complications of infarction. Acute complications easily defined include a ruptured mitral valve, papillary muscle dysfunction or rupture, ventricular septal rupture, cardiac rupture, and pericardial effusion. Chronic complications consist of aneurysm formation and intracavitary clot formation.[34]

It is useful to distinguish between complicated and uncomplicated AMI, since nearly all deaths occur in the former group. Patients in the latter group have an excellent prognosis and are candidates for early mobilization and discharge. Conditions that identify the complicated group include the following:

1. *Persistent pain:* Pain that persists or recurs is frequently associated with unusually high or secondary increases in enzyme elevations and suggests that ischemia persists and infarction is in a process of evolution and extension.

2. *Serious dysrhythmia:* Nearly all patients with acute infarction experience some transient alterations of rhythm. The alterations considered serious include ventricular fibrillation or ventricular tachycardia, second- or third-degree heart block, and new atrial flutter or fibrillation. In addition, sinus tachycardia (greater than or equal to 100 beats/min) that persists for more than 24 hours in the absence of fever should alert those caring for the patient to the possibility of heart failure. Ventricular fibrillation occurs in 5.1% of persons with AMI; the mortality rate is 48.3% in the complicated group but only 1.5% in the uncomplicated group.[6]

3. *Pulmonary edema:* Pulmonary edema produces a sense of breathlessness, wet rales on examination, and typical changes on the chest x-ray film. It is accompanied by a significant rise in PA and wedge pressures and indicates acute left ventricular failure.

4. *Persistent hypotension:* The arterial SBP may drop below 90 mm Hg without accompanying signs of shock. Often this is an early and transient finding associated with bradycardia and other signs of vagal overactivity. Alternatively, it may reflect inadequate blood volume. When hypotension persists despite an adequate HR and central venous pressure, it usually signifies a markedly reduced cardiac output.

MI patients can be further classified according to whether they had nontransmural (non-Q-wave) or transmural (Q-wave) infarcts. In the past, patients with nontransmural infarcts were thought to follow an uncomplicated course. Evidence suggests that patients with nontransmural infarctions are actually at higher risk for complications and sudden death after discharge from the hospital. In view of these findings, survivors of nontransmural infarction are especially appropriate candidates for early functional assessment and arteriography to determine optimal therapy.

Low-level exercise testing before discharge has proved to be of value in predicting patients at high risk for complications. Evidence indicates that patients who develop ST-segment abnormalities, angina pectoris, and abnormal blood pressure responses during low-level exercise testing are at higher risk of developing cardiac complications.[28,43,47]

Treatment

In the early stages of AMI, pain, anxiety, and alterations of rhythm dominate the clinical picture. After a route for intravenous therapy and ECG monitoring are established, morphine should be given in doses that eliminate or greatly reduce chest pain and relieve anxiety. Excessive bradycardia with a pulse rate below 50 beats/min, particularly if accompanied by hypotension and ectopic beats, should be treated with atropine.

The greatest threat to life in the early hours after MI is ventricular fibrillation. In approximately 50% of patients, episodes of ventricular fibrillation are preceded by ventricular premature beats. The high prevalence of premature beats and the fact that fibrillation is sometimes not heralded by these changes has led in recent years to the use of prophylactic antidysrhythmic therapy in some centers. Lidocaine is given as an initial bolus (75 to 100 mg), followed by a continuous intravenous infusion.

Maintenance of normal serum potassium levels is important in the prevention of ventricular ectopy and fibrillation. Recently, attention has turned to magnesium levels.[48-50] The mortality rate from AMI was reduced in patients who received magnesium intravenously in the first 24 hours after admission to the CCU. Furthermore, guidelines for advanced cardiac life support now include the option of magnesium administration.[51]

Because a decrease in arterial oxygen pressure caused by ventilation perfusion inequalities is common, oxygen is administered to all patients. Most physicians also advocate giving routine low doses of heparin subcutaneously to reduce the possibility of thromboembolic complications.[51]

In patients who have persistent or recurrent pain despite therapy, efforts are made to balance the oxygen supply and demand and hence to diminish ischemia. For example, if sinus tachycardia persists and signs of left ventricular failure are absent, propranolol in doses of 0.05 to 0.10 mg/kg can be given to reduce heart rate. Although this treatment eliminates pain and reduces ST-segment elevation, the hemodynamic response needs to be monitored closely.[51] Other patients with persistent or recurrent pain have elevated arterial blood pressure. Reducing blood pressure with propranolol or nitroprusside has a favorable effect in these patients. Finally, in patients with left ventricular failure and elevated PA and wedge pressures, vasodilators such as nitroprusside or nitroglycerin given intravenously "unload" the ventricle and often reduce pain and ST-segment elevation.

Nitroglycerin given intravenously is efficacious in limiting complications (pump failure, chest pain) of an AMI. Nitroglycerin is an excellent coronary vasodilator, whereas nitroprusside sodium may have deleterious effects on the ischemic heart. Nitroprusside dilates the intramyocardial resistance arteries supplying the normal myocardium. Because resistance vessels supplying the ischemic areas are already presumably maximally dilated, dilating other resistance vessels further would shunt blood from the ischemic areas to normal areas, resulting in a "coronary steal" phenomenon. Consequently, nitroglycerin given intravenously is the preferred drug. A review at 10 randomized trials in AMI demonstrated a 35% reduction in the mortality rate with the use of nitroglycerin given intravenously.[52]

MI is a dynamic process in which the fate of ischemic but still viable heart muscle is not determined until several hours after the onset of symptoms. Survival after MI depends on the size of the infarction and residual left ventricular function.[53] The primary objective of therapy after an MI is to reestablish myocardial perfusion and thereby minimize necrosis and ischemic damage. Current revascularization techniques include thrombolytic therapy, PTCA, and CABG (see Chapter 10 for more information on CABG).

The secondary objective of therapy is to reduce the deleterious effects of the remodeling process. Left ventricular dysfunction related to the remodeling process after an MI can lead to heart failure. In the early phase after MI (1 to 10 days), the malleable necrotic area thins, resulting in left ventricular dilatation. This expands the area at infarct and increases left ventricular volume. Antiinflammatory agents have been implicated as agents that can promote expansion of the MI, while control of afterload and hypertension can reduce the effects of this process. Nitroglycerin given intravenously[52] and angiotensin-converting enzyme (ACE) inhibitors are effective in preserving left ventricular size and shape.[53-55] The late phase of remodeling after MI occurs over months and is due to the structural changes in the noninfarcted myocardium that stretches the wall and dilates the chamber even more.[53] Long-term use of ACE inhibitors also reduces this form of dilatation and remodeling.[55]

Thrombolytic therapy

Because most MIs are caused by coronary arterial thrombosis, the goal of thrombolytic therapy is to lyse the intracoronary clot, restore blood flow, and thereby salvage ischemic myocardium, limit the size of the infarction, and preserve left ventricular function.[54,56,57] Four thrombolytic agents are approved for use by the Food and Drug Administration: streptokinase, urokinase, recombinant tissue-type plasminogen activator (rt-PA), and anistreplase.

Thrombolysis can be initiated by the activation of plasminogen, a serum protein that is a precursor of the enzyme plasmin. Plasminogen activators are chemicals that convert plasminogen into plasmin. Plasmin breaks down fibrin, causing the clot to dissolve. This also produces fibrin-degradation products, which are potent anticoagulants (Fig. 8-6).[58]

Streptokinase is a proteolytic enzyme synthesized by streptococcal bacteria. When this enzyme is injected into humans, it combines with circulating plasminogen to form the streptokinase-plasminogen complex, which activates plasminogen to form plasmin. The net effect of the therapy is to produce a hypocoagulable state. Streptokinase can be given via the intravenous or intracoronary routes. The intravenous route allows for quicker administration of the drug. Potential adverse effects include allergic reactions such as fever, rash, and, rarely, anaphylactic shock. Hypotension, sometimes requiring vasopressors, can occur.[58] Streptokinase was used as a thrombolytic agent in many studies.[59] Data from two large clinical trials, the Gruppo Italiano per lo Studio Streptochinase nell'Infarto Miocardico (GISSI) study and ISIS-2, revealed a 50% increase in survival with the use of streptokinase as opposed to traditional medical therapy.[60,61] The GISSI study also showed a higher survival rate in patients who received streptokinase therapy early during the infarct episode. In addition, the ISIS-2 trial demonstrated a higher survival rate with the combination of streptokinase and oral aspirin than with either drug alone.[62]

Urokinase is another proteolytic enzyme; it is made from cultured kidney cells. It also works by converting plasminogen to plasmin, causing a systemic lytic state. Urokinase can be given as an intracoronary infusion or an intravenous bolus.[58] It is nonantigenic, and no adverse effects have been reported. Like streptokinase, it has a more

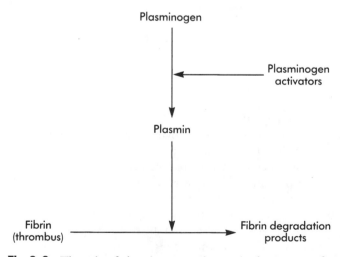

Fig. 8-6 The role of plasminogen activators in the process of thrombolysis.

pronounced effect on the hemostatic system and a longer half-life than rt-PA.[59]

Tissue plasminogen activator (TPA) is a naturally occurring protein with a very high affinity for fibrin. In the presence of fibrin, TPA converts fibrin-bound plasminogen to plasmin at the surface of a clot. The plasmin then breaks down the fibrin, and the clot dissolves. Therefore TPA is clot specific,[57] whereas streptokinase and urokinase have a hypocoagulable effect on the entire circulatory system. This enzyme can now be mass-produced with recombinant deoxyribonucleic-acid (DNA) techniques, and it is called *recombinant tissue-type plasminogen activator (rt-PA)*. Advantages of rt-PA include the fact that it has a short half-life, it is clot specific in its action, and it causes no allergic reactions.[59] A disadvantage is the relatively high cost for the drug, more than 10 times the cost of streptokinase.[63] The incidence of bleeding complications is about the same for rt-PA as for streptokinase. Several studies have shown a 70% to 75% efficacy for rt-PA to successfully lyse a coronary thrombus, and two studies have demonstrated that rt-PA has a higher efficacy than streptokinase.[64,65] GISSI-2 found no difference in the mortality rate between rt-PA and streptokinase, but there was an increased risk of stroke with rt-PA.[66] Global Utilization of Streptokinase or tPA for Occluded Coronary Arteries (GUSTO) again found a higher rate of stroke with rt-PA, but there was a significantly lower mortality rate when compared with streptokinase. When rt-PA was used, 10 more lives per 1000 patients were saved.[67]

Anisolated plasminogen streptokinase activator complex is a combination of streptokinase and plasminogen marketed under the name *anistreplase (Eminase)*. One clinical advantage of anistreplase is that it can be given intravenously in less than 5 minutes, whereas rt-PA must be given intravenously over several hours.[68]

Not all MI patients are candidates for thrombolytic therapy. For such therapy to be beneficial, the drug should be administered 4 to 6 hours from the onset of symptoms; the earlier the treatment is initiated, the greater the benefit derived. Patients must meet the ECG criteria of ST elevation of at least 1.0 mV in two leads. Most centers exclude patients older than 70 because of a higher incidence of intracranial hemorrhage in this population,[69] although some investigators have recommended including high-risk patients such as older adults and patients with pulmonary edema.[11,51] Contraindications are related to an increased risk of bleeding such as recent active internal bleeding, history of cerebrovascular accident, recent history of major surgery or trauma, prolonged cardiopulmonary resuscitation (CPR), hypertension, history of a bleeding disorder, or puncture of a noncompressible vessel.[69-70] In addition, clinical factors such as older age, female gender, low body weight, and low fibrinogen and fibrin-degradation levels are believed to increase the risk of bleeding. In the major clinical trials, the number of bleeding complications reported has been very low. The major bleeding complication is hemorrhagic stroke, which occurs in approximately 1 of every 200 to 250 patients regardless of the thrombolytic agent used.[71]

Thrombolytic therapy is initiated with other pharmacologic agents for AMI.[69-72] A heparin bolus and drip are usually given to prevent further clot formation, with the infusion titrated to keep the partial thromboplastin time 1½ to 2 times normal. Lidocaine is used prophylactically to prevent dysrhythmias caused by the infarction or reperfusion. Antiplatelet drugs such as aspirin, sulfinpyrazone, and dipyridamole have been tried to help prevent reocclusion and infarction. In view of current research and if there are no contraindications, it is recommended that one aspirin a day be given to MI patients.

The definitive method for determining whether reperfusion has been successfully achieved by thrombolytic therapy is by cardiac catheterization. However, certain clinical signs have been associated with reperfusion. These clinical markers include an abrupt cessation or reduction of chest pain, resolution of ST-segment elevation, reperfusion dysrhythmias, and a rapid peaking (within 4 to 12 hours) of CK levels. The most common dysrhythmias associated with reperfusion are ventricular tachycardia, sinus bradycardia, accelerated idioventricular rhythm, and premature ventricular contractions.[69-71]

Frequent complications of thrombolytic therapy are related to bleeding. The use of heparin to prevent further clot formation may also contribute to these complications. Bleeding around the access site for cardiac catheterization can be a problem. Intracranial hemorrhage occurs in 0.5% of patients receiving thrombolytic therapy. There may also be gingival bleeding, epistaxis, hemoptysis, and bleeding from recent cuts and abrasions. Internal bleeding, such as gastrointestinal or retroperitoneal bleeding, occurs less frequently. A serious bleeding episode may necessitate the immediate discontinuation of the thrombolytic agent and heparin infusion. Blood transfusions may be required.[69-71]

Coronary artery reocclusion may be caused by rethrombosis, coronary artery spasms, or incomplete lysis of the thrombus. With coronary artery occlusion, the myocardium is again at risk. Signs and symptoms of ischemia, such as chest pain, nausea, diaphoresis, and ECG changes may occur. Continuous ST-segment monitoring is a useful way to assess for reocclusion.[72] Cardiac catheterization, PTCA, or another dose of rt-PA may be required.

Frequent and careful monitoring of the patient receiving thrombolytic therapy is required. Many of the observations are necessary because of the increased risk of bleeding caused by the thrombolytic agents and concomitant heparin infusion. The partial thromboplastin time should be monitored frequently. The patient's neurologic status should be evaluated frequently and checked for any changes in level of consciousness or complaints of headache that may indicate intracranial bleeding. All puncture and access sites should be checked for bleeding or hematoma formation. The patient's gums and nose should be checked for bleeding, and the skin should be inspected for bleeding, bruises, or ecchymotic areas. In addition, the urine, stool, sputum, and emesis should be checked for blood. Unnecessary arterial and venous punctures should be avoided, and saline-flushed intravenous cannulas should be used for blood sampling. Intramuscular injections should not be given while the patient is in a hypocoagulable state. It is important to assess for signs of internal bleeding such as a drop in hemoglobin levels or the hematocrit, a sudden change in vital signs, restlessness, a rapidly distending abdomen, low back pain, or diminished peripheral pulses. Direct pressure should be applied for at least 30 minutes (or until bleeding stops) to all puncture sites, and then a sterile pressure dressing should be applied. The patient should be handled gently to prevent bruising.[69-71]

During thrombolytic therapy, the nurse observes the patient for any signs of reperfusion such as a cessation of chest pain, resolution of ST-segment elevation, early peaking of CK levels, or dysrhythmias. The patient is closely monitored for signs of myocardial ischemia, including chest pain, nausea, diaphoresis, shortness of breath, or ECG changes. Once their conditions are stabilized, patients in whom reperfusion was successful will usually undergo elective cardiac catheterization to define coronary anatomy and evaluate for possible revascularization procedures.[71,73]

In addition to the intense monitoring of the patient receiving thrombolytic therapy, psychologic support of the patient and family is important. Anxiety and fear are common reactions during an MI. The potential risks of thrombolytic therapy may increase these reactions. It is important to provide a calm, reassuring atmosphere and give clear, simple explanations of treatments and activities.

PTCA

PTCA is a nonoperative procedure that uses a balloon catheter to increase the luminal diameter of stenotic coronary arteries and thereby increase blood flow distal to the stenosis. Improvement in coronary blood flow after PTCA is associated with decreased symptoms and increased exercise tolerance in patients with angina pectoris. PTCA may also prevent reocclusion after thrombolytic therapy for AMI. Finally, emergent PTCA during the acute phase of an MI is a safe and effective alternative to thrombolysis to reperfuse the myocardium.[74] Consequently, PTCA has gained wide acceptance as an effective therapy for selected patients with symptomatic coronary artery disease.

Dotter and Judkins[75] first used a percutaneously introduced catheter in 1964 to dilate peripheral atherosclerotic lesions. In 1977, Gruentzig[76] applied PTCA to a highly selected group of patients with stable angina and discrete proximal, noncalcific stenoses of a single coronary artery. Technical advancements in percutaneous catheters, guidewires, and balloons have expanded the range of indications for PTCA. Patients with unstable angina, multivessel disease, multiple stenoses in single vessels, and stenoses in coronary artery bypass grafts have been successfully treated.

The use of PTCA has increased for several reasons. When compared with CABG, PTCA is psychologically and physically much less traumatic. The recovery period for PTCA is short; less than 24 hours of bedrest is required after the procedure. The patient is usually discharged from the hospital within 1 to 2 days after angioplasty and can resume usual activities within days unless myocardial damage was incurred before the procedure.

Equipment. Basic equipment used during angioplasty includes a balloon, pacing and guiding catheters, and a transducer system for monitoring ventricular and coronary artery pressures. The balloon catheter has two lumens; the central lumen is used for injecting contrast media and for monitoring pressure, and the outer lumen is used for inflating and deflating the balloon. Gold markers, visible under fluoroscopy, are positioned at both ends of the balloon to define its alignment within the lesion. Some catheters have a third lumen that allows for distal perfusion of the coronary artery.

As a precautionary measure, a pacing catheter is placed before angioplasty. If the right coronary artery is to be dilated, third-degree AV block may result while the artery is occluded. If the left anterior descending artery is occluded during angioplasty, an idioventricular rhythm may occur.

The guiding catheter has a large, single lumen and is used to position the balloon catheter. A modern angioplasty catheter system is shown in Fig. 8-7.

Mechanism. Initially, the main mechanism of PTCA was thought to be the compression and relocation of the atherosclerotic plaque. Several human cadaver and animal studies now suggest that balloon inflation during angioplasty causes the plaque to split at its thinnest and weakest point. This split may extend into internal elastic membrane, and further balloon dilatation may stretch the media and adventitia of the vessel, causing an arterial wall tear in the direction of blood flow. The subsequent healing process is not well understood; presently it is thought that some of the plaque may dissolve in the bloodstream. Arterial wall fibers may cause retraction of the split, and endothelial cells may promote healing of the exposed inner surface of the vessel.[34]

Selection of patients. The results of the history, treadmill test, and coronary angiogram are used to determine a patient's suitability for PTCA. Ideally, the stenosis should be less than 10 mm in length, should not involve a major vessel bifurcation, and should be free of angiographic filling defects. The ideal candidate for PTCA has a single proximal, concentric, noncalcific coronary artery lesion in the setting of persistent angina despite medical therapy. When these features are present, a greater than 90% success rate is expected.[37] Patients whose symptoms are controlled by

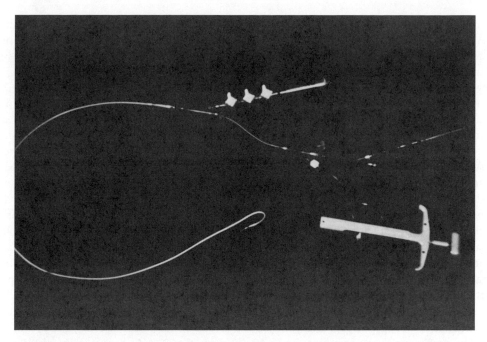

Fig. 8-7   Modern steerable guidewire equipment used for coronary angioplasty.   (Courtesy Dr. Richard Stack, Duke University Medical Center.)

medical therapy may do just as well on medical therapy as they would with PTCA.[34,37] PTCA may be performed in older patients. Although the success rate is lower in this age group than in younger patients, PTCA is less risky than CABG.[77] Persons who develop lesions in saphenous vein grafts may be candidates for PTCA of the bypass graft.[78]

Not all lesions are considered for angioplasty. An increased frequency of coronary occlusion and an inability to localize and effectively use the dilating balloon make high risk any lesions that are excessive in number and length and distal in location. If tortuosity of the vessel precludes easy placement of the steerable guidewire, the patient should not be considered a candidate for angioplasty. In most centers, patients with left main disease are not candidates. Individual coronary arteriograms must be evaluated to make these decisions. The box lists indications and precautions for PTCA.

Procedure. In most cases a diagnostic cardiac catheterization precedes PTCA by at least 1 day. Although the angioplasty procedure is very similar to cardiac catheterization, the patient may express new fears concerning balloon dilatation and possible emergent CABG. Therefore it is important to thoroughly explain the procedure. The family or support system of the patient should be included in the teaching so that they have an understanding of the procedure and can provide the support the patient needs.

The patient is allowed nothing by mouth from midnight until after angioplasty to minimize the risk of emesis and aspiration during the procedure. The groin is cleansed and shaved. Routine laboratory tests obtained before angioplasty include hemoglobin measurements, hematocrit, coagulation studies, electrolyte evaluation, blood urea nitrogen tests, and creatinine measurements. Blood is typed and screened in case that emergency surgery is required.

INDICATIONS AND PRECAUTIONS FOR PTCA

Indications	Precautions
Stenosis that is:	Stenosis that:
Less than 10 minutes in length	Involves a major vessel bifurcation
Proximal	Has angiographic filling defects
Single	Is tortuous
Concentric	Multivessel disease
Noncalcific	CABGs
Angina unresponsive to medical treatment	Excessive number of stenoses
Older person or a patient with a severe general medical problem that would make the person a high-risk surgical candidate	Chronic total coronary artery lesions
Young patient with the possibility of subsequent progression of coronary artery disease	Left main disease (contraindicated in most medical centers)

The operating suite should be notified in advance of all angioplasty cases. A room is often prepared, and a cardio-thoracic team must be mobilized in case of complications of angioplasty that may require immediate surgery.

Because platelet adhesion may be the cause of early restenosis after angioplasty, low-molecular-weight dextran or a combination of aspirin and dipyridamole may be given before the procedure. Diphenhydramine is commonly administered before angiography to reduce the risk of allergic reaction to contrast media. Long-acting nitrates and calcium channel blockers may be given before angioplasty.

Once in the angiography laboratory, the patient is prepared and draped using sterile technique. After the femoral vein is located with a large-bore needle, an introducer sheath is inserted, and the pacing catheter is advanced to the level of the inferior vena cava. A second needle is used to locate the femoral artery. An introducer sheath is placed in the artery, and the guiding catheter is advanced to the level of the coronary ostium. To prevent spasm, 200 to 300 mcg of nitroglycerin given via the intracoronary route, nifedipine given sublingually, or both, may be given. A steering device on the distal end of the guidewire system directs the guidewire into the coronary circulation and across the atherosclerotic lesion. Once in place and verified by fluoroscopy, the balloon is advanced along the guidewire and across the lesion. Gold markers at each end of the balloon assist in determining proper placement within the vessel, and pressure gradients across the lesion may then be measured. The guiding catheter measures proximal pressure, whereas the dilating catheter measures distal pressures; the difference in pressures is termed the *pressure gradient*. A large lesion that significantly obstructs blood flow causes a greater decrease in pressure distal to the lesion and consequently a greater pressure gradient.

The balloon is then inflated at pressures from 2 to 10 atmospheres for 10 to 120 seconds (Fig. 8-8). One or more inflations at varying pressures may be performed. With the guidewire across the lesion in case of sudden reocclusion, the results are assessed by arteriography. The pressure gradient measured after successful angioplasty should be significantly lower. Pressure gradients may be distorted by the presence of the balloon catheter or guidewire across the lesion, contrast media, or collateral blood flow. With these limitations in mind, some investigators do not rely on pressure gradients to determine success after PTCA. Fig. 8-9 shows coronary arteriograms before and after PTCA.

If angioplasty is successful, the catheters are removed. Because heparin is given during angioplasty, clotting times are elevated after the procedure. The sheaths are left in place to prevent bleeding, and the patient is returned to the room. To decrease the risk of sudden arterial reocclusion after PTCA, heparin may also be given intravenously after the procedure. The heparin may be discontinued several hours to 24 hours after PTCA. When coagulation times return to normal, the sheaths may be removed, after which the patient should lie flat for approximately 6 hours to promote healing of the femoral artery puncture site. The patient should be watched closely for signs of bleeding in the groin. Pedal pulses should be checked frequently in case thrombosis of the femoral artery occurs. Blood pressure is taken frequently to monitor for hypotension.

Most important, the patient should be monitored for chest pain, which is common after PTCA and may be

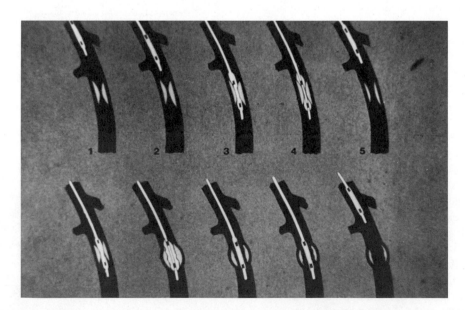

Fig. 8-8   Balloon compression of atherosclerotic lesion.   (Courtesy Dr. Richard Stack, Duke University Medical Center.)

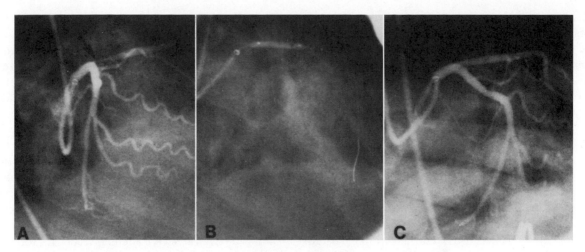

Fig. 8-9   Coronary arteriograms during PTCA. Arrows denote the lesion before (**A**) and after (**C**) dilatation. **B,** The balloon inflated within the lesion.   (Courtesy Dr. Richard Stack, Duke University Medical Center.)

caused by abrupt occlusion or restenosis of the dilated coronary artery, coronary artery spasm, or pulmonary embolism. When chest pain occurs, an ECG should be obtained, and nitrates and calcium channel blockers should be administered. If the ECG reveals ST-segment elevations and chest pain is not relieved by medication, occlusion should be suspected, and emergent repeat PTCA or CABG should be performed. After medication, if ST elevations return to baseline and pain subsides, spasm should be considered and the medication continued. Because ST-segment depressions on ECG indicate possible restenosis, urgent PTCA should be performed again. Pulmonary embolism should be considered if no cardiac source of chest pain is found. The usual source of pulmonary emboli after PTCA is the femoral vein puncture site. When pulmonary embolism is documented, systemic anticoagulation should be initiated. If no organic source of chest pain is found, anxiety is probably the cause, and the patient should be reassured.

Complications. Complications associated with PTCA are similar to those of cardiac catheterization. Dye reaction, hypotension, bradycardia, blood loss, and hematoma may occur. Each of these can usually be treated effectively and results in minor morbidity. Other complications—coronary artery dissection, occlusion, spasm, embolism, perforation, and rupture—result from the angioplasty procedure. An ischemic event, such as an MI or prolonged angina, also may occur during PTCA.

MI, emergency surgery, and in-hospital death occur in 2% to 10% of patients. Minor complications include prolonged angina, bradycardia, transient ventricular dysrhythmias, or excessive blood loss.[73]

Restenosis is a significant long-term complication associated with PTCA. It is a greater than 30% narrowing of the stenotic site at follow-up angiography or a 50% reduction in luminal diameter when compared with the initial improvement obtained at angioplasty.[73] Restenosis occurs in approximately 25% to 30% of patients, but a wide range (13% to 47%) has been reported.[37] The incidence of restenosis is highest in the first 24 hours after PTCA but remains higher for the next 6 months.

Restenosis can be documented only by coronary arteriography, but recurrence of symptoms after PTCA may suggest restenosis. Most coronary restenoses after a successful PTCA occur in the first 6 to 8 months after the procedure. Another PTCA usually results in the same or improved success rate as the first procedure.[73]

Several antiplatelet agents are routinely used to help prevent restenosis, although their effectiveness has not yet been documented. Aspirin alone or with dipyridamole is frequently used to reduce platelet adhesion to the endothelium of the dilated coronary vessel.

Because acute closure and restenosis affect so many patients who have undergone PTCA, research is focused on alleviating these problems. Techniques under investigation include intracoronary stents, atherectomy devices, and laser angioplasty.

Intracoronary stents are metal coil or tubular mesh devices placed in the area of the coronary lesion to keep the vessel open. The device counteracts inwardly directed forces to prevent spasm and provide a scaffold for repair at the vascular wall.[77] The stents are self-expanding or balloon expandable. Chronic anticoagulation is required to prevent thrombus formation. Stabilizing the anticoagulant level may require a longer hospitalization than that required for a PTCA. Restenosis rates at 15% to 30% have been reported for single stents and 46% to 64% for multiple-stent placements.[79,80] Although complication rates are increased when stents are placed after emergent PTCA, these problems can be avoided with careful selection at the stent size.[81]

Atherectomy and rotational devices have been developed to leave a smoother intraarterial surface. The directional coronary atherectomy (DCA) device and the transluminal extraction device physically remove plaque from the inside of the vessel, thereby improving blood flow.[82] The DCA device was developed to excise eccentric lesions using a rotating blade that shaves the plaque and deposits the material in the nose of the catheter.[83] Early reports describe complication and restenosis rates similar to those of PTCA.[84] DCA is recommended for small coronary arteries and calcified and distal lesions. MI occurs in 5.6% of patients undergoing DCA because of embolization of shared material.[83] DCA requires a larger arterial puncture; therefore postprocedure observation of the site is critical.

Laser angioplasty works by vaporizing solid matter, such as an atheromatous plaque, to gas. The continuous- or pulsed-wave laser energy is transmitted through a flexible fiberoptic catheter. Lasers currently under investigation include the argon, neodymium:yttrium-aluminum-garnet (Nd:YAG), excimer, and pulsed dye systems.[79,83]

Complications

A pericardial rub is heard in about 25% of patients with transmural infarction, usually on the third to fifth day. Within 1 to 4 weeks after infarction, pericarditis with effusion and fever develop in about 2% to 5% of patients. This is known as *Dressler syndrome* and is thought to result from an autoimmune response. Pericarditis, early or late, is generally treated symptomatically. The use of aspirin, indomethacin, or even steroids may be required; however, use of these medications may result in worsening at the remodeling process after MI.[53-56] Anticoagulation should be discontinued unless there is an overriding reason to continue its use, such as an overt pulmonary embolus. Pulsus paradoxus is evaluated to detect early signs of potential cardiac tamponade.

Prolongation of the PR interval and Wenckebach periods are common after posterior and inferior infarctions. They usually regress or can be treated with atropine. Third-degree AV block and conditions associated with a high incidence of progression to complete block (for example, Mobitz type II second-degree block or new bifascicular bundle branch block [especially that associated with PR prolongation]) are regarded as indications for insertion of a temporary transvenous pacemaker. Use of the pacemaker is then determined primarily by the ventricular rate and the patient's hemodynamic response (see Chapter 6).

Heart Failure

Heart failure may be defined as a state in which cardiac output is insufficient to meet the metabolic needs of the body. It can occur when cardiac output is normal, in-creased, or decreased. In most cases, patients with heart failure have decreased cardiac output and left ventricular dilatation. Congestive failure is manifested by retention of fluid and the formation of edema. Low output failure occurs when the heart is unable to meet the metabolic demands of tissues, even if they are normal. A number of cardiac disorders can result in low output failure. For example, MI affecting a large area of the left ventricle or stenosis or insufficiency of the cardiac valves can impair the heart's ability to pump. Constrictive pericarditis or pericardial effusion can restrict the ability of the heart to fill and empty.

Less common, heart failure occurs when peripheral demands exceed even the capacity of a normal heart to adequately perfuse the tissues. This is called *high output failure* and can occur in severe anemia, sepsis, thyrotoxicosis, and arteriovenous fistulas.

The usual defect in heart failure is a decrease in the pumping ability of the heart. Patients with early or mild heart disease may show no significant abnormalities at rest because of reserve in cardiac function. Despite a normal cardiac output at rest, cardiac output with exercise is subnormal, and the patient shows a decreased exercise tolerance.

Factors that affect cardiac output are preload, afterload, heart rate, and contractility. Preload is the amount of blood delivered to the ventricles during diastole (venous return). Afterload is the force that the heart pumps against (systemic vascular resistance). Contractility is the force of contraction of the heart (see Chapter 1). As the heart begins to fail, a large number of compensatory mechanisms are set in motion in an effort to maintain cardiac output at a level adequate to meet the metabolic needs of the body. Most of these mechanisms are the same as those used by normal persons during exercise or periods of increased stress. The principal initial adjustments are a reflex increase in sympathetic nerve discharge and a decrease in parasympathetic activity. These autonomic alterations, affecting the heart, arteries, and veins, result in the increase of systemic vascular resistance and arterial pressure (afterload). Venous tone increases, which in turn increases venous pressure and helps maintain venous return (preload).

An increase in heart rate (tachycardia) by itself may increase cardiac output. Above a certain rate, however, cardiac output may begin to decrease. This rate is about 170 to 180 beats/min for most normal young individuals. In trained athletes the rate may be 200 to 220 beats/min, whereas in patients with myocardial disease the rate limit may be 120 to 140 beats/min. A decrease in cardiac output above a certain heart rate is caused by a shortening of diastole, which limits the time for adequate filling of the ventricles and for coronary blood flow. Slow heart rates allow more complete diastolic filling.

When cardiac output falls for whatever reason, the kidney retains salt and water as an early compensatory mechanism. This is caused in part by sympathetic stimulation, which produces renal vasoconstriction and a reduction in renal blood flow. Sympathetically mediated activation of the renin-angiotensin system triggers aldosterone release and causes more sodium retention. Expansion of the intravascular blood volume results in increases in the end-diastolic volume and pressure and ultimately in leaking of fluid from the vascular bed and edema formation (Table 8-2). The current pharmacologic treatment of heart failure includes ACE inhibitors, diuretics, and antihypertensives. In addition, fluid restriction is essential.

A major long-term hemodynamic adjustment to heart failure is ventricular hypertrophy. This is thought to be caused by a chronic increase in the systolic force or tension developed by the myocardial fibers. Although the contractility of hypertrophied myocardium is lower than normal for each unit of muscle and is associated with an imbalance between energy production and usage, the hypertrophied myocardium may maintain compensation because the total mass of myocardium is increased. If the pumping capacity (contractility) of the ventricle is restored by hypertrophy, tachycardia and edema may no longer be present.

Left Ventricular Failure

The heart is composed of two pumps in series, the right ventricle and the left ventricle. Certain events may alter the function of one of these pumps without affecting the other. In AMI, for example, the primary insult is usually to the left ventricle. When the ability of the left ventricle to pump blood is compromised without compromise to the right ventricle, a temporary imbalance in the output of the two sides of the heart results. The right side of the heart continues to pump blood into the lungs. At the same time, the left side of the heart is unable to move the blood adequately into the systemic circulation.

The blood backs up into the left atrium and the pulmonary vessels and increases the pressure in the left side of the heart and the pulmonary vessels. Consequently, one of the first symptoms associated with acute left ventricular failure is dyspnea. If dyspnea occurs when the patient is recumbent, it is called *orthopnea* and is usually relieved by sitting. Dyspnea is the symptomatic manifestation of the increased work of breathing related to pulmonary venous engorgement and increased pulmonary blood volume.

Paroxysmal nocturnal dyspnea, which is a form of acute pulmonary edema, is almost a specific sign of left ventricular failure. The patient awakens suddenly at night, extremely breathless, and seeks relief by sitting or running to an open window for fresh air. When the patient goes to sleep, the metabolic needs of the body may decrease. As a result, the cardiac output that had previously been inadequate may now be adequate to supply the body's needs. Fluid that had been pocketed away is mobilized into the vascular system, thus increasing the blood volume. The blood volume and a redistribution of this volume to the lungs resulting from the recumbent position are major factors in causing nocturnal dyspnea.

As the heart's compensatory mechanisms fail, the already elevated diastolic filling pressure and left atrial pressure continue to increase. To maintain flow, the pressure in the pulmonary veins and capillaries exceeds the intravascular osmotic pressure (approximately 30 mm Hg), and fluid rapidly leaks into the interstitial regions of the lung tissue. Pulmonary edema greatly reduces the amount of lung tissue available for the exchange of gases and consequently results in a dramatic clinical presentation characterized by extreme dyspnea, cyanosis, and severe anxiety. This is called *acute pulmonary edema* and is considered a medical emergency.

In the early stages of pulmonary edema, the patient appears anxious, restless, or vaguely uneasy. Wheezing, orthopnea, diaphoresis, and pallor appear as left ventricular failure progresses. A third heart sound may be heard as the distensibility of the ventricle decreases. Sinus tachycardia and increased systemic arterial pressure are common as

TABLE 8-2	Edema Formation	
Organ	**Edema**	**Description**
Skin	Dependent edema, pitting type	Increased venous pressure forces fluid through capillary walls into subcutaneous tissues; in ambulatory patients, edema is localized in dependent parts of body (hands and feet); patients in bed may lose edema of legs and feet and have it only in presacral region.
Liver	Hepatomegaly	Increased pressure in hepatic veins causes accumulation of fluid in liver, which becomes enlarged and tender.
Pleural cavity	Pleural effusion; hydrothorax	Venous congestion forces fluid into pleural cavity.
Pericardial cavity	Pericardial effusion	Fluid accumulation occurs in pericardial cavity.

neural reflexes attempt to correct the imbalance. If these physiologic compensations fail, hypotension may occur, rales develop from alveolar edema, and copious blood-tinged, frothy sputum is expectorated. As the accumulation of pulmonary interstitial and intraalveolar fluid progresses, arterial hypoxemia and cyanosis occur in varying degrees. Arterial blood gas measurements may show the presence of hypoxia with a drop in the arterial oxygen pressure. The chest x-ray film typically shows mottling from the hilar regions, which may cover both lung fields. With the elevation of the pulmonary venous pressure, diffuse interstitial edema results and is seen as cloudy lung fields. In severe pulmonary edema, Kerley B lines and possibly a total "white out" of the lung fields appear. This deterioration in pulmonary function is reflected in the patient's mental status. Anxiety progresses to mental confusion and eventually to stupor and coma. Patients literally drown in their own secretions. See Table 8-3 for treatment of acute pulmonary edema.

Right Ventricular Failure

Usually right ventricular failure follows left ventricular failure. Right-sided heart failure without left-sided heart failure may be caused by pulmonary hypertension secondary to lung disease or recurrent pulmonary emboli; it is referred to as *cor pulmonale*. In either case, pulmonary hypertension presents an increased resistance to right ventricular ejection and a resulting increase in right ventricular end-diastolic and right atrial pressures. This impedes venous return. Clinical manifestations include: (1) distention of the neck veins, which appear full even when the head is raised (normally these empty when the head is elevated to a 45-degree angle); (2) a distended and often tender liver, and (3) peripheral edema (see Table 8-2). When the accu-

---

TABLE 8-3   Treatment of Acute Pulmonary Edema

Therapy	Principle	Precaution
Supplemental oxygen by face mask, nasal cannula, or, rarely, IPPB	Supplemental oxygen raises oxygen pressure levels.	Patient may not be able to tolerate face mask; high-flow (>4-6 L/min) oxygen must always be administered with humidification to avoid airway drying; IPPB and CPAP may increase patient's work of breathing and anxiety level.
Placement of patient in high Fowler position	Sitting increases lung volume and vital capacity and decreases venous return and work of breathing.	In presence of hypotension, Fowler position is avoided or used cautiously.
Morphine sulfate given intravenously	Morphine decreases anxiety, respiratory rate, and venous return (preload).	Morphine sulfate may cause respiratory depression; it is contraindicated in the presence of severe pulmonary disease
Preload reduction: possible use of vasodilators to reduce preload; use of nitroglycerin (usually drug of choice); possible use of nitroprusside sodium if the patient is extremely hypertensive	Nitroglycerin and nitroprusside sodium cause venous vasodilatation and reduce preload and afterload; nitroglycerin has more pronounced effect on venous system.	Blood pressure should be closely monitored; hypotension and reflex tachydysrhythmias may occur.
Decrease in intravascular volume; use of diuretics such as furosemide, ethacrynic acid, or bumetanide; phlebotomy of 300 to 500 ml	Decrease in intravascular volume improves ability of lungs to exchange gases and decreases cardiac work.	Blood pressure and intake and output should be monitored; diuretics can cause volume and electrolyte depletion.
Aminophylline given intravenously for bronchospasm caused by bronchiolar congestion	Aminophylline dilates bronchioles and is venous vasodilator.	Aminophylline may cause tachydysrhythmias, nausea, vomiting, headache, and hypotension.

IPPB, Intermittent positive pressure breathing; *CPAP,* continuous positive airway pressure.

mulation of fluid becomes extensive and generalized, the patient is said to have *anasarca*. Other consequences of congestive heart failure include pleural effusions, ascites jaundice caused by hepatic engorgement, and ultimately cardiac cachexia.

Treatment of heart failure

Treatment of patients with heart failure requires an understanding of the conditions that lead to this clinical state and of the mechanisms that produce congestion.

When heart failure results from certain specific mechanical problems such as aortic or mitral valve stenosis or insufficiency, persistent and uncontrolled dysrhythmias, severe anemia, hypertension, or a congenital cardiac lesion, therapy is directed at correcting the cause. Regardless of the cause of heart disease, infections, dysrhythmias, anemia, thyrotoxicosis, and pregnancy may place a sufficient added burden on the heart to precipitate heart failure. Thus appropriate treatment of these conditions may convert a patient with heart disease from a decompensated to a compensated state.

Heart failure has previously been defined as a condition in which the cardiac output is not sufficient to meet the metabolic demands of the body. Essentially all of the situations that aggravate heart failure do so by increasing the metabolic demands on a heart that is not capable of responding with an adequate output. A favorable response in patients with heart failure often can be obtained by rest. Defining the level of physical activity that a patient can tolerate without precipitating failure is a major objective of subsequent follow-up and treatment.

A second focus of therapy is improving cardiac performance and output. Obviously if tight aortic stenosis or another structural defect is present, surgery is indicated. On the other hand, digitalis, which increases the contractility of heart muscle, has a favorable effect on cardiac performance and output. In most instances of heart failure, it is used routinely with beneficial results. In AMI with heart failure, the evidence of benefit from digitalis is minimal. Furthermore, because of a potentially increased sensitivity to toxic manifestations of digitalis excess, its use in this situation is still controversial.

In patients with a severely decompensated congestive heart, the renin-angiotensin system is activated, resulting in the maintenance of elevated systemic vascular resistance (afterload). Captopril inhibits this renin-angiotensin mechanism, reducing afterload and resulting in clinical improvement of congestive heart failure.[55,85] Vasodilator agents are an important addition to the treatment of heart failure. This class of agents includes nitrates, nitroprusside, hydralazine, minoxidil, and prazosin.[86,87] Some are designed for intravenous use and some for oral use. Some act predominantly on the arterial system, and others exert significant actions on veins as well. These agents reduce arterial resistance (afterload), which is accompanied by an increase in cardiac output, a decrease in left atrial and pulmonary venous pressure, and a decrease in left ventricular end-diastolic volume (preload) and pressure. These agents have proved very useful in the treatment of acute heart failure in MI, in heart failure associated with severe mitral insufficiency, and in chronic heart failure caused by myocardial disease. The benefits of vasodilator therapy are greatest when left atrial and pulmonary pressures are elevated. Vasodilators are not useful and may even be detrimental in patients with normal or reduced left ventricular filling pressures.

Two additional agents used in the treatment of congestive heart failure are milrinone and amrinone. These are nonadrenergic, nonglycoside agents with combined positive inotropic and vasodilating properties. Amrinone given intravenously causes an increase in cardiac output and a decrease in the pulmonary capillary wedge pressure, right atrial pressure, and systemic vascular resistance. Subsequently, the myocardial oxygen consumption rate is also decreased. No major change in the blood pressure or heart rate is observed. Amrinone is comparable to dobutamine and dopamine as inotropic therapy in heart failure. Milrinone has shown similar results in the treatment of congestive heart failure.[87]

The third focus in the treatment of patients with heart failure is achieving and maintaining an appropriate blood volume. As noted before, the compensatory mechanisms invoked with insufficient cardiac output also affect sodium and water balance by the kidneys. The net effect of these influences is sodium (and water) retention and a diminished ability to excrete a sodium load. A normal sodium intake of 5 to 8 g/day cannot be tolerated by most patients with heart failure and should be reduced to 2 g/day or even less. Diuretics promote the excretion of sodium and hence water by the kidneys through one or more of several specific actions. Thiazide diuretics inhibit sodium transport primarily in the distal or cortical segment of the nephron. Loop diuretics such as ethacrynic acid and furosemide are very potent and act on the cortical and medullary segments of the nephron. Spironolactone is a diuretic that specifically antagonizes the effect of aldosterone on the collecting duct. Triamterene has an action on sodium transport identical to spironolactone, but its action does not depend on blocking aldosterone. In general, thiazides and loop diuretics also cause potassium loss, whereas spironolactone and triamterene do not. These agents vary in potency, but with appropriate selection and dosage they can promote diuresis in patients with edema caused by heart failure and with chronic use can diminish the tendency of patients with heart failure to retain salt and water.

Mild to moderate heart failure in patients with acute infarction is usually managed successfully with limitation of physical activity, oxygen, morphine, careful attention to fluid balance with optimization of PA wedge pressure, and use of vasodilators and diuretics when indicated.

Cardiogenic Shock

When oxygen and other nutrients become unavailable to the cells of the body, shock may occur. *Shock* is a descriptive term denoting a clinical picture that develops in the presence of inadequate tissue perfusion. Cardiogenic shock is shock caused by decreased cardiac output. AMI is the most common cause of cardiogenic shock. Other causes include acute valvular insufficiency, dysrhythmias, and cardiac tamponade. Cardiogenic shock can also occur with tension pneumothorax, pulmonary embolism, and open heart surgery. It occurs in about 15% of patients hospitalized with AMI. The clinical picture is characterized by (1) a systolic blood pressure of less than 90 mm Hg or at least 30 mm Hg lower than the prior base level and (2) signs of impaired tissue perfusion such as pallor; cyanosis of varying degrees, cool and clammy skin, mental confusion or obtundation; and a urine output of less than 20 ml/hr. Cardiogenic shock caused by AMI is thought to evolve over hours or days as more and more myocardium becomes necrosed. With conservative management, the mortality rate is 80% to 90%.[88] Reperfusion therapy and aggressive treatment of heart failure are recommended.

Cardiogenic shock occurs in three stages. In the first stage, compensated hypotension, the body tries to compensate for the fall in cardiac output by increasing the rate and force of contraction of the heart. Constriction of peripheral blood vessels occurs, resulting in shunting of blood to the brain, heart, and kidneys. The second stage, uncompensated hypotension, occurs when these compensatory mechanisms fail. The body cannot maintain an adequate arterial blood pressure or perfusion of vital organs, and cardiac, cerebral, and renal ischemia occur. Further vasoconstriction and hypoperfusion occur, leading to tissue hypoxia and metabolic acidosis. Unless the shock can be reversed, the third and irreversible stage occurs: microcirculatory failure and cellular membrane injury. This results in irreversible organ damage and death.[89]

It is important to quickly and accurately diagnose cardiogenic shock and to institute appropriate therapy to reverse this process. Hemodynamic monitoring is useful, not only in the diagnosis of cardiogenic shock, but also as a means of assessing the effectiveness of treatment.

Hemodynamic assessment

Most CCUs have developed means of measuring hemodynamic status by the bedside without increasing risk or discomfort for the patient. With the aid of fluoroscopy, a pressure recorder, or both, a balloon-tipped, flow-directed catheter is inserted into the subclavian or brachial vein and directed into the right ventricle and PA (Fig. 8-10). A multipurpose flow-directed PA catheter permits monitoring of the PA pressure, pulmonary capillary wedge pressure, central venous pressure, and cardiac output. In addition, the standard thermistor catheter can be modified to include electrodes for atrial, ventricular, and atrioventricular sequential pacing and for recording intraatrial and intraventricular ECGs.

PA pressure

The PA waveform evidences a sharp rise during ejection of blood from the right ventricle after the pulmonary valve opens. This pressure rise is followed by a slow decrease in pressure during the ejection of blood from the right ventricle until the pulmonic valve closes, indicated by the dicrotic notch. The pressure continues to decrease until systole occurs again.

Normal PA systolic pressure is 20 to 30 mm Hg, and normal PA diastolic pressure ranges from 5 to 16 mm Hg. The normal mean PA pressure ranges from 10 to 20 mm Hg. The PA systolic pressure normally equals the right ventricular systolic pressure (Fig. 8-11). The PA end-diastolic pressure should be almost equal to the mean pulmonary capillary wedge pressure in the absence of pulmonary vascular disease.

Elevation of PA pressure may occur during increased pulmonary blood flow, as in a left-to-right shunt resulting from an atrial or a ventricular septal defect; increased pulmonary arteriolar resistance resulting from primary pulmonary hypertension or mitral stenosis; and left ventricular failure resulting from any cause.

Pulmonary capillary wedge pressure

Since there is normally a direct relationship among PA end-diastolic pressure, pulmonary capillary wedge pressure, and left ventricular end-diastolic pressure, an elevated PA end-diastolic pressure or pulmonary capillary wedge pressure reflects the elevated left ventricular end-diastolic pressure that occurs when the left ventricle can no longer adequately pump blood.

The pulmonary capillary wedge pressure reflects the elevated left ventricular end-diastolic pressure that occurs when the left ventricle can no longer adequately pump blood. The pulmonary capillary wedge pressure is normally 4 to 12 mm Hg. Pulmonary capillary wedge pressure exceeding 12 mm Hg may occur as a result of left ventricular failure, mitral stenosis, or mitral insufficiency, in addition to other possible causes.

PA end-diastolic pressure

Since the PA end-diastolic pressure is approximately equal to the pulmonary capillary wedge pressure and because the PA end-diastolic pressure is an accurate reflection of left ventricular end-diastolic pressure (Fig. 8-12), the PA end-diastolic pressure can be used as an alternative measurement of left ventricular end-diastolic pressure in most patients, even in the presence of pulmonary venous hypertension. At the time of catheter insertion, the PA end-diastolic pressure can be compared with the pulmonary capillary wedge pressure. If the difference is less than 5 mm Hg, the PA end-diastolic pressure can be used as an accurate estimation of the left ventricular end-diastolic pressure, eliminating the need for wedging the catheter.[90] A PA end-diastolic pressure or pulmonary capillary wedge pressure

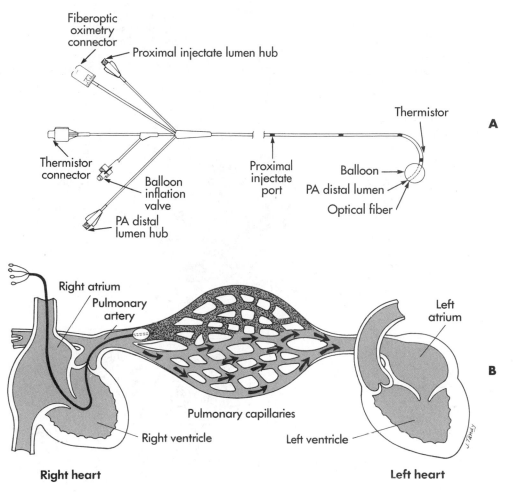

Fig. 8-10 **A,** PA catheter. The proximal injectate lumen hub attaches to a pressure line to measure right atrial central venous pressure. This is also the hub where the solution will be injected to measure cardiac output. The injectate solution will exit at the proximal injectate port in the right atrium. **B,** Representation of the PA catheter in the wedged position. The inflated balloon floats into a segment of the PA. No blood flows distally to the balloon-occluded segment. This creates a nonmoving column of blood that allows the electronic monitoring equipment to "look through" a nonactive segment of the pulmonary circulation to the left atrium. When the mitral valve is open during diastole, the left ventricular end-diastolic pressure is reflected in the PA wedge pressure.   (From Flynn JM, Bruce N: *Introduction to critical care nursing skills,* St Louis, 1993, Mosby.)

measurement of greater than 12 mm Hg is considered abnormal. The balloon-tipped catheter may also aid in establishing the cause of heart failure or shock, as well as in evaluating the effectiveness of the therapy. For example, in a state of hypotension caused by hypovolemia, infusing normal saline, whole blood, or low-molecular-weight dextran elevates the systemic pressure. In this case the PA end-diastolic pressure and pulmonary capillary wedge pressure, initially low, return to normal when the blood volume has been restored. If the PA end-diastolic pressure is elevated because of heart failure, effective therapy should lower the pressure readings that were initially elevated.[85,86,90]

The use of the central venous pressure to measure right atrial pressure is no longer considered sufficiently accurate because the relationship between the right atrial pressure and left ventricular end-diastolic pressure is inconsistent. Therefore PA end-diastolic pressure and pulmonary capillary wedge pressure, rather than central venous pressure, should be used as major guides in the treatment of heart failure and shock.

As the clinical features of heart failure worsen, they are usually accompanied by an elevation of the PA end-diastolic pressure and pulmonary capillary wedge pressure, a drop in cardiac output, a drop in arterial and right atrial

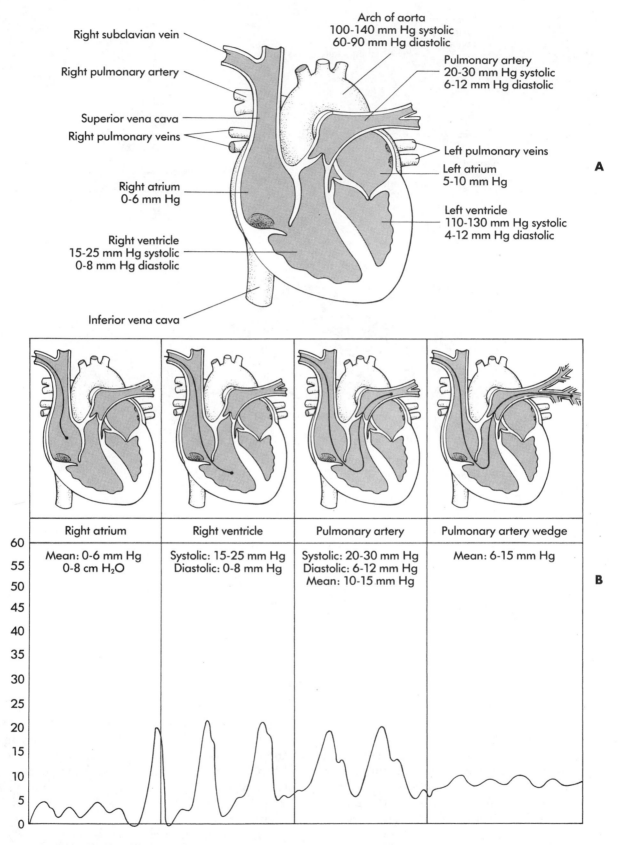

Fig. 8-11   **A,** Representation of the heart showing all four chambers and valves visible in the anterior view. Normal pressures are delineated for each chamber. **B,** PA catheter insertion with corresponding waveforms and pressures.   (From Flynn JM, Bruce N: *Introduction to critical care nursing skills,* St Louis, 1993, Mosby.)

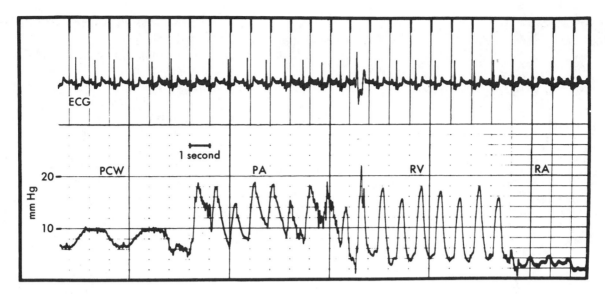

Fig. 8-12 Simultaneous recording of ECG and pulmonary capillary wedge *(PCW),* PA, right ventricular *(RV),* and right atrial *(RA)* pressures. The PA catheter was initially in a wedged position, with the balloon inflated. The balloon was then deflated, and the catheter was slowly withdrawn through the right heart chambers. Note the cyclic respiratory effects in the pressure signals. The pulmonary capillary wedge and PA end-diastolic pressures are equal. (From Mantle JA and others: *Advances in the treatment of heart failure.* In Rackley CF, editor: *Critical care cardiology: cardiovascular clinics,* vol 11, no 3, Philadelphia, 1981, Davis.)

oxygen saturations, and a widening of the oxygen difference between arterial and venous blood samples, commonly referred to as the *A-V oxygen difference.* The drop in arterial oxygen tension is a sign of abnormal lung function and is thought to result, at least in part, from elevation of left atrial pressure. Changes in pulmonary function include abnormalities of diffusion, particularly of oxygen; a redistribution of pulmonary blood flow into the less well-ventilated upper lobes; and intrapulmonary shunting. Not only is the arterial oxygen tension reduced in patients with acute infarction and shock, but it also fails to increase to expected values with the administration of oxygen, until pulmonary congestion has cleared.[90,91]

When right atrial oxygen saturation is reduced, a widened A-V oxygen difference and a low cardiac output can be suspected. If arterial oxygen saturation remains at normal levels, reduced right atrial oxygen saturation reflects increased extraction of oxygen during the passage of blood from the arterial to the venous circulation. A widened A-V oxygen difference reflects this increased extraction and indicates a reduced cardiac output. Right atrial and PA oxygen saturation can be useful indices of circulatory failure in patients with acute infarction. In addition to the bedside techniques for measuring PA pressure and pulmonary capillary wedge pressure, the simple test of determining whether the right atrial or PA oxygen saturation is above or below 65% is a useful guide to therapy. The use of

this variable is based on the Fick equation for measuring cardiac output.

$$\text{Cardiac output} = \frac{\text{Oxygen consumption}}{\text{A-V oxygen difference}}$$

Most PA catheters are equipped with a thermistor (temperature) electrode to measure cardiac output using the principle of thermodilution. The procedure involves the injection of cold or room-temperature solution into the right atrium or superior vena cava.[90,92] The temperature change is perceived by the thermistor electrode in the PA. Cardiac output is inversely proportional to the temperature change; that is, the greater the cardiac output, the less the temperature change. The use of such a catheter facilitates measurement of cardiac output and eliminates the need for a systemic arterial blood sample to determine cardiac output. Normal cardiac chamber oxygen values are found in Fig. 8-13. Normal cardiac output is 4 to 8 L/min. However, in the assessment of cardiac performance, the cardiac index—which is the cardiac output adjusted for body size and is calculated by dividing the cardiac output by the patient's body surface area—is a more useful indicator. The body surface area is calculated by obtaining the patient's height and weight and plotting them on a Dubois body surface area chart. Normal cardiac index is 2.5 to 4.2 L/min/m². In cardiogenic shock, the cardiogenic index is below 2.2 L/min/m².[88,89]

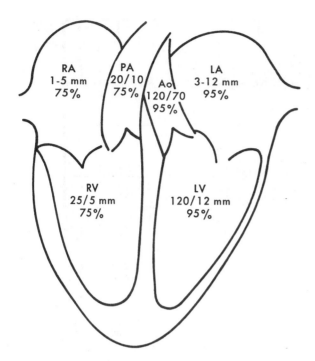

Fig. 8-13 Normal average cardiac pressures (mm Hg) and normal oxygen content (%) in each chamber.

Measurement of PA pressure and pulmonary capillary wedge pressure

The method used to record PA pressure, pulmonary capillary wedge pressure, or both from the standard strain gauge pressure transducer differs among institutions. Special points to consider in maintaining the catheter and measuring pressures include the following:

A. Obtaining measurements
 1. Record pressures at regular intervals as specified by the physician and as necessary. Evaluate changes and report to the physician as appropriate.
 2. Calibrate equipment before each measurement.
 3. Irrigate the line before each measurement by pulling the red rubber Intraflo plunger for 5 seconds (or manually if an Intraflo catheter is not used).
 4. Take measurements using the phlebostatic axis, which is located at the midaxillary line at the sixth intercostal space.
B. Maintaining the catheter
 1. Maintain patency of the catheter.
  a. Irrigate automatically with 3 ml of D5W or 0.9% NaCl or normal saline and heparin solution per hour, using an Intraflo catheter and maintaining the pressure bag at 300 mm Hg.
  b. Flush the catheter using the manual device at the transducer every 2 to 4 hours and as necessary.
  c. Measure irrigating solution used at the end of each shift as part of the intravenous intake.

d. Change the dressing as described in the section on arterial catheters.
 e. Observe for signs of infection, phlebitis, or both at the insertion site.
 2. Observe the complexes for changes in fluctuations.
  a. A flattened complex is caused by a possible wedging of the catheter in a pulmonary arteriole, which could result in pulmonary infarction. Turn the patient and ask the patient to cough and take some deep breaths; this may dislodge a catheter stuck in a wedge position. The physician should be notified so that the catheter can be repositioned.
  b. An irregular complex is an irregular fluctuation with no clear pressure waveform, indicating the need for irrigation with a 10-ml syringe. If this complex continues, the catheter is probably of no value and should be removed.
  c. An unobtainable wedge pattern occurs when the balloon is inflated and no wedge pattern is noted. The balloon is ruptured, or the catheter is out of position. The physician should be notified to reposition or remove the catheter.
  d. For no complex, check all stopcocks for proper position and follow with recalibration if needed.

Care of the Patient and PA Equipment

1. After insertion of the PA catheter, apply a sterile occlusive dressing to the site and change it at least every 48 hours. Note the condition of the site, including the presence of active bleeding and signs of infection.
2. If the femoral or brachial vein is used, immobilize the extremity to prevent accidental dislodgement of the catheter. Tape the catheter to the extremity to stabilize the catheter. A padded armboard or wooden device promotes comfort and immobilizes the extremity.
3. Check the extremity for circulatory insufficiency and bleeding at least every hour.
4. Observe the catheter frequently for leakage and proper stopcock position. Care should be taken to return the stopcock to the *off* position when drawing blood from the catheter.
5. The balloon should always remain deflated with a syringe attached, except when the pulmonary capillary wedge pressure is being read.
6. After the catheter is removed, observe the site closely for bleeding and infection until healing is complete. Apply a sterile dressing to the site.

Potential problems in the use of PA catheters

Several complications may occur from the use of a PA catheter. The major complication, pulmonary hemorrhage, may result if the balloon is inflated when the catheter tip is in a small arterial branch; however, careful adherence to proper procedures for balloon inflation minimizes this risk. The catheter tip may become wedged in a distal branch after repeated inflations, which may lead to a pulmonary infarction. When the catheter tip is withdrawn from the wedged position, it often recoils into the right ventricle or right atrium and must be repositioned.[92] Particular changes in the PA waveform configuration indicate that the catheter has slipped into the right ventricle (see Fig. 8-11, *A*). Other complications associated with PA catheters include dysrhythmias, thrombosis, intracardiac knotting, ruptured balloon, valve damage, and infection.[93]

Measurement of arterial pressure

In addition to hemodynamic monitoring, arterial pressure monitoring is useful for the continuous assessment of blood pressure and rapid access for frequent blood specimens.

When monitoring arterial pressure directly, personnel must carefully observe the following precautions to obtain meaningful values:

1. Standardize, balance, and calibrate the monitoring equipment every 4 to 8 hours and after position changes or movements that might alter the calibration. Instructions for this procedure accompany the manufacturer's equipment.
2. Use a continuous flush device to provide a prescribed flow rate of a solution of D5W or normal saline with or without heparin.[94] Flush the catheter manually to clear the line after blood is drawn or if blood is in the line for any reason. The pulse waveform becomes dampened or flattened somewhat if impairment of flow occurs.
3. Prevent catheter displacement by fastening the arterial catheter securely to the skin. The catheter may be sutured to the skin after insertion. Keep pressure alarm limits set and turned on at all times so that dislodgement at the catheter can be immediately detected.
4. Prevent blood from entering the transducer. Blood in the transducer dampens the pressure reading and may damage the transducer.
5. Observe the extremity in which the catheter is inserted every 1 to 2 hours for bleeding and check for circulatory insufficiency by capillary refill, skin temperature, and distal pulses. Check the arterial catheter frequently for leakage and proper stopcock position.
6. Apply a sterile occlusion dressing to the site, and change it at least once every 48 hours. Avoid the use of antimicrobial ointments at the insertion site. Povidone-iodine ointment at the insertion site is recommended to prevent infection.
7. Immobilize the extremity to prevent accidental dislodgement of the catheter. If an armboard or wooden device is used, proper padding prevents stasis changes of skin and increases comfort.
8. Exercise care when drawing blood from the catheter. The stopcock must be returned to the original position to ensure proper operation and prevent leakage.

9. After removing the catheter, apply direct pressure to the artery for at least 10 to 15 minutes, until bleeding ceases. The site should be covered with a sterile pressure dressing for 24 hours.
10. After the catheter is removed, observe the site for signs of bleeding, infection, and circulatory insufficiency until healing is complete. If any of these are noted, immediate attention should be given to correction of the condition.

Additional Approaches to Hemodynamic Monitoring

Thermodilution cardiac output has been measured by injection of a bolus of room-temperature or cool fluid through a proximal port of a PA catheter. A thermistor at the tip of the catheter measures the change in temperature, displaying a curve that depicts the temperature change over time. From this information, the computer can calculate cardiac output.[92] A new PA catheter provides continuous cardiac output measurement. This catheter has a heating element on its surface at the right ventricular area. The element heats the blood for 3 seconds, and the change in temperature is recognized at the distal thermistor. The advantages of this system are reduced fluid intake, reduced risk of infection from injectate, reduced nursing time, reduced number of measurement errors and errors related to poor injection technique, and update of the cardiac output measurement within minutes to guide therapy[95,96] (Fig. 8-14).

Continuous mixed venous oxygen saturation (O_2) can be performed with another special PA catheter with a fiberoptic sensor at the tip. The fiberoptic emits light across the blood in the PA, illuminating the red blood cells. The light is absorbed by desaturated hemoglobin and reflected by oxyhemoglobin. The fiberoptic sensor records the reflection of the light, and the computer calculates the percentage of saturation of the venous blood. Measurement of venous oxygen saturation provides a continuous analysis that reflects the oxygen supply-demand balance. Normal range is 60% to 80%, reflecting the fact that the body uses the remaining 20% to 40% of oxygen to meet the usual needs.[97] A drop may result from a decrease in oxygen delivery (anemia, hypoxia, decreased cardiac output) or an increase in oxygen demand (fever, shivering, activity). An increase is due to an increase in oxygen delivery (increased fractional inspired oxygen concentration) or a decrease in oxygen demand (anesthesia, paralysis, hypothermia). Venous oxygen saturation monitoring provides an indication of tissue oxygenation and is advantageous when observing a person who has acute or chronic pulmonary dysfunction[91,98] (Fig. 8-15).

Right ventricular volumetric monitoring is the final innovation in hemodynamic monitoring. This device is used to calculate right ventricular ejection fraction to obtain more information about volume load of that chamber.[99,100] Right ventricular ejection fraction is calculated

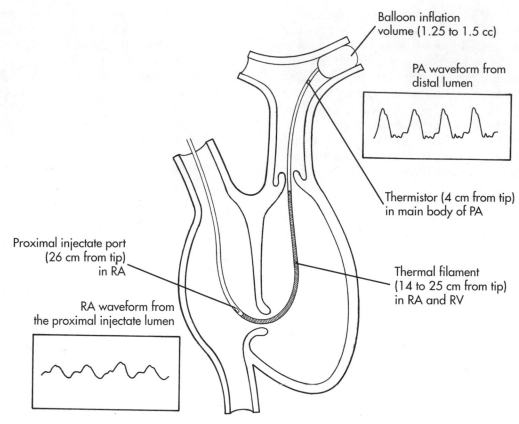

Balloon inflation
volume (1.25 to 1.5 cc)

PA waveform from
distal lumen

Thermistor (4 cm from tip)
in main body of PA

Thermal filament
(14 to 25 cm from tip)
in RA and RV

Proximal injectate port
(26 cm from tip)
in RA

RA waveform from
the proximal injectate lumen

Fig. 8-14   Continuous cardiac output thermodilution catheter characteristics and placement. (Courtesy Baxter Healthcare Corp, Edwards Critical-Care Division, Santa Ana, Calif.)

by comparing the ECG with the thermodilution cardiac output curve. The change in volume marked for each cardiac cycle represents the stroke volume. Right ventricular ejection fraction can be extrapolated from this calculation (Fig. 8-16).

Treatment of shock

The term used to describe the problem of patients in cardiogenic shock with or without congestive heart failure is *pump failure*. Goldberg and others,[101] report a 7.5% incidence of shock with 44% occurring on the first day of the infarct. Most studies indicate a mortality rate of at least 80% in cardiogenic shock during the course of MI; unfortunately, therapeutic measures have not affected these figures.

Although the primary therapeutic goals are to increase cardiac contractility and maintain renal blood flow, there is no clear-cut regimen for the treatment of cardiogenic shock that can be applied to all patients, since therapy depends on the specific findings in the individual. Therefore so that the physician can direct treatment intelligently, as much clinical and hemodynamic information as possible should be available.

Therapy, as well as the natural evolution of the shock state, may change these values; therefore measurements

should be repeated as often as necessary. Clinical management of the patient in cardiogenic shock is divided into general and specific measures as follows:

A. General therapeutic measures
1. Have patient assume a supine position with a pillow. The Trendelenburg position is not recommended for cardiogenic shock.
2. Relieve pain with intravenous doses of morphine (5 to 10 mg initially) just sufficient to be effective. Large doses of morphine sulfate should be avoided if possible. Observe for lowering of arterial pressure.
3. Insert a Foley catheter to measure hourly urine output as an index of kidney function. Maintain urine output at a minimum of 20 ml/hr to prevent renal failure.
4. Insert an intraarterial needle or catheter to monitor arterial blood pressure, blood gas levels, pH, cardiac output, A-V oxygen difference, and peripheral resistance.
5. Insert a balloon-tipped, flow-directed catheter to monitor PA end-diastolic pressure, pulmonary capillary wedge pressure, and cardiac output as a reflection of left ventricular performance.

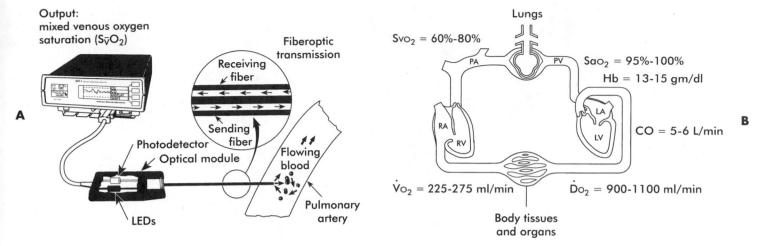

Fig. 8-15 **A,** Continuous monitoring of mixed venous oxygen saturation *(Svo2).* The monitoring system consists of a fiberoptic catheter, an optical module, and an oximeter. Light of selected wavelengths is transmitted down one fiberoptic filament in the catheter body to the blood flowing past the catheter tip. The reflected light is then transmitted back through the second fiberoptic filament to a photodetector in the optical module. Since hemoglobin and oxyhemoglobin absorb light differently at the selected wavelengths, the reflected light can be analyzed to determine the percent of venous oxygen saturation. *LEDs,* Light-emitting diodes. **B,** Simplified diagram of the human circulatory system with normal values. Blood leaves the lungs with an arterial oxygen saturation (SaO$_2$) of 95% to 100%. Hemoglobin *(Hb),* at a concentration of 13 to 15 g/dl, transports the oxygen in the blood. The left ventricle *(LV)* pumps the blood to body tissues at a cardiac output *(CO)* of 5 to 6 L/min. The oxygen delivery *(Do2)* to the tissues is 900 to 1100 ml/min. At rest the body tissues use the oxygen at an oxygen consumption *(Vo2)* rate of 225 to 275 ml/min. The venous blood carrying the remaining oxygen then returns to the heart and is pumped through the PA towards the lungs. The mixed venous oxygen saturation *(Svo2)* is measured in the PA and reflects a mixture of all of the venous blood saturations from many body tissues. The normal Svo$_2$ is 60% to 80%. (Courtesy Baxter Healthcare Corp, Edwards Critical-Care Division, Santa Ana, Calif.)

B. Specific therapeutic goals
  1. Correct dysrhythmias and establish an appropriate heart rate. If the heart rate is above normal but not in the abnormal tachycardia range, no special therapy is necessary. If the rate is abnormally slow, the use of atropine in patients with MI may be considered. For the symptomatic (ventricular ectopic systoles, hypotension) patient with sinus bradycardia, atropine is clearly indicated. For the asymptomatic patient with sinus bradycardia, it would appear best not to administer atropine but to monitor closely. When atropine is indicated, initial doses should be in the range of 0.4 to 0.6 mg intravenously, repeating with 0.2 to 0.4 mg if the initial dose does not produce the desired effect. If atropine does not raise the heart rate sufficiently to eliminate the symptoms accompanying the slower rate or if the cause of the low heart rate is complete heart block, then transcutaneous or transvenous temporary pacing should be considered. Also, isoproterenol (Isuprel) in a continuous infusion may be indicated to increase

heart rate. However, isoproterenol may increase myocardial oxygen consumption.
  2. Correct hypovolemia. Older patients with MIs are prime candidates for relative hypovolemia, especially if they have been receiving diuretics or are on low-sodium diets. The acute stages of AMI are associated with a reduced fluid intake because of pain or resulting from analgesic therapy and nausea and vomiting. Further routes of fluid loss are profuse sweating, diarrhea secondary to medication administration, vigorous treatment with diuretics, and phlebotomy. Consequently, patients showing evidence of low cardiac output with hypotension and oliguria may be given a trial of fluid loading particularly if the PA end-diastolic pressure and pulmonary capillary wedge pressure are low. Patients with evidence of severe pulmonary congestion are not suitable for this therapy. With low PA end-diastolic pressure and pulmonary capillary wedge pressure, normal saline, blood products, or low molecular dextran may be infused until the pulmonary

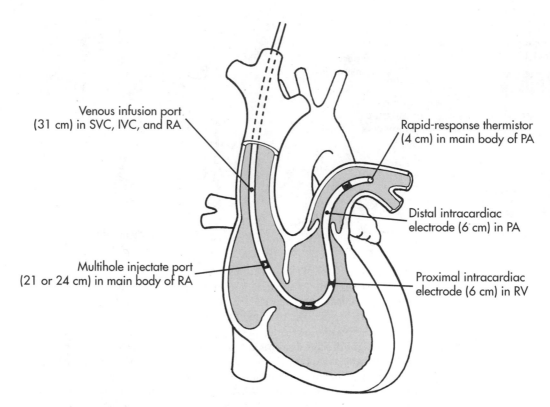

Fig. 8-16 PA, right ventricular *(RV)* ejection fraction/volumetric catheter characteristics and position. *SVC,* Superior vena cava; *IVC,* inferior vena cava; *RA,* right atrium. (Courtesy Baxter Healthcare Corp, Edwards Critical-Care Division, Santa Ana, Calif.)

capillary wedge pressure reaches 15 to 18 mm Hg. Current experience indicates that the pulmonary capillary wedge pressure should be kept slightly elevated in patients with cardiogenic shock.

3. Correct hypoxemia. Hypoxia with arterial oxygen pressure values below the level of 70 to 75 mm Hg while the patient is receiving nasal oxygen indicates that the patient's lungs should probably be intubated and given positive pressure or volume assistance and 100% oxygen.

4. Correct acidosis. When circulatory impairment exists, the metabolic activity of the perfused cells of the body changes, and lactic acid and other metabolic products are released into the vascular system and ineffectively metabolized; as a result, systemic acidosis develops. This state contributes to poor tissue perfusion and is indicated by the blood pH. The complication is treated with sodium bicarbonate given intravenously while taking precautions not to produce sodium overload.

5. Improve cardiac contractility. Use of digitalis in the management of cardiogenic shock is not well supported by existing data. The positive inotropic effect of digitalis preparations improves contractility but significantly increases myocardial oxygen demand. Other agents that enhance the state of cardiac contractility have been used in cardiogenic shock. In patients with adequate filling pressures and normal or increased peripheral resistance, dopamine hydrochloride, dobutamine, or amrinone can cause a significant increase in cardiac output. Dopamine has an inotropic-vasoconstrictor effect and causes renal vasodilatation at low doses. Dobutamine increases contractility, stroke volume, and cardiac output, and decreases systemic vascular resistance. Amrinone has no effect on blood pressure or heart rate but decreases pulmonary capillary wedge pressure, systemic resistance, and myocardial oxygen consumption.[87]

6. Improve circulation. Clinical estimates of the degree of increased peripheral resistance usually present in the shock syndrome can be made from the degree of increased venous pressure, the amount of decrease in pulse pressure, the decrease in cutaneous blood flow with cold and cyanotic extremities, the poorly palpable peripheral pulses in spite of bounding pulsations, urine flow, and the clinical appearance of the patient. If these findings persist, a dangerously in-

appropriate, prolonged period of peripheral vaso-constriction may exist. If the patient exhibits signs of the shock syndrome with a low or normal calculated peripheral resistance, an infusion of a drug with combined α- and β-adrenergic properties may be considered. Norepinephrine (Levarterenol, Levophed) is used to increase arterial blood pressures and improve perfusion of ischemic areas of myocardium that are functionally depressed. The elevated pressure may open existing or latent coronary collateral channels, which require a relatively high pressure to maintain blood flow through them, bypassing concomitant areas of arterial atherosclerosis. Consequently this drug improves myocardial function and increases cardiac output. However, at the same time, it increases cardiac afterload (resistance against which the ventricle pumps) and thus myocardial oxygen consumption. Therefore the use of this agent should be aimed at producing the desired balance between coronary perfusion and afterload.

Vasodilators are used to decrease preload and afterload in patients with cardiogenic shock. A decrease in preload caused by venous dilatation causes a decrease in pulmonary congestive pressure and a decrease in myocardial oxygen consumption. A reduction in afterload improves left ventricular ejection and stroke volume. Commonly used vasodilators include nitroprusside and nitroglycerin given intravenously. Current studies of these drugs show promise in patients with increased pulmonary capillary wedge pressures and signs of left ventricular failure. They should not be used if the arterial pressure is below 90 mm Hg unless they are used with dopamine to maintain an adequate blood pressure.[87]

Intraaortic balloon pumping

In addition to pharmacologic therapy, intraaortic balloon pumping (IABP), also referred to as *counterpulsation,* may be required to treat cardiogenic shock. IABP can improve cardiac output, reduce evidence of myocardial ischemia, relieve pain, and reduce ST-segment elevation. Other indications include severe congestive heart failure, medically refractory ischemia, ventricular septal defects, and left main coronary stenosis. In most instances, the IABP provides additional protection for the myocardium until surgery can be done.

In this procedure the balloon is inserted percutaneously into the femoral artery and positioned in the descending aorta just below the origin of the left subclavian artery. The catheter is connected to a console that controls the inflation and deflation of the balloon with helium. The balloon is inflated and deflated in a cyclic fashion, according to the cardiac rhythm of the patient. An ECG and arterial waveform are used to time the inflations and deflations of the balloon. The balloon is inflated during diastole, increasing aortic diastolic pressure and coronary perfusion, and thus improving myocardial oxygen supply. Balloon inflation during diastole (and the resulting increased pressure) does not affect the left ventricle because the aortic valve is closed. The intraaortic balloon is deflated during ventricular systole and thus partially empties the aorta. The effect is to decrease the resistance to ventricular ejection (afterload), allowing the left ventricle to eject blood with less effort. This decreases myocardial work and myocardial oxygen consumption.

Timing of the inflation and deflation of the balloon are correlated with the ECG, the arterial waveform, or both. On the ECG, the R wave triggers balloon deflation. Inflation is triggered on the downslope of the T wave or a set time interval after the R wave. The arterial waveform may be used for manual adjustment or fine tuning of the balloon pump. Inflation should be adjusted first and should occur at the beginning of diastole, represented by the dicrotic notch on the arterial waveform. Deflation should occur at the very end of diastole or just before ventricular systole. (Fig. 8-17 illustrates timing of the IABP.) Pumping options on the balloon console range from 1:1 (every heartbeat is assisted) to 1:8 (every eighth beat is assisted). The usual therapeutic option is 1:1. Adjustment of timing should be done in the 1:2 mode (or greater) to allow comparison of an assisted beat to an unassisted beat. Timing should be assessed every hour and with any change in the patient's condition.[102]

Complications of IABP therapy include arterial wall injury, compromise of peripheral circulation, bleeding, and infection. Arterial wall injury may occur during insertion of the balloon or as a result of catheter dislodgement and migration. Compromise of the peripheral circulation may be caused by plaque dislodgement, thrombus formation, gas emboli, improper placement or migration of the balloon, or incorrectly timed counterpulsation. It is important to assess pulses, temperature, and sensation of extremities before and at least every hour after insertion of the balloon. The head of the bed should be elevated no more than 30 degrees. The affected leg should not be flexed. The patient should be turned every 2 hours by log-rolling technique. Anticoagulant therapy (usually heparin) is required to prevent thrombus formation on the balloon. Close monitoring of the prothrombin time, partial thromboplastin time, hemoglobin levels, hematocrit, and platelet levels is required, and the insertion site should be observed frequently for bleeding. The patient should be monitored for signs of internal bleeding such as tachycardia, hypotension, a drop in the hemoglobin level or the hematocrit, and low back pain, which may be a sign of retroperitoneal bleeding.[102,103] IABP therapy may cause stress ulcers. For this reason, all stools and nasogastric drainage should be checked for occult blood. Antacids, histamine 2 antagonists, or both may be used to neutralize or block the secretion of excess stomach acids. Strict attention to sterile

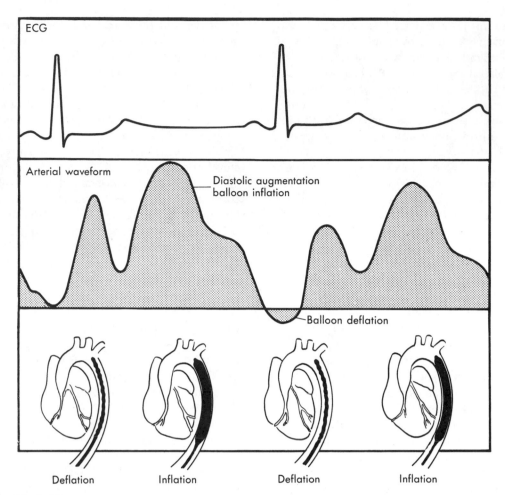

ECG

Arterial waveform

Diastolic augmentation
balloon inflation

Balloon deflation

Deflation   Inflation   Deflation   Inflation

Fig. 8-17 Two counterpulsation cycles. The balloon is inflated during diastole, thus "augmenting" diastolic pressure. Deflation occurs during isovolumetric contraction. Because balloon inflation displaced intraaortic balloon volume, aortic end-diastolic pressure is "lowered" during balloon deflation.   (From Quaal SJ: *Comprehensive intra-aortic balloon counterpulsation,* ed 2, St Louis, 1993, Mosby.)

technique is necessary to prevent infection in an already compromised patient. Dressings should be changed daily and as needed, and the insertion site should be checked for redness, swelling, or drainage. The Foley catheter should be taped to the opposite leg to avoid contamination of the IABP insertion site. The patient's temperature should be monitored every 4 hours. It is also important to provide emotional support to the patient and family. Clear, simple explanations of the equipment and procedures should be given, and the patient and family should be provided with frequent updates on the patient's progress.

Dysrhythmias

Dysrhythmias can compromise cardiac function by reducing cardiac output and coronary blood flow, increasing the myocardial need for oxygen, predisposing the patient to more serious dysrhythmias, and complicating therapy.

Therefore prompt prevention and control of dysrhythmias and the states predisposing to them (acidosis, electrolyte imbalance, early cardiac failure, pain, and anxiety) decrease the incidence of more serious dysrhythmias and should improve the chances for survival after MI. Awareness of these facts underscores the importance of detecting dysrhythmias through cardiac monitoring.

Dysrhythmias can be divided into two categories: acutely life-threatening and potentially life-threatening. Acutely life-threatening dysrhythmias include ventricular fibrillation, ventricular tachycardia without a pulse, and asystole. Potentially life-threatening dysrhythmias include ventricular tachycardia with a pulse and its precursors, supraventricular tachydysrhythmias and bradydysrhythmias. Because of the life-threatening nature of some dysrhythmias, it is necessary that the staff be certified in basic cardiac life support (BCLS) as defined by the American Heart

Association or the American Red Cross. Personnel must also be trained to perform other procedures, including preparing medication, recording times of events and medication given, and assisting as necessary with activities during the resuscitation effort.

Certification in the skills of advanced cardiac life support (ACLS) is also important for coronary care personnel. ACLS includes all the skills of BCLS in addition to the techniques of endotracheal intubation, venipuncture, dysrhythmia interpretation, and drug administration.

Defibrillation and Cardioversion

Transthoracic defibrillation delivers electric energy to the heart by means of metal paddles placed on the intact chest or placed directly on the heart when the chest is opened (for example, during cardiac surgery). This procedure depolarizes the excitable myocardium, thereby interrupting reentrant circuits and discharging automatic pacemaker foci to establish electric homogeneity. Defibrillation successfully restores sinus rhythm if the sinus node becomes the first automatic focus to fire after the electric shock and thus controls the packing function of the heart.

When the capacitor is synchronized to discharge during the downslope of the R wave or with the S wave, the vulnerable period of the ventricle (an interval of 20 to 40 msec near the apex of the T wave) may be avoided. This minimizes but does not completely eliminate the danger of precipitating ventricular fibrillation with the direct-current shock. Defibrillation with synchronization of the R wave is called *cardioversion* and is always used if the patient has a pulse. However, when the patient has no pulse and immediate defibrillation is indicated, the shock is delivered asynchronously. Immediate defibrillation using 200 joules is the mandatory treatment for ventricular fibrillation and ventricular tachycardia without a pulse. If the tachydysrhythmia does not terminate promptly, immediate defibrillation should be performed a second time using 200 to 300 joules. If this is unsuccessful, a third shock is delivered using 360 joules. If defibrillation is unsuccessful, intravenous drug therapy should begin with epinephrine followed by lidocaine, bretylium tosylate, magnesium sulfate, or procainamide.[51] Short, limited bursts of ventricular tachycardia are treated medically. As a general rule, supraventricular tachydysrhythmias that produce signs or symptoms such as hypotension, angina, or congestive heart failure and do not respond promptly to medical therapy should be terminated electrically. CPR is performed during this period as indicated by patient condition. See ACLS algorithms for ventricular tachycardia and fibrillation (Fig. 8-18).

An elective cardioversion may be done wherever resuscitative aids such as suction, intubation equipment, medications, and experienced personnel trained in airway management are available. Cardioversion may be indicated for

ventricular tachycardia in the patient who is alert and/or has a pulse but is unresponsive to medical therapy or who has controlled atrial fibrillation. The cardioversion procedure follows:

1. Explain the procedure to the patient and obtain written *informed* consent.
2. Withhold diuretics and short-acting digitalis preparations for 24 to 36 hours. However, it has been suggested that discontinuing digitalis in nontoxic, normokalemic patients may not be necessary. If indicated, obtain a serum potassium or serum digitalis level. Hypokalemia enhances electric instability and may increase the likelihood of dysrhythmias after cardioversion.[51]
3. Withhold food and drink for 6 to 8 hours before cardioversion.
4. Perform a thorough physical examination, including vital signs, mentation, and palpation of pulse.
5. Obtain a 12-lead ECG before and after cardioversion, as well as a rhythm strip, oscilloscopic monitoring, or both during procedure.
6. Maintain a patent intravenous access.
7. If the patient has dentures, remove them.
8. Allow the patient to breathe oxygen for 5 to 15 minutes before and then immediately after direct-current shock if not contraindicated; this promotes myocardial oxygenation. During cardioversion, the presence of oxygen with electric arcing may encourage combustion.
9. Use the synchronous discharge mode on the defibrillator/cardioverter. The QRS complex recorded on the oscilloscope must be tall to ensure that it alone triggers the capacitor discharge. Determine the accuracy of synchronization by discharging several test shocks before applying the paddles to the patient.
10. Administer diazepam or another medication (such as methohexital [Brevital] or midazolam [Versed] prescribed to produce transient amnesia or light sleep.
11. Apply electrode paste liberally but not excessively to the polished surface of the paddles (or use gel defibrillation pads), and then place them in firm contact with the chest wall at points distant from the monitoring electrodes. The paddles may be positioned anterioposteriorly in the left infrascapular region and over the upper sternum at the third interspace or anteriorly to the right of the sternum at the second intercostal space and in the left midclavicular line at the fifth intercostal space.
12. Using the minimum effective electric energy level reduces complications; therefore the starting level for most dysrhythmias is around 50 joules or less (Fig. 8-19). The energy necessary to terminate some dysrhythmias, such as atrial flutter or ventricular tachycardia, may be considerably less. If unsuccessful, this initial level may be increased to 100 joules and then

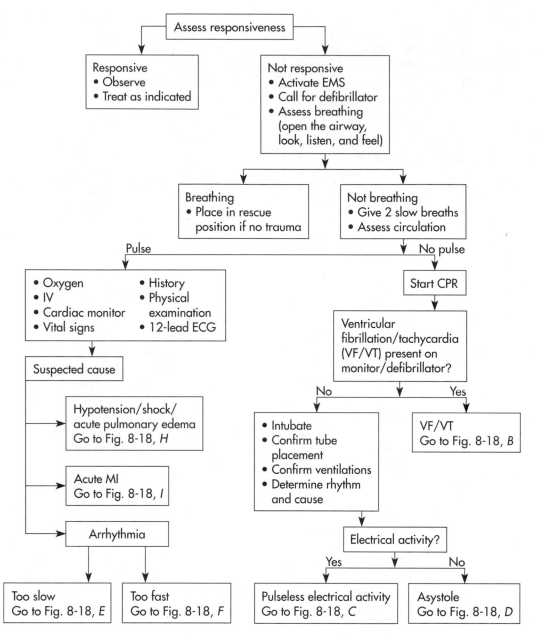

Fig. 8-18   ACLS universal algorithms. **A,** Adult emergency care.   (From American Medical Association: New ACLS guidelines: 1992, *JAMA* 268(16):2216, 1992.)

by 100-joule increments until a level of 360 joules is reached. Make sure that all personnel have moved away from the patient and the bed before discharging the defibrillator, and call out "all clear."

13. Record the postshock rhythm to determine whether the procedure was successful. V_1 or MCL_1 lead recording is preferable. An oscilloscope interpretation is frequently unreliable.

14. Continue rhythm monitoring and close observations of cardiovascular and pulmonary status for 2 to 3 hours until the patient's condition is stable after cardioversion.

15. Precautions
   a. When digitalis excess is suspected, electric cardioversion should be deferred and the dysrhythmia initially treated with medication to prevent pro-

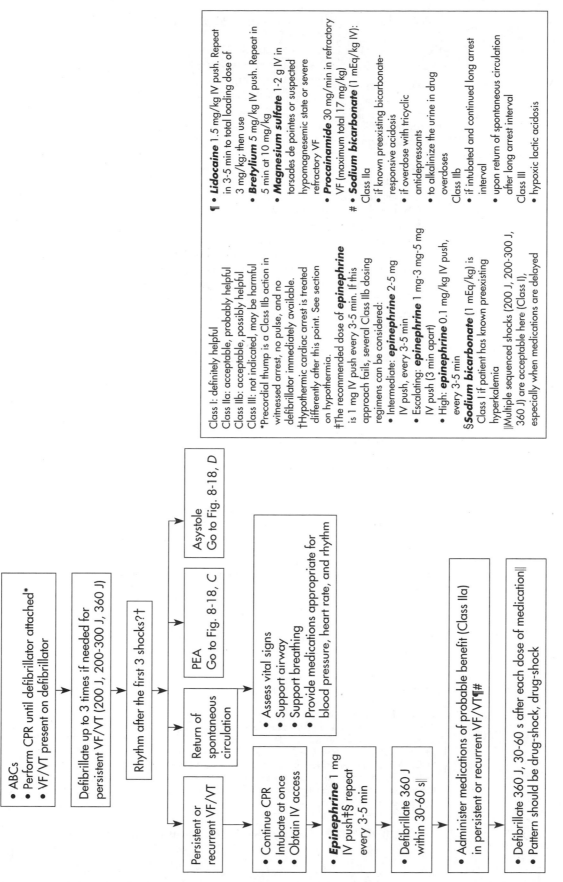

Fig. 8-18, cont'd B, Ventricular fibrillation and pulseless ventricular tachycardia.

PEA includes
- Electromechanical dissociation (EMD)
- Pseudo-EMD
- Idioventricular rhythms
- Ventricular escape rhythms
- Bradyasystolic rhythms
- Postdefibrillation idioventricular rhythms

- Continue CPR
- Intubate at once
- Obtain IV access
- Assess blood flow using Doppler ultrasound

↓

Consider possible causes
(Parentheses=possible therapies and treatments)
- Hypovolemia (volume infusion)
- Hypoxia (ventilation)
- Cardiac tamponade (pericardiocentesis)
- Tension pneumothorax (needle decompression)
- Hypothermia (see hypothermia algorithm, Section IV)
- Massive pulmonary embolism (surgery, ***thrombolytics***)
- Drug overdoses such as tricyclics, digitalis, β-blockers, calcium channel blockers
- Hyperkalemia*
- Acidosis†
- * Massive acute myocardial infarction (go to Fig. 8-18, *I*)

↓

- ***Epinephrine*** 1 mg IV push, *‡ repeat every 3-5 min

↓

- If absolute bradycardia (<60 beats/min) or relative bradycardia, give ***atropine*** 1 mg IV
- Repeat every 3-5 min up to a total of 0.04 mg/kg§

Class I: definitely helpful
Class IIa: acceptable, probably helpful
Class IIb: acceptable, possibly helpful
Class III: not indicated, may be harmful
****Sodium bicarbonate*** 1 mEq/kg is Class I if patient has known preexisting hyperkalemia.
†***Sodium bicarbonate*** 1 mEq/kg:
Class IIa
- if known preexisting bicarbonate-responsive acidosis
- if overdose with tricyclic antidepressants
- to alkalinize the urine in drug overdoses
Class IIb
- if intubated and long arrest interval
- upon return of spontaneous circulation after long arrest interval
Class III
- hypoxic lactic acidosis
‡The recommended dose of ***epinephrine*** is 1 mg IV push every 3-5 min.
If this approach fails, several Class IIb dosing regimens can be considered.
- Intermediate: ***epinephrine*** 2-5 mg IV push, every 3-5 min
- Escalating: ***epinephrine*** 1 mg-3 mg-5 mg IV push (3 min apart)
- High: ***epinephrine*** 0.1 mg/kg IV push, every 3-5 min
§Shorter ***atropine*** dosing intervals are possibly helpful in cardiac arrest (Class IIb).

Fig. 8-18, cont'd   **C,** Pulseless electrical activity (PEA).

- Continue CPR
- Intubate at once
- Obtain IV access
- Confirm asystole in more than one lead

↓

Consider possible causes
- Hypoxia
- Hyperkalemia
- Hypokalemia
- Preexisting acidosis
- Drug overdose
- Hypothermia

↓

Consider immediate transcutaneous pacing (TCP)*

↓

- **Epinephrine** 1 mg IV push,†‡ repeat every 3-5 min

↓

- **Atropine** 1 mg IV, repeat every 3-5 min up to a total of 0.04 mg/kg§∥

↓

Consider
- Termination of efforts¶

Class I: definitely helpful
Class IIa: acceptable, probably helpful
Class IIb: acceptable, possibly helpful
Class III: not indicated, may be harmful
*TCP is a Class IIb intervention. Lack of success may be due to delays in pacing. To be effective TCP must be performed early, simultaneously with drugs. Evidence does not support routine use of TCP for asystole.
†The recommended dose of **epinephrine** is 1 mg IV push every 3-5 min. If this approach fails, several Class IIb dosing regimens can be considered:
- Intermediate: **epinephrine** 2-5 mg IV push, every 3-5 min
- Escalating: **epinephrine** 1 mg-3 mg-5 mg IV push (3 min apart)
- High: **epinephrine** 0.1 mg/kg IV push, every 3-5 min
‡**Sodium bicarbonate** (1 mEq/kg) is Class I if patient has known preexisting hyperkalemia.

§Shorter **atropine** dosing intervals are Class IIb in asystolic arrest.
∥**Sodium bicarbonate** 1 mEq/kg:
Class IIa
- if known preexisting bicarbonate-responsive acidosis
- if overdose with tricyclic antidepressants
- to alkalinize the urine in drug overdoses
Class IIb
- if intubated and continued long arrest interval
- upon return of spontaneous circulation after long arrest interval
Class III
- hypoxic lactic acidosis
¶If patient remains in asystole or other agonal rhythms after successful intubation and initial medications and no reversible causes are identified, consider termination of resuscitative efforts by a physician. Consider interval since arrest.

Fig. 8-18, cont'd   D, Asystole.

duction of serious ventricular tachydysrhythmias and failure to terminate the digitalis-related dysrhythmia.

b. Emergency drugs and equipment needed for pacing, intubation, or suction must be available.

c. If using electrode paste, avoid coating the paddles excessively or placing them too near monitoring electrodes, which may allow a spark to jump and burn the skin. Local skin inflammation caused by the paddles is best treated with a topical steroid preparation.

d. Certain dysrhythmias may occur after cardioversion; therefore monitoring the rhythm must continue for 2 to 3 hours. Other complications may include embolic episodes, which occur in 1% to 3% of patients after the dysrhythmia is converted to sinus rhythm.

Electrophysiologic monitoring

When the modified PA catheter is in the right atrium at the junction of the superior vena cava, stable ECGs of high quality can be obtained. These high-fidelity ECGs allow rapid and accurate diagnosis of various complex dysrhythmias. Because of the limited noise in the ECG signal, con-

tinuous qualitative interval measurements by a computerized system are possible. Moreover, the stable intracavitary electrode position provides a reliable atrial pacing site for converting supraventricular tachycardias, for maintaining an adequate rate during sinus bradycardia, and for suppressing ventricular premature beats by rapid atrial pacing rates. This multipurpose catheter provides safe and convenient monitoring for long periods in patients with unstable cardiopulmonary problems.

Circulatory Arrest

Resuscitation begun during the first 3 to 4 minutes after circulatory arrest usually prevents irreversible cerebral damage. Ventricular fibrillation, rather than ventricular asystole, commonly precipitates the arrest. Defibrillation procedures should be initiated in a CCU within 30 seconds of onset of the arrest. Prompt reversion to sinus rhythm often prevents the biochemical derangements that accompany ventricular fibrillation, eliminates the need for endotracheal intubation, and significantly increases the success rate of resuscitation attempts. After a successful resuscitation, it is important that measures be taken to prevent recurrence of the cardiac arrest. Prophylactic lidocaine and cardiac pacing can be used to prevent extrasystoles, bradycardia, or both,

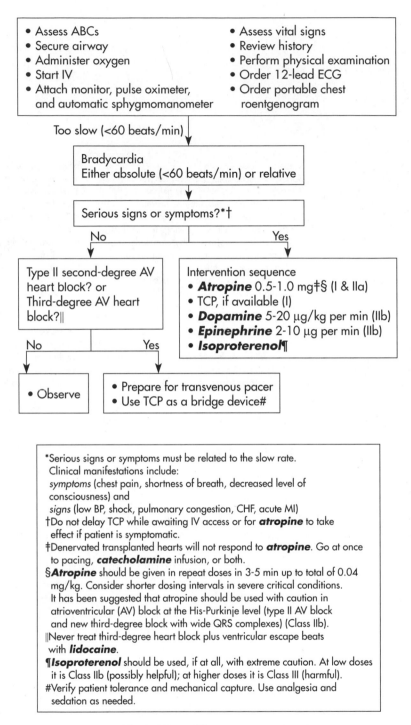

- Assess ABCs
- Secure airway
- Administer oxygen
- Start IV
- Attach monitor, pulse oximeter, and automatic sphygmomanometer

- Assess vital signs
- Review history
- Perform physical examination
- Order 12-lead ECG
- Order portable chest roentgenogram

Too slow (<60 beats/min)

Bradycardia
Either absolute (<60 beats/min) or relative

Serious signs or symptoms?*†

No

Type II second-degree AV heart block? or Third-degree AV heart block?‖

No   Yes

Yes

Intervention sequence
- *Atropine* 0.5-1.0 mg‡§ (I & IIa)
- TCP, if available (I)
- *Dopamine* 5-20 μg/kg per min (IIb)
- *Epinephrine* 2-10 μg per min (IIb)
- *Isoproterenol*¶

- Observe

- Prepare for transvenous pacer
- Use TCP as a bridge device#

*Serious signs or symptoms must be related to the slow rate.
  Clinical manifestations include:
  symptoms (chest pain, shortness of breath, decreased level of consciousness) and
  signs (low BP, shock, pulmonary congestion, CHF, acute MI)
†Do not delay TCP while awaiting IV access or for *atropine* to take effect if patient is symptomatic.
‡Denervated transplanted hearts will not respond to *atropine*. Go at once to pacing, *catecholamine* infusion, or both.
§*Atropine* should be given in repeat doses in 3-5 min up to total of 0.04 mg/kg. Consider shorter dosing intervals in severe critical conditions. It has been suggested that atropine should be used with caution in atrioventricular (AV) block at the His-Purkinje level (type II AV block and new third-degree block with wide QRS complexes) (Class IIb).
‖Never treat third-degree heart block plus ventricular escape beats with *lidocaine*.
¶*Isoproterenol* should be used, if at all, with extreme caution. At low doses it is Class IIb (possibly helpful); at higher doses it is Class III (harmful).
#Verify patient tolerance and mechanical capture. Use analgesia and sedation as needed.

Fig. 8-18, cont'd   E, Bradycardia.

since these dysrhythmias may foreshadow the occurrence of ventricular tachycardia and fibrillation.

When the monitor alarm is activated or the dysrhythmia is observed on the oscilloscope, personnel must correlate the observed rhythm with the patient's clinical status by rapidly evaluating the patient's orientation, respirations, pupils, and carotid or femoral pulses. Loose leads can produce a rhythmic pattern simulating ventricular fibrillation. Moreover, a lidocaine reaction can mimic the disoriented state seen in tachydysrhythmias associated with inadequate

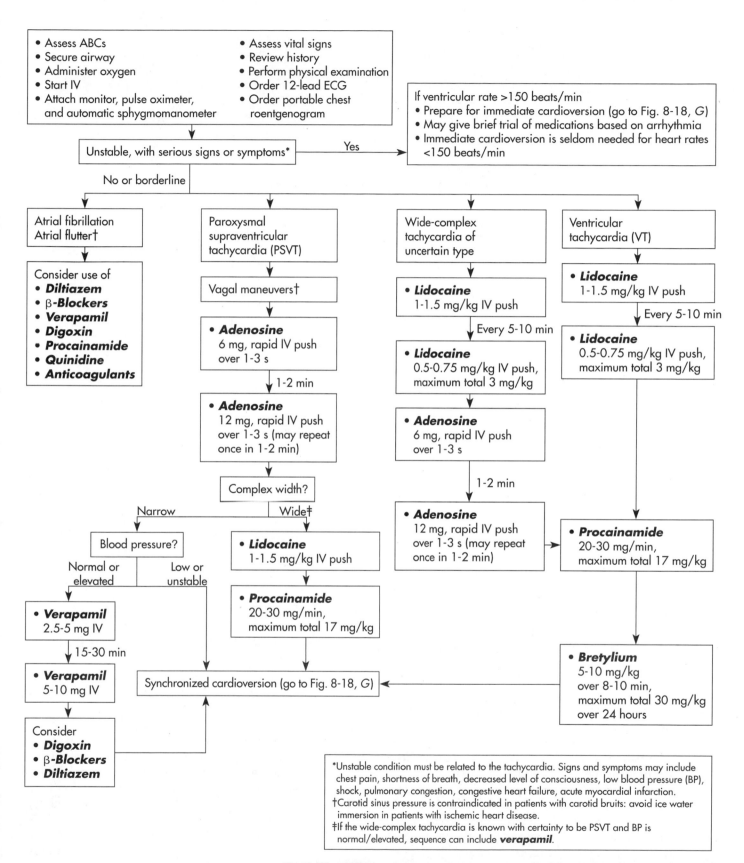

- Assess ABCs
- Secure airway
- Administer oxygen
- Start IV
- Attach monitor, pulse oximeter, and automatic sphygmomanometer

- Assess vital signs
- Review history
- Perform physical examination
- Order 12-lead ECG
- Order portable chest roentgenogram

If ventricular rate >150 beats/min
- Prepare for immediate cardioversion (go to Fig. 8-18, *G*)
- May give brief trial of medications based on arrhythmia
- Immediate cardioversion is seldom needed for heart rates <150 beats/min

Unstable, with serious signs or symptoms*   — Yes →

No or borderline

Atrial fibrillation Atrial flutter†

Consider use of
- ***Diltiazem***
- ***β-Blockers***
- ***Verapamil***
- ***Digoxin***
- ***Procainamide***
- ***Quinidine***
- ***Anticoagulants***

Paroxysmal supraventricular tachycardia (PSVT)

Vagal maneuvers†

- ***Adenosine***
  6 mg, rapid IV push over 1-3 s

  ↓ 1-2 min

- ***Adenosine***
  12 mg, rapid IV push over 1-3 s (may repeat once in 1-2 min)

Complex width?

Narrow — Wide‡

Blood pressure?

Normal or elevated — Low or unstable

- ***Verapamil***
  2.5-5 mg IV

  ↓ 15-30 min

- ***Verapamil***
  5-10 mg IV

Consider
- ***Digoxin***
- ***β-Blockers***
- ***Diltiazem***

- ***Lidocaine***
  1-1.5 mg/kg IV push

- ***Procainamide***
  20-30 mg/min, maximum total 17 mg/kg

Synchronized cardioversion (go to Fig. 8-18, *G*) ←

Wide-complex tachycardia of uncertain type

- ***Lidocaine***
  1-1.5 mg/kg IV push

  ↓ Every 5-10 min

- ***Lidocaine***
  0.5-0.75 mg/kg IV push, maximum total 3 mg/kg

- ***Adenosine***
  6 mg, rapid IV push over 1-3 s

  ↓ 1-2 min

- ***Adenosine***
  12 mg, rapid IV push over 1-3 s (may repeat once in 1-2 min)

Ventricular tachycardia (VT)

- ***Lidocaine***
  1-1.5 mg/kg IV push

  ↓ Every 5-10 min

- ***Lidocaine***
  0.5-0.75 mg/kg IV push, maximum total 3 mg/kg

- ***Procainamide***
  20-30 mg/min, maximum total 17 mg/kg

- ***Bretylium***
  5-10 mg/kg over 8-10 min, maximum total 30 mg/kg over 24 hours

*Unstable condition must be related to the tachycardia. Signs and symptoms may include chest pain, shortness of breath, decreased level of consciousness, low blood pressure (BP), shock, pulmonary congestion, congestive heart failure, acute myocardial infarction.
†Carotid sinus pressure is contraindicated in patients with carotid bruits: avoid ice water immersion in patients with ischemic heart disease.
‡If the wide-complex tachycardia is known with certainty to be PSVT and BP is normal/elevated, sequence can include ***verapamil***.

Fig. 8-18, cont'd   **F,** Tachycardia.

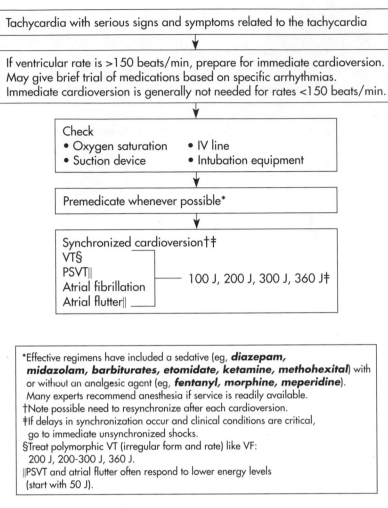

Fig. 8-18, cont'd **G,** Electrical cardioversion.

cardiac output. The importance of careful diagnosis cannot be overemphasized.

Resuscitation*

1. Unresponsiveness is established by shaking the patient and calling his or her name. If there is no response, the rescuer calls for help.
2. The patient is placed in a supine position with a board or firm mattress under the chest.
3. The patient's airway is opened using the head-tilt and chin-lift method or head-tilt and neck-lift method. The chin-lift method is preferred.
4. The rescuer looks, listens, and feels for breathing. If the patient is breathing, the airway is kept open, but other CPR techniques are not begun.
5. If the patient is not breathing, 2 breaths of about 1.5 seconds each are administered into the victim's mouth after the nostrils are pinched and the mouth is sealed.
6. The patient's carotid pulse is checked. If present, only breathing is administered at a rate of 1 breath every 5 seconds.
7. If the patient has no palpable pulse, cycles are begun: 5 external cardiac compressions (at a rate of 80 to 100/min) and 1 breath if two people are resuscitating or 15 compressions (at a rate of 80 to 100/min) and 2 breaths if only one person is resuscitating the patient. Correct hand positioning is essential.
8. After four cycles of ventilation and compression, the rescuer checks for return of the patient's pulse

---

*For further information, refer to the American Heart Association or the American Red Cross guidelines for CPR.

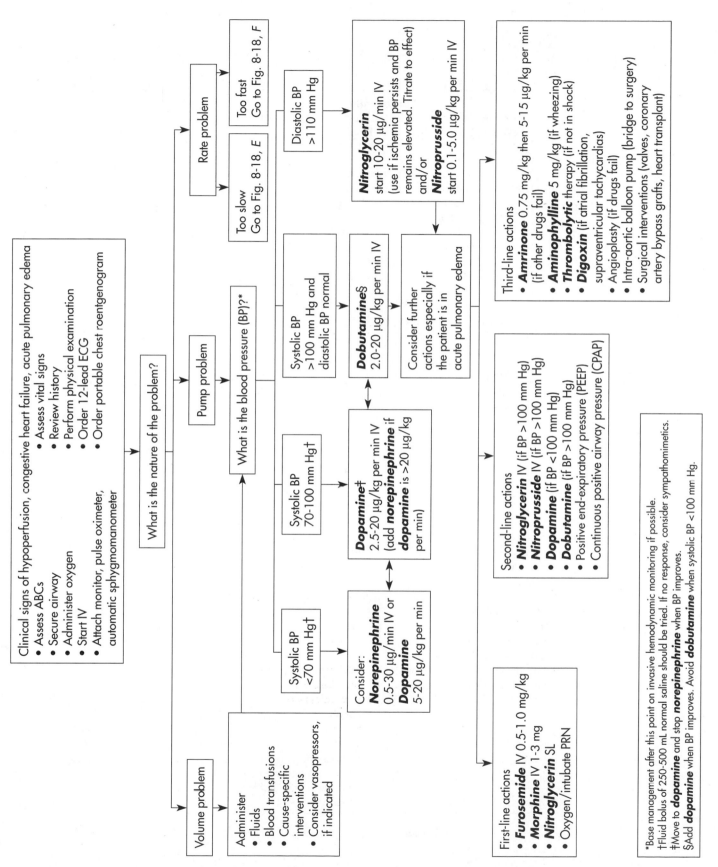

Fig. 8-18, cont'd H, Hypotension, shock, and acute pulmonary edema.

Community
- Community emphasis on "call first/call fast, call 911"
- National Heart Attack Alert Program

EMS System
EMS system approach that should address
- Oxygen-IV-cardiac monitor-vital signs
- *Nitroglycerin*
- Pain relief with narcotics
- Notification of emergency department
- Rapid transport to emergency department
- Prehospital screening for *thrombolytic* therapy*
- 12-lead ECG, computer analysis, transmission to emergency department*
- Initiation of *thrombolytic* therapy*

Emergency Department
"Door-to-drug" team protocol approach
- Rapid triage of patients with chest pain
- Clinical decision maker established (emergency physician, cardiologist, or other)

Time interval in emergency department

Assessment
Immediate:
- Vital signs with automatic BP
- Oxygen saturation
- Start IV
- 12-lead ECG (MD review)
- Brief, targeted history and physical
- Decide on eligibility for *thrombolytic* therapy
Soon:
- Chest roentgenogram
- Blood studies (electrolytes, enzymes, coagulation studies)
- Consult as needed

Treatments to consider if there is evidence of coronary thrombosis plus no reasons for exclusion (some but not all may be appropriate)
- Oxygen at 4 L/min
- *Nitroglycerin* SL, paste or spray (if systolic blood pressure >90 mm Hg)
- *Morphine* IV
- *Aspirin* PO
- *Thrombolytic* agents
- *Nitroglycerin* IV (limit systolic BP drop to 10% if normotensive; 30% drop if hypertensive; never drop below 90 mm Hg systolic)
- β-*Blockers* IV
- *Heparin* IV
- Percutaneous transluminal coronary angioplasty
- Routine *lidocaine* administration is not recommended for all patients with AMI

30-60 min to *thrombolytic* therapy

*Optional guidelines

Fig. 8-18, cont'd   I, Acute myocardial infarction.

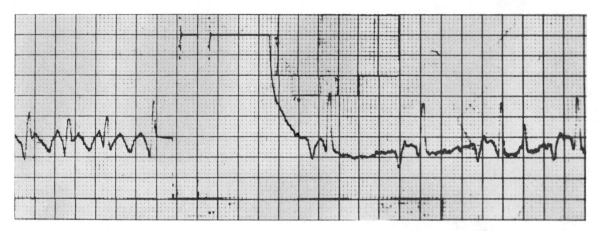

Fig. 8-19 Termination of atrial flutter. Direct current countershock was administered at 50 watt-seconds. The synchronized discharge occurred on R wave and terminated the flutter rhythm.

and spontaneous breathing. If there is no pulse or spontaneous breathing, the process is repeated.

9. CPR must not be stopped for more than 7 seconds once it has begun. The rescuer pauses every four cycles (after the initial pause noted in No. 8) to check for carotid pulse, spontaneous breathing, and pupillary reaction to light.

10. At the same time one or more people provide cardiorespiratory support, someone else sets up the defibrillator if the patient's rhythm is unknown or is known to be ventricular tachycardia or fibrillation. If only one person is present, he or she must decide between instituting CPR and attempting to defibrillate the patient. If the defibrillator is close at hand and the patient can be treated with it in 15 to 30 seconds, it is best for the single resuscitator to choose defibrillation rather than beginning CPR alone. *(It is extremely critical that direct-current shock not be delayed when CPR has begun, an intubation attempted, an ECG recorded, or a physical examination [other than, for example, a brief palpation of pulses] performed. Rapid application of direct-current shock is usually the most important therapeutic maneuver in this situation.)*

11. As soon as the defibrillator is ready (this should take no more than 30 seconds), the paddles are applied for a quick look. Most defibrillators have monitoring capability; their paddles act as electrodes that display and record the rhythm disturbance. The defibrillator is then charged to the appropriate energy level (Fig. 8-20), and the electric countershock is delivered.

12. The hearts of patients with ventricular fibrillation and pulseless ventricular tachycardia are defibrillated immediately at 200 joules. If this shock is unsuccessful, a second shock is delivered at 200 to 300 joules. If the second shock is unsuccessful, a third shock is delivered at 360 joules (see ACLS algorithms). These shocks should be delivered as quickly as possible. Failure to restore an effective rhythm after delivery of a properly administered countershock at high intensity suggests complicating problems such as hypoxia, acidosis, or drug toxicity. If possible, these conditions should be corrected before the next countershock is delivered. Sodium bicarbonate may be given to treat documented acidosis. When time permits, change from the quick look ECG paddles to the ECG leads for continuous cardiac monitoring.

13. Intravenous fluid is started if it is not already running.

14. It helps to have a drug list such as the one shown in Table 8-4 taped to the emergency cart. Medications most likely to be needed are prepared at the first opportunity.

15. Repetitive shocks may not be effective in the presence of fine fibrillatory waves on the ECG. Giving the patient 5 ml of epinephrine, 1:10,000 solution intravenously, may convert these fine waves to large coarse, fibrillatory waves. In some cases, lidocaine alone or with epinephrine may assist in defibrillation. Procainamide given intravenously, bretylium tosylate, or magnesium sulfate, may also be tried.

16. After successful conversion to sinus rhythm, continuous infusion with the antidysrhythmic drug,

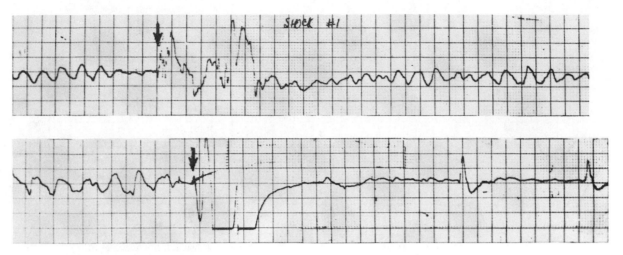

Fig. 8-20 Ventricular fibrillation was treated with application of unsynchronized countershock at 200 joules in top strip *(arrow).* Because countershock was unsuccessful, as noted in continuous strip, countershock was again applied at 300 joules *(arrow).* Rhythm then converted to idioventricular mechanism.

such as lidocaine, procainamide, or bretylium, should be instituted for maintenance therapy.

17. If the rhythm is known to be ventricular asystole, CPR should be initiated immediately (see Nos. 1 to 9 and administer epinephrine. See No. 18.)

18. After establishing intravenous access, epinephrine, 0.5 to 1.0 mg of a 1:10,000 solution, is administered intravenously. If this is unsuccessful, atropine, 1.0 mg, may be administered intravenously. Atropine may be repeated in 5 minutes.

19. The patient's trachea should be intubated. If intubation occurs before intravenous access is established, epinephrine, lidocaine, and atropine may be given by the endotracheal route. Dilution in 10 ml of sodium chloride is recommended to ensure delivery of the medication.

20. External and transvenous pacing may be attempted.

21. Electromechanical dissociation, now referred to as *pulseless electrical activity (PEA),* is also a form of cardiac arrest (see Nos. 1 to 9). The highest priority is to maintain the patient's condition while searching for a correctable cause, such as hypovolemia, cardiac tamponade, tension pneumothorax, hypoxemia, acidosis, or pulmonary embolism. See ACLS algorithm for PEA (see Fig. 8-18).

22. At the first opportunity an episode sheet is completed, and clinical events and a drug tally are recorded.

Control of environment

Regulation of the environment facilitates the rapidity and efficiency of the resuscitation procedure. The corridor to the patient's room must be free from obstacles. The patient's room should have adequate lighting with electric outlets visible from the door. Furniture should not block traffic from the room door to the patient's bed. Flowers, if allowed in the CCU, should be set on a shelf away from the bed so that they will not be knocked off the table during an emergency.

A fully stocked, adequately maintained emergency cart is imperative in every unit. It should include all drugs and equipment needed in an arrest and should not be cluttered with unnecessary items. The emergency cart and equipment should be checked each shift.

Care after resuscitation

In the aftermath of a successful resuscitation it seems natural for CCU personnel to relax; however, meticulous attention to the patient's hemodynamic status, blood gas levels, and electrolyte balance continues to be important in maintaining clinical stability and in preventing recurrence. This is a time too during which the patient's family should be encouraged to visit when appropriate. The family should be prepared for changes in the patient or new equipment in use, such as a ventilator.

Sudden Cardiac Death

Sudden cardiac death is the loss of life occurring within 1 hour of the onset of cardiovascular symptoms in a patient previously free of symptoms who has not suffered circulatory collapse during the preceding 24 hours and in whom no other cause of death is identified either by history or by autopsy. Sudden cardiac death accounts for approximately 1000 deaths in the United States every day.[104]

TABLE 8-4   Drugs Commonly Used in Cardiac Arrest

Drug	Concentration and Volume of Prefilled Syringe	Dose	Infusion Rate	Remarks
Adenosine	3 mg/ml or 2-ml vials (total = 6 mg)	6 mg intravenous push dose of 12 mg at 1-2 min if needed. May be repeated one time.	—	Give rapidly over 3 sec followed by 20-ml bolus of nitroglycerin. Then elevate extremity.
Amrinone	5 mg/ml in 20-ml vials; mix in 0.45 ng to max at 750 mg/250 ml	—	Initial loading dose of 0.75 mg/kg over 10-15 min, then 5-15 μg/kg/min infusion	Know that it can cause tachycardias, hypotension, and thrombocytopenia.
Atropine sulfate	0.1 mg/ml in 10-ml syringe	0.5-1.0 mg = 5-10 ml. Dilute in 10 ml ng for endotracheal administration.	—	Repeat at 5-min intervals to achieve desired heart rate; generally, do *not* exceed 2 mg.
Bretylium tosylate	50 mg/ml in 10-ml ampule	5 mg/kg bolus. Repeat at 10 mg/kg in 5 minutes.	500 mg in 5% dextrose in water (in 250 ml = 2 mg/ml; in 500 ml = 1 mg/ml) Infusion: 1-2 mg/min	—
Calcium chloride 10%	100 mg/ml in 10-ml syringe	50-100 mg = 5-10 ml for hyperkalemia.	—	—
Dobutamine	125 mg/ml in 20-ml vials 500-1000 mg in 250-ml ng or D5W	—	2-20 μg/kg/min	Know that it may cause tachycardia, blood pressure elevations, headache, and nausea.
Dopamine	200 mg in 5-ml ampule	—	200 mg in 250 ml dextrose in water = 800 μg/ml Infusion: 1-5 μg/kg/min "renal dose" 5-10 μg/kg/min "cardiac dose" 10-20 μg/kg/min "pressor dose"	—
Epinephrine 1:10,000	0.1 mg/ml in 10-ml syringe	1.0 mg = 10 ml intravenously per endotracheal tube. May repeat every 3-5 min. Alternative dosing: Intermediate: 2-5 mg intravenous push every 3-5 min.	1 mg in 5% dextrose in water (in 250 ml = 4 μg/ml; in 500 ml = 2 μg/min) Infusion: 1 μg/min for maintenance of blood pressure.	Avoid intracardiac injection; repeat dose every 5 min as needed in cardiac arrest.

Continued.

Adapted from American Heart Association: *Textbook of advanced cardiac life support,* Dallas, 1993, American Heart Association.

TABLE 8-4 Drugs Commonly Used in Cardiac Arrest—cont'd

Drug	Concentration and Volume of Prefilled Syringe	Dose	Infusion Rate	Remarks
Epinephrine—cont'd		Alternative dosing—cont'd: Escalating: 1, 3, 5 mg intravenous push every 3 min High: 0.1 mg/kg intravenously every 3-5 min		
Isoproterenol	0.2 mg/ml in 5-ml ampule	—	1 mg in 5% dextrose in water (in 250 ml = 4 µg/ml; in 500 ml = 2 µg/ml) Infusion: 2-20 µg/min Titrate	Beware of premature ventricular contractions.
Lidocaine	For intravenous bolus: 2% (20 mg/ml) in 5 ml = 100 mg	1-1.5 mg/kg intravenous push; may repeat in 3-5 min to a maximum of 3 mg/kg	2 g in 500 ml 5% dextrose in water (or 1 g in 250 ml) = 4 mg/ml Infusion: 1-4 mg/min	For breakthrough ventricular ectopy; give additional 50-mg bolus every 5 min to suppress to a total of 225 mg; increase drip to 4 mg/min.
Magnesium sulfate	10-ml ampule of 50% = 5 g magnesium	Cardiac arrest: 1-2 g intravenously diluted in 10 ml D5W over 1-2 min AMI: 1-2 g loading dose over 5-60 min, then 0.5-1 g/hr for 24 hours Torsades de pointes: 1-2 g loading dose over 5-60 min, 1-4 g/hr infusion	—	Know that it may cause a fall in blood pressure during administration as well as renal failure.
Procainamide	For intravenous bolus: 100 mg/ml in 10-ml ampule For infusion after bolus: 500 mg/ml in 2-ml ampules	30 mg/min until: a) Dysrhythmia suppressed b) Hypotension c) QRS widens by 50% d) Total 12 mg/kg administered	1 g in 250 ml 5% dextrose = 4 mg/ml Infusion: 1-4 mg/min	Monitor ECG and blood pressure; administer cautiously in patients with AMI.
Sodium bicarbonate	1 mEq/ml in 50 ml = 50 mEq	1 mEq/kg or 75 ml initial dose (average-size adult) according to pH	—	Repeat according to pH; know that it is not recommended for routine use in cardiac arrest.

Ventricular fibrillation is the most common dysrhythmia recorded at the onset of CPR in patients who have out-of-hospital cardiac arrest or in patients who die suddenly.[105] Bradydysrhythmias commonly occur when there has been delay in initiating emergency care, but it is unclear how often they actually cause sudden death. An ECG depicting a cardiac arrest caused by the spontaneous onset of rapid ventricular tachycardia that degenerated into ventricular fibrillation is shown in Fig. 8-21. Ventricular dysrhythmias are the most likely cause of sudden death in patients who have an AMI but die before being hospitalized.

Most patients who have coronary artery disease and develop sudden cardiac death demonstrate no recent thrombi in the coronary arteries at postmortem examination. Moreover, the majority of patients successfully resuscitated from sudden death do not have an AMI.[105] In patients resuscitated from out-of-hospital sudden death, the presence of an AMI has important prognostic significance: of survivors of ventricular fibrillation, the 1-year mortality in patients who had an AMI was 2%, and in patients who did not have an infarction the mortality was 22%.[106] These data confirm the observation that the occurrence of ventricular fibrillation in the CCU in patients who have AMIs does not increase the risk of sudden death in these patients after hospital discharge.

The difference in long-term survival after resuscitation for a patient who had and one who did not have an AMI may be partially explained by the following: The transient electrophysiologic and biochemical alterations that occur in the ventricle during AMI may result in ventricular fibrillation. When the acute phase of the infarction resolves, such patients have a low recurrence rate of ventricular fibrillation, most likely because their hearts no longer have the electrophysiologic and anatomic capability to develop and/or to sustain ventricular dysrhythmias. In contrast, patients who have ventricular fibrillation without infarction have a relatively high risk of recurrent ventricular fibrillation. The high recurrence rate in these patients may be related to the fact that the "arrhythmogenic" area of the ventricle does not become infarcted and remains capable of initiating or sustaining ventricular dysrhythmias.

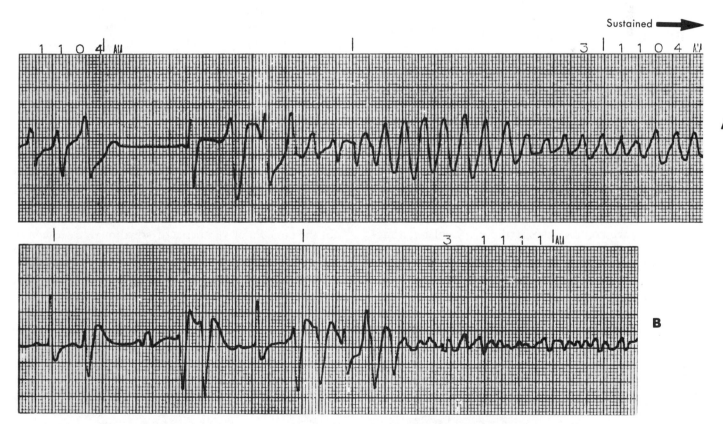

Fig. 8-21 Ventricular fibrillation recorded during ambulatory monitoring. These ECG tracings occurred during an in-hospital, 24-hour, ambulatory recording on a patient who had a previous out-of-hospital cardiac arrest. **A,** The onset of rapid (approximately 300 beats/min) ventricular tachycardia that degenerated into ventricular fibrillation; the patient was successfully defibrillated to sinus rhythm. **B,** Some 7 minutes later a second episode of ventricular fibrillation occurred after a short run of ventricular tachycardia; defibrillation again restored sinus rhythm.

Although sudden cardiac death occurs most often in patients who have coronary artery disease, it also occurs in patients with a variety of other cardiac conditions such as hypertrophic cardiomyopathy, dilated cardiomyopathy, mitral valve disease, heart failure, and primary electric disease (which is the presence of cardiac dysrhythmias with no other cardiac abnormalities found during physical examination, echocardiography, or cardiac catheterization).

Patients who have a prolonged QT interval are at increased risk for sudden cardiac death.[107] The upper limit for QT duration corrected for heart rate (QTc) is usually given as 0.44 seconds. Although a QTc interval of at least 0.44 seconds can occur in patients without dysrhythmias, there is a congenital disorder called *prolonged QT syndrome* that occurs in patients with or without deafness;[108] this disorder is associated with a predisposition to develop ventricular tachycardia or ventricular fibrillation. Sudden cardiac death in patients with an acquired prolonged QT interval may be caused by hypokalemia and quinidine-like antidysrhythmic drugs. A connection between prolonged QT interval and sudden death has been dramatically demonstrated in patients receiving a liquid protein diet.[109]

Risk factors for sudden cardiac death

Risk factors for sudden cardiac death include the presence of complex premature ventricular contractions, ventricular tachycardia, or left ventricular dysfunction. Simple (uniform, infrequent) and complex (multiform, frequent) premature ventricular contractions commonly occur in patients who have coronary artery disease. The prevalence of complex premature ventricular contractions increases directly with the number of diseased coronary arteries and with the severity of left ventricular dysfunction. Although the presence of complex premature ventricular contractions increases the risk of subsequent sudden death, most patients who have complex premature ventricular contractions do not die suddenly. Ventricular fibrillation is often preceded by ventricular tachycardia (Fig. 8-22), but it is not known how frequently ventricular tachycardia degenerates into ventricular fibrillation.

Sudden death also occurs in patients who have nonsustained ventricular tachycardia associated with few or no symptoms. In some cases, nonsustained ventricular tachycardia may progress to sustained ventricular tachycardia, and this may lead to the development of ventricular fibrillation. The occurrence of a sustained ventricular tachycardia may depend on multiple factors such as myocardial ischemia, increased left ventricular dimension, electrolyte disorders, or autonomic disturbances.

Patients who have AMIs are at increased risk of developing subsequent sudden death if they have congestive heart failure while still in the CCU[106] or have a low cardiac ejection fraction (determined by radionuclide angiography) before hospital discharge.[71] As noted in the previous section, complex premature ventricular contractions commonly occur in patients who have myocardial dysfunction, and the two abnormalities compound the risk for sudden death.[34] This risk is greatest in patients who have heart failure and complex premature ventricular contractions but is lower for patients who have only heart failure or complex premature ventricular contractions. Other clinical factors related to an increased risk of sudden death include psychologic stress, increasing age, hypertension, and diabetes.[109]

Diagnosis

Several diagnostic tests are used to determine the cause of the dysrhythmia in survivors of sudden cardiac death. Holter monitoring is commonly used to document the presence of dysrhythmias and to evaluate the effectiveness of antidysrhythmic drugs. The ECG monitor is worn by the patient for 24 hours, and the patient is encouraged to pursue normal activities. Exercise stress testing may also be used to detect dysrhythmias. A third test used to determine the cause of dysrhythmias is the signal-averaged ECG. The signal-averaged ECG is a noninvasive procedure, similar to a standard 12-lead ECG, that can be used to detect late potentials (low-amplitude, high-frequency signals that may occur at the end of the QRS). The presence of late potentials seems to indicate an increased risk of reentrant tachycardias and sudden death.

Treatment of ventricular dysrhythmias

Ventricular tachydysrhythmias may be controlled by a variety of therapies that include drugs, pacemakers, cardioverter/defibrillators, and surgery. Probably the most difficult task in caring for patients who have ventricular dysrhythmias is deciding *whether* to treat them rather than which treatment to use. Since the risk of sudden death is not the same for all ventricular dysrhythmias, treatment to suppress ventricular dysrhythmias should be guided by the relative risks of sudden death in a particular dysrhythmia. The assumption, although often difficult to prove, is that abolition of the dysrhythmia will prevent death; obviously, the decision to treat a patient must be made from the data obtained on the patient and sound clinical judgment. Of the ventricular dysrhythmias, the lowest risk of sudden death occurs in patients who have premature ventricular contractions but no structural heart disease, and the highest risk occurs in patients who have sustained ventricular tachycardia and severe congestive heart failure; as a rule, the former group should not receive antidysrhythmic therapy (assuming that the patient's condition is asymptomatic), whereas the latter group requires therapy. In general, drug therapy is not recommended for any patient with asymptomatic premature ventricular contractions, but patients who have sustained ventricular tachycardia should be

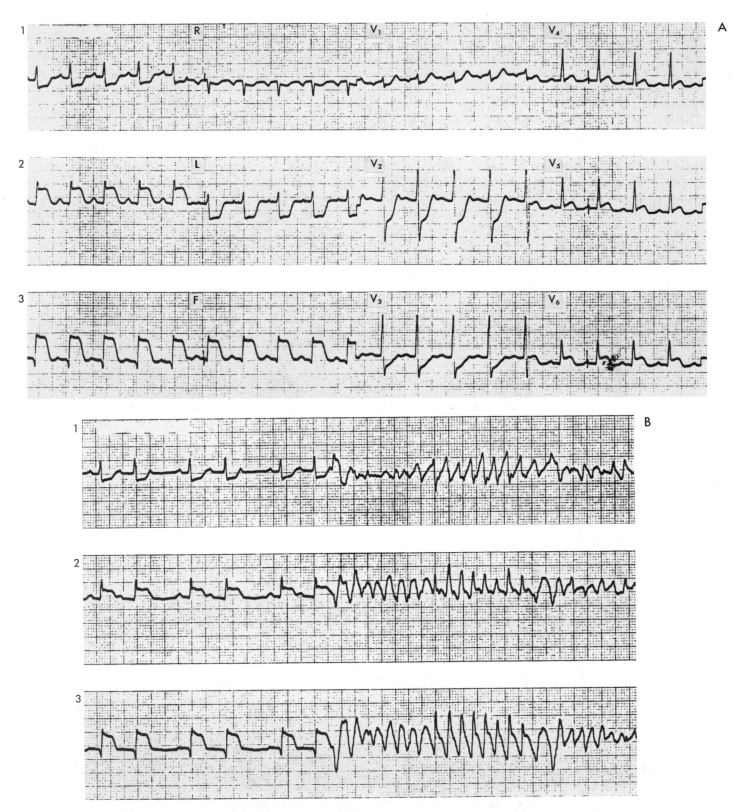

Fig. 8-22 Ventricular fibrillation in the presence of an AMI. **A,** A 12-lead ECG demonstrating a current of injury pattern (that is, ST elevations) in leads II, III, aV$_F$, and V$_4$ to V$_6$. This patient later developed Q waves in these leads. In **A** and **B** the three leads arranged vertically were recorded simultaneously (for example, I, II, and III). **B,** A rhythm strip taken simultaneously for leads I, II, and III. Wenckebach AV block occurs on the left, and rapid ventricular tachycardia that degenerates into ventricular fibrillation is seen on the right.

treated. If nonsustained ventricular tachycardia causes substantial symptoms in patients with or without structural heart disease, it may be desirable to suppress the dysrhythmia; if the dysrhythmia is asymptomatic and occurs in otherwise healthy individuals, treatment may not be necessary, but careful follow-up is suggested.

In studies testing the effectiveness of therapy with β-blocking drugs, a significant decrease in sudden death occurred in patients treated with alprenolol, practolol, timolol, and metoprolol compared with control patients.[110-111] The apparent benefits of β blockers may be caused by their antisympathetic effects, membrane-active properties, antiischemic effects, or a combination of multiple actions. Antidysrhythmic drug therapy is not without risks. Antidysrhythmic drugs commonly cause side effects and in some patients can cause ventricular tachycardia and sudden death. In some patients, administration of type I antidysrhythmic drugs (for example, quinidine, procainamide, or disopyramide) may cause marked prolongation of the QT interval and result in a specific form of ventricular tachycardia, known as *torsades de pointes* (Fig. 8-23).

Electrophysiologic testing

One method used to assess the efficacy of drug therapy in the suppression of spontaneous ventricular tachycardia and fibrillation is to monitor, for variable periods, the patient's heart rhythm during therapy, under normal activity, and during stress testing.[42] If ventricular dysrhythmias are markedly suppressed during monitoring, the patient is discharged, and further follow-up is done out of the hospital. In many patients, ventricular tachydysrhythmias are episodic, which precludes accurate assessment of drug efficacy by noninvasive monitoring techniques only; unfortunately, out-of-hospital sudden death is not an uncommon sequela in these patients.

Electrophysiologic studies with programmed electric stimulation to induce ventricular tachycardia has been used to judge the ability of drugs to prevent ventricular dys-

rhythmias.[112] Thus patients who have ventricular tachycardia induced before but not after drug therapy usually have no recurrence of ventricular tachycardia if they continue to take the dosage of the antidysrhythmic drug that prevented induction of ventricular tachycardia during the electrophysiologic study.

An electrophysiologic study procedure is similar to a cardiac catheterization. Multielectrode catheters are inserted into a vein, usually the femoral, brachial, basilic, subclavian, or jugular, and the electrodes are positioned in various locations within the heart. Arterial cannulation is done only if left ventricular stimulation is required. The catheters are used to make simultaneous recordings of the electrical activity of the heart (similar to ECGs). Pacing electrodes on the catheters are used to stimulate the heart (a process called *programmed electric stimulation* [PES]), and induce dysrhythmias, which are also recorded. The pacing electrodes can also be used to terminate a dysrhythmia by overdrive pacing. Cardioversion or defibrillation may be required if the dysrhythmia causes loss of consciousness or hemodynamic compromise.

The initial study is performed after withholding all antidysrhythmic medications. After obtaining baseline data, an antidysrhythmic drug may be infused, and the programmed electric stimulation is repeated. Plasma drug levels of the antidysrhythmic agent used may be drawn during or after the study.

Many electrophysiologic studies may be required to ascertain which drug or combination of drugs effectively prevent dysrhythmia induction. It also is necessary to ensure that plasma drug levels are in a therapeutic range before initiation of the study. It may be necessary to return the patient to a drug-free state before evaluating the efficacy of the next drug. All of these factors influence the scheduling of repeat studies, which may range from 1 to 14 days.

The care of the patient preparing for electrophysiologic study includes providing psychologic support. The sudden

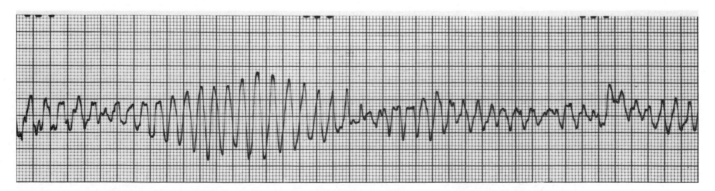

Fig. 8-23 Torsades de pointes. This specific type of ventricular tachycardia usually occurs in the presence of a prolonged QT interval and is characterized by a QRS morphology that appears repeatedly to change its axis by 180 degrees.

appearance of a cardiac dysrhythmia, especially one that is life-threatening, is often devastating to patients and frequently produces feelings of anger, anxiety, and depression. The thought of undergoing an invasive procedure magnifies these emotions.

It is very important for nurses and physicians to realize the emotional upheaval that occurs in patients with dysrhythmias and make attempts to help them cope with their feelings. Although patients may use a variety of coping mechanisms on their own, attempts should be made to make their environment calm, in or out of the electrophysiology laboratory. It is useful to bring patients to the laboratory on the day before the study to familiarize them with the surroundings. Patients and family members often cannot remember what was explained to them in the laboratory at the end of the procedure, possibly because of their heightened emotional state, and therefore it is helpful to go over the study results with them shortly after they have been returned to their room.[113]

Immediate care after electrophysiologic study is similar to that after cardiac catheterization: frequent assessment of vital signs, observation of insertion site, assessment of peripheral pulses, bedrest, and immobilization of the affected extremity. On initiation of antidysrhythmic drug therapy, the patient should be observed for signs and symptoms of drug toxicity or allergy. ECG monitoring is necessary to document rhythm changes.

In summary, electrophysiologic testing in selected patients who have ventricular tachycardia and fibrillation is an important adjunct to testing drug efficacy. Ideally, the patient should be discharged while receiving the antidysrhythmic drug or drugs that totally suppress ventricular tachycardia and fibrillation during electrophysiologic testing. Practically, however, total suppression of ventricular tachycardia during electrophysiologic testing is not accomplished in many cases, and nonsustained or sustained ventricular tachycardia can still be induced. If patients continue to have hemodynamically unstable ventricular dysrhythmias with all drug combinations, they should be considered for an alternative therapy such as surgery or the implantation of pacemakers or other electric devices, such as the automatic implantable cardioverter defibrillator (ICD).

ICD

The ICD is a miniaturized cardioverter-defibrillator that is used to treat ventricular tachycardia and fibrillation. This device has dramatically improved the survival rate of sudden death. Currently, the ICD is used for patients who have survived at least one sudden-death episode not associated with an MI and in whom conventional antidysrhythmic drug therapy has failed. Candidates for ICD implantation should have a life expectancy of at least 6 months. Patients who have frequent episodes of ventricular tachycardia or fibrillation are not candidates for ICD because of early battery depletion.

The initial evaluation for ICD includes documentation of the dysrhythmia and assessment of the cardiac anatomy by echo, multiple-gated (acquisition blood pool) (MUGA) scan, and cardiac catheterization. A baseline electrophysiologic study, serial drug tests, and an exercise test may be done. Psychologic evaluation is also important. Candidates should demonstrate emotional maturity, stability, and a willingness to cooperate during the extensive follow-up required after implantation.[114]

The epicardially placed ICD device consists of a pulse generator and four electrodes (Fig. 8-24). The titanium pulse generator is approximately $11 \times 7 \times 2$ cm and weighs 0.25 kg (about ½ lb). It contains the circuitry, capacitors, and a lithium battery. One set of electrodes is used for sensing the QRS waveform and delivering the shock when required. This set of electrodes can consist of (1) a left ventricular patch electrode sewn onto the epicardium and a spring electrode inserted transvenously into the superior vena cava near the right atrium or (2) a right atrial and a left ventricular patch sewn onto the epicardium. The second set of electrodes is for rate sensing. These electrodes may be inside a single bipolar transvenous lead that is placed in the right ventricle, or they may be inside two epicardial screw-in electrodes (Fig. 8-25).

The ICD has two sensing systems, one for sensing heart rate and one for sensing QRS morphology. The rate-sensing system determines the patient's heart rate. For the cardioverter defibrillator to deliver a charge, the heart rate must exceed a set cutoff rate. The cutoff rate is set by the manufacturer and is usually in the range of 120 to 200 beats/min. Ideally, the cutoff rate should be below the rate of the patient's ventricular tachycardia but greater than the maximum sinus rate. The morphology sensing system allows the ICD to differentiate ventricular tachycardia and

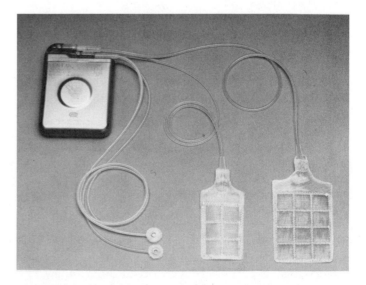

Fig. 8-24 ICD, pulse generator, and electrodes. (Courtesy CPI, St Paul, Minn.)

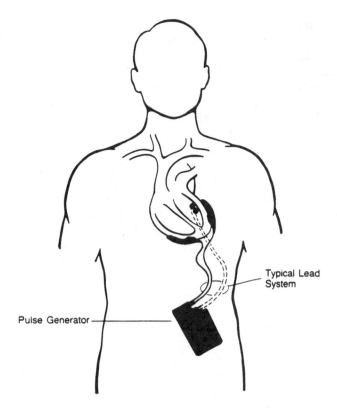

Fig. 8-25   Implanted ICD.   (Courtesy CPI, St Paul, Minn.)

ventricular fibrillation from sinus rhythms. However, some sinus rhythms with wide QRS complexes may be mistaken for ventricular tachycardia by the ICD, but these rhythms should not meet the rate criteria. Some ICD models may be programmed to meet only the rate criteria, whereas other models are required to meet the rate cutoff as well as QRS morphology.

Once the rate cutoff and the morphology criteria, if required, have been met, the ICD takes 10 to 35 seconds to charge and deliver the first shock of approximately 10 to 25 joules. If the dysrhythmia continues, the device charges and delivers second, third, and fourth shocks of 30 joules each. After the fourth shock, the ICD must sense at least 35 seconds of a nonventricular rhythm to reset for the next four-shock cycle. In most instances, the ICD is successful with the first shock. If the ICD is unsuccessful after the cycle of four shocks for a life-threatening dysrhythmia, external countershock must be applied immediately. Some models of the ICD deliver at least a five-shock cycle.

There are four surgical options for the placement of the epicardial and patch leads. A median sternotomy approach is used when patients are undergoing additional cardiac surgery such as CABG. The left lateral thoracotomy, left subcostal, and subxyphoid approaches also can be used. Once the epicardial leads and patches are in place, the wires

are tunneled under the skin and connected to the pulse generator, which is pocketed in the paraumbilical area. Once the system is in place, intraoperative testing is performed to ensure that the ICD can terminate the induced dysrhythmia. The cardioverter/defibrillator electrodes may be repositioned to determine optimal placement.[115]

The ICD can be activated and deactivated with a magnet. The device is implanted in the deactivated mode and then activated for intraoperative testing. The ICD is then deactivated for completion of surgery. For activation of the ICD, a doughnut-shaped magnet is placed over the right corner of the pulse generator for 30 seconds. An audible beeping tone, synchronized to the QRS, should be heard. To deactivate the ICD, the magnet is placed over the pulse-generator. After 30 seconds the beeping should change to a continuous tone. When caring for a patient with an ICD, it is important to note whether the ICD is in the active or inactive mode. A device called an *Aidcheck* is used to determine battery life and the total number of shocks delivered through the lead system. A recent advance is the completely transvenous ICD lead, which eliminates the need for a thoracotomy. Furthermore, many models now also have pacing capabilities. Overdrive pacing may be programmed as the initial treatment for the dysrhythmia, and a shock is delivered only if pacing is not successful.[116]

Potential complications of ICD implantation include infection, subclavian vein thrombosis, lead dislodgement, pericarditis, and pacemaker interactions. Unipolar pacemakers emit large signals that may cause double sensing by the ICD.

Before the patient is discharged, another electrophysiologic study is performed. The dysrhythmia is induced to determine that the ICD is functioning properly. This also allows the patient to experience a shock in a controlled environment. Some patients describe the shock as feeling like a blow or kick to the chest. If someone is touching the patient during a shock, that person may feel a tingling or buzzing sensation. In addition to an electrophysiologic study, exercise testing may be performed to determine that the exercise-induced sinus tachycardia is less than the ICD cutoff rate.

Predischarge instructions after ICD implantation

1. Follow activity limitations: avoid contact sports, which could cause lead fracture; some states have laws prohibiting persons with dysrhythmias from driving.
2. Avoid strong magnetic fields (arc welding, electrocautery, airport metal detectors, radiofrequency transmitters), which may interfere with the functioning of the ICD. If the beeping tone is heard, walk away in the opposite direction. The magnetic field may inactivate the ICD.
3. Observe the incision and report any signs of infection.
4. Avoid restrictive clothing around the waist, which may cause lead fracture.

5. Report a first shock to the physician.

The patient's family should be encouraged to learn CPR, and the patient and family should be instructed about when to notify the physician or call emergency medical services.

PSYCHOLOGIC ADJUSTMENT TO CORONARY HEART DISEASE

The emotional, behavioral, and social impact of a heart attack is often profound and, for many patients, may be even more debilitating than the limitations imposed solely by the physical effects of the disease. Psychologic adaptation begins when symptoms are first noticed and continues throughout hospitalization and the subsequent return home. Three phases of the illness will be discussed: prehospital, hospital, and posthospital.

Prehospital Phase

Probably the most common reaction of patients to the first signs of illness is simply to do nothing and hope that the symptoms go away. The average time between symptom onset and admission to a medical facility is about 3 hours, although patients may delay seeking help for more than 24 hours.[14]

Approximately 55% to 65% of the time between symptom onset and hospital arrival involves what has been termed *decision time*. During this period, patients become aware of their symptoms and may engage in behaviors designed to provide themselves with relief: They may rest, take medication, or discuss the problem with spouse or friends. An additional 25% of the time between symptom onset and entry into the medical facility involves the period of *medical preparation*. During this time, the physician is contacted and arrangements are made for subsequent hospital care. The remaining 10% is time required for transportation to the hospital and is typically referred to as *transportation time*.

Since more than half of all deaths after MI occur within the first 4 hours, it is important that the interval between symptom onset and medical care be reduced. Longer time to respond to symptoms appears to be unrelated to demographic factors such as age, gender, or socioeconomic status. Psychologic factors appear to play a predominant role, especially in the decision time. Denial (that is, the tendency to ignore or minimize the true significance of the symptoms) seems to be the most common reaction and often leads to incorrectly attributing the symptoms to noncardiac factors such as indigestion or dysfunction in other organ systems.[117]

Hospital Phase

Admission to the hospital is an unmistakable sign to the patient that something is wrong and that medical intervention is required. The most important emotional feature of patients in the initial acute phase of their illness is extreme fear and anxiety. The content of anxious thought usually focuses on the realization of the possibility of sudden death, concerns about being abandoned and out of control, and the conscious preoccupation with symptoms such as shortness of breath, chest pain, fatigue, or irregular heart rhythm. Depression, hostility, and agitation also are observed in many patients. Cassem and Hackett[118] have developed a model for the temporal sequence of emotional reactions in patients with coronary heart disease based on reasons for psychiatric referral in the CCU. The sequence is graphically displayed in Fig. 8-26. The patient feels heightened anxiety during the first 2 days of hospitalization and subsequently becomes depressed for a few days. Anxiety and depression decline after 5 or 6 days as a result of the mobilization of two main defense mechanisms: denial and repression. Isolation of affect is a third common defense mechanism that helps the patient cope with the illness. This process involves the acknowledgement of the reality of the situation, but the affective or emotional component of this awareness is unconscious. Although the majority of patients do not require formal psychiatric intervention, a substantial number experience significant emotional distress. Many patients have confronted death for the first time, they are frightened and depressed over the perceived loss of physical health, they are prone to worry about future employment, family relations are disrupted, and financial security may be threatened.

Although patients with coronary heart disease often tend to avoid admitting fears and worries during brief interviews, more intensive contact in which the patient is given an opportunity and permission to discuss feelings and problems in a supportive, nonthreatening environment can be extremely therapeutic. Most patients welcome a chance to "get things off their chest," and the process often promotes feelings of reassurance and relief.

Patient teaching is another important aspect of the hospital phase. Frequently, patients have trouble assimilating and retaining all the information presented to them. However, most want to know about their condition (in varying degrees of detail), so it is often useful to sit down with the patient and spouse to review the important aspects of cardiac care. It is imperative to *listen* as well as to talk with the patient. Patients communicate what they know and what they want to know if given an opportunity. Disguised fears, anxieties, and misconceptions about their illness also can become apparent. For example, the statement "I guess this means I'll never go back to work" may reflect apprehension about remaining autonomous, anxiety about being dependent on others, and uncertainty about the realistic limitations of the illness. Such statements should be explored and discussed with the patient.

Patient instruction is extremely important; it increases the patient's knowledge and improves subsequent psychosocial and medical adjustment. It should be noted, however, that patients differ in their receptivity to health information, and the amount of responsibility and infor-

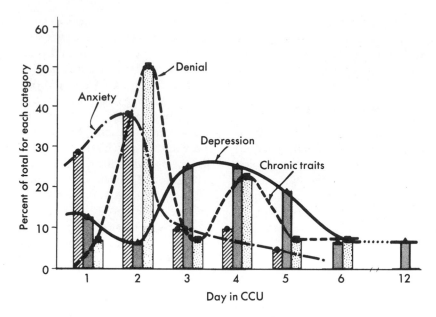

Fig. 8-26 Hypothesized course of emotional behavioral reactions in the CCU. (From Cassem NH, Hackett T: *Ann Intern Med* 75:9, 1971.)

mation given to a patient must be carefully determined by taking into account the patient's ability to comprehend and use the information.

A number of research investigations have attempted to relate stressful experiences in the CCU to subsequent recovery. In general, data suggest that the CCU equipment, activities, and procedures do not result in any long-term maladjustment in coronary patients.

Posthospital Phase

After 1 to 3 days on the CCU, the patient is transferred to a telemetry unit. In some situations, patients with uncomplicated conditions and MI may never go to a CCU and instead be treated on a telemetry unit for their entire hospitalization. This ward has less supervision but intensive medical care for the next 2 to 4 days. The posthospital phase begins with the patient's discharge from the hospital and for all practical purposes continues indefinitely thereafter. During this phase, the responsibility for the patient's care shifts from the hospital team of physicians, nurses, physical therapists, and others to the patient and family.

Psychologic and behavioral factors affect the course of recovery, and psychologic problems are seldom resolved during the acute period of hospitalization. For example, research has documented that at 6 months to 1 year after discharge from the hospital, many patients are anxious or depressed, report disturbed sleep, do not return to work, and complain of excessive weakness. Heart disease also affects the family, and marital conflicts, often centering around medical instructions (concerning such areas as diet, medication, and sexual activity), are common.

Unlike the structured hospital setting, the return home often means that the patient is unsupervised and that no concrete, specific guidelines are made available. The patient may be uncertain about the extent to which physical activity is permissible, and the advice "take it easy" is too often misunderstood or is so general as to be of no real value. Concern about sexual functioning, apprehensiveness about returning to work, and awareness of diminished energy and strength are common.

In general, emotional distress reaches its peak during the patient's convalescence. There appear to be at least five problem areas that affect a substantial number of coronary patients: excessive concerns about health and the fear of dying, organic problems, emotional problems, continuation of personality problems from the time before the illness, and developmental issues and existential concerns.

Excessive concerns about health

Once a person has experienced an MI, good health may no longer be taken for granted. Many patients become sensitized to their bodily functioning. In extreme cases, patients may become preoccupied with their health and overreact to even minor discomfort.

Fear and anxiety about death are common reactions to a heart attack. Most people do not think about their own deaths very much. However, a heart attack is a reminder of mortality and raises a cultural expectation of death. This expectation is founded in clinical fact, since patients with coronary heart disease have higher mortality rates than their healthy age-matched counterparts.

Thus a diagnosis of coronary disease may suggest that death is imminent.

Losses are considered to be less disruptive when they are "scheduled" or when the events are perceived as being subject to schedule.[119] Anxiety about death as a major loss is also related to attitudes about aging. Expectations for decline, loss, or death are far more inconsistent for the later years of life than for the early years. Thus for the young, society expects continued growth, and the pattern of change is predictable. As people grow older, however, the pattern of development becomes ambiguous, and expectations become unclear. The lack of clear positive expectations for development during the adult years also contributes to the attribution of normative loss. However, an MI may be more traumatic for a young person than for an older individual whose MI, which heralds aging, is more often expected. Disability and death are seen as more appropriate to older than to young adults, and public policy decisions predictably follow this attitude.

For many patients, a heart attack represents significant *loss:* of income, family and friends, job, status, and independence, as well as health. As a result of these actual and threatened losses, grief reactions are not unusual and may be a protective coping mechanism.[117] The patient's reactions may parallel the stages observed among patients with cancer: denial, anger, depression and, ultimately, acceptance. These "states of dying" have not been fully confirmed, however, and some of the conceptual and methodologic deficiencies have been described elsewhere. Repeated losses or unresolved loss can eventually lead to morbid grief and depression.[117,119]

In the past, it was felt that health professionals should not talk with cardiac patients about anything that might disturb or excite them. As a consequence, the MI patient's fears and anxieties were often denied or ignored. More recently, however, the importance of effective communication with the coronary patient has been recognized. Specifically, affective empathy is considered extremely important along with acceptance of the patient's feelings.

Cardiac neurosis is a term often used to describe a situation in which the patient has become completely debilitated by the illness. Fear of leaving home or anxiety over physical exertion may be present, and even minor symptoms are thought to be emergencies or precursors of a fatal cardiac event. Encouragement and support, firm and concrete guidelines for progressive physical exercise, and regularly scheduled medical checkups appear to be very therapeutic for these patients.[120]

Organic problems

Impaired cognitive functioning is present in a small number of patients with coronary disease. Patients who undergo bypass surgery have a higher incidence of cognitive changes. In addition to the effects that the disease process may have on cognitive functions, advancing age contributes to a general decline in mental abilities. Aging is associated with a decline in cognitive functioning, and cardiac disease is most common in the latter half of the life cycle. Research has suggested that "crystallized" abilities, such as a person's vocabulary or fund of information, may remain intact, whereas "fluid" abilities, such as problem-solving or verbal reasoning skills may deteriorate more quickly as a result of the combined effects of aging and organic damage.

Emotional problems

Depression is a common complaint often characterized by sadness, crying spells, sleep disturbance (such as early morning awakening), excessive fatigue and weakness, and low energy. Anxiety is also fairly common, although the defense mechanisms of repression, denial, and isolation of affect often protect the patient from consciously experiencing the subjective discomfort associated with anxiety. Most patients do not suffer from significant and debilitating anxiety a year after MI. For patients whose symptoms persist, however, anxiolytic or antidepressant medication (such as doxepin hydrochloride [Sinequan] or alprazolam [Xanax]) often helps to reduce symptoms.

Coronary artery disease may evoke feelings of vulnerability and worthlessness. The patient may become dependent or passive as a result of the socially acceptable role as patient. Encouraging the patient to talk about feelings and to become more physically active are important aids to treatment. The importance of exercise therapy is now widely recognized.

Problems continuing from earlier years

Most patients who develop coronary artery disease are not psychiatric patients. However, patients with significant emotional problems also develop heart disease. Problems that have developed over the course of a lifetime rarely improve after a heart attack. People who are prone to depression can be extremely affected by a sudden decline in health. Similarly, people who tend to act impulsively or who show an inability to tolerate life's frustrations may exhibit a continuation of past behaviors; they may continue to overeat, overdrink, or overindulge themselves in ways that have a negative effect on their health and on those around them.

In brief, individuals who have problems before their illness are likely to have problems after their illness. Marriages are seldom improved when one member becomes sick, and often coronary artery disease may cause additional problems for couples and families.

Developmental issues and existential concerns

Familial, cultural, and spiritual values become more important as one grows older, and illness often brings about a reevaluation of what is meaningful, not only in terms of what happens after death but also in terms of what happens before death. An MI may make a patient seek to avoid feelings of helplessness and hopelessness and may stimulate a renewed interest in people. It is common for patients to review their lives and to reflect on opportunities chosen and neglected. Some patients adopt a new philosophy about life and shift from material to more spiritual interests.

Patients with coronary heart disease are often in their middle years and must face developmental issues common to middle age. The most important issues facing middle-aged and older adults are how to cope with loss; for the MI patient, the most obvious loss is that of physical prowess and functional abilities. This may threaten self-concept and lead to forced dependence on others.

As one gets older, the experience of illness becomes more frequent, and it is more difficult to compensate for lost friends. Patients may feel lonely, isolated, and deserted and experience the loss of shared memories. Retirement also can be traumatic. It means an end of a phase of life, and with the loss of work is often a loss of a sense of autonomy and power. Loss of relationships with co-workers, of social status, and of income are also experienced.

Talking about life requires someone who is willing to listen. Although professional help is often useful, a patient should also be encouraged to talk with a spouse, relatives, and friends.

Treatment considerations

Most published research on the psychologic treatment of MI patients has been about treatment in the form of group psychotherapy. To date, results have been mixed. Several studies have demonstrated improved psychologic well-being in the treatment group compared with that in a no-treatment control group, and at least one study has reported a significantly lower mortality rate in the treated group. However, group treatment of cardiac patients does not follow a process similar to group treatment of psychiatric patients (see review by Gil and Blumenthal[121]). Educational and supportive groups appear to be preferable to self-exploratory or psychoanalytically oriented groups.

Several recent studies have used behavioral techniques, including progressive muscle relaxation training and stress-management techniques.[122] The main behavioral treatments for patients with coronary disease appear to be those that attempt to remove the source of stress or modify the patients' perceptions and reactions to stress. Progressive muscle relaxation, in which the patient is taught to tense and relax muscles, is an example of a technique that counteracts the effects of a stressful environment. Other behavioral techniques for treating stress reactions include cognitive restructuring, in which the patient is taught to reinterpret events to make them less stressful, and systematic desensitization, in which the patient learns to relax to counteract the emotional or physical symptoms during exposure to situations that evoke symptoms. Biofeedback, a treatment designed to teach patients control of autonomic nervous system functions, has been used successfully to treat a variety of cardiovascular disorders, including cardiac dysrhythmias, hypertension, and peripheral vascular disease. However, the effectiveness of behavioral techniques in actually prolonging the life of patients with coronary disease has not been established. Type-A modification has also gained widespread recognition, and recent data have suggested that reductions in type-A behavior may be associated with decreased risk of recurrent events of coronary artery disease.[123]

Recovery from a heart attack is a complex process. Social, psychologic, and medical factors are important and are interrelated. Successful treatment is most likely achieved by the collaborative efforts of nurses, physicians, psychologists, physical therapists, and vocational counselors. The key ingredient is an interest in and commitment to victims of a disease with important psychosocial and physical consequences.

CARE ISSUES
Sociocultural Considerations

Because the United States is a pluralistic society, health professionals must be prepared to work with patients from various cultures and to present health care in ways appropriate for individuals. In addition, when professionals understand factors that influence individual health behaviors, they are in a better position to meet patients' needs. Knowledge of cultural backgrounds can help personnel anticipate differences in values, religion, dietary practices, lines of authority, family life patterns, and beliefs and practices related to health and illness. Total care can only become a reality when patients are seen in the framework of their individual cultural patterns.[124]

A minority culture frequently speaks English only as a second language. Persons who are bilingual may manifest a communication pattern that uses a combination of their native language and English, resulting in idiomatic speech. Because they have difficulty understanding and following medical jargon and staff directions, patients often feel devalued by staff members. Many patients express feelings of inferiority because of the inability to speak English or because they speak English incorrectly. Because of language difficulty, many patients are unable to read and comprehend consent forms or explanations of therapies.

Role expectations for the health professional vary. In general, they are based on gender, age, educational preparation, and the ethnic identity of the staff. Greater courtesy and deference have been accorded to female nurses than to their male counterparts, and disapproval has been expressed by patients when health professionals did not fulfill gender role expectations. Age is an important consideration in providing care. Many subcultures maintain a reverence for older adults that has become minimized in our youth-dominated society. The older patient expects to be treated respectfully and in a formal manner, and the behavior of some younger staff members has been viewed as callous and disrespectful.

In many subcultures, health is not viewed as a high priority. The illness episode is viewed as a small part of a person's life. It is often difficult to gain cooperation for preventive health behaviors such as diet as part of blood pressure control and cessation of smoking to prevent heart and lung disease.

Daily Care

After potential problems have been assessed, daily care of the patient can be based on the data obtained. Important components in daily care include relieving anxiety and pain, monitoring blood gas levels and fluids, decreasing the myocardial workload, continuing dietary recommendations, and preventing and detecting complications.

If the patient experiences pain, it is important to note the frequency, duration, quality, quantity, location, associated factors such as diaphoresis and dyspnea, and alleviating factors. This information should be recorded on the patient's chart, accompanied by an ECG rhythm strip. Furthermore, a 12-lead ECG should be obtained and evaluated for changes from the initial ECG, and the patient's physician should be notified. If the physician has prescribed nitrates and analgesics, they should be given to the patient, and the nurse should monitor the patient's vital signs and respiratory characteristics. If the pain is not relieved, the physician should be notified so that the duration of pain and the increased oxygen demand on the heart can be decreased as soon as possible.

Once established, the need for supplemental oxygen should be evaluated often during the acute phase of the illness. Arterial blood gas samples should be drawn at intervals to evaluate acid-base balance.

Flow sheets that record many values are useful in maintaining a graphic representation of the patient's progress (Fig. 8-27). Some CCUs prefer a separate flow sheet for arterial blood gas levels, especially for people who require frequent arterial blood gas analysis.

Limiting myocardial work continues to be an important component of daily patient care. Activities should be gradually increased according to the plan of rehabilitation and the patient's stage of recovery. Patients are now being mobilized earlier than in previous years, since prolonged bed rest may not only prevent but also promote development of complications after MI. The patient must, however, be assisted in all activities, especially during the acute phase of the illness.

Initial dietary recommendations are usually maintained throughout the acute phase of illness and often throughout hospitalization and convalescence.

As previously discussed, fluid and electrolyte balance is vital during the acute phase of the MI. Accurate measurement of intake and output levels, daily weight readings, evaluation of hydration, presence of pulmonary findings such as crackles, and edema are all important components in the evaluation of fluid and electrolyte balance.

Techniques such as recording daily weight and accurate intake and output measurements are aimed at preventing congestive heart failure or detecting it early. Except in an emergency, all fluids should be administered via microdrip, and drugs such as lidocaine should be placed in a reliable automatic infusion device and checked frequently to determine whether the proper amount of fluid is being delivered. A saline-flushed lock may be substituted when it is necessary to continue intravenous medications.

Each of these components should be evaluated and care planned accordingly. Goals should be set with the patient for care. Reevaluation and further planning are performed in relation to changes in patient status.

Antiembolic hose on the legs also may be used to prevent venous stasis. They must be applied with equal pressure from the foot to above the knee, checked frequently, and removed 2 to 3 times a day. Lotion or powder may be applied to the skin. The patient should be instructed not to cross the legs or ankles to prevent venous stasis. Sometimes the elastic stockings roll down over the knee and create a tourniquet effect on the leg; if this occurs, it should be corrected promptly. The legs should be observed for redness, swelling, heat, red streaks, and a positive Homans sign. This sign occurs as a slight pain at the back of the knee or calf where the ankle is forcibly dorsiflexed and is indicative of incipient or established thrombosis in the veins of the leg. If evidence of embolization is observed, the patient's physician should be notified.

The exercise program is a necessary component of the total rehabilitation effort. An exercise program can help prevent complications engendered by inactivity, such as respiratory complications, venous stasis, joint stiffness from immobility, and weakness resulting from loss of muscle tone. Furthermore, exercise therapy promotes relaxation by decreasing tension and aids the patient psychologically.

An exercise program with appropriate program goals and priorities for implementation should be planned with the patient for use throughout hospitalization and after discharge. Structured in progressive stages, the exercise program should be individualized according to the patient's tolerance. Initially the patient may be assisted in performing passive exercises. A footboard is useful for the patient to exercise leg muscles. Tolerance to exercise at each stage should be observed, evaluated, and recorded. When the patient is out of bed for the first time, medical personnel should record the supine and standing blood pressures and heart rate.

Stamp here with
patient's Addressograph
plate

	Date: Time: 7-3	3-11	11-7	7-3	3-11	11-7
Chest						
Chest pain	No					
R_x and response	-					
Gallops/murmurs	S3					
1 + edema	1+pedal					
Jugular venous distention	No					
Breath sounds	Bilateral					
Crackles	Inspiratory					
Rhonchi	No					
Wheezes	RUL					
Cough	Yes					
Dyspnea	No					
Cyanosis	No					
Other						
Abdomen						
Nausea/vomiting	No					
Appetite/diet	Not hungry					
Bowels/guaiac	No					
Abdominal distention	No					
Hepatomegaly	No					
Other						
Rhythm						
Basic rhythm	NSR					
Arrhythmias	Occ. PVCs					
Conduction defect	No					
Emotional status	Quiet Appears depressed					
Other						
Vital signs	Bed bath/bed rest					
Bath/activity level	up to B.S.C.					
Temperature/weight	99.4°/206 lbs.					
Apical/radial pulse	82/82					
Respirations	20 at rest					
Blood pressure	138/84 R. arm					
Pedal pulses	3+bilateral					
Cardiac output	N.A.					
Right atrial pressure	N.A.					
Pulmonary artery pressure	N.A.					
Pulmonary capillary wedge pressure	N.A.					
Time	7 A.M.					
Laboratory data						
Enzymes	CK-MB-7%, $LDH_1 > LDH_2$					
Blood gases	N.A.					
Other						
I and O						
Intake						
Oral	740 cc					
IV	280 cc					
Total	1020					
Total 24 hours						
Output						
Urine	530 cc					
Emesis/Gomco	N.A.					
Total						
Total 24 hours	530					
Signature						

Fig. 8-27 CCU summary flow sheet.

Transfer from CCU

Patients experiencing minimum or no complications are generally transferred to an intermediate care unit by the first to third day after MI. Adequate preparations are important to minimize emotional or physiologic reactions that may accompany transfer. Because the CCU is viewed by some patients as a safe atmosphere, they may be reluctant to leave. Others may anticipate moving to an environment they view as less restrictive. Whatever the reaction, it is important that the personnel in the CCU provide explanations of the regimens to be followed that can be reinforced by the staff in the intermediate care unit.

Because the actual transfer may be planned or sudden, the patient should be informed about the elements of transfer before the anticipated time of transfer. The patient should be aware that the staff in the intermediate care unit will be given a verbal report concerning the illness, progress, and problems for which they should be alert.

The following suggestions will ease the patient's transition from the CCU to the intermediate care area:

1. Have the intermediate care area prepared with all the equipment needed by the patient.
2. Monitor cardiac activity by telemetry to provide rapid detection of potential dysrhythmic problems.
3. Provide a proposed guideline of educational activities for the patient to participate in during the remainder of hospitalization.
4. Provide the patient and family with information on routines appropriate to efficient operation of the unit, such as visiting policies, educational opportunities, activity routines, and the purpose of specialized equipment.

Several terms have evolved to describe an area designed to allow closely supervised convalescence for patients who have been transferred from the CCU. This area provides more intense observation and care than a routine medical unit but less than that provided in a CCU. Synonyms for this area include *step-down unit, liberalized cardiac unit, telemetry unit,* and *intermediate care unit.* Regardless of the name selected, this unit has the following purposes:

1. Continued patient monitoring to allow for immediate recognition of cardiac dysrhythmias and conduction disturbances
2. Immediate CPR
3. Safe, supervised, early mobilization
4. Reduction in costs
5. Environment conducive to psychologic and physical recovery
6. Education and reeducation concerning abilities and disabilities related to heart disease
7. Continuation of the planned rehabilitation program

Studies have shown that some patients who suffer AMI continue to be at risk even after surviving the first few hazardous days after onset. In fact mortality rates during the later in-hospital phase of the illness, when the patient is usually no longer being cared for in the CCU, may be as high as that in the CCU for some groups of patients. This situation is the basis for the concept of intermediate coronary care, whereby patients can be located in an area that is usually close to the CCU. This unit has monitoring and resuscitative equipment and is staffed with personnel sufficiently prepared to provide routine as well as emergency cardiopulmonary care.

The following groups of patients have been shown to be at increased risk of catastrophic cardiac events during hospitalization and after discharge from the CCU[43]:

1. Patients with anterior infarctions involving large portions of the left ventricle and interventricular septum
2. Patients who while in the CCU exhibit circulatory failure in the form of cardiogenic shock, pulmonary edema, and congestive heart failure
3. Patients with preexisting cardiovascular disease, prior infarction, and fascicular block
4. Patients who exhibit dysrhythmias that are primarily ventricular in origin such as premature ventricular systoles or that are indicative of heart failure such as atrial fibrillation or flutter, persistent sinus tachycardia, or both
5. Patients with severe left ventricular dysfunction
6. Patients with functional abnormalities, such as exercise-induced ischemia noted as at least 2 mm of ST-segment depression or angina at heart rates less than 135 beats/min and exercise intolerance noted as exercise capacity of less than 4 metabolic equivalents (METs)

Although current data indicate that people who fall within the categories listed above have a 2 to 6 times greater chance of late in-hospital sudden death, this cannot be predicted with complete accuracy. However, these patients have had a slightly longer stay in the CCU (1 to 2 days longer) and tend to be 3 to 4 years older than their counterparts who survive hospitalization. These facts alone support the need for accurate assessment and interpretation of data to prevent and treat the complications that contribute to this high late in-hospital mortality.

Priorities During Intermediate Care

During the period of intermediate care, attention is focused on activity tolerance, educational strengths and deficits, and the patient's physical and psychologic status.

One goal of intermediate care is supervised early mobilization. Consistent with this expectation is a gradual increase in physical activity during the remainder of hospitalization, enabling the patient to reach activity levels required for self-care at home. The activities allowed include progressively increased self-care, increasing time spent sitting in a chair, and body motion and strength-building exercises. Ambulation should be increased daily until the patient can walk around the hospital unit without tiring.

These physical activities are alternated with rest periods. Exercise should always be avoided after meals, when a large percentage of cardiac output is diverted to digest food. Criteria for decreasing the level of activity include the following[43]:

1. Chest pain or dyspnea
2. Heart rate exceeding 120 beats/min
3. Occurrence of a significant dysrhythmia
4. Decrease in systolic blood pressure of 20 mm Hg
5. Increased ST-segment displacement on the ECG or monitor

Assessment of the patient's educational strengths and deficits should be determined soon after admission to the intermediate care unit so that planned teaching can be completed before discharge. In many instances, personnel with special knowledge and skill in psychologic evaluation can be of tremendous assistance in determining how best to motivate patients and facilitate learning. For some patients, denial, depression, and despair are patterns of behavior that prevent optimal benefit from educational efforts. Individuals who have psychologic expertise can be of help in dealing with these patients and their families. This period immediately after the CCU experience has been recognized as the time when patients are most receptive to changes in lifestyle. Lifelong habits can be changed at this point more easily than later when the emotional impact of the acute event has subsided. Personnel must take full advantage of this receptive period.

Preparation for Discharge

The past decade has witnessed changes in patterns of referrals from hospitals to home health care. Patients are being released from the hospital earlier in their convalescence. Some patients are being discharged directly from ICU while still requiring respirators, suction machines, nasogastric tubes, urinary catheters, intravenous therapy, and continuous oxygen.[125]

The average length of stay for the patient with an uncomplicated MI has decreased. This shortened hospital stay has impinged on the time available for patient education and comprehension. Written materials are especially useful to patients and families in helping them to understand information given to them by personnel and in reminding them of the information once they are at home. Written materials should cover information needed by the patient to comply with prescriptions related to medications, diet, physical activity, and health behaviors. Although providing such information does not ensure compliance, it is necessary that the patient know how to best contribute to recovery.

Medications

Prescriptions and details of the drug regimen should be explained to the patient and a responsible family member.

Prescriptions should be labeled, and actions and side effects of each drug are noted. The patient should be assisted to adjust the medication schedule to the usual lifestyle at home to ensure maximum adherence to the regimen.

Nutrition

The desired dietary modifications of calories, cholesterol, fats, and sodium should be explained. Demonstration of food preparation consistent with the dietary regimen and the patient's eating preferences and habits is desirable.

Physical activity

An activity prescription should be individualized based on the patient's prior level of activity and job requirements. It is the responsibility of the health team to prescribe and initially supervise the type of exercise, determine its duration and schedule, and warn against overexercising and describe its signs.[42]

Smoking

Patients who smoke should be discouraged from continuing this practice. Many self-help programs are available to assist in smoking cessation. Moreover, health care personnel should set an example by not smoking.[38]

Sexual activity

It is important that the patient and partner receive information about resuming sexual relations. Often patients and their partners do not ask questions because of embarrassment or fear and make false assumptions about returning to previous sexual behavior. The health care team must ensure that this information is provided and that the patient and partner are allowed to express concerns and ask questions. Patients and their partners should learn when it will be safe to engage in sexual intercourse and that sexual activity should commence when the patient is rested and has not had a heavy meal or alcohol consumption.

Follow-up care

Patients should receive information about a follow-up visit to the physician. In addition, the patient should know that chest pain, palpitations, shortness of breath, syncope or presyncope should be reported at once. It is important that family members learn about available community emergency services and ways to obtain help if needed. Moreover, family members should be encouraged to acquire CPR skills.

Community resources

The local heart association, vocational rehabilitation center, Veterans Administration, and other organizations may be of help to the patient. Other people, such as the social worker, public health nurse, dietician, physical therapist, chaplain, occupational therapist, and psychologist may be asked for assistance and advice. Many communities have developed "coronary clubs," in which interested patients, families, and health care workers meet at regular times for guidance in care and education. This offers an opportunity to teach BCLS to the patient and family. Guest speakers may discuss topics such as nutrition, exercise, sexuality, BCLS, and antismoking techniques.

REFERENCES

1. Lynaugh JE, Fairman J: New nurses, new spaces: a preview of the AACN history study, *Am J Crit Care* 1:19, 1992.
2. Meltzer L and others: *Intensive coronary care,* Bowie, Md, 1965, Charles Press.
3. Groeger JS and others: Descriptive analysis of critical care units in the United States, *Crit Care Med* 20:846, 1992.
4. Hofvendahl S: Influence of treatment in a coronary care unit on prognosis in acute myocardial infarction, *Acta Med Scand* 519(suppl):1, 1971.
5. Rogove H, Hughes C: Defibrillation and cardioversion, *Crit Care Clin* 8:839, 1992.
6. Chiriboga D and others: Temporal trends (1975 through 1990) in the incidence and case-fatality rates of primary ventricular fibrillation complicating acute myocardial infarction: a communitywide perspective, *Circulation* 89:998, 1994.
7. McGregor M: Myocardial ischemia: towards better use of the coronary care unit, *Am J Med* 76:887, 1984.
8. Wheeler DJ: Unresolved questions concerning coronary care units, *Clin Invest Med* 4(1):13, 1981.
9. Lee TH and others: Sensitivity of routine clinical criteria for diagnosing myocardial infarction within 24 hours of hospitalization, *Ann Intern Med* 106:181, 1987.
10. Roberts R, Kleiman NS: Earlier diagnosis and treatment of acute myocardial infarction necessitates the need for a "new diagnostic mind set," *Circulation* 89:872, 1994.
11. Gibler WB and others: Rapid diagnostic and treatment center in the emergency department for patients with chest pain, *Circulation* 84(4[suppl 1]):I-15, 1992.
12. Keriakes DJ and others: Time delays in the diagnosis and treatment of acute myocardial infarction: a tale of eight cities, *Am Heart J* 120:773, 1990.
13. Keriakes DJ and others (Cincinnati Heart Project Study Group): Relative importance of emergency medical system transport and the prehospital electrocardiogram on reducing hospital time delay to therapy for acute myocardial infarction: a preliminary report from the Cincinnati Heart Project, *Am Heart J* 123:835, 1992.
14. Dracup K, Moser DK: Treatment-seeking behavior among those with signs and symptoms of acute myocardial infarction, *Heart Lung* 20:570, 1991.
15. National Heart Attack Alert Program Coordinating Committee, 60 Minutes to Treatment Working Group: *Emergency department: rapid identification and treatment of patients with acute myocardial infarction,* NIH Publication No 93-3278, 1993, US Department of Health and Human Services.
16. Cardin S and others: Use of patient care extenders in critical care nursing, *AACN Clin Iss Crit Care Nurs* 3:789, 1992.
17. Katz R: Cluster management, *AACN Clin Iss Crit Care Nurs* 3:743, 1992.
18. McElroy MJ, Campbell S: Case management with the nurse manager in the role of case manager in an interventional cardiology unit, *AACN Clin Iss Crit Care Nurs* 3:749, 1992.
19. Ahrens T: Nurse clinician model of managed care, *AACN Clin Iss Crit Care Nurs* 3:761, 1992.
20. Keane A and others: Critical care nurse practitioner: evolution of the advanced practice nursing role, *Am J Crit Care* 3:232, 1994.
21. National Institutes of Health (NIH): Consensus Development Conference on Critical Care, 4:6, 1983.
22. Spodick DH: The CCRN-CCMD partnership: advancing the quality of patient care, *Heart Lung* 22:381, 1993.
23. Evans SA, Carlson R: Nurse/physician collaboration: solving the nursing shortage crisis, *Am J Crit Care* 1(10):25, 1992.
24. Gordon S: Inside the patient-driven system, *Crit Care Nurse* 74(suppl):1, 1994.
25. Mitchell PH and others: American Association of Critical-Care Nurses Demonstration Project: profile of excellence in critical care nursing, *Heart Lung* 18:219, 1989.
26. Zimmerman JE and others: Improving intensive care: observations based on organizational case studies in nine intensive care units: a prospective, multicenter study, *Crit Care Med* 21:1443, 1993.
27. Mendleson Y: Pulse oximetry: theory and applications for noninvasive monitoring, *Clin Chem* 38:1601, 1992.
28. American College of Sports Medicine: *Guidelines for exercise testing and training,* ed 4, Philadelphia, 1991, Lea & Febiger.
29. Laks M and others: Will relaxing safe current limits for electromedical equipment increase hazards to patients? *Circulation* 89:909, 1994.
30. Furst E: The safe medical device act, *J Cardiovasc Nurs* 8(2):79, 1994.
31. Hickey C: *Advances in the care of the patient with ischemic heart disease: developing new nursing strategies.* In Baas LS, editor: *Essentials of cardiovascular nursing,* Rockville, Md, 1991, Aspen.
32. Bergstrom DL, Keller C: Drug-induced myocardial ischemia and acute myocardial infarction, *Crit Care Nurs Clin North Am* 4:273, 1992.
33. Cheng TO: Variant angina of Prinzmetal with normal coronary arteriograms: a variant of the variant, *Circulation* 47:476, 1973.
34. Cheitlin MD and others: *Clinical cardiology,* ed 6, Norwalk, Conn, 1993, Appleton & Lange.
35. Bashoour TT and others: Unstable myocardial ischemia, *Pract Cardiol* 15:10, 1989.
36. Chou TE: *Electrocardiography in clinical practice,* ed 3, Philadelphia, 1991, Saunders.
37. Chesler E: *Clinical cardiology,* ed 5, New York, 1993, Springer-Verlag.
38. Lowther N, Dunn SC: *Tobacco dependence.* In Baas LS, editor: *Essentials of cardiovascular nursing,* Rockville, Md, 1991, Aspen.
39. Waters D: A practical approach to diagnosis and treatment of unstable angina, *Heart Dis Stroke* 3:159, 1994.
40. Agency for Health Care Policy and Research: *Unstable angina: diagnosis and management.* AHCPR Publication No 94-0602, Rockville, Md, 1994, US Department of Health and Human Services.
41. Reichek N and others: Antianginal effects of nitroglycerin patches, *Am J Cardiol* 54:1, 1984.
42. Baas LS: *Assessing and prescribing activity for the person with cardiac disease.* In Baas LS, editor: *Essentials of cardiovascular nursing.* Rockville, Md, 1991, Aspen.
43. American Association of Cardiovascular and Pulmonary Rehabilitation: *Guidelines for cardiac rehabilitation programs,* Champaign, Ill, 1991, Human Kinetics Books.
44. Creel CA: Silent myocardial ischemia and nursing implications, *Heart Lung* 23:218, 1994.
45. Gerson M: *Cardiac nuclear medicine,* ed 2, New York, 1991, McGraw-Hill.
46. Hochrein MA, Sohll L: Heart smart: a guide to cardiac tests, *Am J Nurs* 92(12):22, 1992.
47. Deedwania PC: Comparison of the prognostic values of ischemia during daily life and ischemia induced by treadmill exercise testing, *Am J Cardiol* 73:15B, 1994.
48. Hix DC: Magnesium in congestive heart failure, acute myocardial infarction and dysrhythmias, *J Cardiovasc Nurs* 8(1):19, 1993.

49. Horner SM: Efficacy of intravenous magnesium in acute myocardial infarction in reducing arrhythmias and mortality: meta-analysis of magnesium in acute myocardial infarction, *Circulation* 86:774, 1992.

50. Woods KL and others: Intravenous magnesium sulphate in suspected acute myocardial infarction: results of the second Leicester Intravenous Magnesium Sulphate Intervention Trial (LIMIT-2), *Lancet* 339:1553, 1992.

51. 1992 National Conference on Cardiopulmonary Resuscitation and Emergency Cardiac Care: New ACLS guidelines—1992, *JAMA* 268:2171, 1992.

52. Yusef S and others: Effects of intravenous nitrates on mortality in acute myocardial infarction: an overview of the randomized trials, *Lancet* 331:1088, 1988.

53. Pfeffer MA, Braunwald E: Ventricular remodeling after myocardial infarction, *Circulation* 81(1):161, 1990.

54. Brown EJ, Pfeffer MA: Ventricular remodeling after MI: a modifiable process, *Heart Dis Stroke* 3:164, 1994.

55. Fara AM: The role of angiotensin-converting enzyme inhibitors in reducing ventricular remodeling after myocardial infarction, *J Cardiovasc Nurs* 8(1):32, 1993.

56. Hugenholtz PG, Suryapranata H: Thrombolytic agents in early myocardial infarction, *Am J Cardiol* 63:94E, 1989.

57. Ostrow CL: Thrombolytics. *AACN Clin Iss Crit Care Nurs* 3:423, 1992.

58. Kleven MR: Comparison of thrombolytic agents: mechanism of action, efficacy and safety, *Heart Lung* 17:6, 1988.

59. Sherry S: Origin of thrombolytic therapy, *J Am Coll Cardiol* 14:1085, 1989.

60. Gruppo Italiano per lo Studio Streptochinase nell'Infarto Miocardico (GISSI): Effectiveness of intravenous thrombolytic treatment in acute myocardial infarction, *Lancet* 1:397, 1986.

61. ISIS Collaborative Group: Intravenous streptokinase given within 0-4 hours of onset of myocardial infarction reduced mortality: ISIS-2, *Lancet* 1:502, 1987.

62. ISIS-2 Collaborative Group: Randomized trial of intravenous streptokinase, oral aspirin, both or neither among 17,187 cases of suspected acute myocardial infarction, *J Am Coll Cardiol* 12:6, 1988.

63. Sun M: The coming competition among clot busting drugs, *Science* 240:1267, 1988.

64. Verstraete M and others: Randomized trial of intravenous recombinant tissue-type plasminogen activator versus intravenous streptokinase in acute myocardial infarction, *Lancet* 1:842, 1985.

65. Topol EJ: Advances in thrombolytic therapy for acute myocardial infarction, *J Clin Pharmacol* 27:735, 1987.

66. Gruppo Italiano per lo Studio della Sopraveivenza nell'Infarto Miocardico: GISSI-2: a factorial randomized trial of alteplase versus streptokinase and heparin versus no heparin among 12,490 patients with acute myocardial infarction, *Lancet* 336:65, 1990.

67. The GUSTO Investigators: An international randomized trial comparing four thrombolytic strategies for acute myocardial infarction, *N Engl J Med* 329:673, 1993.

68. Bassand J and others: Multicenter trial of intravenous anisolated plasminogen streptokinase activator complex (APSAC) in acute myocardial infarction: effects on infarct size and left ventricular function, *J Am Coll Cardiol* 13:988, 1989.

69. Kline E: Clinical controversies surrounding thrombolytic therapy in acute myocardial infarction, *Heart Lung* 19:596, 1990.

70. Aragon D, Martin M: What you should know about thrombolytic therapy for acute MI, *Am J Nurs* 93(9):24, 1993.

71. American College of Cardiology/American Heart Association, Task Force on Assessment and Diagnostic and Therapeutic Cardiovascular Procedures, Subcommittee to Develop Guidelines for the Early Management of Patients with Acute Myocardial Infarction: Guidelines for the early management of patients with acute myocardial infarction, *J Am Coll Cardiol* 16:249, 1990.

72. Bell NN: Clinical significance of ST-segment monitoring, *Crit Care Nurs Clin North Am* 4:313, 1992.

73. Topol E: *Textbook of interventional cardiology,* Philadelphia, 1991, Saunders.

74. Grines CL, for the Primary Angioplasty in Myocardial Infarction Study Group: A comparison of immediate angioplasty with thrombolytic therapy for acute myocardial infarction, *N Engl J Med* 328:673, 1993.

75. Dotter CT, Judkins MP: Transmittal treatment of arteriosclerotic obstruction: description of a new technique and a preliminary report of its application, *Circulation* 30:654, 1964.

76. Gruentzig AR and others: Nonoperative dilatation of coronary artery stenosis: percutaneous transluminal coronary angioplasty, *N Engl J Med* 301:61, 1979.

77. Jeroudi MO and others: Percutaneous transluminal coronary angioplasty in octogenarians, *Ann Intern Med* 113:423, 1990.

78. Webb JG and others: Coronary angioplasty after coronary bypass surgery: initial results and late outcome in 422 patients, *J Am Coll Cardiol* 16:812, 1990.

79. Albert NM: Laser angioplasty and intracoronary stents: going beyond the balloon, *AACN Clin Iss Crit Care Nurs* 5:15, 1994.

80. Foley JB and others: Safety, success, and restenosis after selective coronary implantation of the Palmaz-Schatz stent in 100 patients at a single center, *Am Heart J* 125:686, 1992.

81. Sutton JM and others: Major clinical events after coronary stenting: the multicenter registry of acute and elective Gianturco-Roubin stent placement, *Circulation* 89:1126, 1994.

82. Deelstra MH: Coronary rotational ablation: an overview with related nursing interventions, *Am J Crit Care* 3:16, 1993.

83. Gist HC and others: New interventional techniques for coronary revascularization, *Heart Dis Stroke* 2:198, 1993.

84. CAVEAT Investigators: The coronary angioplasty versus excisional arthrectomy trial: preliminary results, *Circulation* 86:I-374, 1992.

85. Kuhn M: Angiotensin converting enzyme inhibitors, *AACN Clin Iss Crit Care Nurs* 3:461, 1992.

86. Kuhn M: Nitrates, *AACN Clin Iss Crit Care Nurs* 3:409, 1992.

87. Clements JV: Sympathomimetics, inotropics, and vasodilators, *AACN Clin Iss Crit Care Nurs* 3:395, 1992.

88. Alpert JS, Becker RC: Mechanisms and management of cardiogenic shock, *Crit Care Clin* 9(2):205, 1993.

89. Huddleston VB: *Multisystem organ failure: pathology and clinical implications,* St Louis, 1992, Mosby.

90. Gardner PE: Pulmonary artery pressure monitoring, *AACN Clin Iss Crit Care Nurs* 4:98, 1993.

91. Ahrens TS, Rutherford DA: *Essentials of oxygenation,* Boston, 1993, Jones & Bartlett.

92. Sommers MS and others: Issues in methods and measurement of thermodilution cardiac output, *Nurs Res* 42:228, 1993.

93. Daily EK, Schroeder JS: *Techniques in bedside hemodynamic monitoring,* ed 5, St Louis, 1994, Mosby.

94. American Association of Critical-Care Nurses: Evaluation of the effects of heparinized flush solutions on the patency of arterial pressure monitoring lines: the AACN Thunder Project, *Am J Crit Care* 2:16, 1993.

95. Woods SL, Osgulthorpe S: Cardiac output determination, *AACN Clin Iss Crit Care Nurs* 4:81, 1993.

96. Gillman PH: Continuous measurement of cardiac output: a milestone in hemodynamic monitoring, *Focus Crit Care* 19:155, 1992.

97. White KM: Using continuous SVO$_2$ to assess oxygen supply/demand balance in the critically ill patient, *AACN Clin Iss Crit Care* 4:134, 1993.

98. Ahrens TS: Changing perspectives in the assessment of oxygenation, *Crit Care Nurse* 13:78, 1993.

99. Headley JM: Diethorn ML: Right ventricular volumetric monitoring, *AACN Clin Iss Crit Care Nurs* 4:120, 1993.

100. Headley JM, VonReuden K: The right ventricle: significant anatomy, physiology and interventricular considerations, *J Cardiovasc Nurs* 6:1, 1991.
101. Goldberg RJ and others: Cardiogenic shock after acute myocardial infarction: incidence and mortality from a community-wide perspective—1975-1988, *N Engl J Med* 325:1117, 1991.
102. Quaal SJ: *Comprehensive intra-aortic balloon counterpulsation,* ed 2, St Louis, 1993, Mosby.
103. Shinn AE, Joseph D: Concepts of intraaortic balloon counterpulsation, *J Cardiovasc Nurs* 8(2):45, 1994.
104. American Heart Association: *Heart and stroke facts: statistical supplement,* AHA Publication No 55-0515, Dallas, 1993, The Association.
105. Eigenberg MS and others: Cardiac arrest and resuscitation: a tale of 29 cities, *Ann Emerg Med* 19:179, 1990.
106. Moss AJ, Benhorin J: Prognosis and management after a first myocardial infarction, *N Engl J Med* 322:743, 1990.
107. Surawicz B: Electrophysiologic substrate of torsade de pointes: dispersion of repolarization or early after depolarizations? *J Am Coll Cardiol* 14:172, 1989.
108. Ward O: A new familial cardiac syndrome in children, *J Irish Med Assoc* 54:103, 1964.
109. Mark DB: An overview of risk assessment in coronary artery disease, *Am J Cardiol* 73:19B, 1994.
110. Clark BK: Beta-adrenergic blocking agents: their current status, *AACN Clin Issues Crit Care Nurs* 3:447, 1992.
111. Frishman WH and others: Beta adrenergic blockade and calcium channel blockade in myocardial infarction, *Med Clin North Am* 73:409, 1989.
112. Darling ES: Overview of cardiac electrophysiologic testing, *Crit Care Nurs Clin North Am* 6(1)1, 1994.
113. Miracle VA, Hovekamp G: Needs of families of patients undergoing invasive cardiac procedures, *Am J Crit Care* 3:155, 1994.
114. Dougherty CM: Longitudinal recovery following sudden cardiac arrest and internal cardioverter defibrillator implantation: survivors and their families, *Am J Crit Care* 3:129, 1994.
115. Moser SA and others: Updated care guidelines for patients with automatic implantable cardioverter defibrillators, *Crit Care Nurse* 13:62, 1993.
116. Davidson T and others: Implantable cardioverter defibrillators: a guide for clinicians, *Heart Lung* 23:205, 1994.
117. Robinson KR: Developing a scale to measure denial levels of clients with actual or potential myocardial infarctions, *Heart Lung* 23:36, 1994.
118. Cassem NH, Hackett TP: Factors contributing to delay in responding to the signs and symptoms of acute myocardial infarction, *Am J Cardiol* 24:651, 1969.
119. Erickson HC and others: *Modeling and role-modeling: a paradigm for nursing,* Lexington, SC, 1988, Pine Press.
120. Riegel BJ, Dracup KA: Does overprotection cause cardiac invalidism after acute myocardial infarction? *Heart Lung* 21:529, 1992.
121. Gil K, Blumenthal JA: Behavior modification in the primary and secondary prevention of coronary heart disease, *Cardiol Pract* 1:274, 1985.
122. Ornish D: Can lifestyle changes reverse coronary disease? *Lancet* 336:129, 1990.
123. Dossey B: *Holistic nursing,* Rockville, Md, 1990, Aspen.
124. Tripp-Reimer T and others: Cultural assessment: content and process, *Nurs Outlook* 32:78, 1984.
125. Andreoli KG, Musser LA: Trends that may affect nursing's future, *Nurs Health Care* 6:47, 1985.

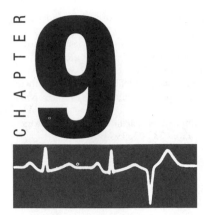

Valvular Heart Disease

Erin L. Abramczyk
Mary-Michael Brown

The heart has four valves: aortic, mitral, pulmonary, and tricuspid. These valves are responsible for ensuring the one-way flow of blood through each heart chamber and for preventing backflow within the heart.

Diseases of these valves result in valvular stenosis, valvular regurgitation, or both. Valvular stenosis is the narrowing of the valve orifice, which hinders the forward flow of blood from a heart chamber. Some causes of valvular stenosis include rheumatic fever, congenital malformations of the valve, idiopathic calcification, myxomas, bacterial vegetations, and thrombus. Valvular regurgitation is the leaking of blood in a backward direction as a result of malformed, floppy, stretched, inflamed, infected, or lesion-lined valve leaflets that prevent tight valve closure. The aortic and mitral valves are most commonly affected by disease. The pulmonary and tricuspid valves are affected less often; however, these valves can be diseased significantly and may even result in death. Pulmonary valve dysfunction, when present, is often associated with congenital malformations. Tricuspid valve disease rarely occurs by itself and usually occurs with mitral valve disease.

Nurses who care for patients with valvular heart disease are challenged to understand the complex nature of these illnesses. Valvular heart disease may be a chronic or an acute problem and may be manifested at any time in life. Nurses must be aware of the different types of valvular heart disease and know which valves are typically affected. Nurses must be knowledgeable about the treatments available to patients, and they must be able to identify the disastrous complications that may accompany valvular heart disease. Finally, nurses must evaluate patients' understanding of their illnesses and the degree of family support available. It is essential that nursing care be based on an understanding of the structure and function of the heart valves and the causes and treatments for the malfunction.

This chapter describes the location and function of each heart valve; discusses manifestations of valvular disease; reviews the physical findings and diagnostic evaluation of valvular disease; and considers the medical, surgical, and nursing care of the patient with valvular heart disease.

STRUCTURE AND FUNCTION OF VALVES

Although there are four valves in the heart, structurally and functionally there are two types: semilunar and atrioventricular (AV). The semilunar valves are the aortic and pulmonary; they are named for their half-moon shape. Each semilunar valve consists of three pocketlike leaflets of equal size. These leaflets are smooth and thin and arise from the arterial wall (see Fig. 1-2).

The mitral and tricuspid valves are called *AV valves* because of their location between the atria and ventricles. The AV valves are composed of four major structures: annulus, leaflets, chordae tendineae, and papillary muscles. These valves originate from the annulus, which is a well-defined ring of fibrous tissue around the AV orifice. The AV valves have two or three leaflets, which are thin, membranous, trapezoid structures. The mitral (or bicuspid) valve has two leaflets: one anterior and one posterior. Each leaflet is composed of three to four cusps. The tricuspid valve has three leaflets: one anterior, one posterior, and one septal.

Chordae tendineae are strong, tendonlike cords that attach the ventricular surface of the leaflets to the papillary muscles and allow the valve leaflets to balloon upward and against each other.[1] The papillary muscles are located at the base of the ventricles and pull the chordae and AV leaflets together and downward at the beginning of ventricular systole. This downward pull on the chordae prevents the eversion of valve leaflets into the atria during ventricular systole.

It is important to keep these basic valve structures in mind because valvular disease affects them. Treatment of valvular heart disease is aimed at modifying or replacing one or more of the dysfunctional structures to alleviate symptoms.

MURMURS OF VALVULAR HEART DISEASE

When the cardiac cycle proceeds normally, the valves open to let blood flow from one chamber to the next and close to keep blood from leaking backward[2] (see Chapter 1). The sound produced as blood flows through a stenotic or regurgitant valve is called a *murmur*. The murmur is a result of the turbulent blood flow through a diseased valve and is characteristic of valvular heart disease.

There are two major types of murmurs: systolic (or ejection) and diastolic. Chapter 2 details the cardiac cycle and the various features of cardiac murmurs. Table 9-1 describes the murmurs associated with each valvular disease.

AORTIC VALVE DISEASE

The aortic valve is located between the left ventricle and the aorta. The aortic valve opens to facilitate the flow of blood during ventricular systole and closes to prevent the backflow of blood from the aorta into the left ventricle during ventricular diastole.

Aortic Stenosis

Aortic stenosis is a narrowing of the aortic valve orifice, which obstructs the ejection of blood from the left ventricle. This obstruction leads to a high-pressure gradient between the left ventricle and aorta during systolic ejection.[3] Isolated aortic stenosis affects men 3 times more often than women.[4]

Etiology

The three major causes of aortic stenosis are congenital abnormalities, rheumatic fever, and leaflet degeneration with calcification. Aortic stenosis of congenital origin, such as unicuspid, bicuspid, multicuspid, or unequal aortic valve leaflets, is generally seen in patients younger than 30 years of age.[3] These congenital aberrations of the aortic valve make the valve leaflets more susceptible to the normal stress of cardiac hemodynamics. This increased stress and turbulent blood flow cause injury, predisposing the valvular leaflets to the development of fibrosis and calcification. The aortic valvular orifice then becomes rigid and narrowed. See Table 9-1 for more information on the causes of aortic stenosis.

Rheumatic disease affects patients from childhood through the seventh decade and causes the commissures of the valve to fuse, retract, and shorten the leaflet edges.[3] Although the aortic valve may be affected by rheumatic disease, the mitral valve is more frequently affected. However, improved treatment of streptococcal sore throat has markedly decreased the incidence of rheumatic valvular disease in the United States. Rheumatic fever is more common in developing countries. Idiopathic calcification most often affects patients in their seventh decade. Calcified deposits cause the valve leaflets to fuse and become fibrotic.[3]

Pathophysiology

Normally, the aortic valve orifice is 2.6 to 3.5 cm^2.[5] A valve orifice acutely narrowed to 0.5 cm^2 requires surgical intervention. If the stenosis develops over several years, the left ventricle may be able to compensate for a time by exerting more pressure against the valve.[6] Hypertrophy of the left ventricle develops concentrically without ventricular wall dilatation, which normalizes the systolic force of the ventricular wall. This concentric hypertrophy results in a near-normal ejection fraction and cardiac output.[3] As the aortic valve orifice continues to narrow and the left ventricle attempts to compensate, a pressure gradient occurs between the aorta and left ventricle. When the aortic valve orifice narrows to 0.4 cm^2 with a peak systolic pressure gradient above 50 mm Hg, a critical obstruction is reached.[5] The left ventricle dilates, and the left atrium enlarges with an increase in pressure to overcome the ventricular dilatation. The higher pressure in the left atrium is reflected backward through the pulmonary vasculature to the right side of the heart. Right ventricular pressure, right atrial pressure, and central venous pressure increase. Eventually, the left side and the right side of the heart fail (Fig. 9-1).

Signs and symptoms

Fatigue, chest pain, syncope, and dyspnea on exertion are the classic manifestations of aortic stenosis. Approximately 50% of patients experience chest pain (exertional angina) caused by underlying coronary artery disease or a disproportion of myocardial oxygen demand and supply during strenuous activities.[3,5] The already thickened and stretched left ventricle cannot meet the challenge of the increasing cardiac demand during exercise.

Syncope affects between 15% and 30% of patients with aortic stenosis because of a dysrhythmia or an abrupt fall in the systemic vascular resistance with a fixed cardiac output.[5] Dyspnea on exertion occurs as a sequela of left ventricular dysfunction. An increase in left ventricular end-diastolic pressure causes an increased left atrial pressure, which is reflected back into the pulmonary vascular system. As left ventricular failure worsens, the patient experiences cough, orthopnea, paroxysmal nocturnal dyspnea, and fatigue. Once patients develop severe symptoms such as angina, syncope, and heart failure, survival becomes extremely limited. Patients who develop angina or syncope may survive another 2 or 3 years, but those with heart failure may live only half as long.[7]

On examination, the patient appears pale and fatigued and has a narrow pulse pressure. The murmur of aortic stenosis is a loud, harsh, crescendo-decrescendo systolic ejection murmur heard best at the second intercostal space at the right sternal border[3,5] (see Table 9-1).

Diagnostic evaluation

The electrocardiogram (ECG) reveals left ventricular hypertrophy, first-degree AV block, and a left bundle

TABLE 9-1   **Physiologic Dynamics of Acquired Valvular Heart Disease**

Causes	Signs	Symptoms
AORTIC STENOSIS		

Rheumatic heart disease
Atherosclerosis
Calcification
	Harsh, systolic, crescendo-decrescendo
	  murmur at second intercostal space,
	  right sternal border
	Increased point of maximum impulse
	  (PMI)
	Paradoxically split second heart
	  sound (S_2)
		Angina pectoris
		Dysrhythmias
		Myocardial infarction
		Syncope
		Fatigue
		Cough
		Dyspnea on exertion
		Orthopnea
		Paroxysmal nocturnal dyspnea
		Pulmonary edema

AORTIC REGURGITATION		

Rheumatic heart disease
Deceleration blunt chest
  trauma
Syphilis
Arthritic disease
Infective endocarditis
Aortic valve sclerosis
Hypertension
Aortic aneurysm
Calcification
Dysfunction of an aortic
  valve prosthesis
Senile dilatation of the
  annulus
	Chronic
	  High-pitched, blowing diastolic decrescendo
	    murmur at third or fourth intercostal space,
	    right sternal border
	  Systolic hypertension
	  Diastolic hypotension
	  Capillary beds flush and pale with each pulse
	  Water hammer pulse
	  Head bob with pulse
	  PMI that is downward and to the left
	  Diastolic thrill at the suprasternal notch
	Acute
	  Soft murmur
	  Tachycardia
	  Third heart sound (S_3)
		Chronic:
		  Palpitations
		  Fatigue
		  Cough
		  Dyspnea on exertion
		  Orthopnea
		  Paroxysmal nocturnal dyspnea
		  Pulmonary edema
		  Angina pectoris
		  Night sweats
		  Headaches
		Acute:
		  Fatigue
		  Cough
		  Dyspnea on exertion
		  Orthopnea
		  Paroxysmal nocturnal dyspnea
		  Pulmonary edema

MITRAL STENOSIS		

Rheumatic heart disease
Tumor
Left atrial thrombus
Bacterial vegetations
Calcification
	Low-pitched, rumbling diastolic murmur at
	  the apex
	Opening snap
	Atrial fibrillation
	Hepatomegaly
	Ascites
	Jugular venous distention
	Peripheral edema
		Dyspnea
		Interstitial and alveolar
		  pulmonary edema
		Orthopnea
		Paroxysmal nocturnal dyspnea
		Hemoptysis
		Hoarseness

MITRAL REGURGITATION		

Rheumatic heart disease
Endocarditis
Prolapse
Dilated left ventricle
Calcification
Trauma
Dysfunction of a mitral
  valve prosthesis
Rupture or dysfunction
  of a papillary muscle
	Chronic
	  High-pitched, blowing systolic murmur at
	    the apex
	  PMI that is downward and to the left
	  Atrial pulsation at the third left intercostal
	    space
	  Atrial fibrillation
	  Jugular venous distention
	  Hepatomegaly
		Chronic:
		  Fatigue
		  Exhaustion
		  Palpitations
		  Atypical chest pain
		  Dysphagia
		  Symptoms of mitral stenosis

Adapted from Schakenbach LH: J Cardiovasc Nurs 1(3):14, 1987.

TABLE 9-1 Physiologic Dynamics of Acquired Valvular Heart Disease—cont'd

Causes	Signs	Symptoms
MITRAL REGURGITATION—cont'd		

	Acute:
	  High-pitched, blowing systolic murmur at
	    the apex
	  Sinus tachycardia
	  Fourth heart sound (S$_4$)
	  Widely split S$_2$
		Acute:
		  Pulmonary edema
		  Symptoms of mitral stenosis

PULMONARY STENOSIS		

Rheumatic heart disease
Previous repair of
  congenital heart defect
Cancer
	Harsh, systolic crescendo-decrescendo murmur at
	  the second intercostal space, left sternal border
	Widely split or absent S$_2$
	Jugular venous distention
	Peripheral edema
	Hepatomegaly
	Ascites
		Dyspnea on exertion
		Fatigue

PULMONARY REGURGITATION		

Infective endocarditis
Tumors
Syphilitic aneurysm of
  the pulmonary artery
  (rare)
Previous repair of right
  ventricular outflow
  tract
	With elevated pulmonary pressures:
	  High-pitched blowing, diastolic murmur at
	    the mid left sternal border
	Jugular venous distention
	Peripheral edema
	Hepatomegaly
	Ascites
	Without elevated pulmonary pressures:
	  Medium-pitched, diastolic decrescendo
	    murmur with inspiration
	Jugular venous distention
		With elevated pulmonary
		  pressures:
		  Dyspnea on exertion
		  Fatigue

TRICUSPID STENOSIS		

Rheumatic heart disease
Atrial myxomas
Cancer
	Low-pitched, rumbling diastolic, decrescendo
	  murmur at the fourth intercostal space
	  (increasing in intensity with inspiration),
	  left sternal border
	Jugular venous distention
	Peripheral edema
	Hepatomegaly
	Ascites
		Fatigue
		Neck pulsations

TRICUSPID REGURGITATION		

Rheumatic heart disease
Infective endocarditis
Right ventricular
  dilatation
Trauma
Myocardial infarction
Tricuspid valve prolapse
Left heart failure
Pulmonary hypertension
Cancer
Right atrial myxoma
	High-pitched, blowing systolic murmur at the
	  fourth intercostal space, left sternal border or
	  at the xyphoid region (increases with
	  inspiration)
	Left parasternal lift
	Hepatomegaly
	Splenomegaly
	Right bundle branch block
	Ascites
	Peripheral cyanosis
		Fatigue
		Jaundice
		Anorexia

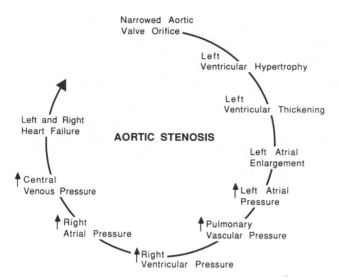

Fig. 9-1   Pathophysiology of aortic stenosis.

branch block pattern.[3,5,6] The chest roentgenogram evidences left ventricular enlargement, a poststenotic dilatation of the aorta, calcification of valve cusps, and pulmonary congestion. The echocardiogram reveals left ventricular wall thickening, reduced mobility, and possible calcification of the valve leaflets. Nuclear scans assess ventricular function and myocardial performance and determine the ejection fraction at rest and after exercise. Cardiac catheterization allows estimates of the severity of obstruction by determining the gradient and evaluation of left ventricular function. This study can determine the presence of valvular lesions as well as the presence or absence of coronary artery disease.

Treatment

Medical treatment consists of antibiotic prophylaxis against infective endocarditis. When patients require dental or other procedures requiring instrumentation (urinary catheterizations, prostatic manipulations, abortions)[3] or surgery, they should receive antibiotic coverage before and after the procedure.

Nitrates, which are used to relieve chest pain, should be administered cautiously because of the potential for syncope and orthostatic hypotension. Digoxin and diuretics may be prescribed for controlling left ventricular dysfunction and dyspnea; however, the best treatment for aortic stenosis is relief of the mechanical obstruction.

Percutaneous aortic valvuloplasty is a nonsurgical procedure available to older adults or to patients whose conditions are high surgical risks. These patients may have severe left ventricular dysfunction, severe coronary artery disease, or chronic pulmonary disease.[5,9] Under fluoroscopy, a balloon-tipped catheter is directed to the aortic valve and inflated and deflated repeatedly. This dilatation may separate fused commissures or fracture calcified valve cusps, thus reducing the stenotic obstruction. If leaflet tearing, valve ring disruption, and restenosis of the valve result from valvuloplasty, emergent valve replacement becomes necessary.[10] Although valvuloplasty may be a viable alternative to surgical valve replacement, aortic stenosis may return in weeks or months.[11]

Surgical treatment is indicated for asymptomatic conditions in patients who develop gradients greater than 50 mm Hg and for patients who develop congestive heart failure, angina, or exertional syncope.[12]

An aortic commissurotomy, or repair of the valve, may be performed for congenital aortic stenosis, particularly in young patients. However, most of these patients eventually require replacement of the valve.[12]

Aortic valve replacement requires the use of extracorporeal circulation and selection of a valvular prosthesis. There are two kinds of prosthetic valves: mechanical and biologic.

Mechanical valves include the ball valve (Starr-Edwards), the tilting disk (Medtronic-Hall), and the bileaflet valve (St. Jude Medical) (Fig. 9-2). Mechanical valves are durable but also thrombogenic, requiring long-term anticoagulation.

Bioprostheses are made from animal tissue (pig or calf) and are called *xenografts*. Bioprostheses may also be harvested from human cadavers and are known as *homografts* (Fig. 9-3). Porcine valves are excised aortic pig valves, which are preserved in glutaraldehyde. Bovine valves are made from calf pericardium, which is cut into three pieces and mounted on a stent to form three valve leaflets.[13] The Carpentier-Edwards valves are available in a porcine valve or as a pericardial graft.

The advantage of a bioprosthesis is the low risk of thromboembolic complications without anticoagulation. The disadvantage is the tendency of the bioprosthesis to degenerate.[11] Approximately 15% to 20% of patients with bioprosthetic aortic valves require second valve replacements within 10 years.[12] However, in the older population, the need for re-operation is less frequent.

Homografts are harvested from the human cadaver shortly after death (within 12 hours is optimal). There are several advantages of selecting a homograft: They have excellent hemodynamic performance, anticoagulation is rarely required because the valves are human, and they are greatly resistant to prosthetic endocarditis.[14] Some of the disadvantages of a homograft are the lack of availability, evolving preservation techniques, and the limitation to only the aortic position.[15] In addition to using cadaver homografts, the Ross procedure is gaining in popularity. This operation involves translocation of the native pulmonary valve into the aortic position and replacement of the pulmonary valve with a cadaver pulmonary homograft.[15a] The

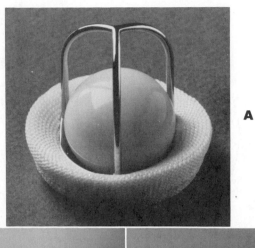

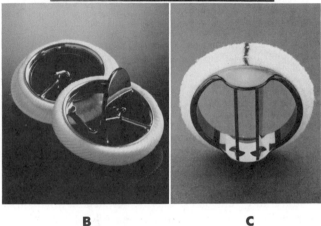

Fig. 9-2 **A,** Starr-Edwards prosthetic valve. **B,** Medtronic-Hall prosthetic valve. **C,** St. Jude Medical heart valve.   (**A** courtesy Baxter Healthcare, Edwards CVS Division, Irvine, Calif.; **B** courtesy Medtronic, Minneapolis; **C** courtesy St. Jude Medical, St Paul, Minn.)

benefits of the Ross procedure are the same as those of single homograft replacements. Currently, pulmonary homografts are more accessible than aortic homografts.

Selection of the type of prosthetic valve is determined by the surgeon who measures the size of the valve orifice during surgery. (See Fig. 9-4 for the instrument used to measure the valve orifice.) Before surgery, the surgeon discusses with the patient the advantages and disadvantages of each type of prosthetic valve. A patient with a life expectancy of more than 10 years generally receives a mechanical valve. A patient with a questionable ability for compliance with anticoagulation, a patient with liver dysfunction, and a woman who expresses a desire to bear children receive bioprostheses.

Nursing treatment is based on a holistic assessment of the patient. The individual's response to aortic stenosis must also be determined. Decreased activity tolerance, alterations in comfort (chest pain, syncope), potential for infection, and anxiety related to knowledge deficit are problems commonly seen in patients with aortic stenosis.

For patients who have had an aortic valve replacement, potential for injury (thromboembolism, hemorrhage), potential for noncompliance, and potential for infection are the major problems requiring nursing therapy. Patients with bioprostheses can expect to take warfarin (Coumadin) for approximately 6 weeks after valve replacement. The blood of patients with mechanical valves is anticoagulated with warfarin for the rest of the patients' lives. Nurses must scrutinize patients' understanding of the necessity for and the hazards of anticoagulation. Nurses must also assess patients' abilities and desires to comply with therapeutic prescriptions.

Antibiotic prophylaxis against infective endocarditis is always indicated for surgical or dental procedures. See Table 9-2 for a list of possible nursing problems and treatment strategies.

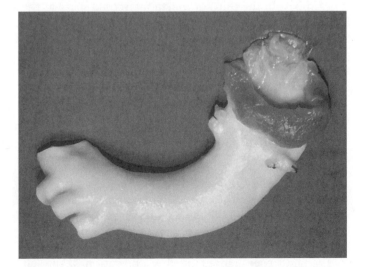

Fig. 9-3   Cryopreserved homograft aortic heart valve with conduit.

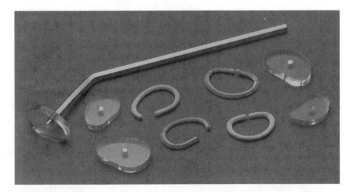

Fig. 9-4   Carpentier-Edwards annuloplasty ring and ancillary equipment.   (Courtesy Baxter Healthcare, Edwards CVS Division, Irvine, Calif.)

Aortic Regurgitation

Aortic regurgitation is the backflow of blood from the aorta into the left ventricle during ventricular diastole.

Etiology

Rheumatic fever and syphilis have previously been identified as the major causes of aortic regurgitation; however, in recent years, antibiotics have controlled this problem.[12] Connective tissue disorders such as Marfan syndrome, rheumatoid arthritis, and ankylosing spondylitis are responsible for changes in the annulus or leaflets causing leaflet malalignment and regurgitation. Aortic stenosis is also capable of causing aortic regurgitation because fixed and stenotic leaflets may allow the backflow of blood.[12]

Aortic dissection, infective endocarditis, trauma, and unsuccessful valvular surgery are causes of acute aortic regurgitation. Chronically elevated blood pressure and arteriosclerosis may cause mild aortic regurgitation.[8,12]

Pathophysiology

Aortic regurgitation, whether developing acutely or as a chronic problem, produces a volume overload for the left ventricle. During ventricular diastole, the backflow of blood from the aorta is added to the blood emptied from the left atrium. When aortic regurgitation develops over several years, the increase in left ventricular end-diastolic volume results in a more forceful left ventricular contraction. The force of contraction is maintained by left ventricular hypertrophy and dilatation. Eventually, the hypertrophied ventricle can no longer support the force of contraction needed to eject blood. Under these circumstances, left ventricular end-diastolic pressure increases and is reflected backward to the left atrium, pulmonary vasculature, and right heart. Pulmonary congestion and right-sided heart failure ensue.

If aortic regurgitation develops acutely, the left ventricle does not have the opportunity to hypertrophy and increase the force of contraction to eject blood from the left ventricle. An increase in left ventricular end-diastolic volume causes an elevated left ventricular end-diastolic pressure. This pressure may exceed left atrial pressure and cause the mitral valve to close prematurely.[8] These hemodynamic changes produce pulmonary venous hypertension and pulmonary edema[12] (Fig. 9-5).

Signs and symptoms

Mild aortic regurgitation may be asymptomatic. Signs and symptoms vary greatly, depending on the severity of the disease. Patients with chronic aortic regurgitation have the signs and symptoms of left ventricular failure: fatigue, dyspnea, and pulmonary edema. Patients may develop palpitations with exercise, neck pulsation, exertional chest pain, skin that appears warm and flushed, diaphoresis, dizziness, and increased systolic blood pressure with an ab-

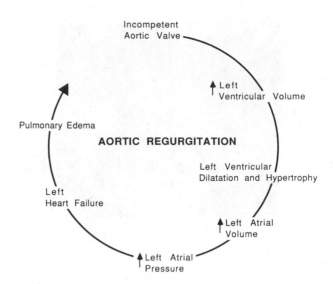

Fig. 9-5 Pathophysiology of aortic regurgitation.

normally low diastolic blood pressure. Depending on cerebral blood flow, patients' neurologic status may vary markedly from alertness to altered mentation and consciousness. Patients may complain of an awareness of their heartbeat, particularly when lying on their left sides. Patients with acute aortic regurgitation develop left ventricular failure and pulmonary edema. Physical abnormalities that may be found are the arachnodactyly of Marfan syndrome and head bobbing with carotid pulsations.[12] A classic finding of aortic regurgitation is the water-hammer pulse, which manifests as a rapid disappearance of the pulse as arterial pressure suddenly falls in late systole and early diastole.

The diastolic murmur auscultated in chronic aortic regurgitation is high-pitched, blowing, and decrescendo and is heard best in the third or fourth intercostal space at the left or right sternal border.[12] If the patient sits forward and exhales, the murmur intensifies. S_3 or S_4 may be heard, depending on the degree of aortic regurgitation. Other murmurs, such as an Austin Flint murmur, may also be auscultated. (See Chapter 2 for a discussion of murmurs.)

In acute aortic regurgitation, the murmur is soft, and S_3 is audible (see Table 9-1).

Diagnostic evaluation

The ECG shows left ventricular hypertrophy (increased amplitude of the QRS and ST-T–wave strain pattern).[12] AV conduction is prolonged. Hypertrophic changes are not evident on the ECG with acute aortic regurgitation, but changes in the ST-T wave are consistent with myocardial ischemia.[12]

The chest roentgenogram shows dilatation of the left ventricle with elongation of the apex inferiorly and posteriorly (as seen in fluid volume overload). A prominent ascending aorta may be seen with Marfan syndrome.

The echocardiogram visualizes vegetation formation on the valve leaflets that results from endocarditis. The amount of valvular regurgitation may also be quantified with this diagnostic study.

The cardiac catheterization allows estimates of the severity of regurgitation and evaluation of the extent of left ventricular failure.[12] Radionuclide studies can demonstrate diminished performance of the left ventricle during exercise.

Treatment

Medical treatment includes antibiotic prophylaxis against infective endocarditis. As with aortic stenosis, patients should receive antibiotics before and after dental or surgical procedures. Congestive heart failure is treated with diuretics, digoxin, vasodilators, and preload and afterload reducers.[12] Hydralazine has been successfully prescribed to control the regurgitant volume and improve the mechanical function of the left ventricle.[12]

Surgical treatment is indicated for patients with chronic aortic regurgitation who have developed symptoms. Patients whose conditions are asymptomatic and who evidence left ventricular failure as well as patients with left ventricular end-systolic dimensions greater than 55 mm also require surgery.[12,16] Surgical treatment is indicated for patients who develop acute aortic regurgitation such as in aortic dissection or infective endocarditis.

Selection of a prosthetic valve for treatment of aortic regurgitation depends on the patient's age, need for anticoagulation and durability. (Please see previous discussion of valve selection with aortic stenosis.)

Nursing treatment of patients with aortic regurgitation is similar to care rendered to patients with aortic stenosis. One point to remember is that aortic stenosis is a pressure overload disturbance, whereas aortic regurgitation is a fluid volume overload problem of the left ventricle. Therefore nurses treat impaired gas exchange caused by fluid volume overload by administering diuretics, vasodilators, and preload- and afterload-reducing agents. Nurses assist patients to manage anxiety by treating dyspnea and by addressing knowledge deficits about the disease process and treatment. Nurses need to anticipate infection, hemorrhage, and thrombus formation in patients treated surgically to correct aortic regurgitation (see Table 9-2).

MITRAL VALVE DISEASE

The mitral valve is located between the left atrium and the left ventricle. During diastole, the mitral valve opens and permits blood to flow from the left atrium into the left ventricle. Immediately before ventricular systole, the mitral valve closes, preventing leakage of blood from the left ventricle into the left atrium during the high-pressure phase of systolic ejection.

There are three types of mitral valve disease: mitral stenosis, mitral regurgitation, and mitral valve prolapse.

Mitral Stenosis

Mitral stenosis refers to the narrowing of the mitral valvular orifice, which produces an obstruction of blood flow from the left atrium, across the mitral valve, and into the left ventricle.

Etiology

Mitral stenosis is primarily a result of rheumatic fever. Approximately two thirds of patients with mitral stenosis of rheumatic origin are women.[17] Myxomas, bacterial vegetations, thrombus, and calcification are less frequent causes.[18] The inflammatory processes of rheumatic fever cause the leaflets of the valve to fibrose and thicken, thus decreasing the surface area of the opening (see Table 9-1).

Pathophysiology

The disease process begins with the formation of fibrous plaques on the mitral valve leaflets. These plaque aggregations lead to thickening, scarring, fusion, and contractures of the leaflets. Eventually, the valve becomes calcified and stenotic. This calcification and fusion process decreases the valvular orifice and impedes blood flow through the mitral valve.

The chordae tendineae, which provide secondary channels for blood flow from the left atrium to the left ventricle, also become inflamed and diseased in mitral stenosis. The chordae fuse and further obstruct blood flow across the mitral valve.[3]

The normal mitral valve orifice is 5 cm². In mitral stenosis, the valvular opening may decrease to 1.5 cm². This narrowed opening causes an increased pressure in the left atrium, resulting in dilatation of the chamber.

A "backward" heart failure increases pressure in the pulmonary veins, capillaries, and arteries. Pulmonary artery hypertension, which serves as a compensatory mechanism, may develop. As the pressure in the pulmonary capillaries exceeds the oncotic pressure, pulmonary edema develops. Eventually, the right ventricle hypertrophies, fails, and produces jugular venous distention, liver enlargement, ascites, and peripheral edema. Fig. 9-6 provides a summary of the sequelae of mitral stenosis.

Signs and symptoms

In acquired mitral stenosis, the symptoms appear gradually over approximately 20 years.[3] Mitral stenosis affects primarily women in their third or fourth decade. The most frequently occurring symptoms of mitral stenosis are dyspnea, fatigue, palpitations, cough, and hemoptysis. These are all signs of the "backward" failure into the pulmonary system and the right side of the heart. Less common symptoms include dysphagia, hoarseness, chest pain, embolic events, seizure, and cerebrovascular accident.

The decrease in cardiac output and cardiac reserve that results from mitral stenosis is directly proportional to the

TABLE 9-2   Nursing Treatment of Valvular Heart Disease

Problem	Treatment
1. Anxiety, related to dyspnea	Apply oxygen as needed. Administer diuretics and vasodilators as prescribed. Place patient in a comfortable position such as semi-Fowler. Use relaxation techniques as needed.
Anxiety related to knowledge deficit	Explain the function of the diseased valve and the cause of the dysfunction. Carefully review the medical and/or surgical plan. Clarify the patient's misconceptions and answer the patient's questions.
Anxiety, related to alterations in comfort (chest pain, syncope)	Discuss reasons for chest pain and syncope. Discuss avoidance measures (minimizing strenuous activities and exertion). Assist patient to rise slowly from a supine to an upright position to avoid syncope and orthostatic hypotension. Carefully administer diuretics and vasodilators. Administer antidysrhythmic medication to maintain sinus rhythm.
2. Decreased activity tolerance, related to decreased cardiac output	Assist patient in activities of daily living. Instruct patient to alternate periods of activity and rest. Consult cardiac rehabilitation specialist for reconditioning exercises. Administer antidysrhythmic medications, diuretics, and vasodilators as prescribed.
3. Fluid volume excess, related to dysfunctional valve	Provide bedrest. Administer prescribed diuretics. Monitor intake and output, daily weight, and laboratory values for electrolyte imbalances.
4. Impaired gas exchange, related to fluid volume excess	Auscultate breath sounds frequently. Monitor chest roentgenogram for fluid volume excess. Notify physician of absent, unequal, or diminished breath sounds; crackles; or wheezing. Notify physician for changes in the patient's baseline arterial blood gas levels. Provide supplemental oxygen or mechanical ventilation as needed. Administer diuretics as prescribed. Position patient comfortably (semi-Fowler or high Fowler).
5. Potential for infection, risk factors: congenitally misshaped valve, intravenous drug abuse	Administer antibiotics as prescribed. Instruct patient about the necessity of antibiotic prophylaxis with invasive procedures and about signs and symptoms of infection. Instruct intravenous drug abusers about the fatality of infections in valve replacement recipients; instruct about cleaning used needles with bleach.
6. Potential for injury, risk factors: anticoagulation, thrombus formation	Explain the use of warfarin and dipyridamole to patient. Administer warfarin as prescribed. Determine that the prothrombin time is 1.5 times greater than the control. Alert the physician of subtherapeutic prothrombin times. Instruct the patient to refrain from activities that may precipitate bleeding (use soft-bristled toothbrush and electric shaver; refrain from intense contact sports such as football, soccer, and skiing). Instruct women of child-bearing age to contact their physician before attempting to become pregnant. Instruct patients to have their laboratory studies (blood work) done according to their scheduled appointments.
Potential for injury, risk factor: improperly seated prosthetic valve	Auscultate heart sounds after surgery. Notify physician for changes in heart sounds or the presence of a new murmur. Monitor vital signs per the critical care unit's routine. Notify the physician for abrupt changes (increased heart rate, decreased blood pressure, and decreased cardiac output).
7. Potential noncompliance, risk factors: knowledge deficit; lack of economic resources	Review therapeutic regimen with the patient. Answer all questions; clarify misconceptions. Carefully explain the consequences of not adhering to the prescribed medical regimen. Ascertain the patient's ability to comply with the therapeutic plan. Note any discrepancies in subtherapeutic prothrombin times and verify that the patient is taking medication as prescribed.

severity of the stenosis.[19] Generally, symptoms of mitral stenosis are not experienced at rest. However, the symptoms are worsened by exercise and are evidenced as dyspnea and pulmonary edema.

The murmur associated with mitral stenosis is a result of turbulent blood flow through and around the stenotic mitral valve. It is appreciated best at the apex. An opening snap may be auscultated followed by a low-pitched diastolic rumble that may be intensified when the patient is placed in the left lateral recumbent position.

Diagnostic evaluation

The ECG evidences characteristically wide, notched P waves.[18] Atrial fibrillation occurs in 40% to 50% of patients

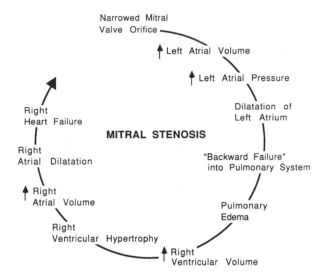

Fig. 9-6 Pathophysiology of mitral stenosis.

with mitral stenosis. In atrial fibrillation, the atrium does not contract as completely or forcefully as it does in normal sinus rhythm. The loss of proper atrial contraction in atrial fibrillation increases the risk of thrombus formation and subsequent embolic events.

Chest roentgenograms of patients with mitral stenosis may reveal left atrial, right ventricular, and pulmonary artery enlargement.[18] Pulmonary capillary and alveolar wall thickening and fibrosis may be detected. Oxygen use is inhibited, and eventually lung capacity decreases.

The most useful noninvasive method for detection of mitral stenosis is the echocardiogram. The stenotic mitral valve appears thick and shows diminished motion and posterior leaflet movement. Valvular gradient data may be obtained by cardiac catheterization.[18]

Treatment

Medical therapy includes diuretics for symptoms of heart failure, a low-sodium diet, avoidance of exertion (which may invoke symptoms), and anticoagulation. Digoxin, quinidine, or synchronized cardioversion are indicated for atrial fibrillation. Caution should be taken when performing cardioversion on any patient who has been in atrial fibrillation for a prolonged period because of the possibility of mobilizing thrombi. Prophylactic antibiotic therapy is indicated to reduce the risk of recurrent rheumatic fever and endocarditis. Patients with mitral stenosis must receive antibiotics before an invasive procedure or dental surgery.

Balloon valvuloplasty is used in patients with mitral stenosis who are considered at high operative risk (for example, older adults with ischemic heart disease). Balloon valvuloplasty does not repair the stenotic valve; rather it alleviates the symptoms associated with the mitral stenosis.[17] Complications of valvuloplasty such as bleeding, inadver-

tent creation of atrial septal defects with the balloon catheter, and restenosis require more extensive evaluation.

Surgical intervention is the only permanent method of reducing obstruction of a stenotic mitral valve. Valve replacement or valve repair are two surgical alternatives. Currently, attempts are made to surgically repair the stenotic mitral valve instead of replacing it. There are two types of surgical repair procedures: commissurotomy and annuloplasty. Generally, commissurotomy involves surgical trimming and reconstruction of the posterior leaflet of the valve. In patients with pure mitral stenosis (those who develop mitral stenosis in their third decade), a mitral valve commissurotomy is the treatment of choice. Annuloplasty entails implantation of a ring to narrow the annulus, thereby reducing the regurgitation (see Fig. 9-7 for examples of prosthetic valvular rings).[20] If reconstruction of the valve is not appropriate, replacement of the stenotic mitral valve is indicated. (Refer to the section on surgical treatment of aortic stenosis for a discussion of selection of a valve prosthesis.) The transesophageal echocardiogram (TEE) may be used intraoperatively to assess the degree of success of the valvular reconstruction. If the TEE demonstrates inadequate repair, the valve is usually replaced.

Generally, younger patients receive mechanical valve replacements. Long-term anticoagulation is indicated with these prostheses and is generally acceptable in young, otherwise healthy adults. Mechanical valves function for a longer time than bioprostheses before requiring replacement. Patients over 50 years old receive bioprosthetic valves.

Nursing treatment primarily includes reduction of anxiety related to occurrence of symptoms of right-sided heart failure, impaired gas exchange, and lack of knowledge of diagnosis. Counseling for activity intolerance and coping with the diagnosis are also important features of nursing intervention (see Table 9-2).

Mitral Regurgitation

Mitral valve regurgitation is the backward leakage of blood from the left ventricle into the left atrium during ventricular systole. The incompetent or regurgitant mitral valve fails to provide a secure seal between the left atrium and left ventricle.

Etiology

Historically, an overwhelming number of the cases of mitral regurgitation were attributed to rheumatic fever; however, research indicates that mitral valve prolapse and coronary artery disease are the principal causes of mitral valve regurgitation.[18] Less common causes of acquired mitral regurgitation include Marfan syndrome, calcification of the mitral valve annulus, Ehlers-Danlos syndrome, ischemic heart disease, myocardial infarction, ventricular aneurysm, papillary muscle damage, and endocarditis.[18] Mitral regurgitation may also be congenital.

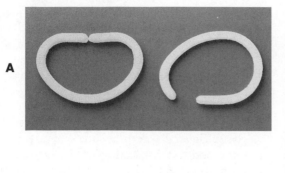

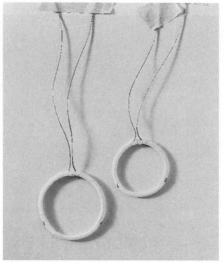

Fig. 9-7   **A,** Carpentier mitral and tricuspid rings. **B,** Sorin Puig Massana annuloplasty ring. (**A** courtesy Baxter Healthcare, Edwards CVS Division, Irvine, Calif; **B** courtesy Sorin Biomedical, Irvine, Calif.)

Cardiomyopathy or any other disease process that causes the left ventricle to hypertrophy may increase the valvular orifice, thus disrupting the anchoring function of the papillary muscles. Mitral regurgitation may also be caused by calcification of the mitral ring. This calcification is common in older women.[19] The majority of patients with acquired mitral regurgitation are women.[3]

Pathophysiology

Mitral regurgitation results in an increased blood volume in the left ventricle and left atrium. Because the diseased mitral valve does not close tightly during systole, blood leaks into the left atrium, resulting in a smaller volume of blood being ejected into the aorta during left ventricular systole.[9] The inflammation and scarring from rheumatic fever produce rigidity and contraction of the valvular leaflets, fusion of the valve commissures, and shortening of the chordae tendineae. All of these changes culminate in a leaky, incompetent mitral valve.

As mitral regurgitation progresses, the increased volume in the left atrium creates left atrial enlargement. The posterior leaflet of the mitral valve is shifted posteriorly and loses its full range of motion, thus invoking an incompetent closure of valvular leaflets.[18]

Increased volume from the left atrium to the left ventricle results in left ventricular dilatation and hypertrophy. Despite attempts to adjust, the left ventricle fails, and this failure is reflected into the left atrium and the pulmonary system. The pulmonary system attempts to compensate for the greater volume by increasing lymphatic flow, thus increasing pulmonary pressures. If the left atrial pressure reaches 30 to 40 mm Hg, pulmonary edema usually ensues.[19]

Over time, pulmonary edema may lead to pulmonary hypertension and failure of the right side of the heart. Pulmonary edema may also create a "backward" failure on the right side of the heart. The right ventricle enlarges to compensate for higher blood volumes and fails. Right ventricular failure causes right atrial failure, which culminates in ascites and peripheral edema. See Fig. 9-8 for a synopsis of mitral regurgitation.

Signs and symptoms

Fatigue, weakness, exhaustion, and cachexia occur when the cardiac output is significantly decreased from mitral regurgitation. Atrial fibrillation is a common symptom of mitral regurgitation. As the atrium dilates, a greater surface area is created, thus increasing the distance the cardiac conduction impulse must travel. The increased distance enhances the potential for the impulse to become abnormal and for atrial fibrillation to develop. In the presence of atrial fibrillation, the heart's ability to function as a strong pump decreases, which further reduces cardiac output.[19] Other signs of mitral regurgitation include tachypnea, hypotension, and pulmonary edema.

The murmur associated with mitral regurgitation is a blowing, systolic sound appreciated best at the apex and radiating to the left axilla. In mitral regurgitation, the first heart sound (S_1) is difficult to auscultate and may be absent. S_2 is split, and occasionally, S_3 or S_4 may be noted.[3]

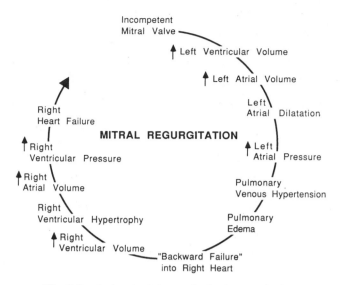

Fig. 9-8 Pathophysiology of mitral regurgitation.

Diagnostic evaluation

The ECG of the patient with mitral regurgitation evidences altered P waves and QRS-complex amplitude. Atrial fibrillation is usually seen. Q waves from previous myocardial infarctions may also be noted if the mitral regurgitation is the result of coronary ischemia. Several nonspecific ST-segment changes may also be exhibited on the ECG. The chest roentgenogram demonstrates left ventricular and left atrial enlargement. The echocardiogram evidences decreased ventricular wall motion, and the echo Doppler provides data for estimating the severity of the regurgitation.[19] Cardiac catheterization is useful in measuring the left ventricular end-diastolic pressure and demonstrating wall motion.

Treatment

Medical treatment is aimed at alleviating the symptoms. The presence of symptoms is directly related to the severity of the disease. Medications prescribed include diuretics, digoxin, quinidine, and vasodilators to alleviate the symptoms associated with right-sided heart failure. Anticoagulation therapy may also be prescribed to decrease the risk of thrombus and subsequent embolus caused by atrial fibrillation. Restriction of symptom-producing activity is recommended, and a low-sodium diet is also prescribed. Surgical treatment of mitral regurgitation is similar to surgical intervention for mitral stenosis.

Nursing treatment focuses on relieving anxiety related to the diagnosis of mitral regurgitation. Because the symptoms of mitral regurgitation may not be evidenced for many years, the patient needs to know about the signs and symptoms of mitral regurgitation. Nursing intervention for treating the symptoms of decreased cardiac output is also

necessary for the patient with mitral regurgitation. Using the interdisciplinary health care team is essential in providing holistic care (see Table 9-2).

Mitral Valve Prolapse

Mitral valve prolapse, also known as *Barlow syndrome* or *floppy valve syndrome,* occurs when one or more valvular leaflets become thickened and protrude into the left atrium during ventricular systole. The posterior leaflet is most commonly involved. Mitral valve prolapse is the most widespread valvular disease in adults, occurring in 2.5% to 5% of the population. The syndrome occurs in all age groups; however, it is most frequently found in women between 20 and 50 years of age. This abnormality tends to occur in families and is probably carried in an autosomal dominant genetic pattern.[3]

Etiology

Mitral valve prolapse is hereditary, and it may also be a result of atrial and ventricular septal defects, patent ductus arteriosus, skeletal abnormalities, or Marfan syndrome. Acquired mitral valve prolapse may be the result of endocarditis, myocarditis, coronary artery disease, cancer with myocardial metastases, muscular dystrophy and acromegaly, or collagen vascular diseases such as systemic lupus erythematosus.[18]

Pathophysiology

Regardless of the etiology, the posterior leaflet of the mitral valve thickens and protrudes into the left atrium during ventricular systole.

Signs and symptoms

The most common symptom is chest pain. This pain may be related to the myocardial ischemia that may result from the tremendous pull that must be exerted by the papillary muscles on the damaged leaflet. Coronary artery spasm may also occur as a result of this force.[18] Other symptoms include dizziness, panic attacks, palpitations, dyspnea, and syncope. Patients with mitral valve prolapse also have an increased incidence of transient ischemic attacks and stroke.[21] Skeletal abnormalities such as a pigeon breast, funnel chest, scoliosis, kyphosis, or straight back syndrome may be exhibited.

The murmur associated with mitral valve prolapse is a systolic click that is best appreciated at the apex along the left sternal border. The literature suggests that dysautonomia (dysfunction of the nervous system) may be linked to mitral valve prolapse. Patients have significantly elevated levels of epinephrine and norepinephrine. These high levels of catecholamines may suggest why mitral valve prolapse patients have panic attacks, are susceptible to stress-induced dysrhythmias, and demonstrate altered blood pressure and pulse responses to position changes.[22] Mitral valve prolapse rarely involves lethal dysrhythmias resulting in sudden death. In some patients, mitral valve prolapse may progress to mitral valve regurgitation and require repair or surgical replacement of the regurgitant valve.

Diagnostic evaluation

Dysrhythmias are evident in the ECGs of 60% of patients with mitral valve prolapse. The most frequently occurring rhythm disturbances include supraventricular tachycardias, premature ventricular contractions, and premature atrial contractions. There may be ST-segment and T-wave alterations and QT prolongation. The chest roentgenogram shows a normal cardiac silhouette. Echocardiogram evidences a floppy posterior mitral valve leaflet.

Treatment

Medical treatment includes propranolol for chest pain and dysrhythmias. All patients with mitral valve prolapse and any degree of mitral regurgitation should receive prophylactic antibiotics before procedures involving instrumentation. Medical therapies for dyspnea and palpitations may be prescribed. Low doses of barbiturates may be indicated for hypervagal patients. Psychotherapy may also be prescribed for patients with panic attacks. Patients with asymptomatic mitral valve prolapse may not require treatment. However, refractory dysrhythmias, persistent regurgitation, and increasing pulmonary congestion secondary to mitral regurgitation may be indications for surgery.

The goal of nursing treatment is alleviation of anxiety related to the diagnosis of mitral valve prolapse and the symptoms of dysautonomia. Nursing treatment must also include educating persons about the etiology and treatment of the condition (see Table 9-2).

TRICUSPID VALVE DISEASE

The tricuspid valve is located between the right atrium and right ventricle and is closed during right atrial diastole to allow blood to collect in the right atrium. The tricuspid valve opens as pressure in the right atrium exceeds that in the right ventricle. As right ventricular diastole is completed, the tricuspid valve again closes in preparation for right ventricular systole. The closure of the tricuspid valve prevents backflow of blood from the higher-pressured right ventricle into the lower-pressured right atrium during ventricular systole.

Tricuspid Stenosis

Tricuspid stenosis is the narrowing of the tricuspid valve orifice; this narrowing obstructs blood flow across the valve during the diastolic filling of the right ventricle.[23]

Etiology

The cause of tricuspid stenosis is usually rheumatic fever. Primary tricuspid stenosis is rare. Generally, tricuspid stenosis occurs with mitral or aortic valvular disease.[23]

Pathophysiology

The hemodynamic effects of tricuspid stenosis, including increased right atrial pressure and reduced cardiac output, are worsened by the usually coexistent mitral stenosis (Fig. 9-9).

Signs and symptoms

The major signs and symptoms are dyspnea and fatigue. Patients may have peripheral edema and neck pulsations as the internal jugular veins become distended.[24]

The murmur of tricuspid stenosis is a low-pitched diastolic rumble best heard at the fourth intercostal space at the left sternal border. The murmur increases in intensity with inspiration as intrathoracic pressure is reduced and right ventricular filling increases.[8] The murmur is caused by turbulent blood flow across the narrowed valvular orifice (see Table 9-1).

Diagnostic evaluation

The ECG reveals large P waves in the absence of right ventricular enlargement.[24] The chest roentgenogram shows a prominent right atrium. The echocardiogram can identify fibrosis, calcifications, and obstruction of the valve. The echo Doppler can estimate the diastolic gradient across the valve. Cardiac catheterization confirms a gradient of greater than 1 mm Hg between the right atrium and right ventricle.

Treatment

In the absence of symptoms, no treatment is indicated for mild tricuspid stenosis. Antibiotic prophylaxis to prevent infective endocarditis is indicated. Peripheral edema may not respond to diuretics, digitalis, and preload or afterload reduction, since the edema is a result of not the fluid volume overload but a pressure overload.[24] Surgical

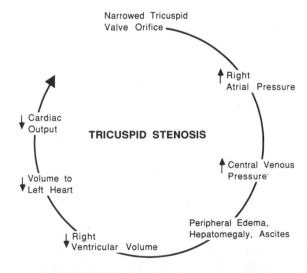

Fig. 9-9 Pathophysiology of tricuspid stenosis.

treatment is indicated if tricuspid stenosis is severe. Because of the high thrombogenic rate associated with tricuspid valve replacement, anticoagulation with warfarin is warranted. Long-term anticoagulation therefore negates the benefit of a bioprosthesis; hence, mechanical valves are often used to replace a diseased tricuspid valve. Preferred valves include the St. Jude Medical bileaflet valve, a tilting-disk valve, or a ball-valve device.[24]

Nursing treatment is directed toward alleviation of anxiety. Such anxieties result from a lack of knowledge about valvular disease and treatment. Similarly, anxiety may be precipitated by dyspnea. Patients may suffer from decreased activity tolerance, which is a consequence of low cardiac output. Ankle edema is typically present. The potential for valve infection is a persistent problem; infective endocarditis may strike a dysfunctional valve or a prosthetic replacement. Patients undergoing anticoagulation therapy are at risk for injury (hemorrhage) and must be instructed about safety precautions; they must also be responsible for self-administration of warfarin or antiplatelet medications (see Table 9-2).

Tricuspid Regurgitation

Tricuspid regurgitation is the backflow of blood from the right ventricle into the right atrium through an incompetent valve during right valvular contraction.

Etiology

The most common reason for tricuspid regurgitation is right ventricular dilatation and failure, which develop as sequelae to left ventricular failure, pulmonary hypertension, or both. Concomitant aortic and mitral valvular disease are frequently responsible for this left ventricular failure and pulmonary hypertension. Right ventricular dilatation causes the valve orifice and annulus to stretch and enlarge, thus preventing the valve leaflets from closing completely (Fig. 9-10).[18]

Infective endocarditis causes the tricuspid valve leaflets to malalign because of vegetations along the cusps. Intravenous drug abuse is a major cause of infective endocarditis.[23] Other causes include myocardial infarction, blunt trauma to the chest (steering wheel injuries in automobile accidents or external compressions from cardiopulmonary resuscitation), carcinoid syndrome, and congenital anomalies (see Table 9-1).

Pathophysiology

The backflow of blood into the right atrium increases right atrial pressure, which in turn increases systemic venous pressure. Because some blood escapes backward into the right atrium during right ventricular systole, not all blood reaches the left side of the heart. Therefore cardiac output is reduced. The right ventricle dilates and hypertrophies in an effort to eject more blood, but this dilatation and hypertrophy can worsen the tricuspid regurgitation.

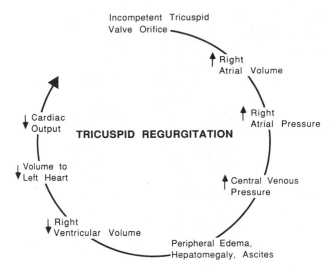

Fig. 9-10 Pathophysiology of tricuspid regurgitation.

The right atrium then enlarges, and frequently, atrial fibrillation ensues, further reducing the cardiac output. This course is often complicated by pulmonary hypertension and left-sided heart failure, which initially may have caused the tricuspid regurgitation.

Signs and symptoms

Patients experience dyspnea, orthopnea, peripheral edema, and fatigue. Atrial fibrillation is common. Patients with infective endocarditis causing tricuspid regurgitation may have a fever. Other signs and symptoms include hepatomegaly, anorexia (from liver and intestinal venous congestion), and peripheral cyanosis (from a low cardiac output).[8]

The murmur of tricuspid regurgitation is high pitched, blowing, and holosystolic; it is heard best at the fourth intercostal space at the left sternal border or xiphoid area. The murmur intensifies with inspiration.

Diagnostic evaluation

The ECG frequently shows atrial fibrillation or right bundle branch block caused by right ventricular hypertrophy. The chest roentgenogram evidences right atrial and right ventricular enlargement. The echocardiogram facilitates recognition of vegetative lesions, ruptured chordae and papillary muscles, and the back-and-forth movement of the valve.[24] The echo Doppler estimates the severity of the regurgitation. The cardiac catheterization reveals a prominent cv wave in the right atrium that suggests tricuspid regurgitation.

Treatment

Medical treatment is directed toward alleviation of right ventricular failure. A low-sodium diet, digitalis, diuretics, and vasodilators are used to treat right- and left-sided heart failure. If pulmonary hypertension and left heart failure are present, adding prostaglandin E, dobutamine, and dopamine to the regimen may help dilate the pulmonary vasculature and increase cardiac output.[24]

Surgical treatment is based on the extent of concurrent mitral valvular disease. If mitral stenosis is critical, a mitral valve replacement is performed.[24] Intraoperatively, after the mitral valve surgery, the surgeon determines whether the tricuspid regurgitation has significantly improved. The surgeon also inspects the right atrium and venae cavae for moderate enlargement, an indication of the severity of tricuspid regurgitation. A tricuspid valve repair or replacement may ensue.

A repair or reconstruction of the valve leaflets (valvuloplasty) and the valve annulus (annuloplasty) is preferred, since long-term results of these procedures are more favorable than complete valve replacement.[24] However, if the leaflets are hopelessly deformed, which may be seen with infective endocarditis, a tricuspid valve replacement is indicated.

As discussed in the surgical management of tricuspid stenosis, thrombogenesis remains a problem. Hence, the more durable mechanical valves may be favored, since anticoagulation will still be necessary. The St. Jude Medical bileaflet, tilting-disk, and ball-valve prostheses are frequently used. A total tricuspid valvotomy may be performed in the case of infective endocarditis from intravenous drug abuse. Although there is a risk of congestive heart failure, if the cessation of intravenous drug abuse is remote, implanting a mechanical valve will likely result in a fatal infection.

Nursing treatment is aimed at improving gas exchange, related to the fluid volume overload. Patients may also suffer from decreased activity tolerance related to a decrease in cardiac output; potential for infection, anxiety from dyspnea and knowledge deficit about the disease process and treatment; and potential for injury related to anticoagulation (see Table 9-2).

PULMONARY VALVE DISEASE

The pulmonary valve is located between the right ventricle and the pulmonary artery; it prevents blood flow from the pulmonary artery into the right ventricle during diastole.[13] It is a semilunar valve with three similarly shaped leaflets. Although the pulmonary valve may become diseased, the symptoms are generally not life threatening because of the low pressures in the area where the valve is located.

Pulmonary Stenosis

Pulmonary valve stenosis refers to the obstruction of blood flow across a narrowed pulmonary valve during systole.

Etiology

Stenosis of the pulmonary valve is usually congenital. Acquired pulmonary stenosis rarely occurs, although it may be caused by rheumatic fever, cancerous valvular lesions, syphilis, endocarditis, and tuberculosis.

Pathophysiology

The inflammatory changes that occur from rheumatic fever and endocarditis cause a fibrous thickening of the leaflets of the pulmonary valve, resulting in a decreased valvular orifice. The reduced opening of the stenotic valve causes a backflow of blood into the right ventricle. Right-sided heart failure ensues from the increase in right heart volume and pressure. As the right side of the heart fails, a diminished cardiac output results. The pressure and volume in the right atrium also increase, resulting in venous engorgement, most notably hepatomegaly, jugular venous distention, and peripheral edema.[3] See Fig. 9-11 for the sequelae of events of pulmonary stenosis.

Signs and symptoms

Pulmonary stenosis may be asymptomatic for many years. The appearance of symptoms is directly proportional to the severity of the disease. The most frequently occurring symptoms are dyspnea, fatigue, and syncope.

The murmur auscultated in pulmonary stenosis is a sharp, systolic crescendo-decrescendo sound; it is best appreciated at the left sternal border at the second or third intercostal space. S_2 is widely split or may be absent (see Table 9-1).

Diagnostic evaluation

Obtaining a thorough medical history of the patient is important in determining the cause of pulmonary stenosis (see Chapter 2). No definitive ECG abnormalities are

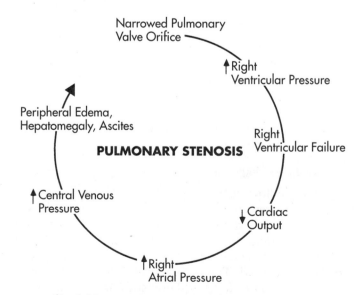

Fig. 9-11 Pathophysiology of pulmonary stenosis.

associated with pulmonary stenosis. However, if pulmonary hypertension is present, the ECG evidences right axis deviation because of right ventricular hypertrophy and P-wave morphologic changes related to right atrial enlargement.[25]

The chest roentgenogram reveals poststenotic dilatation, prominence of the pulmonary artery, and right ventricular hypertrophy. Echocardiography is the most valuable noninvasive tool for diagnosing pulmonary stenosis. The echo Doppler can ascertain the severity of the stenosis. Cardiac catheterization is not specifically useful in the diagnosis of pulmonary stenosis; however, a right-sided heart injection demonstrates the outline of the pulmonary valve.[25]

Treatment

Medical treatment generally includes prophylactic antibiotics against recurrent endocarditis. If pulmonary emboli are suspected, anticoagulation is indicated. Vasodilator therapies, including nitroglycerin and prostaglandin E, are used to decrease the severity of pulmonary hypertension. Treatment of the symptoms of congestive heart failure may also be undertaken; such treatments include digoxin, diuretics, and a low-sodium diet.

Surgical replacement of a congenitally stenotic pulmonary valve is rare. However, a commissurotomy may be performed to alleviate the stenosis. Balloon valvuloplasty of the stenotic pulmonary valve is also widely used.[26] Because of the high incidence of emboli associated with the mechanical valve prosthesis in the pulmonary valve position, bioprostheses are used when valves require replacement. Currently, a valvotomy, or removal of the valve, and antibiotic prophylaxis seem to be the preferred treatments.[25]

Nursing treatment focuses primarily on patient education related to the diagnosis of acquired pulmonary stenosis. The symptoms of pulmonary stenosis usually remain dormant for many years; therefore a patient requires knowledge of the cause of the stenosis and preparation for the appearance of the symptoms. Nursing intervention to decrease anxiety related to the diagnosis of stenosis is also indicated (see Table 9-2).

Pulmonary Regurgitation

Pulmonary regurgitation is the backward leakage of blood from the pulmonary artery into the right ventricle during diastole. The regurgitant pulmonary valve leaflets become scarred, do not close tightly, and allow blood to leak back into the right ventricle.

Etiology

Pulmonary regurgitation mainly occurs as a congenital defect. Acquired pulmonary regurgitation occurs more frequently than pulmonary stenosis, and it may result from any condition causing pulmonary hypertension; such conditions include mitral stenosis, chronic obstructive pulmonary disease, pulmonary embolism, endocarditis, valvotomy as treatment for pulmonary stenosis, sarcoma or myxoma tumors, and rarely, rheumatic fever or tuberculosis.[25]

Pathophysiology

In pulmonary regurgitation, the leaflets of the valve do not close firmly as a result of various disease processes. With endocarditis and cancerous tumor involvement, the leaflets of the valve thicken, scar, and contract, permitting blood to flow through the gaps between the diseased leaflets. Elevated right ventricular pressure and hypertrophy ensue.[8] Eventually, the right ventricle fails, and a diminished quantity of blood is pumped into the pulmonary system. Increased volume and pressure back up into the right atrium, which causes right atrial hypertrophy and failure manifested by an elevated central venous pressure, jugular venous distention, and peripheral congestion and edema. Fig. 9-12 summarizes the sequelae of pulmonary regurgitation.

Signs and symptoms

The symptoms of pulmonary regurgitation are not evidenced unless pulmonary hypertension exists concurrently. The patient may be asymptomatic for many years, depending on the extent of the underlying disease.

The cardiac murmur associated with pulmonary regurgitation is high pitched with and moderately pitched without pulmonary hypertension. The murmur is a blowing sound most optimally auscultated at the fourth or fifth intercostal space at the left sternal border. It is often difficult to distinguish the murmur of pulmonary regurgitation from the murmur of aortic regurgitation (see Table 9-1).

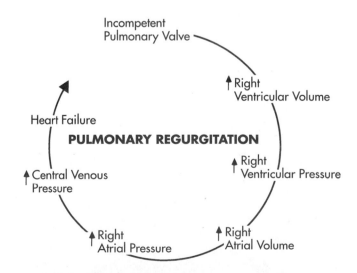

Fig. 9-12   Pathophysiology of pulmonary regurgitation.

Diagnostic evaluation and treatment

The diagnostic tools for pulmonary regurgitation are similar to those of pulmonary stenosis. A complete medical history to delineate the cause of the regurgitation is paramount (see Chapter 2). Treatment is based on alleviating symptoms, usually with a medical regimen of diuretics, digoxin, and a low-sodium diet.

SUMMARY

Valvular heart disease may affect one or more of the cardiac valves, producing stenosis, regurgitation, or both. The most frequent causes of dysfunction of the heart valves are rheumatic heart disease and infective endocarditis. Valvular heart disease occurs in all age groups, and symptoms may develop suddenly or over many years.

REFERENCES

1. Schlant RC and others: *Anatomy of the heart.* In Hurst JW et al, editors: *The heart,* ed 7, New York, 1990, McGraw-Hill.
2. Miracle VA: Anatomy of a murmur, *Nursing* 16:26, 1986.
3. Cavallo GAO: *The person with valvular heart disease.* In Guzzetta CE, Dossey BM, editors: *Cardiovascular nursing: holistic practice,* St Louis, 1992, Mosby.
4. Thibault GE and others: *Aortic stenosis.* In Eagle KA et al, editors: *The practice of cardiology,* ed 2, Boston, 1989, Little, Brown.
5. Vitello-Cicciu J, Lapsley DP: *Valvular heart disease.* In Kinney MR and others, editors: *AACN's clinical reference for critical-care nursing,* ed 3, St Louis, 1993, Mosby.
6. Netter FH: *The CIBA collection of medical illustrations: the heart,* vol 5, Summit, NJ, 1978, CIBA Pharmaceutical.
7. Braunwald E: *Heart disease: a textbook of cardiovascular medicine,* ed 4, Philadelphia, 1992, Saunders.
8. Schakenbach LH: Physiologic dynamics of acquired valvular heart disease, *J Cardiovasc Nurs* 1:1, 1987.
9. Ohler L and others: Aortic valvuloplasty: medical and critical care nursing perspectives, *Focus Crit Care* 16:275, 1989.
10. Ventola CA: Nursing grand rounds: aortic and mitral valvuloplasty, *J Cardiovasc Nurs* 1:70, 1987.
11. Ronan J Jr: *Aortic stenosis in adults.* In Hurst JW, editor: *Current therapy in cardiovascular disease,* ed 3, Philadelphia, 1991, Decker.
12. Rackley CE et al: *Aortic valve disease.* In Hurst JW et al, editors: *The heart,* ed 7, New York, 1990, McGraw-Hill.
13. Seifert PC: Surgery for acquired valvular heart disease, *J Cardiovasc Nurs* 1:26, 1987.
14. Hopkins RA: Cardiac reconstruction with allograft valves, New York, 1989, Saunders.
15. Starr A, Grunkemeir G: *Selecting a prosthetic valve.* In Hurst JW, editor: *Current therapy in cardiovascular disease,* ed 3, Philadelphia, 1991, Decker.
15a.McKay R and others: Primary repair and autotransplantation of cardiac valves, *Ann Rev Med* 44:181, 1993.
16. Treasure CB: *Aortic regurgitation.* In Hurst JW, editor: *Current therapy in cardiovascular disease,* ed 3, Philadelphia, 1991, Decker.
17. Schlant RC: *Mitral stenosis.* In Braunwald E, editor: *Heart disease: a textbook of cardiovascular medicine,* ed 4, Philadelphia, 1992, Saunders.
18. Rackley CE and others: *Mitral valve disease.* In Hurst et al, editors: *The heart,* ed 7, New York, 1990, McGraw-Hill.
19. Guyton A: *Textbook of medical physiology,* ed 8, Philadelphia, 1991, Saunders.
20. Baue AE et al: *Glenn's thoracic and cardiovascular surgery,* ed 5, vol 2, Norwalk, Conn, 1991, Appleton & Lange.
21. Plehn JF: Mitral valve prolapse: state-of-the-art evaluation, *Consultant* Oct 1991, p 66-77.
22. Anderson UK: Mitral valve prolapse: a diagnosis for primary nursing intervention, *J Cardiovasc Nurs* 1:26, 1987.
23. Kirklin JW: *Cardiac surgery,* ed 2, New York, 1993, Churchill Livingstone.
24. Rackley CE et al: *Tricuspid valve disease.* In Hurst JW et al, editors: *The heart,* ed 7, New York, 1990, McGraw-Hill.
25. Rackley CE et al: *Pulmonary valve disease.* In Hurst JW et al, editors: *The heart,* ed 7, New York, 1990, McGraw-Hill.
26. Sabiston DC, Spencer FC: *Surgery of the chest,* Philadelphia, 1990, Saunders.

10

Surgical Management of Heart Disease

Flerida Imperial-Perez
Darlene A. Rourke

As the U.S. population ages, heart and blood vessel diseases will likely affect more people in varying degrees. Although considerable advances have been achieved in medical treatment, many patients do not respond well to pharmacologic approaches, which makes them candidates for aggressive surgical interventions. Consequently, health care providers are exposed to challenges in the treatment and management of this patient population. This chapter describes the surgical interventions and management of patients undergoing cardiac surgery for myocardial revascularization; postoperative care is the focus.

MYOCARDIAL REVASCULARIZATION

Myocardial revascularization in the form of coronary artery bypass graft (CABG) is the surgical strategy used in the treatment of coronary artery disease (CAD). It is estimated that 600,000 CABGs are performed annually.[1] Risk-adjusted outcomes are used to make clinical decisions in the selection of patients for myocardial revascularization procedures.[2] The predicted risk has risen since 1988 to 5.3%.[3] Despite increasing risks, there has been an insignificant increase in the observed mortality rate, which was 2.4% in 1988 and 3% in 1992.[3] The explanation for the relatively constant mortality rate is that factors, such as increased use of the internal mammary artery, improved pharmacologic and myocardial protection techniques, and the use of various assist devices, have contributed significantly to maintaining a low mortality rate despite an increasingly older population.

Risk factors and indications for surgery among older patients are also being examined. About 3% of the population in the United States was at least 80 years old in 1990. By the year 2010, this number may increase to about 4.3%, representing about 12 million people.[4] The risk parameters in the older patient are projected to increase as people live longer and older patients undergo surgery.

In general, patients with unstable angina have better long-term outcomes with revascularization than with medical therapy. The amount of myocardium at risk, the severity of symptoms, and the age of the patient are considered in the decision for revascularization therapy.[5] Revascularization therapy is indicated primarily in patients with significant lesions in the left main coronary artery, in patients who have large amount of myocardium supplied by one or more chronically occluded vessels, and in patients with acute myocardial infarction. Indications for myocardial revascularization are summarized in the box.[5,6]

Guidelines for surgical intervention for CAD are now being defined in several clinical trials in the United States (for example, Bypass Angioplasty Revascularization Investigation [BARI] and Emory Angioplasty Surgery Trial [EAST]) and in Europe (for example, Randomized Interventional Treatment of Angina [RITA] and Coronary Angioplasty versus Bypass Revascularization Investigation [CABRI]), which will provide data useful in decision making regarding management of CAD. These data will also complement the studies being done on the changing clinical characteristics of cardiac surgery patients.

INDICATIONS FOR MYOCARDIAL REVASCULARIZATION ANGINA PECTORIS[5,6]

Unstable angina with decreased exercise tolerance
Angina occurring at rest that is associated with transient ST-segment elevation
Chronic stable angina refractory to medical management
CAD (even in the presence of stable angina)
   Severe three-vessel CAD
   Significant left main coronary obstruction of greater than 50%
   Late vein graft disease
Significant myocardial ischemia from one or more chronically occluded vessels causing:
   Depressed ventricular function (cardiogenic function or congestive heart failure)
   Intractable myocardial irritability
   Myocardial infarction (acute or delayed)
Unsuccessful percutaneous transluminal coronary angioplasty

In particular, there is uncertainty regarding the relative efficacy of surgical intervention in men compared with women.[7] Data demonstrate a higher mortality rate in women vs. men.[3,7] This higher rate was attributed to older age, diabetes, more emergent surgery, and the presence of three-vessel disease or left main disease. However, Rahimtoola and others[8] noted that the difference in the operative mortality and long-term survival rates between men and women was small. The study also suggested that patient-related factors rather than gender were independent predictors of poor survival. Therefore according to this study, surgical intervention should not be delayed or denied to women who have the usual indications for surgery.[8]

Chronologic age alone may not be a valid basis for treatment decisions, but careful consideration of the presence or absence of clinical risk factors is needed to make the best treatment decisions.[9] With careful consideration of operative risk among older adults, the decision to proceed with surgical intervention is based on the hope that the patient's cardiac symptoms will improve and that the patient will have a more active lifestyle. However, this high-risk population demands expeditious and expert technical resources to manage postoperative care. Postoperative mortality and morbidity rates for CABG surgery is high at 6% to 15% among this age group.[4] Clinicians are now faced with the challenge of reducing the operative morbidity and mortality rates.

PREOPERATIVE CONSIDERATIONS

CAD is usually first suspected with the development of angina pectoris. The conservative diagnosis is made through assessment of the precise nature of chest pain and the electrocardiogram (ECG). To identify and quantitate the extent of CAD, chest x-ray studies, echocardiography, and coronary arteriography are performed. Associated factors such as hypertension, diabetes, history of smoking, lifestyle, and history suggesting transient ischemic attack should also be considered in the diagnosis of CAD.

Assessment (for example, x-ray studies, laboratory examinations, anesthesia consent) is usually done 2 to 5 days before elective surgery in an outpatient setting, and then the patient is admitted the morning of surgery. Since the patient's length of stay in the hospital is decreasing, it is imperative to start patient and family education even before the patient is admitted to the hospital. Patient and family education include information about medications, the operative procedure, anesthesia, postoperative care, and discharge needs.

Knowledge of autologous blood donation should also be included in educating cardiac surgery patients. Since cardiac surgery is associated with perioperative and postoperative bleeding, the potential need for blood and blood products is well recognized. The risks of donor transfusion–acquired disease have focused attention on encouraging autologous blood donation in patients undergoing elective cardiac surgery. Members of the family and significant others may also be designated blood donors.

Careful evaluation of the patient's health history is needed to determine patients at risk related to surgery. Recent aspirin intake should be investigated, and the medication usually is withheld for at least 7 days. Aspirin inhibits thromboxane formation and platelet aggregation, which can increase the patient's risk for postoperative bleeding. A history of coagulopathy and warfarin sodium (Coumadin) intake should also be included in the evaluation. Warfarin sodium should be withheld at least 4 days before surgery, and if anticoagulation is necessary, heparin should be used instead. Antidysrhythmic agents are usually taken until the morning of surgery. Preoperative prophylactic antibiotics using first- and second-generation cephalosporin (cefazolin or cefamandole) or vancomycin if the patient is allergic to penicillin are usually administered immediately before surgery.

Carotid bruits and other neurologic symptoms need to be evaluated to rule out concomitant carotid disease that may require carotid endarterectomy before CABG surgery. Insulin-dependent diabetes, alcohol abuse, and a history of urologic or respiratory problems need to be considered in planning for intraoperative and postoperative management. Preoperative evaluation of pulmonary function is an effective tool for predicting the degree of postoperative pulmonary complications and the need for prolonged ventilatory support.[10] Thus it would be beneficial to include pulmonary function evaluation, especially in high-risk patients.

INTRAOPERATIVE EVENTS

The intraoperative event significantly affects the patient's postoperative management. Therefore it is imperative for clinicians to understand intraoperative events. Cardiopulmonary bypass (CPB), cardioplegia, and the surgical procedure will be briefly reviewed as part of the intraoperative event.

CPB

CPB is a technique used to divert blood from the heart and lungs into an external heart-lung machine to provide the ventilatory and pumping functions of these organs (Fig. 10-1).[11] This extracorporeal circulation permits a controlled cardiac arrest and provides a dry, motionless heart on which to operate. Before CPB, the patient receives a full dose of heparin, usually 3 to 4 mg/kg. Heparinization has occurred when the activated clotting time is over 500 seconds.

CPB is established using a single venous cannula, the aortic cross-clamp, and the aortic cannula (Fig. 10-1).[11] All blood returning to the right atrium is removed from the body by siphon drainage through one or two venous cannulations via the superior or inferior vena cava or right atrium. Coronary blood flow returning to the right atrium

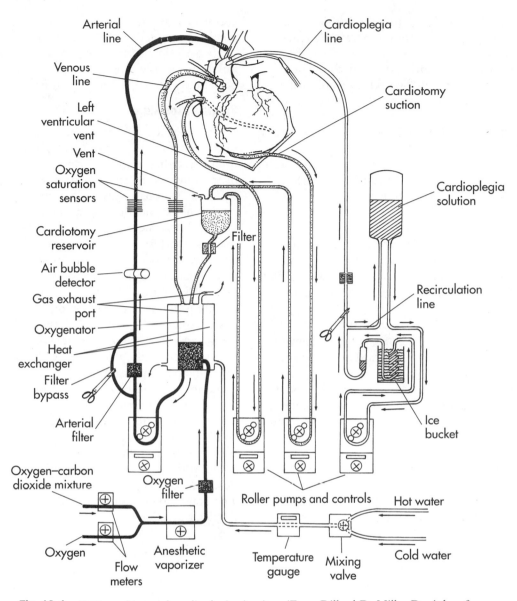

Fig. 10-1 CPB machine and cardioplegia circuit.   (From Dillard D, Miller D: *Atlas of cardiac surgery,* New York, 1983, Macmillan.)

through the coronary sinus is removed by a cardiotomy suction catheter. During CPB, the blood from the bronchial arteries, thebesian veins, and the coronary system returns to the left atrium. The left ventricle is vented when the heart is in full arrest to avoid ventricular distention, which could cause ventricular failure.

Venous blood drains into a bubble or membrane oxygenator, where oxygen and carbon dioxide gas exchange occurs. The oxygenated blood is returned to the systemic circulation via aortic cannulation. Arterial perfusion is provided by a constant-output blood pump. This blood flow is nonpulsatile, unlike normal cardiopulmonary circula-

tion, and is acceptable for the relatively short time required for CPB. A flow rate of 2.4 L/min/m² is generally used for CPB.

Most bubble or membrane oxygenators have a built-in heat exchanger, where blood is cooled or warmed as it passes the oxygenator. The temperature is regulated to maintain a body temperature of 18° to 37° C (64.4° to 98.6° F). The patient's temperature is cooled rapidly by lowering the water temperature in the heat exchanger to 10° C (50° F) or lower. Oxygen requirements are minimized by systemic hypothermia, which reduces cellular oxygen consumption by 50% at 30° C (80° F) and up to 80% at 20° C (68° F).[12] Rewarming is accomplished by slowly raising the water temperature in increments of 10° C.

Weaning from bypass is initiated when the patient's body temperature and heart function return to normal, all suture lines are hemostatically intact, no ischemic changes are noted on the ECG, and mechanical ventilation is resumed. Discontinuation of bypass is initiated by slowly occluding the venous return line. As the patient's heart fills and systemic pressure rises, bypass flow is progressively decreased and then stopped. Protamine sulfate is used to reverse the heparin effect on completion of CPB.

Cardioplegia

When coronary blood flow is interrupted, ischemic injury is avoided through adequate myocardial preservation techniques. Cardioplegic fluids are used throughout CPB. The objectives of cardioplegia are to arrest the heart, create an environment of continued energy production, and counteract ischemia. Potassium, 20 to 30 mEq/L, and coldness, approximately 4° C (39.2° F), are the two major cardioplegic components used in myocardial preservation during ischemic arrest.[12]

Cardioplegic solution is infused into the aortic root via a catheter during bypass immediately after the ascending aorta is clamped (Fig. 10-1).[11] The heart is bathed and covered entirely with cold saline slush at 0° to 1° C (32° to 33.8° F). Myocardial temperature is continuously monitored through a septal thermometer and is maintained below 18° C (64.4° F) during ischemic arrest. Cardioplegic infusion may be given intermittently every 20 minutes or continuously. The cardioplegic solution returns to the coronary sinus and drains to the venous reservoir. Cardioplegia can be accomplished through antegrade or retrograde perfusion. Antegrade perfusion is done through cannulation of the coronary ostia, whereas retrograde perfusion is accomplished via coronary sinus cannulation.[13]

Surgical Procedure

The goals of surgery are to restore myocardial perfusion, prevent further myocardial ischemia, and maintain or improve ventricular function. The conduit, or material used to bypass the stenotic coronary artery, is usually autologous venous or arterial grafts. Venous grafts (most commonly saphenous) require anastomosis to the distal vessel and to the aorta, whereas arterial grafts (internal mammary artery, right gastroepiploic artery, and inferior epigastric arteries) may be anastomosed directly to the vessel or detached and used as described for venous grafts.

CABG is initiated by making a median sternotomy and initiating donor graft harvesting. The greater saphenous vein is removed (Fig. 10-2).[14] If the internal mammary and gastric arteries are used, they are completely mobilized before the pericardium is opened. The pericardium is then opened, and stay sutures and purse-string sutures are applied, including those required for CPB cannulation and infusions of cardioplegia.

After the grafts are prepared, CPB is established, and cold cardioplegia is initiated. With the heart retracted upward and toward the head, the first anastomosis is usually made to the distal right coronary artery or the posterior descending artery using a reversed saphenous vein graft. The graft is then distended gently with a cold blood cardioplegic solution and transected at a point that will permit

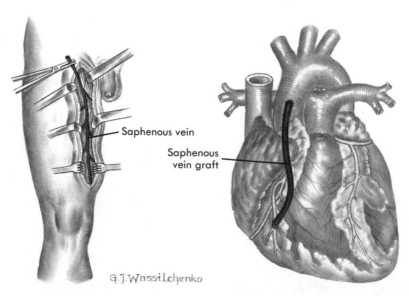

Saphenous vein

Saphenous vein graft

G.J.Wassilchenko

Fig. 10-2   Saphenous vein graft.   (From Thelan L and others: *Critical care nursing: diagnosis and management,* ed 2, St Louis, 1994, Mosby.)

a smooth course without kinks or tension; the end is then spatulated (that is, cut to lie flat). The proximal end of the graft is tacked temporarily to the pericardium.

The next distal vein anastomosis is made to one or more marginal branches of the circumflex coronary artery. The vein graft is pulled gently (that is, made distended by injection of cardioplegic solution), transected at an appropriate point, spatulated, and tacked to the pericardium. The final vein anastomosis is made to one or more diagonal branches, after which the vein is brought beneath the aorta and handled exactly as the marginal branches.

The internal mammary artery is freed, occluded with a clip, transected, and brought through a generous window in the pericardium anterior to the phrenic nerve. The distal end of the internal mammary artery is spatulated and anastomosed to the left anterior descending coronary artery (Fig. 10-3).[14] When the left internal mammary artery does not reach the left anterior descending artery or if it is unavailable, a free graft of the left or right internal mammary artery is used to revascularize the left anterior descending artery. A side-biting clamp is made to the ascending aorta, and punched-out openings are made to connect the venous and free artery grafts to the aorta.

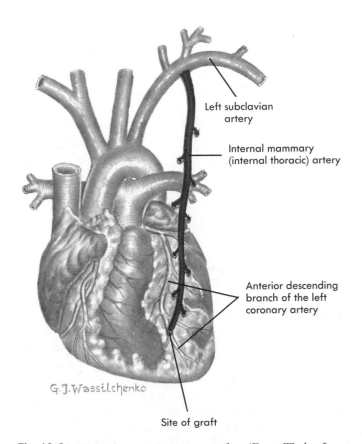

Left subclavian
artery

Internal mammary
(internal thoracic) artery

Anterior descending
branch of the left
coronary artery

G. J. Wassilchenko

Site of graft

Fig. 10-3 Internal mammary artery graft. (From Thelan L and others: *Critical care nursing: diagnosis and management,* ed 2, St Louis, 1994, Mosby.)

After the residual air is removed from the ascending aorta and the side-biting clamp is removed, controlled aortic reperfusion is begun. After the hyperkalemic phase has ended, the light clamp is removed from the internal mammary artery. Rewarming is then begun. Once the heart is beating well, the cross-clamp has been removed, and the chest tubes and epicardial pacing wires have been placed, CPB is discontinued, and decannulation is initiated. Hemostasis of the suture lines and hemodynamic stability are achieved before sternal closure.

POSTOPERATIVE MANAGEMENT

An understanding of the pathophysiologic principles that affect cardiovascular performance and adequacy in tissue perfusion are crucial for managing changes in the cardiopulmonary hemodynamics after cardiac surgery. Patient management after CABG is accomplished through continual clinical assessment, monitoring and evaluation of hemodynamic parameters and laboratory values, and intervention.

Admission to the Unit

The surgeon and anesthesiologist transport the patient from the operating room to the recovery room or intensive care unit. A systematic approach should be used to admit and assess the patient quickly and thoroughly. Prioritized nursing responsibilities are outlined in the box. During the immediate postoperative period, a head-to-toe assessment is performed to establish the patient's baseline condition and identify potential nursing diagnoses. A subsystem approach is used to achieve the primary goal: maintenance of adequate tissue perfusion.

Cardiovascular Subsystem

Cardiac output (CO), the volume of blood ejected per minute by the ventricles, reflects the ability of the heart to pump sufficient blood through the body to meet its metabolic demands. Because of variations in patient size, the cardiac index (CI) is often used in the clinical setting using the formula, CI = CO/Body surface area in square meters, to assess the adequacy of CO. CO is regulated by heart rate and rhythm, preload, afterload, and contractility. The postoperative management of cardiac surgery patients is based on these four parameters. Furthermore, pathophysiologic changes and patient management are described after cardiac surgery.

Heart rate and rhythm

CO is the product of stroke volume and heart rate. A normal heart rate and rhythm contribute significantly to ventricular filling (stroke volume) and thus optimize CO. Cardiac dysrhythmias commonly seen after cardiac surgery significantly disturb normal ventricular filling, thus predisposing patients to allow cardiac output states. The heart's compensatory response to a decrease in CO is to increase

---

NURSING RESPONSIBILITIES ON ADMISSION

Primary Nurse

1. Position self on transducer side of bed.
2. Assess rhythm and blood pressure on portable monitor.
3. Attach ECG monitor to patient.
4. Listen to breath sounds and confirm position of endotracheal tube.
5. Place transducer plate on holder and level transducers.
6. Connect applicable (left and right atrial and pulmonary artery) equipment to monitor nontransduced pressures during transport. Assess waveform, set to zero, and calibrate.
7. Connect arterial line and turn off portable monitor.
8. Assess waveform, check for blood return, and intervene for abnormal blood pressure.
9. Set to zero and calibrate all lines. Run strip on monitor.
10. Call out vital signs to secondary nurse for documentation.
11. Obtain CO. Intervene.
12. Obtain report from anesthesiologist.

Secondary Nurse

1. Connect chest tube to suction; note total drainage.
2. Raise head of bed 30 degrees; have respiratory therapist stabilize endotracheal tube.
3. Correlate cuff blood pressure to arterial line.
4. Empty Foley bag and record total amount.
5. Ask anesthesiologist for last serum potassium level. If it is low, start bolus of potassium chloride.
6. Communicate vital signs and outputs (that is, chest tube and urine) to primary nurse.
7. Connect pacing wires to pacemaker.
8. Turn on warming lights if temperature is less than 36.5° C (97.7° F).
9. Record vital signs on flow sheet. Draw blood for admission laboratory tests.
10. Check placement of gastric tube. Connect to low, continuous suction.
11. Monitor patient while primary nurse gets report from anesthesiologist.
12. Call for portable chest x-ray films. Obtain 12-lead ECG.

---

the heart rate, with a proportionate increase in stroke volume. However, with a high heart rate, there is less time for ventricular filling, causing a decrease in the amount of blood ejected. This causes a decrease in CO and blood pressure. If the heart rate is decreased significantly, CO also decreases.

The most common dysrhythmia seen after cardiac surgery is atrial fibrillation, with a reported incidence ranging from 32% to 64%.[15] Postoperative atrial fibrillation is usually transient and is believed to be caused by a nonuniform dispersion of refractoriness in atrial regions where short refractory regions lie adjacent to areas with a much

longer refractory period.[15] Another hypothesis is that profound myocardial hypothermia and electromechanical arrest achieved in the ventricle are absent from atrial myocardium.[16] The resulting intraoperative atrial ischemia can cause the atrial refractory period distribution to be nonuniform, which can trigger postoperative atrial fibrillation. Atrioventricular (AV) conduction defects after cardiac surgery have been recognized since the introduction of cold potassium cardioplegia.[17] The incidence of postoperative AV conduction defect in one report was 16%.[18] Persistent AV conduction defect (more than 6 hours) may be associated with a higher incidence of postoperative low CO and perioperative myocardial infarction.[18] Although conduction defects are transient in nature, they may persist 2 weeks or longer after cardiac surgery.[19] Factors related to the development of postoperative AV conduction defect follow: (1) The high concentration of potassium in cardioplegic solution decreases the excitability, automaticity, and conductivity in the myocardial AV nodal cells; (2) there is inadequate flow to the AV node artery when right coronary artery grafting is involved; and (3) surgical damage to the sinus node or its artery occurs.[18,19]

Ventricular dysrhythmias often occur in patients with ventricular irritability, intraoperative myocardial ischemia, or electrolyte imbalance. Common dysrhythmogenic electrolyte imbalances that occur after surgery are hypokalemia, hypocalcemia, and hypomagnesemia. Hypokalemia increases automaticity, potentiates the effect of digoxin, and predisposes the patient to premature ventricular contractions.[20] Hypocalcemia is associated with large infusions of citrated blood. The sodium citrate used as a blood preservative binds with serum calcium, which may cause the myocardial tissue to become hypocalcemic. The hypocalcemic state of the myocardium may then intensify the ischemic injury caused by depressed myocardial function, leading to ischemia-related dysrhythmias. Magnesium decreases the outflow of potassium from the cell, an important consideration in maintaining normal serum magnesium levels, since as many as 15% of dysrhythmias have been observed in patients with hypokalemia.[21]

Prompt and accurate recognition is essential in the early treatment of dysrhythmias. Use of the bedside atrial electrogram is indispensable for rapid and accurate recognition and interpretation of cardiac dysrhythmias. The atrial electrogram is useful in diagnosing atrial flutter, atrial fibrillation, and junctional rhythm and for differentiating between ventricular tachycardia and supraventricular tachycardia with aberrant conduction.[22]

Management and treatment

The cause of the alteration in heart rate and rhythm and the patient's clinical status determine the aggressiveness of treatment. Increases in the heart rate may be caused by hypovolemia, sympathetic response to painful stimuli, or a chronotropic response from vasoactive drugs. The treatment is geared toward maintaining fluid and electrolyte balance, providing adequate pain management, and titrating vasoactive support with consideration of the chronotropic side effects of drugs.

Pharmacologic treatment of supraventricular tachydysrhythmias is initiated when the probability of hemodynamic compromise is high. Digoxin, class II and III antidysrhythmic drugs, verapamil, and adenosine are usually indicated.[23] Prophylactic use of procainamide for the prevention of postoperative atrial fibrillation reduces the incidence of dysrhythmias after surgery.[24]

Class IV antidysrhythmic drugs are usually indicated for suppression of ventricular dysrhythmias. However, the preliminary findings of the Cardiac Arrhythmia Suppression Trial (CAST)[25] indicate no improvement in dysrhythmia suppression when antidysrhythmic drugs are used after surgery. Several clinical trials have shown a 49% reduction in dysrhythmias when magnesium sulfate infusions are used for prophylactic treatment of cardiac dysrhythmias precipitated by electrolyte imbalances.[21,26,27] In the immediate postoperative period, treatment of premature ventricular contractions is recommended despite hemodynamic stability when more than six contractions occur in 1 minute, when they occur in couplets or triplets, or when ventricular tachycardia persists for more than 1 minute. Treatment includes lidocaine or procainamide, propranolol, diphenylhydantoin, and bretylium. Mechanical cardioversion is initiated when hemodynamic compromise occurs with sustained ventricular tachycardia.

Epicardial pacing wires placed during surgery can be used for external pacing to manage dysrhythmias. Rapid atrial or overdrive pacing is used for burst suppression or interruption of re-entrant pathways. AV sequential pacing is the preferable mode of treatment for AV dissociation. For suppressing ventricular dysrhythmias, AV sequential pacing with a shorter AV delay in the range of 100 to 150 ms may be preferable. However, the AV delay must be individualized when treating dysrhythmias or attempting to improve CO. If heart block persists for more than 1 week, permanent pacemaker insertion is usually considered.

Preload

Preload is the volume of blood in the ventricles before contraction (that is, ventricular end-diastolic volume), which establishes the stretch and resting muscle length of the myocardial fiber. When the atria are functioning normally as reservoirs, ventricular end-diastolic pressure is similar to the mean pressure in the corresponding atrium. Thus atrial pressure is used after surgery to assess ventricular preload or ventricular end-diastolic pressure. Atrial pressure is measured using a transvenous central venous catheter (central venous pressure) or a transthoracic right or left atrial catheter. In the absence of pulmonary vascular disease, pulmonary artery diastolic pressure or pulmonary capillary wedge pressure is a reasonable approximation of left atrial pressure.

Postoperative low CO associated with decreased preload occurs in conditions in which there is an inadequate circulating blood volume. A decrease in circulating blood volume may be caused by inadequate volume replacement in the presence of hemorrhage, an increased intravascular space from abrupt return to normothermia after a hypothermic episode, third spacing secondary to hemodilution on CPB, and aggressive diuresis. Acute pericardial tamponade decreases preload by mechanically restricting venous return to the heart.

Management and treatment

Decreased preload is managed with volume replacement. In the presence of bleeding, aggressive surveillance and replacement of blood volume is needed. Close monitoring of the patient's coagulation studies and activated clotting time is also important. Careful evaluation of intake and output is critical when replacing volume to prevent fluid overload. Guidelines for volume replacement are described in Table 10-1.

The goal for volume replacement is to maintain a preload status that will achieve adequate systemic perfusion. Attainment of normothermia can also normalize the clotting cascade and augment clotting factor transfusions. Autotransfusion of blood shed from the mediastinum and predonated autologous blood is effective in postoperative volume replacement.[28] Surveillance of chest drainage and prevention of clot formation in the mediastinal chest tube are needed to prevent pericardial tamponade. If pericardial tamponade occurs, immediate removal of the clots in the mediastinal chest tube is considered in patients who are hemodynamically stable. An emergency median sternotomy may be needed if the patient's status starts to deteriorate.

In patients admitted from the operating room in a hypothermic and hypertensive state, the goal is a gradual increase in body temperature and careful titration of vasodilating drugs (nitroprusside) to avoid sudden hypotension when dilatation of intravascular space occurs with rewarming. Patients who have hypothermia and hypertension with low right and left atrial pressures need vasodilating drugs with volume replacement to prevent acute hypotension; this is known as *rewarming shock.* Clinically, a patient who has episodic hypotension during the period of hypertension, known as the *roller coaster effect,* while receiving vasodilators for blood pressure control is likely to have an inadequate volume status. Judicious monitoring of right and left atrial pressures and pulmonary artery diastolic pressure is critical to avoid this period of hemodynamic instability. A right atrial pressure of 18 mm Hg or less should be maintained to optimize the ascending limb of the Frank-Starling curve. An elevated right atrial pressure predisposes patients to pleural effusions, ascites, and anasarca. A left atrial pressure of at least 20 mm Hg puts the patient at risk for developing pulmonary edema.

TABLE 10-1   Treatment Guidelines for Volume Replacement

Cause	Treatment	Note
Bleeding:		
Hematocrit of 25% or less	Packed red blood cells	Administer 1.0 mg of calcium chloride with each milliliter of blood or blood product.
Elevated prothrombin and partial thromboplastin times	Fresh frozen plasma	
Elevated activated coagulation time (greater than 150)	Protamine sulfate	Administer protamine sulfate, 50 mg over 20 minutes, via intravenous piggyback and watch for hypotension.
Low platelet count with bleeding or platelet count less than 40,000/mm³	Platelets	
Third-space fluid	Mannitol Hetastarch (Hespan)	Administer mannitol dose per physician's orders.
	5% albumin	Know that 5% albumin is equivalent to the same volume of plasma
	25% albumin	Know that 25% albumin is equivalent to 5 times its volume of plasma.

A decreased preload 24 hours after surgery is usually related to aggressive diuresis or third spacing as a response from CPB. After CPB, levels of serum protein are decreased with a concomitant decrease in osmotic pressure and an increase in capillary permeability. This results in the shift of intravascular fluid to the interstitial space, depleting the circulating intravascular volume.[29] The goal of management is to pull fluids from the tissue into the intravascular space to optimize preload without administering extra volume, thereby avoiding an increase in third-space fluids. Mannitol or 25% albumin followed by loop diuretics (for example, furosemide) usually improves the preload status without a large volume infusion. Increases in preload that are unresponsive to diuresis are usually associated with renal dysfunction.

Afterload

Afterload is the force that resists ventricular ejection and is largely determined by impedance. Factors that influence impedance include pulmonary vascular resistance (PVR) and aortic systemic resistance, mass, and the viscosity of blood in the blood vessels. An increase in afterload or impedance to ventricular flow results in increased myocardial stress. Afterload reduction alleviates myocardial stress and augments stroke volume and CO. Calculation of the systemic vascular resistance (SVR) and PVR are used to assess left and right ventricular afterload respectively.

Management and treatment

Right ventricular afterload reduction. The goal of reducing right ventricular afterload is to optimize right ventricular function and to reduce PVR through pharmacologic or mechanical afterload interventions. In the presence of increased PVR, nitroglycerin and prostaglandin E_1 via intravenous infusions are used. If pulmonary vascular reactivity is present, bronchodilators, hyperoxygenation, hyperventilation, and sedation are used to decrease vascular reactivity, which could trigger an increase in PVR. Positive inotropic supports such as dopamine, dobutamine, and isoproterenol (Isuprel) are used to support right ventricular function in the presence of increased PVR. Right ventricular assist devices (VADs) and/or extracorporeal membrane oxygenation (ECMO) can be used to mechanically unload the right ventricle. PVR is calculated using the formula:

$$PVR = \frac{PAP - PCWP}{CO} \times 80$$

Normal value = 50 to 250 dyne-seconds-cm^{-5}/m^2

where *PAP* is the pulmonary artery pressure and *PCWP* is the pulmonary capillary wedge pressure.

Left ventricular afterload reduction. The goal of therapy is to maintain systemic pressure after surgery with the least ventricular workload. Control of hypertension and systemic vasoconstriction decrease the impedance against which the left ventricle must work. Prudence is exercised in the control of hypertension in patients with preoperative systemic hypertension and CAD. These patients may require a higher systemic pressure for adequate cerebral perfusion. SVR is the parameter used in afterload reduction. The formula is calculated as:

$$SVR = \frac{Mean\ arterial\ pressure\ -\ Right\ atrial\ pressure}{CO} \times 80$$

Nitroprusside is usually the drug of choice to reduce ventricular afterload because of its potent vasodilating effect and short half-life in the arterial system and, to a lesser extent, the venous system. Calcium channel antagonists such as nifedipine and diltiazem have the same arteriolar vasodilatation effect. However, despite the indirect effect of calcium channel antagonists in reducing the potential for coronary spasm, the myocardial depressant effect and prolonged half-life make nitroprusside a better choice for afterload reduction. If the patient has hypothermia and vasoconstriction, gradual rewarming should be achieved. Rapid rewarming may cause severe hypotension because of a volume-depleted intravascular space. The hypotension is usually responsive to a volume challenge; however, a fluid overload may occur when the intravascular space equilibrates. Patients who receive large volumes in fluid challenges should be considered for early aggressive diuresis to prevent serious third spacing of fluids. Systemic vasoconstriction can be caused by residual hypothermia from the operating room or may be a compensatory response to hypovolemia. Identification of the etiology of systemic vasoconstriction helps the clinician determine the appropriate intervention.

Intraaortic balloon counterpulsation (IABC) is used in the mechanical support of left ventricular afterload (balloon deflation). In addition, diastolic augmentation (balloon inflation) is used to support contractility. Indications for IABC insertion include intraoperative pump failure, unstable angina, preoperative prophylaxis, preoperative shock, and postoperative support.[30] The use of IABC before (36%), during (53%), and after surgery (12%) is associated with mortality rates indicating that earlier use of other supportive measures such as left VADs is needed.[31]

IABC is begun in a 1:1 augmentation frequency. A positive response to this intervention is noted by immediate improvement in the patient's CO. If hemodynamic improvement is obtained, weaning from pharmacologic support should be pursued. After pharmacologic supports are weaned to a therapeutic level with stable hemodynamics (usually 24 to 72 hours), weaning from IABC is initiated. The frequency of augmentation is decreased gradually from 1:1 to 1:2 and finally 1:3. The decrease in balloon augmentation accompanied by hemodynamic stability suggests successful weaning and is an indication for removal of the catheter. Failure to achieve hemodynamic stability results in an inability to wean and is exhibited by increased filling pressures, recurrence of ventricular ectopy, and signs of decreased tissue perfusion.

Serious complications associated with IABC include thrombosis that may lead to limb ischemia, bleeding, dissection of one or more blood vessels, and infection. Balloon entrapment was reported by one author after the balloon catheter was in place for 10 days.[32] The incidence of vascular complications was reported to be 11% in one study.[30] Emphasis on vascular assessment and surveillance of the affected limb should be incorporated in the management of this patient population.

Contractility

Contractility is defined as the strength of cardiac muscle contraction or as the inherent inotropic state of the heart. Alteration in contractility after cardiac surgery is associated with myocardial stunning.[33] Myocardial stunning is reversible ventricular dysfunction in the absence of myocardial necrosis. It is induced by brief periods of regional or global myocardial ischemia, reoxygenation of previously ischemic myocardium, and a prolonged low CO.[33] Cardioplegic arrest during CPB has been suggested as one example of predictable global ischemia, with the potential for subsequent myocardial stunning lasting up to 48 hours.[34] The volume displacement (or third spacing) that occurs after CPB may occur in myocardial tissue, resulting in myocardial edema.[35] The occurrence of edema in the postperfusion period has been attributed to injury to the myocardial cells, including damage to the cell membranes and sodium pump, and to the breakdown of complex carbohydrate molecules and adenosine triphosphate, with secondary increases in intracellular osmolarity.[35] Accumulation of myocardial edema can lead to myocardial stiffness and to a low CO. Confounded by a severely compromised coronary blood flow, myocardial edema further worsens cardiac function.

Management and treatment

Patients for whom weaning from CPB is difficult are assisted with maximum inotropic support such as, dopamine, dobutamine, IABC, or another circulatory device. If myocardial edema is severe, sternal closure may be impossible. Even attempting to approximate the edges of the sternum may produce mechanical tamponade. When this occurs, closure of the sternum is delayed, and sternal stents are used to keep the sternum separated and to promote cardiac decompression. As many as 20% of these patients may require circulatory cardiac assist devices to support ventricular dysfunction.[36]

Circulatory assist devices. Partial or complete support of cardiac output is possible with a circulatory assist device, commonly referred to as a ventricular assist device (VAD). VADs can be used in one ventricle (that is, an RVAD or LVAD), or it may be biventricular (that is, a BVAD). An ECMO circuit can also be connected to the system, providing CPB without arresting the heart. When an RVAD is used, the right ventricular circulation is bypassed when the superior or inferior vena cava or the right atrium is cannulated to drain venous blood into the pump (RVAD) and the pulmonary artery is cannulated to return venous blood into the pulmonary circulation for oxygenation. When an LVAD is used, the left atrium cannulation drains the oxygenated blood into the pump (LVAD) and back to the aorta via aortic cannulation (left ventricular bypass). To optimize ventilation and oxygenation in the presence of severe pulmonary dysfunction, a membrane oxygenator may be connected to the system after the RVAD circuit.

VADs are indicated for patients who cannot be weaned from CPB or who are unresponsive to maximum doses of inotropic medications. VADs are also indicated in patients with postcardiotomy cardiogenic shock unresponsive to medical management. Medical management includes aggressive volume intervention, inotropic support, cardiac pacing, and IABC.

Usually, a cardiac assist device is initiated in the operating room, but the procedure may be performed at the bedside in emergency conditions. The collective effort of the unit staff and perfusionist can expedite the insertion procedure. In the patient who has had a cardiotomy, ventricular dysfunction is thought to be reversible, and the device is used until appropriate ventricular function resumes. The use of VAD has produced satisfactory clinical outcomes and postoperative survival.[37,38] VADs also may be used as bridges to transplantation when the return of ventricular dysfunction is not expected. The care of patients with altered CO is summarized in the standards of care (see box).

Pulmonary Subsystem

Studies of pulmonary function after cardiac surgery have shown that a restrictive change occurs immediately after surgery, with recovery after 6 to 16 weeks.[39,40] Older patients and those with preexisting obstructive lung disease are more susceptible to pulmonary complications after cardiac surgery. Restrictive pulmonary changes are attributed to the absence of pulmonary blood flow during CPB, resulting in low sheer stress in the pulmonary capillaries; leukocyte activation, which incites an inflammatory response in the pulmonary vasculature; increased permeability of the alveolar-capillary barrier; entry of macromolecules into the pulmonary interstitium, and ultimately the alveoli, leading to the development of pulmonary edema; and development of atelectasis (either segmental or lobar), particularly of the left lower lobe, which has a strong tendency to atelectasis because of loss of lung volume.[41,42]

Atelectasis, pleural effusion, pneumothorax, and a large alveolar-arterial oxygen difference are the most common pulmonary complications after CPB. Factors that contribute to the development of these complications are direct trauma to the lungs, retention of secretions, phrenic nerve injury, mechanical obstruction of the lower trachea and bronchi, and ventricular dysfunction.[43]

Mild pulmonary dysfunction, which is manifested by noncardiogenic edema in patients with normal preoperative pulmonary function, slowly improves with coughing, deep-breathing exercises, and progressive ambulation. In patients with marked ventricular dysfunction before surgery, pulmonary dysfunction may persist beyond 5 to 6 days of postoperative convalescence. These patients usually respond to diuretic management and an aggressive pulmonary hygiene regimen. The hypothesis for fluid retention in these patients follows: The fluid that has accumulated in the interstitial space early after CPB returns to the vascular space 24 to 72 hours after surgery (third spacing).

Tracheobronchial secretions that occur 48 to 72 hours after surgery are thought to result from mobilization of protein-rich fluid that has been in the alveoli or interstitium of the lung since CPB. This fluid is moved by cilia out of the terminal bronchioles and into the larger airways; it can be cleared from these structures by aggressive chest physiotherapy.[41] Lung volumes, particularly the vital capacity and the total lung volume, are usually decreased early after cardiac surgery. This is probably the result of the effects of multiple areas of atelectasis, occasionally left lower lobe collapse, occult pulmonary edema and pleural fluid, and reduced inspiratory effort. These changes usually resolve within 3 to 6 months after surgery.[41,42]

If pulmonary dysfunction is not resolved, adult respiratory distress syndrome (ARDS) may ensue. ARDS is manifested by hypoxemia, pulmonary infiltrates, and prolonged intubation. Preoperative treatment with amiodarone therapy can predispose patients to restrictive pulmonary disease. Greenspon and others[44] reported a 50% incidence of ARDS in patients receiving amiodarone therapy 6 to 14 days before surgery.

Pneumothorax is an infrequent complication but can be life threatening after cardiac surgery, with a 1.4% reported incidence.[45] Patients who have chronic obstructive pulmonary disease are predisposed to pneumothorax. This complication is often preventable with conservative management of chest tube drainage. Surveillance of changes in oxygenation status, ventilation, and chest x-ray films is crucial in preventing this complication. Phrenic nerve paralysis may occur as a result of nerve damage from cold cardioplegia or from inadvertent dissection during the operation. In one report, 6.9% of patients developed phrenic nerve paralysis after cardiac surgery, resulting in an ineffective breathing pattern.[46] This complication leads to prolonged intubation and possibly to tracheostomy intervention at more than 14 days if attempts to wean the patient are unsuccessful.

Management and treatment

The goal of treatment is the early return of the patient to spontaneous breathing and ambulation. The resulting hemodynamic changes from early extubation benefits the patient through a decline in intrapleural pressure, an in-

STANDARD FOR DECREASED CO

Decreased CO related to dysrhythmia

Decreased preload secondary to hemorrhage, diuresis, and third-space fluid

Increased afterload secondary to hypertension, hypothermia, and pulmonary edema

Decreased contractility secondary to ventricular dysfunction and cardiac tamponade

Outcome

Patient will maintain a CO adequate for perfusion of body tissues as evidenced by a CI greater than 2.5 L/min, a blood pressure of greater than 90/60 mm Hg, mentation, warm and dry skin, urine output greater than 30 ml/hr, and lack of acidosis.

Assessment

Assess for signs and symptoms of decreased CO:

Hypotension

Low filling pressures

Dysrhythmias

Decreased urine output

Weak peripheral pulses

Cool, clammy skin

Changes in mental status

Assess for possible etiologies of decreased CO.

Interventions

Related to Dysrhythmia

Provide continuous ECG monitoring and evaluation:

Document rhythm every hour.

Document rhythm strip and waveforms every shift and as necessary.

For unstable rhythms, follow hospital protocols and protocols for advanced cardiac life support.

Administer antidysrhythmic agents per physician's order:

Observe for effects of antidysrhythmic agents.

Record dosage every hour and any necessary changes.

Check electrolyte levels.

Connect pacing wires to pacemaker.

Administer potassium boluses for low potassium levels.

Related to Preload

Monitor and evaluate pulmonary artery and right and left atrial pressures every hour.

Monitor and evaluate CO and CI every hour for 4 hours and then every 4 hours and as necessary.

Related to Preload—cont'd

Monitor and evaluate chest tube drainage every hour:

Note consistency of chest tube drainage.

Maintain patency of chest tube. (Gentle milking is recommended.)

Notify physician if chest tube output is more than 200 ml/hour

Monitor spun hematocrit on admission, every 6 hours for 4 times, and as necessary.

Monitor coagulation profile as ordered.

Administer type-specific volume replacement.

Related to Afterload

Monitor systemic pressures and body temperature:

Continuously evaluate blood pressure and calculate SVR and PVR with CO.

Evaluate core temperature every hour until it is stable and then monitor it every 4 hours.

Begin warming measures on arrival to the unit:

Use warming lights and warm blankets to maintain core temperature at 37° C (98.6° F) (no less than 37.5° C [99.5° F]). If core temperature is less than 35° C (95° F), use a heating blanket.

Treat shivering per physician's order.

Administer vasodilator agents per physician's order:

Record rate and dose every hour and any necessary changes.

Evaluate response to vasodilator agents.

For patients on IABC, refer to hospital protocol.

Related to Contractility

Monitor and evaluate acid-base balance according to arterial blood gas analyses.

Administer and titrate vasoactive and inotropic agents per physician's order to maintain adequate CO:

Record rate and dose every hour and any necessary changes.

Evaluate response to vasoactive agents.

Wean patient from vasopressor and inotropic agents gradually, continuously observing blood pressure, heart rate, CO, CI, and venous oxygen saturation.

For patients on VADs, see hospital protocol.

Patient and Family Teaching

Inform patient and family of treatment plan and interventions.

---

creased left ventricular end-diastolic diameter or volume, an increased ventricular systolic function because of increased preload associated with shifting of some of the blood volume toward the chest, and an increased CO.[41]

As soon as hemodynamic stability is attained, weaning from the ventilator and extubation should be initiated. Patients with normal pulmonary function before surgery usually tolerate weaning and extubation 12 to 24 hours after surgery. A delay in extubation usually occurs in the presence of pulmonary dysfunction, high doses of pharmacologic and mechanical inotropic support, neurologic com-

plications, persistent chest tube drainage, or residual cardiac dysfunction with a possibility of returning to the operating room. Weaning from inotropic support to a therapeutic dose should be initiated first to provide an opportunity to increase dosages to compensate for the increased demand in CO during weaning and extubation.

Prolonged intubation (more than 48 hours after surgery) can predispose patients to pulmonary infectious complications, which may cause ARDS. ARDS in cardiac surgery patients usually occurs with sepsis that is exacerbated by noncardiogenic pulmonary edema from CPB.[43,47]

Management of ARDS after surgery is similar to conventional therapy and includes diuresis, optimal ventilator support, and support of oxygenation. However, a strategy for aggressive diuresis and fluid restriction pursued as early as possible, while careful monitoring and supporting perfusion of other organ systems occurs, improves patient outcomes.[48] If conservative medical management fails, ECMO is an effective alternative treatment.[49] The rationale for using ECMO is that mechanical ventilation is disadvantageous in the ARDS lung and lung rest provides a better environment for healing. One recently developed method of supporting the lung during this period is an implantable intravascular oxygenator.[50]

The intravascular oxygenator is a device placed within the vena cava. Venous blood returning to the right atrium flows over and around the device. Blood gas exchange is through the process of diffusion, in which oxygen transfer occurs in the venous blood and carbon dioxide is eliminated in an outer conduit of the double-lumen gas transport tube. This tube is attached to a gas controller unit, where adjustments can be made in the rate of oxygen flow and amount of outlet pressure. When this device is used, ventilator settings such as airway pressure, oxygen concentration, positive end-expiratory pressure, and minute volume can be reduced. These reductions may decrease the potential for oxygen toxicity and barotrauma, which often occur in ARDS, thus optimizing management for pulmonary recovery (see box).

Renal Subsystem

According to Corwin,[51] the incidence of mild to moderate renal insufficiency after cardiac surgery is 20% to 30%. Acute renal failure (ARF) associated with cardiac surgery is associated with prerenal causes such as decreased intravascular volume or decreased renal perfusion with resultant ischemic injury during and after CPB. ARF occurs in 1% to 2% of adults undergoing CPB, even in the absence of preexisting risk factors.[52]

If ARF is ischemic in origin symptoms, it can occur as early as 12 to 18 hours after surgery.[52] The patient has oliguria or anuria, which may be unresponsive to diuretics or dopamine. Thus patients are at risk for severe volume overload. The blood urea nitrogen and creatinine levels may slowly increase, and potassium levels may markedly increase, which may also be related to hemolysis during CPB. Patients may even develop ARF 3 to 4 days after surgery. The patient is usually nonoliguric but tends to have a rapid rise in levels of blood urea nitrogen and creatinine. If ARF persists for more than 5 days with symptoms of uremia, hemodialysis may be considered.

In general, treatment of ARF includes administering aggressive diuresis and optimizing hemodynamics to maintain adequate tissue perfusion. High doses of loop diuretics and renal dose dopamine at 1 to 3 mcg/kg/min promote diuresis and may delay or avoid dialysis while awaiting the return of renal function.[53]

Neurologic Subsystem

The brain is the most oxygen- and perfusion-sensitive organ in the body. The incidence of neurophysiologic injury alone ranges from 0.7% to 3.8% in retrospective studies and from 4.8% to 5.2% in prospective studies and increases to 9% with advancing age (greater than 75 years).[54] The brain receives 15% of the total CO and uses 20% of the body's oxygen supply.[55] Aerobic metabolism occurs in the brain, fueled primarily by glucose and oxygen. During periods of decreased perfusion, embolism, hypoglycemia, and hypoxemia during and after surgery can lead to severe neurologic injury. The cause of injury has been attributed to hypothermic circulatory arrest and may be the result of inadequate nonuniform cooling or embolization of air or microaggregates. Adjunctive techniques in cardioplegia are now being studied to decrease the incidence of embolic brain injury.[56]

Clinical manifestations
Neuropsychologic deficits

Neuropsychologic deficit is defined as a change in cognitive functions. The most frequently reported deficits after cardiac surgery are decreased concentration, memory and learning, and speed of visual responses.[54] Factors contributing to postoperative neuropsychologic changes include age, preexisting cerebrovascular disease, previous stroke, aortic atherosclerosis, cardiac valve operation, and CPB time. The incidence of this complication is 60% to 80% at 1 week after surgery and 20% to 40% at 8 weeks after surgery.[54]

Identification of risk factors before surgery can decrease the likelihood of postoperative neuropsychologic deficits. Postoperative delirium or psychosis that may transiently occur after cardiac surgery usually resolves, and recovery from the symptoms is achieved before discharge. Manifestations of postoperative delirium and psychosis are similar to those of sensory-perceptual alteration related to neuropsychologic deficits, including confusion, agitation, disorientation, short span of attention, and impaired problem-solving capability.[57] Management is geared toward prevention of injury and ongoing reality orientation for the confused and agitated patient, frequent reorientation to environment, and repetitive teaching at short intervals.

Neurophysiologic deficits

Neurophysiologic deficits generally become apparent after recovery from anesthesia and paralytic agents. Most patients regain consciousness 2 to 6 hours after surgery. Prolonged unresponsiveness from anesthesia after CPB may result in irreversible coma. Thus when the level of consciousness is altered, immediate investigation needs to be initiated. The diagnosis of injury is made through physical examination to assess neuroresponsiveness. An electroencephalogram is useful in determining whether there are neurologic deficits and in distinguishing between metabolic and focal lesions. Computerized tomography of the brain helps localize focal lesions. The use of an ob-

STANDARD FOR IMPAIRED GAS EXCHANGE

Impaired gas exchange related to:
  Pulmonary interstitial edema
  Atelectasis, pneumothorax or hemothorax, and pleural effusion
  Sedative-induced respiratory depression
  Pain
  Immobility

Outcomes

Absence of subjective feelings of dyspnea
Respiratory rate within normal limits for the patient (approximately less than 30 and greater than 10)
Vital signs and arterial blood gas levels within normal limits
Lungs clear (on auscultation and chest x-ray film) and equal breath sounds bilaterally
Peak airway pressures within normal limits for the patient
Absence of use of accessory muscles with respiration
Patient ability to use incentive spirometer, to perform effective coughing and deep breathing, and to express understanding of the importance of chest physiotherapy procedures within 4 hours of extubation

Assessment

Assess for signs and symptoms of respiratory failure:
  Arterial blood gas levels: pH of less than 7.35 or greater than 7.45, arterial oxygen pressure of less than 50 mm Hg, arterial carbon dioxide pressure of greater than 50 mm Hg, and oxygen percent saturation of 90% on room air
  Respiratory rate of 30 breaths/min (or above or below patient's baseline)
  Dyspnea accompanied by tachycardia or nasal flaring
  Altered level of consciousness
  Use of accessory muscles, intercostal retraction, and paradoxical breathing
  Cyanosis, pallor, decreased or increased skin temperature, or moisture on the skin
  Adventitious breath sounds
  Thick, viscous secretions
  Fluid overload
  High peak airway pressures
Assess for possible etiologies of respiratory failure.

Interventions

Assess patency of airway, including lack of wheezing, snoring sounds, and ability to pass suction catheter through endotracheal tube.
Maintain mechanical ventilatory support:
  Assess breath sounds and position of endotracheal tube.
  Secure endotracheal tube; consider use of airway or bite block to prevent occlusion from biting.
  Endotracheal suctioning with lavage every 1 to 2 hours and as necessary.
  Provide chest physiotherapy every 2 to 4 hours.
  Initiate ventilator weaning per physician's orders.
Assess respiratory parameters hourly:
  Monitor arterial blood gas levels as ordered and as necessary.
  Check ventilator settings at the start of each shift and with changes.
  Assess tidal volume and rate of spontaneous ventilation.
  Assess hemodynamic changes in response to suctioning, weaning, and turning.
Evaluate factors to maximize oxygen delivery and minimize oxygen consumption, including oxygen consumption, pain, anxiety, shivering, seizures, and fever.
Turn patient side to side every 2 hours for optimal drainage and lung expansion.
Decrease patient and family anxiety:
  Keep patient and family informed of status and plan of care.
  Allow family at bedside as much as possible.
  Assist with communication (alphabet board or slate).
  Keep call bell accessible.
  Ask patient yes-no questions.
Check parameters after extubation:
  Check pulmonary hygiene, chest physiotherapy, and incentive spirometry every 1 to 2 hours.
  Perform nasotracheal suctioning if unable to expectorate secretions.
  Administer supplemental, humidified oxygen and wean to room air per physician's order.
  Initiate out-of-bed activities when hemodynamics are stable.
  Administer diuretics and obtain chest x-ray study per physician's order.
Monitor fluid and nutritional status, including intake and output, daily weight, protein and albumin levels, and calorie count.
Prevent or intervene in complications, pneumothorax, pleural effusion, and atelectasis.

---

jective measurement tool such as the Glasgow coma scale is very helpful in assessing neurophysiologic and neuropsychologic deficits.[58] The Glasgow coma scale is often used with other measurement tools such as the Ramsay objective measurement of the effects of sedation, which guides clinicians in determining the appropriate time to perform neurologic evaluation in the absence of sedation and analgesia.[59]

Another neurologic complication after CABG surgery is cerebrovascular accident, which is defined as any focal deficits continuing for more than 24 hours with a variable degree of neurologic deficits.[60] Older patients and patients with carotid vessel disease are considered high risk for postoperative cerebrovascular accident. Occasionally, after car-

diac surgery patients develop seizures, which may be caused by an ischemic event. Measures to decrease cerebral swelling help prevent further brain injury if hemorrhage has occurred. Anticoagulant therapy is contraindicated from hemorrhagic cerebral infarction after surgery because of the possibility of extending the infarct. Anticonvulsant therapy is initiated at this time. Close monitoring of serum electrolyte, calcium, magnesium, blood urea nitrogen, creatinine, blood glucose, and arterial blood gas levels is necessary. Abnormalities in these values may indicate the likelihood of seizure activity.

Pharmacologic intervention is the most promising intervention for prevention of cerebral injury. Thiopental decreases the incidence of neurologic deficits in patients undergoing CPB at normothermia with bubble oxygenators and no filters. Prostacyclin has been used to minimize platelet aggregation. However, its effect on systemic pressure has reduced its usefulness. Nimodipine is the most promising pharmacologic intervention available. It is a lipophilic calcium channel blocker that crosses the blood-brain barrier in substantial concentrations. Nimodipine is a potent cerebral vasodilator and increases cerebral blood flow at doses that do not alter the systemic blood pressure.[54]

Pain

Pain is "an unpleasant sensory and emotional experience associated with actual or potential tissue damage or described in terms of such damage" and is always subjective.[61] Clinicians need to know as much as possible about the patient's pain experience because of its impact on emotional and physiological well-being. Pain can cause reflex motor activity, sympathetic nervous system activation, and activation of an endocrine stress response. Reflex motor activity can result in contraction of abdominal wall muscles, resulting in rigidity that leads to hypoventilation, avoidance of deep breathing, coughing, and movement. Thus pain may lead to respiratory complications, including atelectasis, pneumonia, and hypoxemia. When the sympathetic nervous system is activated, heart rate and systemic pressure may increase. Therefore pain can increase the myocardial workload and compromise the myocardial oxygen supply. When the endocrine stress response is activated by pain, cortisol, catecholamine, and antidiuretic hormone release are increased. This may lead to fluid retention, protein catabolism, lipolysis, and hyperglycemia.[62]

Few studies focus on the subject of pain management in the cardiac surgical patient population. Gift and others[63]

STANDARD FOR ALTERATION IN COMFORT

Alteration in comfort related to
  Surgical incision
  Intubation
  Drainage tubes or cannula

Outcomes

Patient will have minimum pain as evidenced by the ability to cough and deep breathe; the ability to turn, get out of bed, and ambulate; a heart rate and respiratory rate within normal limits; the ability to rest and sleep; the absence of grimacing, restlessness, and agitation; and verbalization of effective pain relief from medication.

Patient and family are aware of importance of notifying staff members about pain and can verbalize techniques that may be useful in relieving pain.

Assessment

Assess for possible etiologies of pain:
  Procedures and treatments
  Intubation or mechanical ventilation
  Immobility
  Trauma (surgery and ischemia)
Assess for evidence of pain:
  Behavioral responses to pain:
  Facial grimaces
  Hypoventilation
  Moaning and crying
  Restlessness and sleeplessness
  Splinting of incisional area
Physiologic responses to pain:
  Tachypnea
  Tachycardia
  Hypertension
Subjective responses to pain:
  Verbalization of pain
  Description of location, intensity, and other characteristics
  Requests for pain medications

Assessment—cont'd

Patient's response to analgesia:
  Notify physician if prescribed dose does not adequately alleviate the pain or if it causes significant respiratory depression.
  Use acute pain-management assessment scale: *Pain level:* Scale from 0 to 10. 0 = no pain; 10 = worst pain possible. *Sedation level:* 0 = none; 1 = drowsiness present, easy to arouse; 2 = somnolent, difficult to arouse.

Interventions

Assess for and eliminate etiologies of pain when possible.
Assess history of pain and pain management.
Handle patient gently, supporting limbs and trunk:
  Position patient for comfort.
  Support incision and chest tubes or cannulation sites when positioning patient.
Organize activities around medication regimen and vice versa.
Administer analgesia as ordered:
  Suggest continuous narcotic drip for patients with severe pain or those requiring pain medications every 1 to 2 hours.
  Suggest patient-controlled analgesia for patients able to regulate their own pain needs.
Evaluate effectiveness of alternative pain-relief measure, including relaxation, distraction, and guided imagery.
Consult with appropriate referrals as needed.

Patient and Family Teaching

Teach patient and family to describe presence of pain with analogue scale.
Instruct patient and family to request pain medication when pain first occurs and before it increases in intensity.
Teach and assist patient with splinting of incision with pillow when coughing, deep breathing, and moving.
Reassure patient that the incision is stable and that it is safe to move and cough.
Teach patient other pain-relief measures as appropriate.

studied sensations on chest tube removal and found that pain was the second most common sensation. Further study by Puntillo[64] showed that chest tube pain was significantly more intense than the pain associated with endotracheal suctioning or tonic pain. Patients received relatively little analgesia, but the amount of analgesia was the primary and significant indicator of pain. Katz[65] found that preemptive analgesia followed by an epidural saline bolus 15 minutes after incision prevented noxious neural impulses from entering the central nervous system from the incision.

Management and treatment

The goal of postoperative pain management is to provide adequate relief of pain via sedation and analgesia. Pain management after cardiac surgery can be effectively managed by opioid and nonopioid analgesic agents. The most common analgesic agent given after surgery is morphine sulfate and fentanyl in intravenous boluses. After extubation, nonopioid analgesic agents such as nonsteroidal antiinflammatory drugs arc used for mild pain. Severe to moderate pain is usually managed by patient-controlled analgesia or intermittent intramuscular injections of morphine sulfate. If sedation is required, a benzodiazepine such as midazolam is usually administered. Medication before painful procedures such as line removal should be considered a part of pain management.

With advances in technology, clinicians are increasingly exposed to acute hemodynamic instability in patients requiring complex technical interventions. Patients can be sustained in borderline hemodynamic states for prolonged periods. Consequently, pain management is dealt with as a lesser priority, and patients may be undermedicated and thus in pain.[66] Also, the clinician's experience, beliefs, and biases can affect pain management. Clinicians must recognize the physiologic and psychologic consequences of pain and address them with other physiologic issues. Therefore the emphasis on development of multidisciplinary assessment and intervention for pain, education for effective management, and use of a standardized pain assessment tool are of utmost importance. The box on p. 372 summarizes the standard of care for patients with alteration in comfort.

STANDARD FOR INFECTION

Infection related to
  Sternotomy incision
  Donor graft site incision
  Transthoracic line insertion site
  Intravenous line site (central or peripheral)
  Foley catheterization
  Retained pulmonary secretions

Outcomes

  Patient's incisions or wounds will be free of infection as evidenced by approximation of wound edges and a dry, nonreddened, nonecchymotic site.

  There will be an absence of infection as evidenced by an afebrile condition, a white blood cell count within normal limits, negative cultures, an absence of adventitious breath sounds, and an absence of purulent drainage and secretions.

Assessment

Assess for signs of infection:
  Increased white blood cell count
  Increased temperature
  Positive cultures
  Purulent drainage and secretion
  Yellow-green, foul-smelling secretions
Assess for risk factors and etiologies:
  Invasive procedures and interventions
  Antibiotic therapy
  Age
  Immobility
  Malnutrition
  Mechanical ventilation
  Liver and renal disease

Interventions

Use infection-prevention techniques:
  Use aseptic technique.
  Adhere to hospital standards for dressing and line changes.
  Ensure optimal nutrition.
Monitor vital signs and temperature:
  Initiate cooling measures for temperature above 38.5° C.
    Give a tepid sponge bath every 4 hours and as necessary.
    Administer antipyretics as ordered.
    Provide a cooling blanket for temperature above 39° C.
Monitor culture results and white blood cell count as ordered.
Monitor intravenous and wound sites for redness, warmth, swelling, and tenderness; amount, color, and odor of drainage; separating wound edges, and increased tenderness and a firm, ecchymotic area.
Monitor pulmonary system for amount, color, and consistency of secretions and adventitious breath sounds and findings on chest x-ray film.
Monitor for signs and symptoms of urinary tract infection.
Administer antibiotics per physician's order.
Change incision dressing per hospital policy.
Initiate infection-control measures as needed.
Consult nurse epidemiologist or infection-control nurse as needed.

Patient and Family Teaching

Teach patient and family about handwashing, precautions, infection process, and treatment plans.

OTHER CONSIDERATIONS
Infection

Infections after CABG can be systemic or operative or involve any body system. Meticulous attention must be paid to aseptic technique while all care routines, especially wound care, suctioning, and maintenance of the multiple invasive lines, are performed. Maintenance of an open sternotomy after a complicated cardiac surgery is an adjunct in the severely impaired heart. As described earlier, myocardial edema, hemodynamic instability, uncontrolled mediastinal bleeding, intractable dysrhythmia, and placement of a VAD can occur during surgery, which makes it surgically difficult to close the sternum. The reported incidence of mediastinal infection is low, ranging from 3%[67] to 5%,[68] with an increased incidence in patients in whom internal mammary grafts are used (11%).[69] Signs and symptoms of infection such as fever, leukocytosis, and an unstable sternum with purulent discharge are usually noted.

Mediastinal needle aspiration is usually performed to provide a definitive diagnosis for mediastinitis. Medical management of mediastinitis includes systemic antibiotics directed by drug-sensitivity studies. Sternal exploration for drainage and debridement in the advanced stage of sternal infection is usually performed. Povidone-iodine (Betadine) sternal irrigation administered through the mediastinal chest tube may also be indicated as a topical antiseptic. In extreme cases in which infection is extended to the manubrium, sternectomy with plastic surgery reconstruction may be performed. The box summarizes the standard of care for patients with potential for infection.

Nutrition

Although the incidence of gastrointestinal (GI) complications after cardiac surgery is low, there is a reported mortality rate of 14.8% associated with this complication alone.[70] Cardiac surgical patients are particularly susceptible to GI complications resulting from CPB. CPB causes gastric mucosal acidosis associated with splanchnic hypoperfusion during intraoperative nonpulsatile circulatory support.[70] GI hypoperfusion can lead to ileus, delayed initiation of postoperative nutrition, and sepsis. Advances in GI monitoring such as gastric pH monitoring using a tonometer is a useful adjunct in the management of this complication. If GI nutrition cannot be initiated, total parenteral nutrition should be considered to avoid postoperative nutritional deprivation.

REFERENCES

1. American Heart Association: *Heart and strokes facts*, Dallas, 1992, The Association.
2. Grover FL and others: Factors predictive of operative mortality among coronary artery bypass subsets, *Ann Thoracic Surg* 56:1296, 1993.
3. Clark RE: The Society of Thoracic Surgeons National Database Status Report, *Ann Thoracic Surg* 57:20, 1994.
4. Piffare R: Open heart operations in the elderly: changing risk parameters, *Ann Thoracic Surg* 56:S71, 1993.
5. Hollman JL: Myocardial revascularization, *Med Clin North Am* 76(5):1083, 1992.
6. Coleman B and others: *Patients undergoing cardiac surgery*. In Clochesy JM and others, editors *Critical care nursing*, Philadelphia, 1993, Saunders.
7. Weintraub WS and others: Changing clinical characteristics of coronary surgery patients: differences between men and women, *Circulation* 88:79, 1993.
8. Rahimtoola SH and others: Survival at 15 to 18 years after coronary bypass surgery for angina in women, *Circulation* 88:71, 1993.
9. Aranki SF and others: Aortic valve replacement in the elderly: effect of gender and coronary artery disease on operative mortality, *Circulation* 88:17, 1993.
10. Durand M and others: Pulmonary function tests predict outcome after cardiac surgery, *Acta Anesthes* 44(1):17, 1993.
11. Dillard DH, Miller DW: *Equipment used for extracorporeal circulation*. In Dillard DH, Miller DW, editors: *Atlas of cardiac surgery*, New York, 1983, Macmillan.
12. Edmunds LH and others: *Cannulation for cardiopulmonary bypass, cold cardioplegia, and air maneuvers*. In Edmunds LH and others, editors: *Atlas of cardiothoracic surgery*, Philadelphia, 1990, Lea & Febiger.
13. Ihnken K and others: The safety of simultaneous arterial and coronary sinus perfusion: experimental background and initial clinical results, *J Thoracic Cardiovasc Surg* 9:15, 1994.
14. Thelan L and others: *Critical care nursing: diagnosis and management,* ed 2, St Louis, 1994, Mosby.
15. Creswell LL and others: Hazards of postoperative atrial arrhythmias, *Ann Thoracic Surg* 56:539, 1993.
16. Cox JL: A perspective of postoperative atrial fibrillation in cardiac operations, *Ann Thoracic Surg* 56:405, 1993.
17. Michaelson EL and others: Postoperative arrhythmias after coronary artery and cardiac valvular surgery detected by long-term electrocardiographic monitoring, *Am Heart J* 97:442, 1989.
18. Caspi J and others: Frequency and significance of complete atrioventricular block after coronary artery bypass grafting, *Am J Cardiol* 63:526, 1989.
19. Otaki M: Permanent cardiac pacing after cardiac operations, *Artificial Organs* 17(95):346, 1993.
20. Strong A: Nursing management of postoperative dysrhythmia, *Crit Care Nurs Clin North Am* 3(4):709, 1991.
21. Dykner T: Relation of cardiovascular disease to potassium and magnesium deficiencies, *Am J Cardiol* 65:44K, 1990.
22. Lombness PM: Taking the mystery out of rhythm interpretation: atrial electrograms, *Heart Lung* 21(5):415, 1992.
23. Hilleman DE, Mohiuddin SM: Update on the use of new antiarrhythmic drugs, *J Pract Nurs* 9:39, 1991.
24. Laub GW and others: Prophylactic procainamide for prevention of atrial fibrillation after coronary artery bypass grafting: a prospective, double blind, randomized, placebo-controlled pilot study, *Crit Care Med* 21:1474, 1993.
25. Bigger TJ: Implications of the Cardiac Arrhythmia Suppression Trial for antiarrhythmic drug treatment, *Am J Cardiol* 65:3D, 1990.
26. Woods KL and others: Intravenous magnesium sulphate in suspected acute myocardial infarction: results of the Second Leicester Intravenous Magnesium Intervention Trial (LIMIT-2), *Lancet* 339:1553, 1992.
27. Iseri LT: Role of magnesium in cardiac tachyarrhythmias, *Am J Cardiol* 65:47K, 1990.
28. Khan RMA and others: Blood conservation and autotransfusion in cardiac surgery, *J Cardiovasc Surg* 8:25, 1993.
29. O'Brien M, Norris S: Managing low cardiac output states: maintaining volume after cardiac surgery, *AACN Clin Iss Crit Care Nurs* 4(2):309, 1993.
30. Makhoul RG and others: Vascular complications of the intra-aortic balloon pump, *Am Surg* 59:564, 1993.

31. Creswell J and others: Intra-aortic balloon counterpulsation: patterns of usage and outcome in cardiac surgery patients, *Ann Thoracic Surg* 54(1):11, 1992.

32. Horowitz MD and others: Intra-aortic balloon entrapment, *Am Thoracic Surg* 56:368, 1993.

33. Gardner TJ: Reversible postischemic ventricular dysfunction: biochemical insights, *J Cardiothoracic Surg* 8(suppl):271, 1993.

34. Leone BJ, Spahn DR: Is post cardiopulmonary bypass dysfunction a special form of stunning? *J Cardiothoracic Surg* 8(suppl):235, 1993.

35. Sponitz HM, Hsu DT: *Myocardial edema: importance in the study of left ventricular function*. In Karp RB, editor: *Advances in cardiac surgery*, St Louis, 1994, Mosby.

36. Golding LAR: Postcardiotomy mechanical support, *Semin Thoracic Cardiovasc Surg* 3:29, 1991.

37. Lee WA and others: Centrifugal assist device for support of the failing heart after cardiac surgery, *Crit Care Med* 21(8):1186, 1993.

38. Guyton RA and others: Postcardiotomy shock: clinical evaluation of the BVS 500 biventricular support systems, *Ann Thoracic Surg* 56:346, 1993.

39. Wahl GW and others: Effect of age and preoperative airway obstruction on lung function after coronary artery bypass grafting, *Ann Thoracic Surg* 56:104, 1993.

40. Shapira N and others: Determinants of pulmonary function in patients undergoing coronary bypass operation, *Ann Thoracic Surg* 50:268, 1990.

41. Kirklin JW, Barratt-Boyes BG: *Postoperative management*. In Kirklin JW, Barratt-Boyes BG, editors: *Cardiac surgery*, New York, 1993, Churchill Livingston.

42. Macnaughton PD and others: Changes in lung function and pulmonary capillary permeability after cardiopulmonary bypass, *Crit Care Med* 20(9):1289, 1992.

43. Anderson DR and others: *Management of complications of cardiopulmonary bypass: complications of organ system*. In Waldhausen J, Orringer MB, editors: *Complications of cardiothoracic surgery*, St Louis, 1991, Mosby.

44. Greenspon AJ and others: Amiodarone-related postoperative acute respiratory distress syndrome, *Circulation* 84(5 suppl):407, 1991.

45. Urschell JD and others: Pneumothorax complicating cardiac surgery, *J Cardiovasc Surg* 33(4):492, 1992.

46. Sakagoshi N and others: Phrenic nerve palsy after open heart surgery: problems in postoperative respiratory management, *J Jpn Assoc Thoracic Surg* 40(10):1859, 1992.

47. Hyers TM: Prediction of survival and mortality in patients with adult respiratory distress syndrome, *New Horizons* 1(4):466, 1993.

48. Schuster DP: The case for and against fluid restriction and occlusive pressure reduction in acute respiratory distress syndrome, *New Horizons* 1:478, 1993.

49. Gattioni L and others: Role of extracorporeal circulation in acute respiratory distress syndrome: syndrome management, *New Horizons* 1:603, 1992.

50. Vaca KJ and others: Nursing care of the patient with an intravascular oxygenator, *Am J Crit Care* 2:478, 1993.

51. Corwin HL and others: Acute renal failure associated with cardiac operations, *J Thoracic Cardiovasc Surg* 98:1107, 1989.

52. Salehmoghaddan S, Jacobson EJ: *Renal failure in the perioperative patient*. In Karp RB and others, editors: *Advances in cardiac surgery*, St Louis, 1993, Mosby.

53. Flanchbaum L and others: Quantitative effects of low dose dopamine on urine output in oliguric surgical intensive care patients, *Crit Care Med* 22:56, 1994.

54. Mills S: Cerebral injury and cardiac operations, *Ann Thoracic Surg* 56:86, 1993.

55. Hickey J: Cerebral circulation demystified, *AACN Clin Iss Crit Care Nurs* 2(4):657, 1991.

56. Kouchoukos NT: Adjuncts to reduce the incidence of embolic brain injury during operations on the aortic arch, *Ann Thoracic Surg* 57:243, 1994.

57. Leahy NM: Neurologic complications of open heart surgery, *J Cardiovasc Nurs* 7(2):41, 1993.

58. Crippen DW: Neurologic monitoring in the intensive care unit, *New Horizons* 2:107, 1994.

59. Bastos PG and others: Glasgow coma scale score in the evaluation and outcome in the intensive care unit: findings from the Acute Physiology and Chronic Health Evaluation III Study, *Crit Care Med* 21:1459, 1993.

60. Mravinac CM: Neurologic dysfunction following cardiac surgery, *Crit Care Nurs Clin North Am* 3(4):691, 1991.

61. Mersky H and others: Pain terms: a list with definitions and notes on usage, *Pain* 6(3):249, 1979.

62. Puntillo KA: The physiology of pain and its consequences in critically ill patients, In Puntillo KA, editor: *Pain in the critically ill: assessment and management*, Rockville, Md, 1991, Aspen.

63. Gift AG and others: Sensations during chest tube removal, *Heart Lung* 20:131, 1991.

64. Puntillo KA: Dimensions and predictors of pain in critically ill thoracoabdominal surgical patients, *Doctoral Dissertation* UCSF.

65. Katz J: Preemptive analgesia: clinical evidence of neuroplasticity contributing to postoperative pain, *Anesthesiol* 77:439, 1992.

66. Maxam-Moore VA and others: Analgesics for cardiac surgery patients in critical care: describing current practice, *Am J Crit Care* 3:31, 1994.

67. Ulciny KS and others: Sternotomy infection: poor prediction by acute phase response and delayed hypersensitivity, *Ann Thoracic Surg* 50(6):949, 1990.

68. Funary AP and others: Prolonged sternotomy and delayed sternal closure after cardiac operations, *Ann Thoracic Surg* 54(92):233, 1992.

69. Halzerig SR and others: Wound complications after median sternotomy, *J Thoracic Cardiovasc Surg* 98:1096, 1989.

70. Gaer JA and others: Effect of cardiopulmonary bypass on gastrointestinal perfusion and function, *Ann Thoracic Surg* 57:371, 1994.

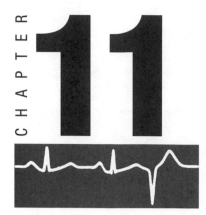

Connie White-Williams

Cardiomyopathy

The cardiomyopathies are a group of heart muscle diseases of unknown cause that affect primarily the structural and/or functional capacity of the myocardium.[1,2] The classification and the nomenclature of the cardiomyopathies continue to create controversy among experts in the field. According to the World Health Organization, the etiology of disease is unknown. Once a cause has been identified, the condition becomes a specific disease. The definition given here differentiates cardiomyopathy from specific heart muscle disease such as valvular heart disease or coronary heart disease in which the myocardial involvement is part of a systemic disease process.[1,2] Others believe that the disease etiologies leading to the cardiomyopathy present the same clinical and pathologic features; thus the cardiomyopathy can be classified according to the structural and/or functional abnormality of the disease. For example, ischemic heart disease resulting in ischemic cardiomyopathy would be considered a cardiomyopathy.[1,2]

CLASSIFICATION

Cardiomyopathies can be classified as primary or secondary.[3] Primary cardiomyopathies are conditions in which the etiology of the heart disease is unknown. In these instances, the myocardium is the only portion of the heart involved, and the valves and other cardiac structures are unaffected. In secondary cardiomyopathy the myocardial disease is known and is secondary to another disease process. Common causes of secondary cardiomyopathy are ischemia, viral infections, high alcohol intake, and pregnancy. See the box for a more comprehensive list of causes of secondary cardiomyopathy.

More commonly, cardiomyopathies are divided into three functional classifications: dilated, hypertrophic, and restrictive.[1,3] Dilated cardiomyopathy is characterized by ventricular dilatation. Hypertrophic cardiomyopathy is associated with an increase in myocardial mass without ventricular dilatation. Restrictive cardiomyopathy is recognized by an impairment of ventricular diastolic filling and

a decrease in cavity size. These three types are illustrated in Fig. 11-1.

Even though the three types of cardiomyopathies are pathophysiologically different, they have several similarities. Primary cardiomyopathies are heart muscle disorders of unknown cause. The disease process affects primarily the myocardium and can often be associated with endocardial or pericardial involvement. All three types of cardiomyopathy can lead to cardiomegaly and congestive heart failure. Similarities and differences among the three types of cardiomyopathy are presented in Table 11-1.

DILATED CARDIOMYOPATHY

Dilated cardiomyopathy is the most common form of cardiomyopathy. Although in many cases the etiology is not known, many factors appear to be associated with its etiology (for example, alcohol, inflammation, myocarditis, infiltrative disorders, metabolic disorders, and pregnancy). The course of dilated cardiomyopathy is one of progressive deterioration, with three fourths of patients dying within 5 years of diagnosis.[3,4] Dilated cardiomyopathy usually occurs between 30 and 40 years of age in the adult population.[4] In the 1993 International Heart and Lung Transplantation Registry, cardiomyopathy was the indication for cardiac transplantation in over 50% of the almost 25,000 cardiac transplants performed throughout the world.[5]

Pathophysiology

Dilated cardiomyopathy is characterized by four dominant features: cardiomegaly with ventricular dilatation, impairment of systolic function, atrial enlargement, and stasis of blood in the left ventricle.

Cardiomegaly is the result of dilatation of the heart chambers; greater dilatation occurs in the ventricles than in the atria. The comparison of the increased cavity size of dilated cardiomyopathy with a normal heart can be seen in Fig. 11-1. The second characteristic of dilated cardiomyopathy is decreased ventricular contraction, which leads to impaired systolic function. Poor contractility results in a decreased stroke volume and thus a reduced ejection fraction. In dilated cardiomyopathy a 15% to 20% decrease in the ejection fraction is common.[6] The inadequacy of the systolic function leads to an elevated end-diastolic volume (EDV), which may progress to pulmonary congestion. The elevation in EDV is a compensatory mechanism (Frank-Starling law) by the heart to maintain the stroke volume in the presence of the decreased ejection fraction.

The body continues to compensate by further increasing EDV and stroke volume and by increasing catecholamine circulation with augmentation of contractility and heart rate.[7] Also, the kidneys begin to retain sodium and water in an effort to maintain cardiac output. Sodium and water retention may be one of the first signs of cardiac impairment.[6] Activation of the renin-angiotensin mechanism further increases ventricular filling through its vasoconstrictive properties. When these compensatory mechanisms fail, congestive heart failure (CHF) progresses. In the decompensated heart, increasing the venous return and systemic vascular resistance increases left ventricular stroke work, leading to left ventricular and left atrial dilatation. Left heart failure (pulmonary venous hypertension) is a common occurrence; however, biventricular failure (pulmonary and systemic venous hypertension) occurs in many patients.

Atrial enlargement also occurs in dilated cardiomyopathy. With the ventricles holding more blood (increased EDV) and the poor ventricular contractility, increased work is required of the atria to eject blood into the ventricles. This increased work results in atrial stretch and di-

---

CAUSES OF SECONDARY CARDIOMYOPATHY

Dilated

Ischemia
Valvular diseases
Infectious diseases
Pregnancy
Metabolic conditions
Hypertension
Cardiotoxic diseases
   Alcohol
   Adriamycin
   Cobalt

Hypertrophic

Genetic factors
Hypertension
Obstructive valvular disease
Thyroid disease
Glycogen storage disease
Friedreich ataxia
Infants of parents with diabetes

Restrictive

Amyloidosis
Endomyocardial fibrosis
Löffler disease
Sarcoidosis
Neoplastic tumor
Ventricular thrombus

Modified from Wynne J, Braunwald E: *The cardiomyopathies and myocarditides.* In Braunwald E, editor: *Heart disease: a textbook of cardiovascular medicine,* Philadelphia, 1988, Saunders; personal notes of Robert C. Bourge.

TABLE 11-1   Characteristics of the Three Cardiomyopathies

Characteristics	Dilated	Hypertrophic	Restrictive
Myocardial mass	↑ > ↑↑	↑↑↑	nl > ↑
Ventricular cavity size	↑↑ > ↑↑↑↑	↓↓ > nl	↓
Dilated atrial cavities	+	+	+
Asymmetric septal hypertrophy	0	+	0
Myocardial fiber disorientation	0	+	0
Contractile function	↓↓↓	↑↑ > ↓	nl > ↓
Ventricular inflow resistance	0	+ +	+
Ventricular outflow obstruction	0	0 ⇌ +	0
Left ventricular filling pressure	↑↑	nl	↑
Intracardiac thrombi	+	0	+

From Wenger NK and others: *Cardiomyopathies and myocardial involvement in systemic disease.* In Hurst JW and others: *The heart,* New York, 1986, McGraw-Hill.
nl, Normal.

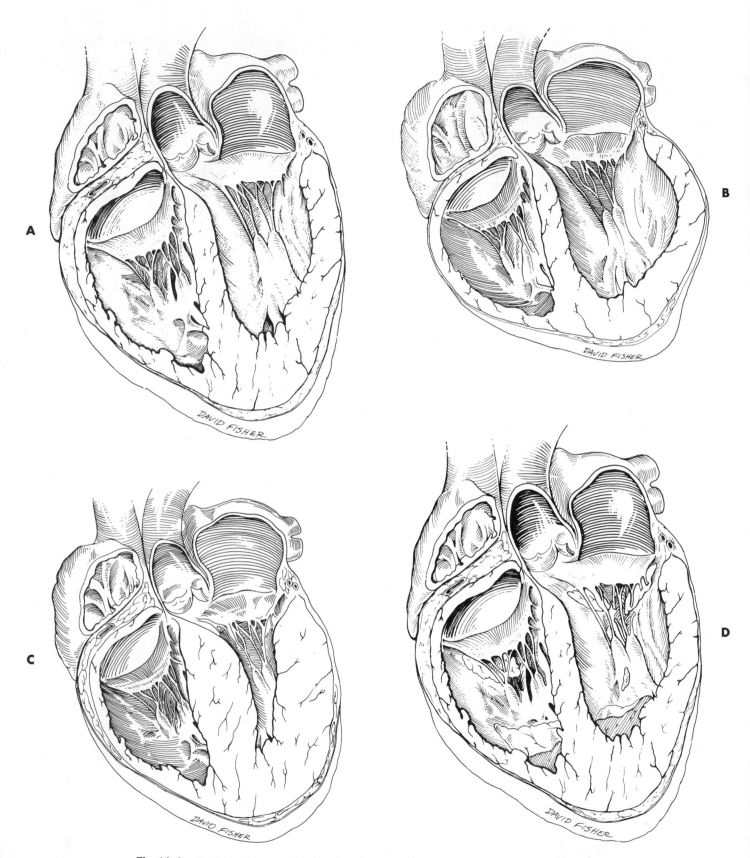

Fig. 11-1   **A,** Normal heart. **B,** Dilated cardiomyopathy. **C,** Hypertrophic cardiomyopathy. **D,** Restrictive cardiomyopathy.   (By David Fisher, Photography and Graphics, University of Alabama at Birmingham.)

latation and ultimately a decrease in the rate of myofibril shortening. According to the Laplace law, dilatation coincides with greater wall tension, which in turn results in a greater metabolic demand and increased myocardial oxygen consumption.

Finally, because of the reduced ejection fraction, stasis of blood in the ventricle occurs, leading to an increased incidence of thrombus formation. The most frequent sites of thrombus formation are the left ventricle, right ventricle, right atrial appendage, and left atrial appendage.[1,2]

Pathology

On postmortem examination, both ventricles are dilated, with one more dilated than the other. The atria are also dilated. The cardiac valves and coronary arteries are usually normal. Minimal left ventricular hypertrophy is present and appears to have a protective role in dilated cardiomyopathy, since it may reduce wall stress and further dilatation. Intracavity thrombi are commonly seen as previously described. Histologic findings reveal interstitial and perivascular fibrosis, especially in the left ventricular subendocardium.[2] Dilated cardiomyopathy may be associated with loss of functioning myofibrils and contractile elements. Unfortunately, histologic findings of dilated cardiomyopathy are relatively nonspecific.[1] See Fig. 11-2 for a cross-sectional view of dilated cardiomyopathy.

Clinical Presentation

The signs and symptoms of dilated cardiomyopathy develop insidiously. Some patients may have asymptomatic left ventricular dilatation for years. Patients with symptoms have fatigue, weakness, and/or dyspnea because of low cardiac output. Over time the body has compensated for the decreased ventricular contractility and decreased stroke volume by increasing EDV and circulating catecholamines. However, as the cardiomyopathy progresses, the body may no longer be able to compensate, particularly with exertion. Consequently, early symptoms include dyspnea on exertion, changes in exercise tolerance, and palpitation. These symptoms progress to orthopnea, paroxysmal nocturnal dyspnea, and dyspnea at rest. With continued deterioration, the body begins to decompensate and CHF ensues.

The precordial examination reveals a laterally displaced apical impulse caused by the ventricular dilatation. A fourth heart sound may precede the development of CHF, whereas a third heart sound is auscultated after decompensation occurs. A summation gallop is often appreciated with tachycardia.

The systolic blood pressure is normal or low with a narrow pulse pressure. Pulsus alternans is common with severe failure. Also, distended jugular neck veins, peripheral edema, and ascites with liver enlargement are present with severe failure.

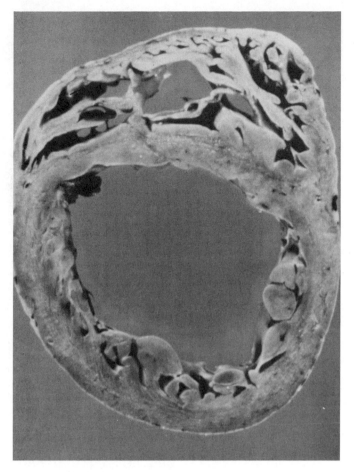

Fig. 11-2 Cross-sectional view of dilated cardiomyopathy. (Courtesy Shirley Smith, Department of Pathology, University of Alabama at Birmingham.)

Diagnostic Tests

The chest roentgenogram shows cardiomegaly caused by left ventricular enlargement. Signs of pulmonary venous hypertension may be present. Finally, pleural effusions may be evident because of the progressive left ventricular dysfunction. See Fig. 11-3 for an example of a chest x-ray film of a patient with dilated cardiomyopathy.

The electrocardiogram (ECG) usually reveals sinus tachycardia. Tachycardia manifests as a compensatory mechanism to compensate for the reduced cardiac output. Dysrhythmias are common manifestations of dilated cardiomyopathy.[3]

Atrial and ventricular tachydysrhythmias, conduction disturbances, and left bundle branch block may be seen in dilated cardiomyopathy. When left ventricular fibrosis is present, Q waves may appear. It is important, however, to rule out myocardial infarction in these cases. ST-segment and T-wave abnormalities are common in patients with dilated cardiomyopathy.[3,8]

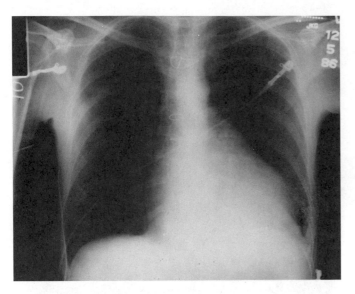

Fig. 11-3 Chest x-ray film of dilated cardiomyopathy.

Echocardiography is a useful diagnostic test in distinguishing dilated cardiomyopathy from other abnormalities. With M-mode, two-dimensional or Doppler echocardiography, the size of the ventricular cavity can be assessed, the thickness of the heart muscle walls can be measured, and the cardiac valves can be evaluated.[9] In addition, the ventricular ejection fraction can be estimated to assess left ventricular impairment. See Fig. 11-4 for a comparison of dilated and hypertrophic cardiomyopathy on echocardiogram.

Invasive cardiac catheterization and coronary angiography is limited in differentiating the manifestations of dilated cardiomyopathy. The coronary arteries are usually normal. Pulmonary artery wedge, left atrial, and left ventricular end-diastolic pressures are elevated, manifesting poor contractility and diminished cardiac output.[8]

If the risk of the dye load is not present, left ventriculography can reveal abnormal wall motion, cavity size, and the presence and degree of mitral regurgitation. Endomyocardial biopsy may be performed but rarely provides information that is significant for the treatment of dilated cardiomyopathy.

Holter monitoring for ventricular ectopy may be important in the prognosis of the patient. Some studies report that high-grade ectopy portends a grave prognosis or higher incidence of sudden cardiac death.[10]

Medical and Surgical Interventions

The goal of medical intervention in dilated cardiomyopathy is to reduce the workload of the heart and improve symptoms of CHF. Thus the treatment is more palliative than curative. In patients in whom a cause has been identified, the treatment is directed toward that cause. For example, in alcoholic cardiomyopathy, abstinence from alcohol is an absolute requirement. Ceasing alcohol consumption may limit or reverse the progressive course of cardiomyopathy.[3,11] Demakis and others[12] studied 57 patients with cardiomyopathy associated with alcohol. Patients who abstained from alcohol and had a short duration of symptoms before the initiation of therapy experienced a more favorable course; 30 of the 57 patients experienced deterioration of their disease, and 26 of the 30 patients continued to drink heavily.[12] Of the 30 patients, 24 had a mean survival time of 36 months.[12]

Corticosteroids may be used in the treatment of cardiomyopathy occurring secondary to sarcoidosis and in postviral cardiomyopathy. However, these therapies remain controversial.

In idiopathic dilated cardiomyopathy the treatment is nonspecific. Moreover, a cluster of medical interventions is directed toward the pathophysiologic manifestations. Pharmacologic treatment, nutritional instruction, and cardiac rehabilitation may help alleviate the symptoms of CHF and improve cardiac output.

The initial therapy for treatment of CHF secondary to dilated cardiomyopathy includes agents such as digitalis and diuretics.[8,13,14] Digitalis is a positive inotropic agent that increases myocardial contractility and slows the renin-angiotensin response in CHF.[13] Since digitalis has a relatively narrow therapeutic range, caution should be taken to avoid life-threatening dysrhythmias.[7] Diuresis can exacerbate problems of hypokalemia and hypomagnesemia; therefore potassium or magnesium should be supplemented if indicated. A new positive inotropic agent, Vesnarinone, is under clinical trials. Vesnarinone is a quinolinone derivative that decreases the outward and inward flow of potassium channels and increases intracellular sodium. It is proposed that Vesnarinone will have a significant impact on the morbidity and mortality rates and quality of life of patients with heart failure.[15]

Specific vasodilator therapy consisting of nitrates, hydralazine, nitrate-hydralazine combinations, or prazosin may improve ventricular performance. Nitrates act by producing venous dilatation and arteriolar relaxation, with a subsequent decrease in preload and afterload. Hydralazine works effectively to decrease afterload by producing arterial dilatation. The nitrate-hydralazine combination therapy provides a more balanced preload and afterload reduction.[13] A Veterans Administration study of over 600 patients with congestive heart failure indicated that the nitrate-hydralazine combination improved survival by increasing the ejection fraction.

Inactivation of the renin-angiotensin system by angiotensin-converting enzyme (ACE) inhibitors such as captopril or enalapril is useful in patients with dilated cardiomyopathy and CHF. ACE inhibitors decrease vascular resistance and ventricular afterload, thus increasing cardiac output. Also, ACE inhibitors increase sodium and water excretion, which decreases venous return to the heart.

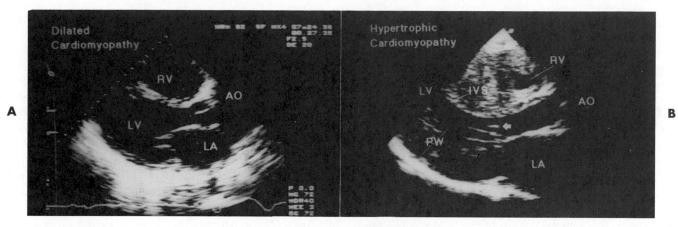

Fig. 11-4   Echocardiograms. **A,** Dilated cardiomyopathy. **B,** Hypertrophic cardiomyopathy. (Courtesy Po Fang, Department of Medicine, University of Alabama at Birmingham.)

The use of β-adrenergic antagonists has been reported as helpful in the treatment of dilated cardiomyopathy. These agents reduce myocardial oxygen demand, improve ventricular filling, and inhibit sympathetic vasoconstriction.

Antidysrhythmic agents may be used in the treatment of symptomatic dysrhythmias associated with dilated cardiomyopathy. However, caution is required, since some of these drugs decrease myocardial contractility. Rhythm control may be accomplished by inserting an automatic implantable pacemaker for the appropriate candidate. Because of the high incidence of thromboemboli in patients with dilated cardiomyopathy and CHF, anticoagulation is desirable.

As a last resort, after medical therapy has failed, the patient may be considered for cardiac transplantation. The candidate for transplantation is generally younger than 60 years of age, is in a New York Heart Association class III or IV, and has a life expectancy from 6 months to 1 year (see Chapter 12).

HYPERTROPHIC CARDIOMYOPATHY

Over the years, hypertrophic cardiomyopathy has also been known as *idiopathic hypertrophic subaortic stenosis* and *hypertrophic obstructive cardiomyopathy.* Although the etiology of hypertrophic cardiomyopathy is unknown, it is speculated that it is genetically transmitted as an autosomal dominant trait. Hypertrophic cardiomyopathy occurs less commonly than dilated cardiomyopathy and is more often seen in men than in women.[7,8] Hypertrophic cardiomyopathy is usually diagnosed in young adulthood and is often seen in active, athletic individuals; it is classically defined as a disease of unknown origin with a greatly hypertrophied, nondilated ventricle, which is manifested in the absence of other cardiac or systemic disease.

Pathophysiology

Four main abnormalities are found in hypertrophic cardiomyopathy: ventricular hypertrophy, rapid contraction of the left ventricle, impaired relaxation, and intracavity systolic pressure gradients. These characteristics determine the signs, symptoms, and prognosis of the patient with this cardiomyopathy. Unlike dilated cardiomyopathy in which systolic function is impaired, the most characteristic abnormality in hypertrophic cardiomyopathy is diastolic dysfunction.[3] Ventricular hypertrophy is associated with a thickened intraventricular septum and ventricular free wall. The hypertrophy is commonly symmetrical but can have varying patterns. The hypertrophy can occur only in the anterior portion of the septum, or it can affect all of the regions in the left ventricle except the basal anterior septum. The ratio of the thickness of the septum to the free wall is usually greater than 1:3 to 1:5. This ratio contrasts with that in the normal heart, which is usually 1:0 and always less than 1:3.[3] With the increased thickness of the free wall and septum, the ventricular cavity is decreased, leading to abnormal left ventricular stiffness during diastole. The result is impaired ventricular filling as the ventricle becomes noncompliant and unable to relax and receive blood from the atrium. This abnormality in relaxation manifests in an elevation of the left ventricular end-diastolic pressure. This elevated pressure contributes to high atrial, pulmonary venous, and pulmonary capillary wedge pressures, all of which lead to dyspnea. Tachycardia, a compensatory mechanism, further impedes ventricular filling time, thus reducing ventricular volume. The most controversial characteristic is the dynamic systolic pressure gradient and the etiology of this gradient. The pressure gradient is found in approximately 40% of patients with hypertrophic cardiomyopathy.[1] Initially, the pressure gradient was thought to be caused by the hypertrophy and the powerful muscle action during ejection. In contrast, many propose that the pressure gradient is the result of the further narrowing of an already small outflow tract produced by the systolic anterior motion of the mitral valve on the septum.[2,3] As a result of the abnormal motion, the mitral valve becomes thickened and develops plaque and may become incompetent. However, the question remains whether the pressure gradient is related to the displacement of the mitral valve or to the powerful contraction of the hypertrophied heart.

The hypertrophic cardiomyopathic heart at necropsy (Fig. 11-5) shows a normal or small left and right ventricular cavity, dilated atrial cavities, abnormal intramural coronary arteries, greater thickening of the ventricular septum than of the ventricular free wall, mural fibrous plaque, a thickened mitral valve, and myocardial fiber disarray.[1]

On histologic examination, disorganization of myocardial fibers and the cell-to-cell arrangement (disarray) are distinctive characteristics of hypertrophic cardiomyopathy. This disorganization and disarray have been found in other diseases; however, in hypertrophic cardiomyopathy, the abnormality is more extensive. In fact, patients with hypertrophic cardiomyopathy with large pressure gradients tend

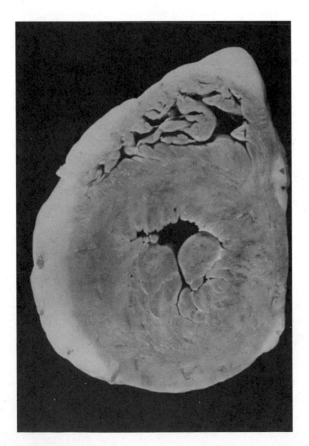

Fig. 11-5   Hypertrophied heart.   (Courtesy Shirley Smith, Department of Pathology, University of Alabama at Birmingham.)

to have more myofibril disarray than those without systolic pressure gradients.

Clinical Presentation

The most common symptom of hypertrophic cardiomyopathy is dyspnea, which is largely a result of elevated left ventricular diastolic pressure. Angina pectoris, fatigue, and syncope also are reported. Angina pectoris is caused by decreased oxygen availability for the increased demand of the hypertrophied heart, narrowing of the transmural coronary arteries, and impaired diastolic relaxation with subendocardial ischemia. Syncope is caused by decreased ventricular filling and thus a decrease in cardiac output. Some patients may have an asymptomatic condition, whereas in others the first manifestation may be sudden cardiac death. Physical exertion exacerbates the symptoms. In addition, the physical signs and symptoms depend on the magnitude of the pressure gradient in the left ventricle. With a pressure gradient, three predominant physical findings emerge. First, a typically harsh, crescendo-decrescendo systolic murmur is heard best between the apex and the left sternal border. This murmur may radiate to the axilla or base of the heart, but it rarely radiates to the neck. Also, the murmur is increased by standing and by performing the Valsalva maneuver, and it is decreased by squatting. This systolic murmur reflects mitral regurgitation and the late onset of the ventricular outflow gradient. Thus this murmur is more holosystolic and blowing at the apex and midsystolic and harsher at the lower sternal border.[3] Second, the arterial pulse is abrupt and ill-sustained. The jerky quality results from the powerful contraction of the left ventricle. Finally, a prominent cardiac apical impulse is formed by the interruption of ejection by the outflow gradient in the left ventricle. A presystolic apical impulse is formed by the forceful atrial contraction in an effort to eject blood into a poorly compliant ventricle.

The first heart sound is usually normal and the second heart sound is often split. The third and the fourth heart sounds can commonly be auscultated.

Diagnostic Tests

The chest roentgenogram is usually normal in hypertrophic cardiomyopathy except in patients with severe disease in which the cardiac silhouette is enlarged.

The most common abnormalities on the ECG are an increased voltage and duration of the QRS complex and T-wave inversion, which reflect hypertrophy. Other features are a short PR interval, Q waves in the inferior and precordial leads, and a P-wave abnormality that is usually caused by left atrial enlargement.[1,3] Ventricular dysrhythmias are common in patients with hypertrophic cardiomyopathy: One fourth of patients experience ventricular tachycardia, and one fourth to one half experience supraventricular tachycardia.[16] It has been reported that patients with asymptomatic ventricular tachycardia recorded on Holter monitors have a higher incidence of sudden death than patients who do not have ventricular tachycardia[17]; 5% to 10% of the patients experience atrial fibrillation.[16,18]

The echocardiogram is the primary diagnostic tool revealing the classic feature of hypertrophic cardiomyopathy, which is left ventricular hypertrophy (see Fig. 11-4). Two-dimensional echocardiography can measure septal and free wall orientation and thickness. The echocardiogram can also detect the narrowing of the left ventricular outflow tract. Color Doppler nicely reveals mitral regurgitation.

Radionuclide image techniques are also used in the diagnosis of hypertrophic cardiomyopathy. Gated radionuclide ventriculography with labeling of the blood depicts the size and motion of the septum and left ventricle. Abnormal diastolic function can be observed by analysis of the blood pool scan. Thallium-201 imaging confirms the thickness of the septum and the free wall.

Cardiac catheterization can also help in diagnosing hypertrophic cardiomyopathy, revealing decreased diastolic left ventricular compliance and abnormal pressure gradients, if present.

Medical and Surgical Interventions

Interventions for hypertrophic cardiomyopathy are directed toward decreasing the force of ventricular contraction (increasing ventricular volume) and decreasing the outflow obstruction.

Of the β-adrenergic blockers, propranolol is the most commonly used in hypertrophic cardiomyopathy. β-adrenergic agents have negative inotropic and chronotropic effects, which reduce myocardial oxygen demand. Furthermore, β-blocking agents decrease the force of contraction and increase diastolic filling time by slowing the heart rate. By decreasing contractility and increasing filling time, the outflow obstruction is reduced.[1,3]

Calcium antagonists (verapamil, diltiazem, nifedipine) are alternatives to β-blocking agents in the treatment of hypertrophic cardiomyopathy. Verapamil, the most common agent used in hypertrophic cardiomyopathy, improves diastolic filling time by promoting relaxation, resulting in an increased exercise tolerance. Also, by decreasing myocardial contractility, verapamil can diminish the left ventricular outflow gradient. Adverse effects of verapamil include suppression of the sinus node, atrioventricular (AV) conduction inhibition, negative inotropic effects, and vasodilatation.[3,19] These side effects may manifest as hypotension, pulmonary edema, and death.[19] Nifedipine is a more potent vasodilator than verapamil but has fewer AV conduction inhibition effects.[20] A combination of nifedipine and propranolol is beneficial in the treatment of hypertrophic cardiomyopathy.[21] Diltiazem improves diastolic function by increasing relaxation and prolonging filling time.[22]

For patients who experience ventricular tachycardia, amiodarone has been used effectively to treat supraventric-

ular and ventricular tachycardias.[23] Atrial fibrillation should be treated as an emergency and should be electrically converted before hemodynamic compromise develops. Anticoagulants are recommended in patients with chronic atrial fibrillation.

Strenuous exercise should be avoided because of the risk of sudden cardiac death. Competitive sports are contraindicated if left ventricular hypertrophy, evidence of outflow gradient, significant ventricular dysrhythmias, or a history of sudden death are present.[24]

A variety of surgical treatments may be used for hypertrophic cardiomyopathy. The most common surgical operation is excision of a part of the hypertrophied septum (septal myotomy-myectomy). This procedure reduces the outflow tract obstruction and mitral regurgitation.

Antibiotic prophylaxis is indicated before invasive procedures to protect against infective endocarditis. The infection usually develops on the mitral or aortic valve.

RESTRICTIVE CARDIOMYOPATHY

Restrictive cardiomyopathy is a heart muscle disease in which the diastolic ventricular volume and stretch are impaired by fibrotic lesions. Systolic function remains relatively unimpaired. Of the three cardiomyopathies, restrictive cardiomyopathy is the least common.

Pathophysiology

Although the specific etiology of restrictive cardiomyopathy is unknown, a number of pathologic processes may result in restrictive cardiomyopathy. Myocardial fibrosis, hypertrophy, and infiltration produce stiffness of the ventricular wall and decreased ventricular filling with subsequent diastolic dysfunction. Secondary causes of restrictive cardiomyopathy include amyloidosis, endocardial fibrosis, glycogen deposition, hemachromatosis, sarcoidosis, and myocardial fibrosis of diverse etiologies.[25]

The principal characteristic of restrictive cardiomyopathy is cardiac muscle stiffness, which is caused by the fibrotic or infiltrative changes in the heart muscle. These changes restrict ventricular filling and lead to reduced cardiac output.

Clinical Presentation

The patient with restrictive cardiomyopathy has symptoms similar to those of dilated cardiomyopathy. Angina pectoris, syncope, fatigue, and dyspnea on exertion are commonly reported. Exercise intolerance is the most frequent symptom, since the heart cannot increase cardiac output by tachycardia without compromising ventricular filling.[3]

In advanced disease, peripheral edema, elevated central venous pressure, and ascites may be present.[25] On physical examination, a third heart sound, a fourth heart sound, or both may be auscultated. Also, jugular vein distention and a palpable apical impulse may be evident.

TABLE 11-2   Functional Classification of the Cardiomyopathies

Dilated	Restrictive	Hypertrophic
SYMPTOMS		
CHF, particularly left-sided	Dyspnea, fatigue	Dyspnea, angina pectoris
Fatigue and weakness	Right-sided CHF	Fatigue, syncope, palpitations
Systemic or pulmonary emboli	Signs and symptoms of systemic disease (for example, amyloidosis, iron storage disease)	
PHYSICAL EXAMINATION		
Moderate to severe cardiomegaly; third and fourth heart sounds	Mild to moderate cardiomegaly; third and fourth heart sounds	Mild cardiomegaly
AV valve regurgitation, especially mitral	AV valve regurgitation; inspiratory increase in venous pressure (Kussmaul sign)	Apical systolic thrill and heave, brisk carotid upstroke
		Common fourth heart sound
		Systolic murmur that increases with Valsalva maneuver
CHEST ROENTGENOGRAM		
Moderate to marked cardiac enlargement, especially left ventricular	Mild cardiac enlargement	Mild to moderate cardiac enlargement
Pulmonary venous hypertension	Pulmonary venous hypertension	Left atrial enlargement
ECG		
Sinus tachycardia	Low voltage	Left ventricular hypertrophy
Atrial and ventricular dysrhythmias	Intraventricular conduction defects	ST-segment and T-wave abnormalities
ST-segment and T-wave abnormalities	AV conduction defects	Abnormal Q waves
Intraventricular conduction defects		Atrial and ventricular dysrhythmias
ECHOCARDIOGRAM		
Left ventricular dilatation and dysfunction	Increased left ventricular wall thickness and mass	Asymmetrical septal hypertrophy
Abnormal diastolic mitral valve motion secondary to abnormal compliance and filling pressures	Small or normal-sized left ventricular cavity	Narrow left ventricular outflow tract
	Normal systolic function	Systolic anterior motion of the mitral valve
	Pericardial effusion	Small or normal-sized left ventricle
RADIONUCLIDE STUDIES		
Left ventricular dilatation and dysfunction	Infiltration of myocardium	Small or normal-sized left ventricle
	Small or normal-sized left ventricle	Vigorous systolic function
	Normal systolic function	Asymmetrical septal hypertrophy
CARDIAC CATHETERIZATION		
Left ventricular enlargement and dysfunction	Diminished left ventricular compliance	Diminished left ventricular compliance
Mitral and/or tricuspid regurgitation	Square root sign in ventricular pressure recordings	Mitral regurgitation
Elevated left- and often right-sided filling pressures	Preserved systolic function	Vigorous systolic function
Diminished cardiac output	Elevated left- and right-sided filling pressures	Dynamic left ventricular outflow gradient

From Wynne J, Braunwald E: *The cardiomyopathies and myocarditides.* In Braunwald E, editor: *Heart disease: a textbook of cardiovascular medicine,* Philadelphia, 1988, Saunders Co.

Diagnostic Tests

The chest roentgenogram may be normal or show cardiomegaly. Pleural effusions and pulmonary congestion may be evident in conditions that have progressed to CHF.

The ECG shows sinus tachycardia. The most characteristic feature is the diffusely decreased voltage seen in amyloidosis. AV conduction abnormalities are also seen frequently in amyloidosis. Atrial fibrillation and complex ventricular dysrhythmias are common features of restrictive cardiomyopathy.

The clinical features of restrictive cardiomyopathy and constrictive pericarditis are similar but not the same. The echocardiogram is helpful in distinguishing between them. The echocardiogram reveals thickened ventricular walls, small ventricular cavities, and dilated atria in restrictive cardiomyopathy; however, these findings are not evident in constrictive pericarditis. In addition, endomyocardial biopsy, computerized tomography, and nuclear imaging are useful in differentiating between constrictive pericarditis and restrictive cardiomyopathy. A characteristic hemodynamic feature in both conditions is a deep and early decline of ventricular pressure at the onset of diastole with a rise to a plateau.[26] This dip and plateau is called the *square root sign* (Fig. 11-6). Right and left filling pressures may display the dip and plateau. However, the left ventricular end-diastolic pressure is usually greater than the right in restrictive cardiomyopathy, whereas the pressures are equal in constrictive pericarditis. Also an M or W waveform may be apparent on the pulmonary capillary wedge tracing.

Medical and Surgical Intervention

The treatment of restrictive cardiomyopathy is palliative and is similar to that of dilated cardiomyopathy and CHF. Medical intervention focuses on diuretic therapy, sodium and water restriction, anticoagulation, and treatment of dysrhythmias. A pacemaker is inserted to treat AV conduc-

tion blocks. Surgical intervention includes excision of the thickened endomyocardial plaque or mitral or tricuspid valve replacement, if needed.

CONCLUSION

The cardiovascular nurse will encounter the patient with cardiomyopathy often during the course of the disease. Frequent hospitalizations and clinic visits will be required for treatment of CHF and monitoring of the disease process. Some nurses may care for patients awaiting cardiac transplantation.

In this chapter, the pathophysiology and clinical presentation of dilated, hypertrophic, and restrictive cardiomyopathy have been presented. A comprehensive functional classification of the cardiomyopathies is presented in Table 11-2. It is important for cardiovascular nurses to understand the pathology and manifestations of this group of cardiac diseases. This understanding will enable the nurse to direct care toward minimizing the complications and discomforts of the cardiomyopathy. Education of the patient and family is imperative during the disease process. The goal of nursing care for patients with cardiomyopathy is an improvement in their quality of life while they live with the disease.

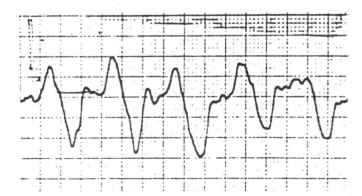

Fig. 11-6 Square root sign of a patient with restrictive cardiomyopathy. (Courtesy Robert Bourge, Department of Medicine, University of Alabama at Birmingham.)

REFERENCES

1. Wenger NK and others: *Cardiomyopathies and myocardial involvement in systemic disease.* In Hurst JW and others, editors: *The heart,* New York, 1986, McGraw-Hill.
2. Goodwin JK: *Overview and classification of the cardiomyopathies.* In Shaver JA, editor: *Cardiovascular clinics,* Philadelphia, 1988, Davis.
3. Wynne J, Braunwald E: *The cardiomyopathies and myocarditides.* In Braunwald E, editor: *Heart disease: a textbook of cardiovascular medicine,* Philadelphia, 1988, Saunders.
4. O'Connell JB, Gunnar RM: Dilated-congestive cardiomyopathy: prognostic features and therapy, *Heart Transplant* 2:7, 1982.
5. The registry of the International Society for Heart and Lung Transplantation: *Tenth official report—1993, Heart Lung Transplant* 12:241, 1993.
6. Gravanis MB, Ansari AA: Idiopathic cardiomyopathies, *Arch Pathol Lab Med* 3:915, 1987.
7. Francis GS, Pierpont GL: *Pathophysiology of congestive heart failure secondary to congestive and ischemic cardiomyopathy.* In Shaver JA, editor: *Cardiovascular clinics,* Philadelphia, 1988, Davis.
8. Miller DH, Borer JS: The cardiomyopathies: a pathophysiologic approach to therapeutic management, *Arch Intern Med* 143:2157, 1983.
9. Uretsky BF: *Diagnostic considerations in the adult patient with cardiomyopathy or congestive heart failure.* In Shaver JA, editor: *Cardiovascular clinics,* Philadelphia, 1988, Davis.
10. Meinertz T and others: Significance of ventricular arrhythmias in idiopathic dilated cardiomyopathy, *Am J Cardiol* 53:902, 1984.
11. McHugh MJ: The patient with alcoholic cardiomyopathy, *J Cardiovasc Nurs* 2:13, 1987.
12. Demakis JG and others: The natural course of alcoholic cardiomyopathy. *Ann Intern Med* 80:293, 1974.
13. Leier CV, Unverferth DV: *Medical therapy of end-stage congestive and ischemic cardiomyopathy.* In Shaver JA, editor: *Cardiovascular clinics,* Philadelphia, 1988, Davis.

14. Johnson RA, Palacios I: Dilated cardiomyopathies of the adult, *N Engl J Med* 307:105, 1982.

15. Feldman AM and others: Effects of Vesnarinone on morbidity and mortality in patients with heart failure, *N Engl J Med* 329:149, 1993.

16. Maron BJ and others: Prognostic significance of 24-hour ambulatory electrocardiographic monitoring in patients with hypertrophic cardiomyopathy: a prospective study, *Am J Cardiol* 48:252, 1981.

17. McKenna WJ: Arrhythmia and prognosis of hypertrophic cardiomyopathy. *Eur Heart J* 4(suppl F):225, 1983.

18. McKenna W and others: Syncope in hypertrophic cardiomyopathy, *Br Heart J* 47:177, 1982.

19. Epstein SE, Rosing DR: Verapamil: its potential for causing serious complications in patients with hypertrophic cardiomyopathy, *Circulation* 64:437, 1981.

20. Lorell BH and others: Modification of abnormal left ventricular diastolic properties by nifedipine in patients with hypertrophic cardiomyopathy, *Circulation* 65:499, 1982.

21. Landmark K and others: Hemodynamic effects of nifedipine and propranolol in patients with hypertrophic cardiomyopathy, *Br Heart J* 48:19, 1982.

22. Suwa M, Hirota Y, Kawamura K: Improvement in left ventricular diastolic function during intravenous and oral diltiazem treatment in patients with hypertrophic cardiomyopathy: an echocardiographic study, *Am J Cardiol* 54:1047, 1984.

23. McKenna WJ and others: Amiodarone for long-term management of patients with hypertrophic cardiomyopathy, *Am J Cardiol* 54:802, 1984.

24. Maron BJ and others: Task Force III: hypertrophic cardiomyopathy, other myopericardial diseases and mitral valve prolapse, *J Am Coll Cardiol* 6:1215, 1985.

25. Siegel RJ and others: Idiopathic restrictive cardiomyopathy, *Circulation* 70:165, 1984.

26. Benotti JR, Grossman W, Cohn PF: The clinical profile of restrictive cardiomyopathy, *Circulation* 61:1206, 1980.

Cardiac Transplantation

Connie White-Williams

Cardiac transplantation, once a mere dream to a few, is now a widely accepted treatment for patients with end-stage heart disease. Although there was a 60-year history of experimentation in the field (Table 12-1), it was not until 1967, when the first successful human orthotopic transplant was performed by Christian Barnard, that the era of cardiac transplantation began. During the next decade, many became discouraged by poor results. However, by the 1980s, with the availability of new immunosuppressive therapies, advances in organ preservation and operative technique, development of endomyocardial biopsy sampling, and the recognition of risk factors affecting survival of the transplanted heart, cardiac transplantation emerged from an experimental procedure to a treatment option to improve survival and quality of life.

Over 25,600 cardiac transplants have been performed worldwide since 1981. The Registry of the International Society for Heart and Lung Transplantation reports 2709 transplants in 1992 with a 1-year survival rate of 79.1%. The number of cardiac transplants have increased annually from 700 in 1984 to 2709 in 1992 (Fig. 12-1).[1]

Cardiac transplantation is not an absolute cure for end-stage heart disease and thus requires scrutinizing long-term management by the transplant team and commitment of the recipient to ensure successful outcome. This chapter addresses issues concerning cardiac transplantation along a continuum from recipient selection, donor selection, and operative procedure to postoperative management of the cardiac transplant recipient.

RECIPIENT SELECTION

Selection of heart transplant recipients is based on which patients are most likely to have the greatest improvement in symptoms, functional ability, and quality of life after transplant. Potential candidates are most likely to be New York Heart Association functional class III or IV, be younger than 65 years, and have a life expectancy of 6 months to 1 year. Fig. 12-2 shows the typical characteristics

TABLE 12-1 Historic Events in Cardiac Transplantation

Year	Researcher	Event
HETEROTOPIC		
1905	Carrel and Guthrie	First canine cardiac transplant
1933	Mann and others	Improved technical aspects of surgery
1951	Marcus and others	Focus on organ preservation
1962	Emikhov	Work in technical aspect of surgery
ORTHOTOPIC		
1958	Goldberg and others	First canine orthotopic transplants
1960	Lower and Shumway	Recipient operation techniques
1965	Lower and others	Rejection monitoring

of cardiac transplant recipients. The heart transplant recipient population is predominantly male (81%) with an average age of 45 years (range is from newborn to 75.3 years).

Because of the limited number of donors that prevent transplantation to all candidates, criteria have been established to assist clinicians in determining the need for transplantation. Clinicians must decide whether the patient is ready for transplantation. Patients with severely depressed left ventricular ejection fractions (less than 20%) are at greater risk for death than patients whose ejection fraction is greater than 20%.[2] Also patients with impairment of exercise tolerance (maximum volume of oxygen use greater

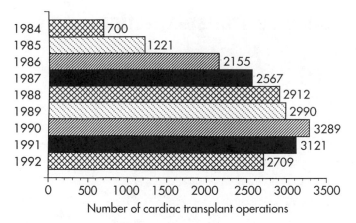

Fig. 12-1 Depiction of growth of heart transplants performed. (Adapted from Registry of the International Society for Heart and Lung Transplantation: Tenth Official Report—1993, *J Heart Lung Transport* 12:541, 1993, UAB Photography and Graphics.)

CONTRAINDICATIONS FOR CARDIAC TRANSPLANTATION

Absolute

Active infection
Malignancy
Autoimmune disorders
Any systemic disease that would limit survival
Irreversible kidney, liver, or pulmonary disease
Pulmonary vascular resistance above 6 Wood units

Relative

Pulmonary infarction
Peptic ulcer disease
Cerebrovascular accident
Peripheral vascular disease
Insulin-dependent diabetes
Current smoking and alcohol use
Morbid obesity

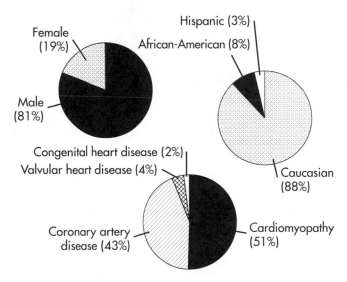

Fig. 12-2 Common characteristics of heart transplant recipients.   (Adapted from Registry of the International Society for Heart and Lung Transplantation: Tenth Official Report—1993, *J Heart Lung Transport* 12:541, 1993, UAB Photography and Graphics.)

than 14 ml/kg/min) who are ambulatory and functional class III elicit a poor prognostic sign.[3] Once all medical and surgical options for management of the cardiac disease have been exhausted, the referral for transplantation is indicated.

Ischemic heart disease with left ventricular dysfunction, dilated cardiomyopathy, and congenital heart disease are the most common disease etiologies leading to transplantation. Patients with left ventricular dysrhythmias not responsive to medical therapy or automatic implantable car-

dioverter devices may also benefit from transplant. Other diseases that may improve after cardiac transplantation are valvular heart disease, hypertropic and restrictive cardiomyopathy, sarcoidosis, amyloidosis, myocarditis, and cardiac tumors.[4-6]

Additional criteria have been established to assist in identifying the best cardiac transplant recipient. From the use of these criteria, absolute and relative contraindications for transplantation have evolved (see box). The best cardiac transplant recipient is one with no other systemic dysfunction that could limit survival. Active infection and malignancy are absolute contraindications to transplant. Immunosuppression required after surgery may accelerate infections and malignancies, leading to premature morbidity and/or mortality. Recent pulmonary infarction may lead to infection after transplantation.[7] Many centers treat patients with recent pulmonary infarctions for 6 to 12 weeks with anticoagulant agents or until documentation of radiographic improvement. Elevation of pulmonary vascular resistance of more than 4 to 6 Wood units may cause right heart failure after transplant.[8] An elevated transpulmonary gradient (greater than 15 mm Hg) may also lead to right-sided heart failure.[9] Pulmonary vascular resistance and transpulmonary gradient should be reduced by pharmacologic intervention (nitroprusside, dobutamine, prostaglandin E); however, if treatment fails, heterotopic (piggyback) or heart-lung transplantation may be a viable option. Right-sided heart catheterizations may need to be repeated to assess changes in pulmonary vascular resistance.[10]

Patients with irreversible liver or kidney disease have generally been excluded from cardiac transplant consideration because of the expected limitation in survival. Once again, immunosuppression received after cardiac transplantation may cause additional damage to these organs. Moderate obstructive lung disease is a relative contraindication because of decreased survival and increased risk of lung infections. A forced expiratory volume in 1 second less than 1.5 L or forced vital capacity less than 50% is considered high risk.[11] Consequently whether an active smoker should have a transplant remains a controversial issue.

Another controversial contraindication is older age. Historically, older age has been a primary contraindication to transplantation. Most transplant centers limit candidates to under 55 years of age; although in select candidates, patients older than 55 years can benefit from transplantation.[12,13]

Diabetes mellitus is a relative contraindication for transplantation.[14-16] Chronic corticosteroid therapy usually used in immunosuppression may increase the difficulty in managing blood glucose levels. Many patients whose diabetes is controlled by diet or oral agents require insulin after transplant. Some transplant centers attempt to reduce or taper steroids to reduce potential complications after surgery. Even though many centers have had successful transplantations in persons with insulin-dependent diabetes, important end-stage organ disease should be carefully evaluated before transplantation.

Other relative contraindications include peptic ulcer disease, diverticulosis, obesity, and cachexia.[17,18] Active peptic ulcer disease and diverticulosis may be aggravated by steroid use after surgery and thus lead to life-threatening consequences. Morbid obesity is associated with higher postoperative morbidity, and on the opposite extreme, cachexia may slow wound healing and increase the risk of infection after surgery. Establishing and maintaining an ideal body weight is important before transplantation.[19,20]

Referral and Cardiac Transplant Evaluation

The cardiac transplant evaluation process begins when a patient is referred to the transplant center. The purpose of the evaluation is to define the disease etiology if unknown, identify medical and/or psychosocial contraindications to transplantation, and determine whether cardiac transplantation will be beneficial to the patient and improve the quality of life.

The evaluation is performed on an inpatient or outpatient basis and lasts 3 to 5 days. During this time, extensive testing is completed, and the patient and family meet members of the transplant team, including the surgeon, cardiologist, transplant coordinator, nurses, psychologist, and social worker. The box shows routine procedures performed during the evaluation process. These procedures may vary from center to center.

It is important for nurses to understand the evaluation process, to be aware of indications and contraindications for transplantation, and to recognize and report any sig-

---

ROUTINE TESTS AND PROCEDURES PERFORMED DURING CARDIAC TRANSPLANT EVALUATION

Complete history and physical examination
Laboratory studies
    Electrolyte and metabolic profile, liver function studies, hematologic profile, fasting cholesterol and lipid profile, arterial blood gas levels
    Urinalysis
    Creatinine clearance
    ABO blood type, antibody screen, histocompatibility leukocyte antigen (HLA) tissue typing, panel reactive antibody
    Virologic and microbiologic profile: cytomegalovirus (CMV) antibody; *Toxoplasma gondii* antibody; human immunodeficiency virus; hepatitis A, B, and C serology; Epstein-Barr virus, Venereal Disease Research Laboratory; purified protein derivative with controls
Radiologic and nuclear studies
    Pulmonary artery and lateral chest x-ray study
    Sinus and panorex films
    Radionuclide angiogram
    Pulmonary function tests
    Ventilation and perfusion lung scans
    Magnetic nuclear resonance imaging (nuclear magnetic resonance)*
    Computerized tomography*
    Abdominal ultrasound
    Exercise testing with oxygen consumption*
Cardiac catheterization
Two-dimensional echocardiogram
Electrocardiogram
Tests for female patients*
    If age is greater than 35: Papanicolaou smear
    If age is greater than 35: mammogram

*When indicated.

---

nificant problems the potential recipient may encounter during the evaluation. Preoperative patient education is also an important responsibility for the nurse (Table 12-2). The goal is to provide the patient and family with factual information such as the procedure, intensive care, usual recovery, changes in diet, exercise, and the impact of immunosuppressive therapy. The associated risks of infection and rejection also need to be clearly explained. The patient uses this information to make a decision to have a transplant. Often, it helps for the candidate to meet a transplant recipient. Many centers have transplant support groups who volunteer to see patients while they are being evaluated. Emotional support is vital in maintaining the hope and integrity of the family unit at this time.

Listing for Transplantation and Waiting for a Donor Organ

When the evaluation is completed, the transplant team discusses the potential candidate's medical and psychosocial data. Based on these data, a decision is made whether the patient is a transplant candidate. Once the patient is ac-

TABLE 12-2   Nursing Management Before Transplantation

Nursing Diagnosis	Outcome	Interventions
Knowledge deficit related to end-stage organ disease, impending surgery, and expectations after transplantation	Patient will demonstrate an understanding of the natural history of the disease process, verbalize knowledge of the information needed to be known during the waiting period, and demonstrate understanding of posttransplant expectations.	Use written materials for preoperative transplant teaching if available. Explain tests and procedures needed during transplant evaluation. Introduce patient to an organ-transplant recipient, if possible. Teach patient about the disease (organ-specific), including the need to conserve energy, dietary concerns, reporting of signs of worsening organ failure, and difficulty concentrating. Educate patient on how to wait for a donor: Give patient telephone numbers. Explain purpose of beeper. Encourage patient to plan for transportation to hospital. Instruct patient on how to deal with stress. Emphasize importance of clinical visits. Explain sequence of events on day of surgery, including notification, nothing by mouth, admission to the hospital, surgery preparation, and waiting room for significant others. Provide emotional support and answer questions.

cepted for transplantation, the patient's name, weight, and ABO blood type are placed in the national organ computer according to urgency of need. The United Network of Organ Sharing (UNOS) is a nationwide system dedicated to the equitable sharing and distribution of donor organs. Contrary to years ago, cardiac transplantation is limited by organ availability. Patients may wait months to years for a heart. The median waiting time for patients 45 to 64 years of age in 1991 was 244 days.[21] Stable patients wait at home or close to the institution. Telephone numbers and a beeper system allow the patient to be reached at any time. Unstable patients wait in the hospital on the cardiovascular nursing unit or in the intensive care unit. Patients who become hemodynamically unstable may require inotropic agents, balloon counterpulsation, and/or ventricular assist devices to maintain their hemodynamic status until a donor organ becomes available.

Waiting for a donor organ is difficult for the patient and family. As waiting times increase, uncertainty about the future and fear of dying before a donor is found are predominant feelings. Currently, 2800 patients are waiting for heart transplantation. Congestive heart failure and fatal dysrhythmias are the leading cause of death in the pretransplant population.[22] According to UNOS, 778 patients died in 1991 while awaiting a donor.[23]

DONOR SELECTION AND OPERATIVE PROCEDURE

Federal law now requires that all health care institutions have policies for identifying potential donors and referring them to organ procurement centers. The individual being considered for donor selection must exhibit irreversible and total cessation of brain function. When a potential organ donor is identified, a cardiac donor evaluation must be completed. Medical history, physical examination, and procedures such as chest x-ray study, echocardiogram, electrocardiogram, central venous pressure measurements, and coronary arteriography, if indicated, will be performed. Criteria have been developed to assist clinicians in evaluating cardiac donors (see box). The goal of donor management is to maintain hemodynamic stability. Donor heart allocation is based on ABO blood compatibility, weight of donor and recipient, waiting time, and severity of illness.

DONOR SELECTION CRITERIA

Brain death
Consent
Age less than 40 years
ABO blood type compatibility
Compatible donor-recipient weight
Absence of active infection
Absence of malignancy except primary brain tumor
Absence of preexisting heart disease or cardiac trauma
Negative serologic test for human immunodeficiency virus and
    hepatitis B virus
Acceptable left ventricular function
If indicated, negative prospective cross-match
Anticipated ischemic time of less than 4 hours

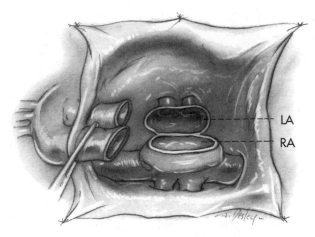

Fig. 12-3 Surgical field after cardiectomy. (From *Primary cardiomyopathy and cardiac transplantation.* In Kirklin JW, Boyes B, editors: *Cardiac surgery,* vol 2, New York, 1993, Churchill Livingstone, courtesy John W. Desley, Rochester, Minn.)

When the donor heart meets criteria for acceptable donation, the organ-procurement organization coordinates activities involved in organ procurement. Multiple organ procurement is usually performed on most donors; thus crucial timing of several organ transplant teams is anticipated. In heart transplantation, the operation is timed to synchronize cardiectomy with arrival of the donor heart. Donor heart ischemia time should be kept to 4 hours or less to reduce the risk of posttransplant morbidity and mortality.[23]

The nurse caring for the recipient should recognize that this is a time of mixed emotions for the recipient and family. Excitement and fear of the unknown predominate before the much anticipated surgery. The recipient is prepared for surgery and awaits word from the procurement team. Once the donor heart is physically seen and approved by the procurement team, the recipient is taken to surgery.

When the donor heart arrives in the operating room, it is prepared on a separate table. Orthotopic transplantation involves median sternotomy, dissection, initiation of cardiopulmonary bypass, and cardiectomy. This procedure involves transection of the main pulmonary artery and aorta and partial removal of the recipient atria, leaving the posterior walls intact (Fig. 12-3). The donor heart is implanted into the pericardium by placing it toward the patient's left side and anastomosing the recipient and donor left atrium, right atrium, aorta, and pulmonary artery (Fig. 12-4). It is important to protect the donor sinoatrial node to ensure normal pacemaking action.

At the conclusion of the grafting, it is critical to evacuate air from all the heart chambers. When the transplanted heart is warmed, it often resumes sinus rhythm. If it does not resume its pumping function, electric defibrillation is required. Epicardial pacing wires, chest tubes, atrial and arterial lines, and venous access are placed as is usual with open-heart surgery. Inotropic drugs (dopamine, dobutamine) and vasodilators (nitroprusside) may be used to increase cardiac output or to maintain renal perfusion. Isoproterenol may be started to maintain the heart rate between 100 and 120 beats/min. The patient is transferred to the intensive care unit when the operation is completed.

POSTOPERATIVE CARE AND LONG-TERM FOLLOW-UP

The immediate postoperative care of the transplant patient is very similar to that of any patient undergoing open-heart surgery. The main differences in cardiac transplant recipients are the effects of denervation in the transplanted heart, management of immunosuppression, rejection surveillance, evaluation of heart function, and diagnosis and treatment of adverse effects. Transplant patients must adhere to lifelong medical management, since complications may occur at any time.

Immediate Postoperative Concerns

Immediate postoperative care focuses on stabilizing hemodynamics. The first 24 to 48 hours are critical to the transplant patient. Low cardiac output may result from a number of early postoperative complications. Intraoperative or immediate postoperative hemorrhage is a serious problem. The risk of hemorrhage is increased by pretransplant anticoagulation therapy and previous cardiac surgery. Cardiac tamponade is another complication. The recipient's pericardial space is usually quite large because of long-term cardiomyopathy; thus after transplantation, there is an increased risk of concealed bleeding. Other complications that may decrease cardiac output are preservation injury, hypovolemia, dysrhythmias, and cardiac rejection. Low cardiac output is managed by the careful titration of inotropic and chronotropic support and temporary atrial pacing. If cardiac output remains unacceptable (less than 2.0 L/min), intraaortic balloon counterpulsation, ventila-

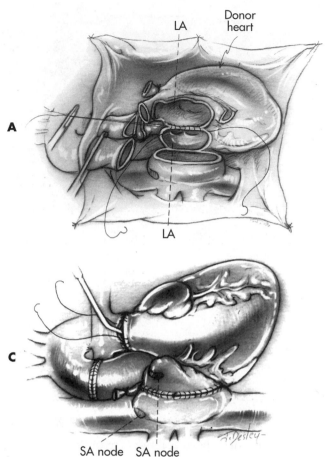

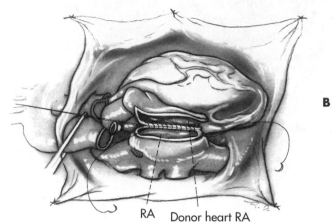

Fig. 12-4 **A,** Insertion of the transplanted heart begins with the anastomoses of donor and recipient left atrium. **B,** The right atria of donor and recipient are then anastomosed. **C,** After the atrial anastomosis is completed, the pulmonary artery and aorta anastomoses are completed. (From *Primary cardiomyopathy and cardiac transplantation.* In Kirklin JW, Boyes B, editors: *Cardiac surgery,* vol 2, New York, 1993, Churchill Livingstone, courtesy John W. Desley, Rochester, Minn.)

tion, or ventricular assist devices may be necessary to improve circulation.

Unique to the cardiac transplant recipient are the physiologic effects of denervation. After cardiac transplantation, there is no longer direct neural control of the conduction system. Thus the adrenal hormones exert primary stimulation of the heart by exciting the adrenergic receptors of the donor myocardium with circulating catecholamines. Epicardial pacing wires placed on the right atrium and ventricle may be used to override atrial or junctional bradycardia in the early postoperative period. An isoproterenol infusion also may be used to augment the heart rate and cardiac output. The denervated donor heart may be less sensitive to drugs such as atropine and digoxin and more sensitive to drugs such as adenosine; therefore all drugs given to affect cardiac performance should be carefully evaluated and adjusted to achieve the desired response.

Also after transplantation, the ECG shows the appearance of activity from sinoatrial nodes of the recipient and donor hearts. Thus there are two P waves in the ECG complex. The recipient's own sinoatrial activity does not propagate an impulse because it is isolated from any conducting pathways. Only the sinoatrial node of the donor heart can propagate an impulse in the donor heart. The presence of an additional P wave should be remembered during rhythm interpretation to avoid misidentification of a dysrhythmia.

Immunosuppression

Immunosuppression has evolved through the understanding of how the immune system works and the availability of ways to alter this system. When a foreign material (antigen) gains access to the tissues of a living host, an immune response (antibody) is mounted to destroy the offending material and maintain homeostasis. This response can occur by humoral immune mechanisms or by cell-mediated immune mechanisms. Both are derived from different types of lymphocytes. Lymphocytes are continually exported from the bone marrow and differentiate into T and B lymphocytes. B lymphocytes are responsible for humoral immunity and develop into plasma cells. These cells produce and secrete antibodies. The result of the antibody-antigen reaction may be a precipitate (an agglutination that renders the cell easily phagocytosed) or a neutralization of the toxin. The humoral response produces vascular damage to the transplanted heart. Sensitized T lymphocytes, important in cellular immunity, are capable of attacking and destroying the invading antigen. Damage to the heart from this response is evident by platelet aggregation and thrombosis.

Immunosuppressive therapy requires a delicate balance of immune-altering therapies to prevent acute allograft cardiac rejection without the development of adverse effects of the immunotherapy itself. Optimal individualized immune therapy is crucial to long-term patient survival. Excessive immunosuppression increases the risk of infection, kidney and liver dysfunction, and malignancies after transplantation, whereas inadequate immunosuppression may lead to rejection.

Cyclosporine

Cyclosporine is a cyclic endocapeptide that inhibits the activation of T lymphocytes and interleukin-2 production.[24] Cyclosporine is usually given immediately before surgery. Doses are individualized according to trough levels and serum creatinine after surgery. Cyclosporine is available in oil-based liquid, gel capsules, and intravenous solution. Cyclosporine is more potent in the intravenous than the oral route and should be administered intravenously at one third the oral dosage. Side effects associated with cyclosporine include hypertension, hyperkalemia, nephrotoxicity, hepatotoxicity, seizures, headaches and tremors. Careful monitoring of cyclosporine, blood urea nitrogen (serum BUN), creatinine, and total bilirubin levels and recognition of drug interactions (Table 12-3) are warranted.

Corticosteroids

Corticosteroids inhibit gene transcription and thus cause inhibition of T lymphocyte growth factor, lymphokine production, antibody synthesis, and release of interleukin by macrophages.[25] Usually corticosteroids are used with cyclosporine and azathioprine; however, many centers have successfully withdrawn steroids from their program.[26] Maintenance steroid dosage is 0.2 mg/kg/day or less. Many centers use high doses of methylprednisolone (1 g/day or 15 mg/kg if the patient weighs less than 50 kg) for 3 days as the first treatment of acute allograft rejection. Adverse effects of corticosteroids are numerous, as noted in Table 12-3.

Azathioprine

Azathioprine is a purine antimetabolite that impairs the immune response by inhibiting lymphocyte proliferation.[27,28] Azathioprine is usually used with cyclosporine and corticosteroids. The dosage is titrated to maintain a WBC count of 4000 to 5000/mm³. The main side effect is leukopenia; therefore the dose may need to be adjusted accordingly. Other side effects are anemia, thrombocytopenia, and drug-induced hepatitis.

Monoclonal and polyclonal antibodies

Polyclonal antibodies (ATG, antilymphocyte globulin [ALG], antilymphocyte gamma globulin [ATGAM]) act by coating T lymphocytes, making them susceptible to phagocytosis. Variations in the quality and potency are major disadvantages of polyclonal antibodies; however, many centers use these drugs for induction therapy or treatment of rejection.[29] ATG is usually administered intramuscularly, whereas ATGAM and ALG are administered intravenously through a central venous line. Common side effects are fever, chills, arthralgia, myarthsia, and thrombocytopenia.

Muromonab-CD3 is a highly potent monoclonal antibody that recognizes and blocks the activity of T lymphocytes. Muromonab-CD3 can be used prophylactically or for the treatment of acute rejection.[30] Some transplant centers report good results with prophylactic therapy, whereas others report increased risk of malignancies and other complications.[31] Adverse effects include hypotension, dyspnea, influenza-like syndrome, fever, and chills.

Cyclophosphamide

Cyclophosphamide (Cytoxan) may become an immunosuppressive agent for the treatment of humoral rejection. Cyclophosphamide is an antineoplastic drug that has identified action on B lymphocytes.[32] One of the major side effects is leukopenia; therefore WBC and platelet counts and liver and renal function tests should be monitored closely during drug administration.

Mycophenolate mofetil

Mycophenolate mofetil is a derivative of mycophenolic acid that inhibits de novo purine synthesis of activated lymphocytes.[33-35] This promising new immunosuppressive agent selectively inhibits Ionosine monophosphate dehydrogenase; therefore global bone marrow suppression is not seen with mycophenolate mofetil as it is with azathioprine and methotrexate. Clinical trials in human heart transplant recipients are under way.

Methotrexate

Methotrexate is a folic acid analog that inhibits dehydrofolate reductase and thus inhibits DNA synthesis and cell division. This agent has known antiinflammatory and antineoplastic activities when used in high doses and has been successfully used in low doses for the treatment of recurrent cardiac allograft rejection.[36-38] The most common side effect is leukopenia.

Total lymphoid irradiation

Total lymphoid irradiation is an immunosuppressive therapy for the treatment of recurrent rejection after cardiac transplantation.[39,40] Total lymphoid irradiation is low-dose radiotherapy that targets the major lymph node regions. Areas of nonlymphoid tissue are shielded during treatment. Radiation causes damage to DNA in susceptible lymphocytes, resulting in cell death. The treatment dose is 80 centigrays (cGy) twice weekly for 5 weeks. A total of 800 rads (1 cGy = 1 rad) is the treatment goal. Common adverse effects are leukopenia, thrombocytopenia, and anemia.

TABLE 12-3   Immunosuppressive Drugs Used in Cardiac Transplantation

	Cyclosporine (Sandimmune)	Corticosteroids	Azathioprine (Imuran)	Antithymocyte globulin (ATG)	Muromonab-CD3 (Orthoclone OKT3)
MECHANISM OF ACTION	Acts selectively on T lymphocytes, preventing production of effector T lymphocytes; does not depress bone marrow like antimetabolites (Immune activity is specific and reversible.)	Has antiinflammatory properties that reduce capillary permeability, vasodilatation, and edema. May also inhibit movement of T lymphocytes from blood to graft	Is an antimetabolite that competes for and blocks specific receptors, affecting deoxyribonucleic acid (DNA) and ribonucleic acid (RNA) synthesis and interfering with protein synthesis	Is prepared by immunizing rabbits or horses with human lymphocytes, binds to T lymphocytes and reduces their number in circulation	Is monoclonal antibody that blocks regeneration and functioning of T3 lymphocytes, effectively blocks cellular and humoral immune responses
SIDE EFFECTS	Nausea, vomiting, diarrhea Hepatotoxicity (elevated liver enzymes and alkaline phosphatase levels) Nephrotoxicity (elevated BUN level and creatinine clearance) Hypertension	Infection Diabetes Gastrointestinal bleeding Cushingoid appearance Steroid psychosis	Bone marrow depression, resulting in leukopenia, thrombocytopenia, and anemia (Rapid recovery of bone marrow occurs after withdrawal or reduction of drug.) Pancreatitis Muscle-wasting (with steroid use)	Chills, fever Hypotension Anaphylaxis	Fever, chills, nausea, vomiting, diarrhea, tremors, arthralgia, hypotension
SPECIFIC NURSING CARE	Pay careful attention to functioning of renal and hepatic systems. Punctually draw blood for laboratory to monitor for trough and peak levels. Be aware of effects from other drugs.	Anticipate multiple adverse effects of steroid therapy and plan care accordingly.	Monitor white blood cell (WBC) and platelet count. Provide good oral hygiene.	Perform skin test before injection. Use Z-tract technique for intramuscular injections. Apply heat, massage, and exercise to site before and after injection to lessen pain and inflammation from injection. Administer acetaminophen and diphenhydramine before injection to minimize anaphylactic response.	Administer preoperative and postoperative medications: steroids, acetaminophen, and antihistamines. Watch for signs of volume overload or pulmonary edema.

TABLE 12-3 Immunosuppressive Drugs Used in Cardiac Transplantation—cont'd

Cyclosporine (Sandimmune)	Corticosteroids	Azathioprine (Imuran)	Antithymocyte globulin (ATG)	Muromonab-CD3 (Orthoclone OKT3)
DRUG INTERACTIONS				
Drugs that increase the level of cyclosporine are diltiazem, ketokonazole, and erythromycin. Drugs that lower the levels of cyclosporine are rifampin, phenobarbital, phenytoin, and isoniazid.	—	Allopurinol potentiates the action of azathioprine; thus, the dose of azathioprine should be decreased to a fourth of usual when the patient is also on allopurinol.	—	—

Photopheresis and plasmapheresis

Ultraviolet-A radiation photopheresis (UVARP) is a new immunosuppressive therapy for the treatment of recurrent cell-mediated or vascular rejection.[41-43] UVARP involves the extracorporeal photoirradiation of lymphocytes pretreated with 8-methoxypsoralen (8-MOP), a photosensitive drug. Studies suggest that reinfusion of the irradiated WBCs produces a down regulation of the immune response, thus suppressing cells responsible for rejection.

UVARP treatments may be performed once or on two consecutive days every 3 to 6 weeks. The exact length of the most effective treatment course is unknown. A large-bore catheter such as a vascular catheter or 16-gauge angiocatheter is required for treatments. To prevent side effects of oral 8-MOP, the patient should wear wrap-around ultraviolet sunglasses and keep the skin covered for 48 hours.

Plasmapheresis removes antibodies circulating in the blood that result from an immune response against the donor organ. This therapy may reduce the incidence of fatal rejection of patients with high antibody levels after transplant. Although several centers are using these therapies, further research is warranted to investigate the efficacy of photopheresis and plasmapheresis.

Other agents

Many immunosuppressive agents are in clinical trials. FK-506 is a new immunosuppressive agent that inhibits cell-mediated immunity by blocking cytokine production.[44,45] 15-Deoxyspergudin suppresses rejection in animal models.[46] This agent suppresses the generation of cytotoxic T cells from antigen stimulated precursors.[47] Rapamicin inhibits lymphocyte responses to cytokines and will soon be evaluated in clinical trials.[48]

Complications

Short- and long-term survival rates have increased in cardiac transplantation because of the improvements in immunosuppression, recipient selection, and identification of risk factors. However, complications do occur, and rejection and infection continue to be the leading causes of death.

Rejection

Cardiac allograft rejection is a natural response when antigens on the transplanted heart are recognized as foreign. Despite all the advances in immunosuppressive therapy, rejection remains one of the leading causes of death after transplantation.

Traditionally, cardiac rejection has been classified into three types: hyperacute, acute, and chronic. With increased knowledge and better understanding of the immune response, rejection is now more commonly classified as cell-mediated (acute rejection) or antibody-mediated (humoral or vascular rejection). *Chronic rejection* is a term used to describe coronary artery disease in the transplanted heart;

however, presently this form of vasculopathy is not considered a type of rejection by most investigators.

Acute rejection

Acute rejection (cell mediated response activated by T lymphocytes) is most common in the first 3 months after transplantation; however, it can occur at any time.[49] Rejection is usually detected by endomyocardial biopsy sampling during routine surveillance visits. Endomyocardial biopsies are performed in the cardiac catheterization laboratory. A bioptome is inserted via the internal jugular vein and passed into the right ventricle for sampling (Fig. 12-5). Biopsies are usually done weekly for the first 2 months then tapered to every 3 or 4 months. Rejection is histologically characterized by evidence of interstitial and perivascular infiltrates that can lead to cellular necrosis if untreated.[50] In 1989, several cardiac pathologists formulated a standardized scale for grading cardiac rejection on the endomyocardial biopsy (Table 12-4).[50] Most patients remain asymptomatic during rejection episodes; however, fever, malaise, dyspnea, reduced exercise tolerance, and decreased blood

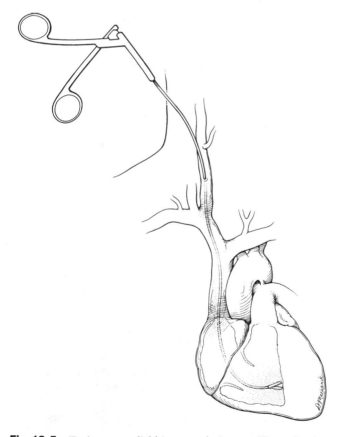

Fig. 12-5 Endomyocardial biopsy technique. (From Registry of the International Society for Heart and Lung Transplantation: Tenth Official Report—1993, *J Heart Lung Transport* 12:541, 1993, UAB Photography and Graphics.)

pressure may occur. The development of increased jugular venous distention and a third heart sound also may signify rejection. The choice of treatment depends not only on the grade of the biopsy but also on the signs and symptoms present. Usually class 1 (mild) rejection is not treated. Class 3 and 4 (moderate and severe) rejection are usually treated aggressively with corticosteroids, polyclonal or monoclonal antibodies, or both.[51] Other immunosuppressive therapies are discussed in the immunosuppression section of this chapter.

Humoral rejection

Humoral rejection is diagnosed by immunofluorescent staining of biopsy samples. Findings include deposition of immunoglobulin and complement on the vascular endothelium along with evidence of endothelial cell swelling.[52] Humoral rejection has been associated with a higher incidence of fatal rejection, development of transplant vasculopathy, and decreased overall survival.[53] Treatment is controversial; however, cyclophosphamide, plasmapheresis, and photopheresis have been used with variable success.

Hyperacute rejection is another form of humoral rejection caused by preformed cytotoxic antibodies in the recipient. It is relatively uncommon today because of ABO compatibility testing and preoperative screening for preformed cytotoxic antibodies. Patients with hyperacute rejection have a poor prognosis.

Cardiac transplant vasculopathy

This accelerated form of coronary artery disease has become one of the leading causes of death later than 1 year after transplantation. The disease is believed to be primarily immune-mediated.[54] Other factors that may

TABLE 12-4	Cardiac Biopsy Grading Scale
Grade	Definition
0	No rejection
1A	Focal infiltrate without necrosis
1B	Diffuse infiltrate without necrosis
2	One focus with aggressive infiltration or myocyte damage
3A	Multifocal infiltrates
3B	Diffuse infiltrates with necrosis
4	Diffuse aggressive infiltrate with necrosis with hemorrhage, edema, and vasculitis

Adapted from Billingham ME and others: A working formulation for the standardization of nomenclature in the diagnosis of heart and lung rejection: Heart Rejection Study Group, *J Heart Transplant* 9:587, 1990.

contribute to this disease are humoral rejection, obesity, hyperlipidemia, HLA mismatch, or CMV infection.[55-57] Because of denervation of the transplanted heart, angina is not a reliable warning signal for the development of disease.

The diagnosis of transplant vasculopathy is made by coronary angiograms. Baseline angiograms should be performed soon after surgery and yearly thereafter. The unique characteristic of this disease in the posttransplant patient is the diffuse concentric, longitudinal obliteration of the distal branch vessels. Retransplantation is the treatment of choice for severe disease. Percutaneous coronary angioplasty has been used as palliative treatment with varying degrees of success.[58] Because of the diffuse nature of the disease, coronary artery bypass grafting is usually not a suitable option of treatment. Medical therapies such as exercise, cessation of smoking, antiplatelet and anticoagulant drugs, antihypertensive drugs, cholesterol-lowering drugs, methotrexate, and calcium channel blockers have not greatly influenced the clinical course of this disease.[59,60]

Infection

Infection continues to be the leading cause of death after cardiac transplantation.[1] Because of the use of nonspecific immunosuppressive agents to prevent rejection, an increased risk of infection is present. Therefore immunosuppressed posttransplant patients are predisposed to infection at any time; however, they are most susceptible during the first month for nosocomial infections, and after 2 to 5 months for opportunistic infections such as CMV infection, pneumocystitis, and candidiasis.[61] The lungs are the primary site for these infections, followed by the blood, urine, and gastrointestinal tract.[61] Many centers use prophylactic regimens of acyclovir, trimethoprim and sulfamethoxazole, and nystatin for 6 months to 1 year to prevent infection.

Malignancy

The development of malignant neoplasms is a potential adverse effect of chronic immunosuppression. Posttransplant lymphoproliferative disease is the most common tumor in cyclosporine-based immunosuppression.[62] The tumor is usually of B cell origin and is associated with the Epstein-Barr virus. It typically occurs 12 to 18 months after transplantation and has a variable to poor prognosis.[63] Reduction in immunotherapy with chemotherapy, radiation, or surgical reduction, if indicated, is a treatment option.

Basal and squamous cell skin carcinomas are commonly seen in azathioprine-treated patients.[62] Squamous cell is more common than basal cell carcinoma in transplant patients and has a higher incidence of metastatic disease.

Complications of immunosuppressive drugs

Complications of immunosuppression result from a specific agent or a combination of the effect of agents. Adverse effects of each agent are discussed in the section on immunosuppression.

Long-Term Follow-Up

Before the cardiac transplant patient is discharged from the hospital, pertinent information such as signs and symptoms of rejection and infection, diet and exercise plan, medication dosages, and any other instructions (blood pressure readings, diabetes teaching) are reviewed (Table 12-5). Many institutions have developed teaching booklets that serve as references for the patient and family. At some centers, patients must remain close to the hospital for approximately 6 weeks before returning to their home, which may be a long distance from the transplant center. This time allows the transplant team to assess the patient frequently. It also allows the patient to gradually become more independent. Meticulous surveillance of these patients is essential for a successful long-term outcome.

Quality of life

In recent years, quality of life has become an increasingly important outcome measure in the heart transplant population. In 1985, Lough and others[64] examined life satisfaction and quality of life in 75 heart transplant recipients 6 months to 14 years after transplant; they determined that patients were highly satisfied with their quality of life after surgery. A long-term multiinstitutional study at the Loyola University Medical Center and University of Alabama at Birmingham is now examining quality of life before and after transplantation.[65-67]

CONCLUSION

Cardiac transplantation is a widely accepted treatment for patients with end-stage heart disease. Pretransplant selection criteria have been developed to assist clinicians in determining the need for transplantation. Once the patient is listed for transplantation, issues of organ donation, allocation, and candidate survival become priorities.

Long-term medical follow-up includes monitoring of immunosuppressive regimens and the prompt diagnosis and treatment of complications. The delicate balance of adjusting immunosuppression remains a challenge for the transplant team. Rejection and infection continue to be leading complications after transplantation. Coronary allograft vasculopathy and malignancies are complications affecting long-term survival of heart transplant recipients.

Despite the complications of immunosuppression and transplantation itself, cardiac transplantation is a viable treatment option for patients with end-stage heart disease to improve survival and quality of life.

TABLE 12-5   Nursing Management for the Cardiac Transplant Recipient

Nursing Diagnosis	Outcome	Interventions
Knowledge deficit related to posttransplant regimen	Recipient will demonstrate knowledge and understanding of routine postoperative course.	Assess patient's readiness to learn. Provide written teaching booklet and verbal instruction. Use resources: pharmacist, dietician, physical therapist, social worker, and clergy. Reinforce teaching throughout immediate hospital stay in the following areas: signs and symptoms of rejection and infection, diet, medications, vital signs (how to take blood pressure and pulse), physical activity, signs and symptoms that require notification of the transplant team, and instruction on monitoring of diabetes, wound care if indicated
Altered immunologic response related to immunosuppression required after organ transplantation	Recipient will remain free from immunosuppressive complications as evidenced by maintaining skin integrity and/or optimal wound healing, demonstrating a normotensive status, remaining free from nephrotoxicity, and remaining free from leukopenia.	Assess incision and wound healing. Dress incisions according to institutional protocol. Teach patient the importance of skin hygiene and reporting new skin lesions, warts, rashes, acne, and easy bruising. Monitor blood pressure and administer antihypertensives if ordered. Monitor renal function tests and cyclosporine levels. Assess intake and output. Monitor WBC count and differential. Monitor immunosuppressive regimen (that is, prednisone and azathioprine).
Potential for rejection of transplanted organ related to impaired immunocompetence	Recipient will remain free from organ rejection and be optimally immunosuppressed as evidenced by lack of fever, dyspnea, dysrhythmias, worsening hemodynamics (blood pressure and cardiac index), fatigue and weakness, and no evidence of rejection will be seen on endomyocardial or transbronchial biopsy.	Assess organ system function: renal and liver function tests, intake and output, bile drainage, cardiac hemodynamic tests, left ventricular function via echocardiogram, venous oxygen saturation. Administer immunosuppressive agents as indicated. Report any sign or symptom of rejection to the transplant team. Monitor cyclosporine levels. Reinforce recipient's understanding of signs and symptoms of rejection and the importance of prompt reporting of these signs to the transplant team.

TABLE 12-5   Nursing Management for the Cardiac Transplant Recipient—cont'd

Nursing Diagnosis	Outcome	Interventions
Potential for infection related to impaired immunocompetence	Recipient will remain free from infection as evidenced by afebrile state, lack of redness and drainage at wound site, lack of leukopenia or elevated WBC, lack of productive cough, clear lung sounds on auscultation, lack of infiltrate on chest x-ray film, and lack of burning on urination.	Use good hand-washing techniques. Maintain protective isolation as indicated. Assess for signs and symptoms of infection: Monitor temperature. Assess wound sites. Auscultate lungs. Monitor WBC output. Monitor urinalysis. Obtain appropriate routine cultures (blood, urine, sputum, CMV shell vial cultures). Teach recipient signs and symptoms of infection and to report these to the transplant team. Encourage optimal caloric intake. Administer antibiotics if indicated. Monitor immunosuppression. Administer prophylactic agents (acyclovir, trimethoprim and sulfamethoxazole, nystatin, ganciclovir) according to institutional protocol.
Alteration in nutrition: potential for less than body requirements related to increased caloric needs after transplant OR potential for more than body requirements related to side effects of immunosuppressive agents	Recipient will demonstrate understanding of appropriate dietary regimen as evidenced by maintaining baseline weight, selecting correct foods, and keeping the cholesterol and lipid profile within normal limits.	Consult dietician. Weigh patient daily. Instruct recipient to count calories. Administer dietary supplements (Ensure, Sustocal, snacks), give total parental nutrition or nasogastric tube feedings as indicated. Restrict certain foods or place patient on prudent diet as indicated. Monitor fasting cholesterol and lipid profiles. Instruct recipient to monitor intake and output.
Alteration in comfort related to postoperative transplant surgery	Recipient will remain free from discomfort.	Provide comfort measures. Encourage deep breathing and relaxation. Administer pain medication as indicated. Assess recipient's pain tolerance level. Offer emotional support.
Potential for ineffective coping after transplantation related to increased stress, anxiety, potential dependency, fear of rejection and/or death, body image disturbance, and lifestyle changes	Recipient will use effective coping, remain free from anxiety, and be able to perform activities of daily living.	Establish rapport with recipient and significant others. Assess recipient's level of anxiety. Explain tests and procedures and provide a plan of care with choices. Consult social worker, clergy, or psychologist if indicated. Reinforce postoperative teaching throughout hospital stay. Provide ways to deal with body image changes (for example, hair remover, diet, and exercises). Set priorities and goals with recipient. Encourage recipient to return home and establish a "normal routine."

REFERENCES

1. Registry of the International Society for Heart and Lung Transplantation: Tenth Official Report—1993, *J Heart Lung Transplant* 12:541, 1993.
2. Keogh AM and others: Prognostic guides in patients with idiopathic or ischemic dilated cardiomyopathy assessed for cardiac transplantation, *Am J Cardiol* 65:903, 1990.
3. Mancini DM and others: Value of peak exercise oxygen consumption for optimal timing of cardiac transplantation in ambulatory patients with heart failure, *Circulation* 83:778, 1991.
4. Valantine HA and others: Cardiac sarcoidosis: response to steroids and transplantation, *J Heart Transplant* 6:244, 1987.
5. Hosenpud JD and others: Successful intermediate-term outcome for patients with cardiac amyloidosis undergoing heart transplantation: results of a multicenter survey, *J Heart Transplant* 9:346, 1990.
6. O'Connell JB and others: Results of heart transplantation for active lymphocytic myocarditis, *J Heart Transplant* 9:351, 1990.
7. Young JN and others: The influence of acute preoperative pulmonary infarction on the results of heart transplantation, *J Heart Transplant* 5:20, 1986.
8. Kirklin JK and others: Pulmonary vascular resistance and the risk of heart transplantation, *J Heart Transplant* 7:331, 1988.
9. Erickson KW and others: Influence of preoperative transpulmonary gradient on late mortality after orthotopic heart transplantation, *J Heart Transplant* 9:526, 1990.
10. Kormos RL and others: Utility of preoperative right heart catheterization data as a predictor of survival after heart transplantation, *J Heart Transplant* 5:391, 1986.
11. Levine AB, Levine TB: Patient evaluation for cardiac transplantation: *Prog Cardiovasc Dis* 33:219, 1991.
12. Carrier M and others: Cardiac transplantation in patients over 50 years of age, *J Am Coll Cardiol* 8:285, 1986.
13. Olivari MT and others: Heart transplantation in elderly patients, *J Heart Transplant* 7:258, 1988.
14. Munoz and others: Long-term results in diabetic patients undergoing cardiac transplantation, *J Heart Transplant* 10:189, 1991.
15. Rhenman MR and others: Diabetes and heart transplantation, *J Heart Transplant* 7:356, 1988.
16. Ladowski J and others: Heart transplantation in diabetic recipients, *Transplant* 49:303, 1990.
17. O'Connell JB and others: Cardiac transplantation: recipient selection, donor procurement and medical follow-up, *Circulation* 86:1061, 1992.
18. Mudge GH and others: Task Force 3: recipient guidelines/prioritization, *J Am Coll Cardiol* 22:21, 1993.
19. Frazier OH and others: Nutritional management of the heart transplant recipient, *J Heart Transplant* 4:450, 1985.
20. Grady KL and others: Obesity and hyperlipidemia after heart transplantation, *J Heart Lung Transplant* 10:449, 1991.
21. UNOS: Trends in organ transplantation, *UNOS Update* 10:3, 1994.
22. McManus RP and others: Patients who die awaiting heart transplantation, *J Heart Lung Transplant* 12:159, 1993.
23. Young JB and others and the Cardiac Transplant Research Database Group: Matching the heart donor and transplant recipient: clues for successful expansion of the donor pool, *J Heart Lung Transplant* 13:353, 1994.
24. Borel JK: Cyclosporine A: pharmacological properties in vivo, *Pharmacol Rev* 41:259, 1989.
25. Snyder DA, Unanve ER: Corticosteroids inhibit murine macrophage Ia expression and interleukin 1 production, *J Immunol* 129:1803, 1982.
26. Renlund DG and others: Feasibility of discontinuation of corticosteroid maintenance therapy in heart transplantation, *J Heart Transplant* 6:71, 1987.
27. Elion GB: Pharmacologic and physical agents: immunosuppressive agents, *Transplant Proc* 9:975, 1978.

28. McCormack JJ, Johns DG: *Purine antimetabolites*. In Chabner B, editor: *Pharmacologic principles of cancer treatment*, Philadelphia, 1982, Saunders.
29. Kirklin JK and others: Prophylactic therapy for rejection following cardiac transplantation: a comparison of RATG vs. OKT3, *J Thoracic Cardiovasc Surg* 99:716, 1990.
30. Bristow MR and others: Use of OKT3 monoclonal antibody in cardiac transplantation, *J Heart Transplant* 7:1, 1988.
31. Swinnen LJ and others: Increased incidence of lymphoproliferative disorder after immunosuppression with the monoclonal antibody OKT3 in cardiac transplant recipients, *N Engl J Med* 323:1723,. 1990.
32. Wagoner LE and others: Cyclophosphamide as an alternative immunosuppressive agent in cardiac transplant recipients with recurrent rejection, *J Heart Lung Transplant* 11:199, 1992.
33. Sollinger HW and others: RS-61443, a new, potent immunosuppressive agent, *Transplantation* 15:27, 1990.
34. Sollinger HW and others: RS-61443: mechanism of action, experimental and early clinical results, *Clin Transplant* 5(spec. issue):523, 1991.
35. Morris RE and others: Mycophenolic acid morpholinoethylester (RS-61443) is a new immunosuppressant that prevents and halts heart allograft rejection by selective inhibition of T- and B-cell purine synthesis, *Transplant Proc* 22(4):1659, 1990.
36. Costanzo-Nordin MR and others: Reversal of recalcitrant cardiac allograft rejection with methotrexate, *Circulation* 78:47, 1988.
37. Hosenpud JD and others: Methotrexate for the treatment of patients with multiple episodes of acute cardiac allograft rejection, *J Heart Lung Transplant* 11:739, 1992.
38. Bourge RC and others: Methotrexate pulse therapy in the treatment of recurrent acute heart rejection, *J Heart Lung Transplant* 110:1116, 1992.
39. Hunt SA and others: Total lymphoid irradiation for the treatment of intractable cardiac allograft rejection, *J Heart Lung Transplant* 10:211, 1991.
40. Salter MM and others: Total lymphoid irradiation in the treatment of early or recurrent heart rejection, *J Heart Lung Transplant* 11:902, 1992.
41. Costanzo-Nordin MR and others: Reversal of heart transplant rejection with photopheresis, *J Heart Lung Transplant* 10:177, 1991.
42. Rose EA and others: Photochemotherapy in human heart transplant recipients at high risk for fatal rejection, *J Heart Lung Transplant* 11:746, 1992.
43. Meiser BM and others: Reduction of the incidence of rejection by adjunct immunosuppression with photochemotherapy after heart transplantation, *Transplantation* 57:563, 1994.
44. Fung JJ and others: KF506 in clinical organ transplantation, *Clin Transplant* 5:517, 1991.
45. Thomas J and Thomas F: The immunosuppressive action of FK506, *Transplantation* 49:390, 1990.
46. Amemiya H and others: A novel rescue drug, 15-deoxyspergualin, *Transplantation* 49:337, 1990.
47. Morris RE: ±15 deoxyspergualin: a mystery wrapped within an enigma, *Clin Transplant* 5:530, 1991.
48. Kahan BD and others: Preclinical evaluation of a new potent immunosuppressive agent, Rapamycin, *Transplantation* 52:185, 1991.
49. Kobashigawa JA and others and the Cardiac Transplant Research Database Group: Pretransplantation risk factors for acute rejection after heart transplantation: a multiinstitutional study, *J Heart Lung Transplant* 12:355, 1993.
50. Billingham ME and others: A working formulation for the standardization of nomenclature in the diagnosis of heart and lung rejection: Heart Rejection Study Group, *J Heart Transplant* 9:587, 1990.
51. O'Connell JB, Renlund DG: *Diagnosis and treatment of cardiac allograft rejection, in cardiac transplantation*, Philadelphia, 1990, Davis.

52. Hammond EH and others: Vascular (humoral) rejection in heart transplantation: pathologic observation and clinical implications, *J Heart Transplant* 8:430, 1989.

53. Hammond EH and others: Vascular rejection and its relationship to allograft coronary artery disease, *J Heart Lung Transplant* 11:111, 1992.

54. Billingham ME: Graft coronary disease: the lesions and the patients, *Transplant Proc* 21:3665, 1989.

55. McDonald K and others: Association of coronary artery disease in cardiac transplant recipients with cytomegalovirus infection, *Am J Cardiol* 64:359, 1989.

56. Costanzo-Nordin MR: Cardiac allograft vasculopathy: relationship with acute cellular rejection and histocompatibility, *J Heart Lung Transplant* 11:S90, 1992.

57. Winters GL and others: Posttransplant obesity and hyperlipidemia: major predictors of severity of coronary arteriopathy in failed human heart allografts, *J Heart Transplant* 9:364, 1990.

58. McBride W and others: Restenosis after successful coronary angioplasty: pathophysiology and prevention, *N Engl J Med* 318:1734, 1988.

59. Schroeder JS and others: A preliminary study of diltiazem in the prevention of coronary artery disease in heart transplant recipients, *N Engl J Med* 328:164, 1993.

60. deLorgerile M and others: Low dose aspirin and accelerated coronary disease in heart transplant recipients, *J Heart Transplant* 9:449, 1990.

61. Miller LW and others (including the Transplant Cardiologists Research Database Group): Infection following cardiac transplantation: a multi-institutional analysis, *J Heart Lung Transplant* 13:1, 1994.

62. Penn I: Lymphomas complicating organ transplantation, *Transplant Proc* 15:2790, 1983.

63. Armitage JM and others: Posttransplant lymphoproliferative disease in thoracic organ transplant patients: ten years of cyclosporine-based immunosuppression, *J Heart Lung Transplant* 10:877, 1991.

64. Lough ME and others: Life satisfaction following heart transplant, *J Heart Transplant* 4:446, 1985.

65. Grady KL and others: Symptom distress in cardiac transplant candidates, *Heart Lung* 21:434, 1992.

66. Grady KL and others: Perception of helpfulness of health care provider interventions by heart transplant candidates, *Cardiovasc Nurs* 29:33, 1993.

67. Jalowiec A, Grady KL, White-Williams C: Stressors in patients awaiting heart transplant, *Behav Med* 19:145, 1994.

13

Cardiac Rehabilitation: Management of the Patient After Myocardial Infarction

Nancy Houston Miller

Technologic advances in the management of patients suffering cardiovascular diseases over the past 2 decades have virtually revolutionized care. Innovations in medical and surgical management, including the introduction of thrombolytic therapy and angioplasty, have been accompanied by a significant reduction in early mortality in patients after myocardial infarction (MI). Moreover, although there has been a burgeoning of technological advances, the public also has become increasingly aware of the importance of changes in health behaviors to reduce their risk of cardiovascular disease or future heart problems.

With such changes in the early care of cardiovascular patients has come a shift and advancement in the rehabilitation of these patients. No longer are patients kept in bed and restricted from activities as they were for almost 30 years; no longer are they prevented from formally participating in moderate- to high-level activity until 8 to 12 weeks after the infarction; and no longer are physicians and nurses questioning the advice they give about resumption of normal activities: All of these decisions are based on scientific evidence of the safety of resuming such tasks early in the course of recovery for the majority of patients.

Since the goal of cardiac rehabilitation is to restore patients to their optimal physical, medical, psychologic, emotional, vocational, and economic status, it is important to review how recent changes in management and rehabilitation have affected and will continue to affect patients treated over the next decade.

Changes in medical management have been dramatic. One such change has been the increasingly widespread application of therapies designed to restore coronary blood flow in the early hours of MI, thereby limiting the extent of infarcted myocardium. This approach has added a new dimension to coronary care, which previously was limited to therapies designed to treat the complications of an infarct rather than the underlying process. The rationale for such intervention comes from evidence that acute coronary thrombosis occurring at the site of a preexisting arteriosclerotic plaque is usually the immediate event that pre-

cipitates an MI,[1] and by restoring blood flow within a critical period of time (1 to 6 hours), myocardium that would otherwise have become infarcted can now be salvaged.[2] Interventions such as thrombolytic agents (for example, streptokinase and tissue plasminogen activator), mechanical dilatation of an occluded or stenotic coronary vessel by percutaneous transluminal coronary angioplasty, and acute surgical coronary artery bypass grafting have all been used for this purpose. Thus the result of salvaging myocardium has had a major impact on in-hospital survival and potential long-term survival in the months after infarction.

A second important change in management has been the recognition that clinical variables and exercise test results performed early in the course of recovery provide important prognostic information about the patient's risk of future events in the year after MI.[3] Such recognition has led to earlier interventions for high-risk patients and recommendations for low-risk patients to resume normal activities earlier. Formerly, patients who were identified as low risk would have been managed in an identical manner to those patients identified as high risk. The management of these patients is discussed in the next section.

A shift in clinical management has also precipitated a shift in cardiac rehabilitation. From the 1930s until the 1960s, physicians severely restricted the activities of coronary patients, especially after MI. Patients were kept on bedrest for many days, hospitalized up to 3 to 4 weeks, and restricted from resuming normal activities, often until 3 months after the event. These recommendations were based on concerns that even routine activities would cause undue stress on a damaged heart and might precipitate further life-threatening cardiac events. Decisions were based on subjective information, with little consideration given to the patient's course of recovery or to exercise testing, which was thought to be unsafe early in the postinfarction period.

In the early 1970s, however, a change in the management of these patients occurred as more information became available. Researchers began to question earlier studies, believing restrictions on activity levels to be excessive and questioning the belief that all patients were at high risk after the event. Early exercise testing provided the impetus for this change in rehabilitation management. After it was determined to be safe in this population, early treadmill testing performed 3 weeks after MI and then at discharge became the standard of care. Such testing provided physicians with important information about the degree of myocardial ischemia, the patient's functional capacity, and the ability of patients to resume physical activities. Likewise, hospitalization stays decreased to 7 days for many patients with uncomplicated disease, and rehabilitation programs began enrolling patients at 3 to 4 weeks after the event rather than at 8 to 12 weeks. This timing facilitated the patient's return to usual activities at a much earlier period after the cardiac event.

Although formal rehabilitation programs were developed in hospitals and community centers around the country beginning in the 1970s, it was apparent that the number of available programs was insufficient to meet the needs of the large numbers of patients with coronary heart disease. As a result, the advent of home rehabilitation for low-risk patients occurred in the 1980s. Methods for enhancing compliance to exercise training and to modification of coronary risk factors, the cornerstone of rehabilitation efforts, continue to be explored for patients involved in home rehabilitation programs.

What is the direction for cardiac rehabilitation now and into the year 2000? As the population ages, health care professionals in rehabilitation programs are caring for an older, sicker population. Although this group is faced with increased co-morbidity, studies indicate that the benefits of exercise training and cardiovascular risk reduction are as beneficial in this population as in their younger counterparts.[4,5] Rehabilitation personnel are learning the best ways to optimize exercise programs for these patients to improve their function and potential quality of life and to manage other medical conditions that may interfere with or limit their capabilities.

In addition, in this era of health care reform, consideration is now being given to the cost and types of services being offered to patients. Rehabilitation programs are looking at restructuring; as was the case in the 1970s and 1980s, rather than receiving a comprehensive package of services offered to all patients, higher-risk patients will continue to receive a very formal, structured program of medically supervised training, psychologic counseling, and risk-factor intervention. Those at lower to moderate risk are exercising at home and undertaking self-help methods to modify the behaviors of smoking, dietary change, weight loss, and other risk factors.

Finally, the focus of rehabilitation programs, which has primarily been exercise, has and hopefully will continue to shift toward intensive health-behavior change directed at cardiovascular risk reduction. New scientific evidence based on providing multiple risk-factor interventions clearly indicates that cardiovascular disease may regress, with a reduction in the morbidity and mortality rates in patients with established disease.[6]

The process of cardiac rehabilitation involves three basic principles. First, the patient must be evaluated early and repeatedly. Evaluation is often provided through treadmill testing. The purposes of evaluation are to provide the basis for recommending specific activities and to identify patients in need of medication therapy or surgical treatment of complicating problems such as angina pectoris. Second, programs of exercise training must be individually prescribed to augment functional capacity. Third, intensive risk-factor intervention and vocational and psychologic assessment and evaluation must be provided by members of the health care team. The remainder of this chapter focuses on these principles.

REHABILITATION PERIODS

The rehabilitation of patients must be viewed as a continual and logical process that begins in the hospital, most often in the coronary care unit (CCU) or intensive care unit (ICU), and extends to a lifetime program of prudent activity and risk-factor control. The efficacy of the process is compromised when such efforts are delayed weeks or months after the patient's discharge from the hospital.

For patients involved in traditional, structured cardiac rehabilitation programs, management has been divided into phases or stages of rehabilitation. These stages have included the in-hospital course, immediate outpatient sessions (normally 10 to 12 weeks), a conditioning stage of 1 to 6 months, and a maintenance stage that continues indefinitely.[7] Although these stages may have been beneficial for exercise training in the 1970s and 1980s, shortened hospitalizations, decreasing reimbursement for rehabilitation activities, and managed care may substantially change the need for defined phases or stages. For patients who may not have access to formal structured programs, it is important to consider the necessary components of rehabilitation during hospitalization and in the outpatient recovery stage.

In-Hospital Rehabilitation
Activity guidelines

Rehabilitation begins after the patient has been stabilized and is free from life-threatening complications. For patients with uncomplicated disease, the use of the bedside commode, short walks to a private bathroom, and self-care activities such as bathing, shaving, and dressing are appropriate even in the first 24 hours. Range-of-motion exercises and chair-sitting counteract the deleterious effects of bedrest[8] and may forestall unwarranted fears that patients have about physical activity; such fears may otherwise persist for extended periods after infarction. Early activity also minimizes the risk of venous thrombosis and pulmonary embolus.[9]

For most patients, gradual walking about the room and in-hospital corridors occurs by the second or third day after the event. The goal at this stage of rehabilitation is not to undertake aerobic training but to minimize physical deconditioning, prevent venous thrombosis, and enhance the overall psychologic well-being of the patient. These goals can best be accomplished through early ambulation.

Walking sessions within the hospital should be short (5 to 20 minutes) and of low intensity. Often the guideline for exercise intensity is a heart rate not exceeding 20 beats/min above the resting heart rate. Multiple short walks throughout the day may be preferable to a single, longer walk. Monitoring heart rate and blood pressure, electrocardiographic (ECG) abnormalities, and symptoms in response to early ambulation becomes important in detecting problems such as myocardial ischemia or dysrhythmias that may require immediate attention or a reduction in activity levels. Activity schedules need to be modified for patients who experience a more complicated course involving postinfarction angina, heart failure, or severe atrial or ventricular dysrhythmias. For patients who experience complications such as ventricular fibrillation or other transient dysrhythmias within the first 24 hours after MI, management is often similar to that for patients with uncomplicated disease.

Because most patients are discharged so quickly after angioplasty, MI, and other cardiovascular events, the goal should be to ambulate patients as quickly as possible to prepare them for a return to normal activities.

Educational and psychologic needs

Shortened hospitalizations prevent nurses, physicians, or a rehabilitation team from spending a great deal of time providing patient education; often, such education is left to the outpatient stage of recovery. Educational efforts, however, routinely begin in the hospital and should include information that is individualized and directed to patients' needs. Most often in the CCU and in the transition unit, information is provided about anatomy and physiology, procedures, and treatments. It is important to provide the following specific information before hospital discharge: instructions about medications, their proper administration, and side effects; activity guidelines with a written prescription for exercise training; recommendations for resumption of sexual activity and issues related to return to work; and an introduction to coronary risk-factor modification, including dietary modification and treatment of hyperlipidemia, smoking cessation, and management of hypertension, diabetes, and stress. Evidence suggests that behavioral counseling to prevent relapse of smoking after discharge is a critical component of education about risk factors.[10] Educational videotapes and pamphlets are often available to supplement teaching efforts. These issues will be discussed in more detail later.

Critical to the rehabilitation of the patient in any stage of recovery is the family and especially the spouse. The spouse should be involved in all educational sessions, and attention should be paid to concerns and questions that may be quite different than those of the patient. Insufficient information about dietary management, permissible activity, and sex have all been found to be sources of concern for spouses.[11] In one study, spouses reported that more information at the time of hospitalization might have helped them to respond more appropriately to patients' needs.[12]

Attention to the patient's psychologic recovery is also important. Patients respond to a cardiac event with diverse coping mechanisms. Some patients deny the crisis event, and others exaggerate the problem, never returning to normal activities despite minimal limitations on cardiac function. For the patient suffering an MI, however, there is a normal sequence of emotional responses similar to that in Kübler-Ross' theory of grief and loss.[13] The patient may suffer anxiety, denial, depression, and anger over the event. Moreover, the spouse and family may respond with similar psychologic reactions. Such reactions should be acknowledged by rehabilitation personnel; individual interviews in the hospital with a psychologist or psychiatrist may contribute a great deal to patient management. In considering the varied responses and adaptation for patients suffering coronary heart disease (CHD), a more detailed review of psychosocial recovery is noted in Chapter 7.

Risk stratification

A major goal of rehabilitation in the early phase of recovery is risk stratification. Establishing a patient's prognosis based on the results of clinical and historical information, including the physical examination and ECG findings, and performing an exercise test alone or with radionuclide scintigraphy or ventriculography provide the bases for important management decisions. Such information is useful because the majority of second events occur early in the course of recovery, most often within 3 to 6 months.[14]

Severe left ventricular dysfunction, myocardial ischemia, and ventricular dysrhythmias are important predictors of outcome. Failure to identify these predictors may deny patients potentially life-saving therapies or may result in inappropriate decisions concerning early rehabilitation. Likewise, failure to identify low-risk patients may result in unnecessary restrictions on physical activity or delayed return to work.

DeBusk and others[15] reviewed data on a cohort of patients followed for 32 months to determine medical events, including death, recurrent MI, congestive heart failure, and unstable angina. Risk in the 6 months after MI was increased (8.6% vs 4.4%) for patients who had histories of previous MI or angina for 2 to 3 months before the MI and recurrent chest pain within 24 hours after admission but before discharge or who had clinical characteristics that were primarily contraindications to symptom-limited treadmill testing (that is, congestive heart failure; angina at rest; severe cardiovascular, pulmonary, or orthopedic disease). The best treadmill test predictor was 0.2 mV or more of ST-segment depression at a heart rate of less than 135 beats/min. Patients with such an abnormality had an event rate of 9.6% over 6 months.[15]

Identifying (stratifying) the risk of additional cardiac events allows high-risk patients with significant abnormalities to be considered for aggressive medical or surgical therapy and patients at low-risk to be cleared for early resumption of work and rehabilitation. In most reported studies, at least 50% of conditions are uncomplicated, with an overall event rate of less than 5% in the year after MI. In this population, it is doubtful that any surgical or medical intervention will improve outcome. However, 25% to 30% of all patients are high risk, and those with compromised left ventricular function are most often treated medically, requiring greater attention to rehabilitation efforts. Fig. 13-1 provides an overview of the prognostic stratification of patients after acute MI from 10 acute care centers. In this more recent era of thrombolytic therapy, early revascularization, and antiplatelet therapy, an even higher proportion of patients may be of lower risk. This will also vary based on the type of patient population for a given hospital.

Treadmill test

To stratify risk, a treadmill exercise evaluation is performed before discharge or soon thereafter (1 to 2 weeks) in patients recovering from acute MI. More important than timing of the test are patient selection criteria. Clinical evidence of heart failure, unstable angina, or other limiting medical conditions such as severe obesity, peripheral vascular disease, or ECG abnormalities of atrial fibrillation or left bundle branch block is a contraindication to testing. As noted in Fig. 13-1, however, a large percentage of patients (80%) are eligible for exercise testing early in the course of recovery.[15] The treadmill test not only provides important prognostic information but also serves as a guide for decisions about resumption of physical activity, including occupational tasks, and forms the basis for an exercise prescription. Moreover, patients' confidence in their ability to perform usual activities is often reduced after an MI.[16] The treadmill test and counseling thereafter may enhance patients' perceptions of their capabilities, which in turn may affect their earlier return to normal activities.

Exercise testing elicits various ECG (ST-segment depression and dysrhythmias), hemodynamic (peak blood pressure and workload), and symptomatic (angina, fatigue, and dyspnea) responses.[17] During the test, a 12-lead ECG should be recorded every 2 to 3 minutes, the blood pressure measured, and the patient's clinical status monitored.

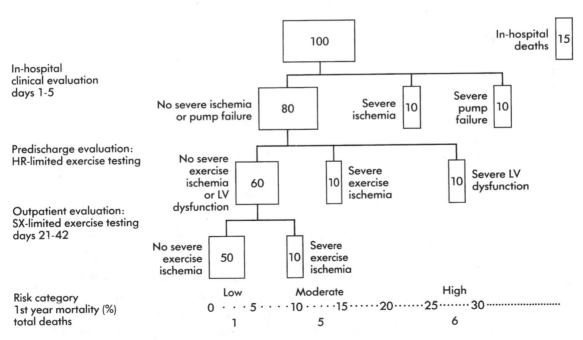

Fig. 13-1   Prognostic stratification of patients into three risk categories (low, moderate, and high) after acute myocardial infarction. The size of each patient subset is indicated by the numbers in boxes. The stratification of patients is based on the extent of myocardial ischemia, and left ventricular *(LV)* dysfunction. *HR,* Heart rate; *SX,* symptom.   (From DeBusk R and others: *N Engl J Med* 314(4):161, 1986.)

Exercise test endpoints include limiting fatigue or dyspnea; severe chest discomfort (3 on a scale of 4); a fall in systolic blood pressure of 10 mm Hg or more on a successive stage; high-grade ventricular dysrhythmias, especially three or more consecutive beats (ventricular tachycardia); and other ECG abnormalities such as second- or third-degree heart block, atrial fibrillation, or rate-related bundle branch block. Although ischemia (ST-segment depression) has prognostic significance, it is not normally an endpoint for terminating a test.

The metabolic equivalent (MET) is used to quantify treadmill workloads, or an individual's physical capacity.[18] Standing quietly at rest requires 1 MET, or 3.5 ml O_2/kg/min. The average patient after an uncomplicated MI can complete about 7 to 8 METs of work on a symptom-limited test performed within the first 3 weeks of recovery.[19] This MET capacity is above the capacity required for almost all occupational and recreational tasks performed by patients. Thus the treadmill workload, in conjunction with other test variables, can be used to determine the safety of a return to various activities. For patients showing prognostically significant treadmill abnormalities (that is, low workload of less than 5 METs, greater than 2 mm ST-segment depression, abnormal fall in systolic blood pressure, or severe angina), further diagnostic testing and evaluation can be prescribed. For the patient who has had an uncomplicated course, a recommendation for moderate exercise can be provided.

On discharge from the hospital, it is recommended that patients be given explicit information about resumption of routine activities. An ideal prescription for activity includes the type, intensity, duration, and frequency of exercise; early warning signs and signals; and the components of an exercise session, which are discussed in the section on exercise training.

Outpatient Recovery Period

The first few weeks after hospital discharge are an important time for the patient and are a critical period in rehabilitation. Not only is this the period of highest mortality rates, but patients are vulnerable to anxiety over the safety of routine activities, and psychologic depression may occur in regard to the future. During this stage of recovery, rehabilitation should address the following:

1. Monitoring the patient's symptoms of angina, dysrhythmias, or severe ventricular dysfunction
2. Allaying psychologic fears and anxieties and fostering a positive outlook
3. Facilitating early return to work and leisure activities based on the patient's clinical status
4. Extending educational efforts with an emphasis on behavior change that was begun in the hospital

It is essential that patients have frequent contact with health care personnel, whether by telephone or face-to-face in a formal rehabilitation setting during this stage of recovery.

If cardiac rehabilitation programs exist within the hospital or community, patients should be enrolled in them immediately after hospital discharge. Such programs provide close medical supervision, which allows prompt identification of complicating medical events, facilitates patients' proper interpretation of new symptoms, and provides reassurance to patients and their families. Specific attention can also be given to the spouse in this difficult time of adjustment. Although patients are given educational instructions during hospitalization, they usually do not have the time for or receptivity to the amount of information provided. The outpatient recovery period is a better time for learning. Therefore adequate provision of information about cardiovascular risk reduction is critical to help patients modify behavior during the outpatient recovery period.

In addition to providing an adequate environment for exercise training, all of the features of rehabilitation can be handled adequately when a patient has access to a formal program. If outpatient cardiac rehabilitation programs do not exist in hospitals or the community, consideration must be given to alternative methods for rehabilitation to address patient needs. Home rehabilitation programs using nurses and other health care personnel to manage by telephone patients with uncomplicated conditions are effective in the outpatient recovery period.[20] The use of group educational classes, frequent contact by the physician's office staff, and transtelephonic ECG monitoring have also proved helpful when formal programs are unavailable.[21]

As patients move beyond 8 to 12 weeks in their recovery process, the focus of rehabilitation shifts from the adoption of health-related behaviors to the maintenance of these behaviors. If patients have been engaged in formal rehabilitation programs, they often graduate to exercising on their own. Before this time, they may return to work and achieve an optimal functional capacity (8 to 9 METs is often a threshold). All rehabilitation personnel must ensure, however, that patients are provided with adequate training to help them maintain the lifestyle change they have adopted in the early weeks after hospital discharge. This training includes knowing what to do if they relapse and smoke a cigarette, discontinue their exercise program, or fail to maintain a low-fat, low-cholesterol diet. Helping patients learn self-motivation skills will provide a better opportunity for success in maintenance.

EXERCISE BENEFITS AND TRAINING

Exercise training has a number of beneficial effects for the patient with CHD who suffers an MI. Exercise aids in the management of hypertension[22] and obesity[23] and may improve glucose tolerance in patients with diabetes mellitus.[24] Moreover, exercise may improve the plasma lipid-lipoprotein profile by increasing levels of high-density lipoprotein (HDL) fraction and HDL subfractions and by reducing triglyceride levels.[25]

Various randomized controlled trials of exercise training in patients with CHD have shown some improvement in psychologic function. Using standard psychologic questionnaires, a reduction in depression and anxiety are seen most commonly in those involved in exercise.[26,27] The psychologic benefits, however, appear to be short-term, with little benefit seen at 1 to 2 years of follow-up.

Although there is evidence that exercise reduces initial CHD events and mortality rates, the benefits of exercise training in reducing morbidity and mortality rates in those with established CHD remain controversial. Two meta-analyses documented a reduction in the mortality rate in randomized controlled trials of cardiac rehabilitation.[28,29] However, these studies were conducted before the more modern and aggressive medical and surgical treatments now being applied to patients after MI. Early intervention has resulted in an extremely low rate of events as noted previously. These interventions have had a far more powerful effect on survival than exercise training. In addition, the reduction in the reinfarction rate as a result of exercise training has shown only modest benefit. Although there is an absence of conclusive evidence regarding the effects of exercise training on longevity, the beneficial effects of improving functional capacity and the independent effects of exercise on other risk factors provide a persuasive case for exercise in cardiac rehabilitation.

Exercise Prescription

To achieve cardiovascular conditioning, an exercise prescription considering the patient's age and past exercise history and preferences should be developed. Exercise prescriptions are normally based on the results of the graded exercise test, taking into account the workload attained, maximum heart rate achieved, blood pressure response, symptoms and signs of ischemia, and dysrhythmias. The level of intensity of exercise should be low enough in the first few weeks of training to prevent undue muscle soreness or orthopedic problems.

A written exercise prescription should include information about the type, intensity, frequency, and duration of exercise and indicate warning signs and symptoms of overexertion. In addition, patients should be aware of various medications that may affect their response to exercise.

Activities that promote cardiovascular conditioning are those involving the large dynamic muscles of the body. Such activities include brisk walking, jogging, stationary and regular cycling, swimming, stair-climbing, and selected others. These types of exercises allow the heart rate to be sustained in an appropriate intensity range to achieve cardiovascular conditioning. Once patients have achieved cardiovascular conditioning through aerobic exercise, consideration may also be given to the benefits of muscle strengthening through weight or resistance training. Data suggest that in selected low-risk patients, these types of exercises may be carried out with safety. Resistance training produces fewer episodes of ischemia, angina, and serious ventricular dysrhythmias compared with maximal exercise testing.[30-32]

Activity intensity

The intensity of exercise is determined by the most recent treadmill test. Although many studies in normal and coronary patients suggest that an ideal training range is an intensity sufficient to increase oxygen consumption to between 70% and 85% of maximum,[33] even patients exercising at 60% of maximum oxygen uptake achieve conditioning benefits.[34]

One can determine the heart rate range for conditioning by adding 70% to 85% of the increment between the resting and maximum heart rates to the resting heart rate. For example, if the resting heart rate is 80 beats/min and the peak exercise heart rate is 180 beats/min, 70% of the maximum heart rate is 150 beats/min (70% of [180 − 80] + 80). When patients count their pulse rates, they should use a 10-second interval and multiply by 6.

If patients have angina or severe ischemia (ST-segment depression of 2 mm or greater) on an exercise test, exercise intensity should be decreased by 10 to 15 beats below the onset of angina or ischemic abnormalities.

Patients should begin an exercise program at the lower-intensity threshold (that is, 60% to 70%) for a few weeks, especially if they have not previously exercised. The patient should watch for signs and symptoms of overexertion; these include excessive fatigue and shortness of breath. Any change in symptoms such as the development of angina pectoris should be reported to the physician.

Another method of monitoring the intensity of exercise is by using the Rating of Perceived Exertion (RPE) Scale or Borg Scale, which corresponds to the patient's level of fatigue with increasing heart rate.[35] This 15-point scale ranging from 6 to 20 is most often used during exercise testing to measure level of comfort. Because the scale corresponds so closely to actual heart rate and is a good indicator of fatigue, it can also be used to monitor exercise training intensity, provided that patients are introduced appropriately to this method.

Activity duration

To achieve cardiovascular benefit, the duration of activity equates to a period of 20 to 40 minutes in which the heart rate is sustained in the target zone. Most exercise sessions begin with a warm-up period of 5 to 10 minutes during which the heart rate gradually increases, 20 to 30 minutes of a conditioning phase in the intensity threshold range, and 5 to 10 minutes of cool down, when the metabolic and circulatory systems gradually return to baseline. A cool-down period is essential. In formal rehabilitation programs, most occurrences of exercise-related ventricular fibrillation have developed during exercise or in the cool-down phase, often in patients who were exercising beyond prescribed intensities.[36,37]

Activity frequency

Exercise must be performed on a regular basis for patients to achieve optimal cardiovascular benefit. Usually 3 to 5 days per week are optimal and may prevent risks of musculoskeletal or orthopedic injuries. If patients are exercising at a lower intensity of effort, five exercise sessions per week are preferable. Scheduling this number of exercising days also helps patients who may have problems complying with exercise sessions.

In helping the patient create an exercise prescription, appropriate consideration needs to be given to the patient's exercise preferences, goals, and personal safety. Often, people begin exercise programs undertaking activities they do not necessarily enjoy and at intensities too high to permit exercise to be enjoyable. Allowing patients to become involved in planning exercise prescriptions often ensures that appropriate choices will be made, which in turn will enhance compliance and satisfaction.

Supervised vs. Unsupervised Exercise

Unfortunately formal rehabilitation programs are available to only 10% to 15% of patients suffering cardiovascular disease.[38] Most programs are located in large metropolitan areas, and the majority are hospital based. These programs provide ongoing supervision of patients during exercise conditioning, facilitate patient education opportunities, and provide medical surveillance of patients' clinical status through contact with health care professionals.

Although the risk of exercise training in cardiovascular patients is extremely low (less than 1 death per 783,927 million patient hours in a supervised setting),[37] serious problems such as ventricular fibrillation and MI do occur. In supervised programs, most cardiac arrest victims are successfully resuscitated, whereas outside this setting, such events may be uniformly lethal.

Because of a lack of availability of programs, however, or for economic and logistical reasons, not all patients choose to attend a formal rehabilitation program. Patients who are not in a program need to be provided with appropriate risk-factor education and exercise guidelines similar to those developed for a structured formal program.

The American College of Physicians and American College of Cardiology,[39,40] among others, have formulated guidelines based on research findings to indicate which patients are at particularly high risk and should require intensive surveillance in cardiac rehabilitation programs. High-risk patients include those:

1. With left ventricular ejection fractions less than 30%
2. With complex dysrhythmias
3. Who demonstrate the appearance of increasing ventricular dysrhythmia with exercise
4. Whose systolic blood pressure falls 15 mm Hg or more during exercise
5. Whose graded exercise tests show ischemia indicated by anginal pain or 2 mm or more of ST-segment depression
6. Whose recent MI was complicated by serious ventricular dysrhythmia
7. Who are survivors of sudden cardiac death

It is estimated by these groups that approximately 25% of patients fall into this high-risk category.[15] For patients who do not exhibit these characteristics, unsupervised activity in the home may be an alternative to a formal rehabilitation program. The efficacy and safety of such programs for patients who have suffered uncomplicated infarctions or who have undergone coronary artery surgery has been documented in the literature.[20,41] Experience with these patients exercising at home indicates that both functional capacity achieved at 6 months after the event and adherence are similar to that of patients enrolled in supervised cardiac rehabilitation programs.[21] The safety of home training is enhanced through patient selection, symptom-limited exercise testing before provision of an exercise prescription, teaching of patients about cautionary symptoms, and use of heart rate monitors during the first few weeks of the program to help patients learn to monitor exercise intensity. Ongoing surveillance of patients is also provided through telephone follow-up by health care professionals such as nurses. In addition, patient adherence to exercise training and risk factors at home can be enhanced through the use of activity logs, self-monitoring charts, contracts, and self-test methods undertaken to determine improvement in exercise conditioning.

According to studies, using nurses to deliver multiple risk-factor interventions to CHD patients in the years after hospitalization may be highly effective.[42] Widely used in managed care settings, such programs offer education and behavioral counseling to patients beginning in the hospital. Patients are followed in the outpatient stage of recovery primarily by telephone contact rather than through face-to-face visits. By managing patients at home, these systems can provide convenient, individualized care at low cost and extend rehabilitation to a larger number of patients. Nurses not only teach patients to manage cardiovascular risk factors such as exercise, smoking, and diet and drug treatment of hyperlipidemia, but also provide initial close surveillance of patients' medical conditions.

MODIFICATION OF LIFESTYLE
Managing Coronary Risk Factors

Although exercise is an important component of rehabilitation, recent evidence suggests that modification of coronary risk factors (for example, smoking, diet, lipids) may help regress atherosclerosis in patients with established CHD.[6,43,44] In addition, modification in these lifestyle behaviors may reduce recurrent MI and CHD deaths.[44] Therefore risk-factor modification becomes a critical component of rehabilitation efforts.

Some programs use a multidisciplinary team to provide education and behavioral counseling about risk-factor management; this team includes exercise physiologists, clinical nutritionists, physical and occupational therapists, and psychologists, whereas in other programs only physicians and nurses are used to provide these services, referring to ancillary personnel when necessary. The high prevalence of coronary-prone lifestyles, maladaptive behavioral responses to environmental stress, and the number of patients exhibiting multiple risk factors warrants the inclusion of a well-developed lifestyle-change program for each patient, whether services are offered by a multidisciplinary team or physicians and nurses. Although education and counseling to help the patient begin lifestyle changes may be difficult during hospitalization, attention must be given to the timing of certain educational interventions to enhance their effectiveness. Early adoption of certain behaviors paves the way for patients to develop self-control strategies for maintaining changes in behavior patterns. The management and timing of modifications in diet, smoking, obesity, stress, alcohol intake, and medications for hyperlipidemia are highlighted in the next section.

Diet

A change in dietary habits may promote a reduction in serum cholesterol and triglyceride levels, blood pressure, and total body weight.[45] Moreover, patients suffering diabetes and CHD may have an improvement in blood glucose levels.[46] Although there is no indication that a change in dietary intake of saturated fat and cholesterol alone has a significant impact on morbidity and mortality rates in patients with established CHD, diet may significantly reduce the need for high doses of lipid-lowering and antihypertensive medications.[47]

In the second report of the National Cholesterol Education Program (NCEP) Adult Treatment Panel (ATP II), dietary therapy remains the first line of treatment for high blood cholesterol. For patients with CHD and a low-density lipoprotein (LDL) cholesterol level greater than 100 mg/100 ml, the NCEP recommends a step-two diet. This diet includes a reduction in total fat to less than 30% of total daily calories (less than 7% saturated fat and 10% polyunsaturated fat and up to 15% from monounsaturated fatty acids); cholesterol is reduced to less than 200 mg/day. Because of the high degree of risk in these patients, an evaluation of their response to this diet is generally made in 6 weeks to 3 months or less. If LDL cholesterol remains elevated after this short intervention period, patients can be treated with lipid-lowering medications.[48] In addition to a diet with low saturated fat and low cholesterol, some patients require sodium restriction for management of hypertension or heart failure, and others may need to limit their total caloric consumption to maintain ideal body weight.

Dieticians and other health care professionals can contribute to the rehabilitation of patients by analyzing dietary patterns and making specific suggestions that allow the diet to remain palatable, affordable, nutritionally adequate, and capable of achieving the desired effects. Ongoing assessment of dietary patterns at follow-up intervals provides a method to determine whether patients are able to maintain suggested dietary changes. Individual or group sessions designed to help patients with label reading, grocery shopping, recipe modification, and cooking techniques also support needed changes in health behavior.

One dietary change important for many cardiac patients is restricting total calories to control obesity. In addition to the deleterious effects obesity has on lipoprotein levels, hypertension, and diabetes, some obese patients may experience great functional impairment and may have cardiac complications such as angina pectoris and heart failure. Good body weight is a body mass index (BMI) (BMI = body weight in kilograms ÷ height in meters, squared) between 19 and 25 kg/m^2 for men and women between 19 and 34 years and between 21 and 27 kg/m^2 for those over 35 years.[49] A BMI greater than 30 kg/m^2 is associated with obesity. Patients who are overweight or obese should embark on calorie restriction and regular exercise. Even 5- to 10-lb weight losses can substantially reduce LDL cholesterol.[50] A reasonable weight-reduction program involves reducing caloric intake by 500 calories/day and achieving a gradual weight loss of 0.5 to 1 lb/week. Severe calorie restriction diets (500 to 800 calories/day) are normally not recommended for most patients.[51]

Serum cholesterol levels

The NCEP ATP II recommends that most patients with CHD should be treated to lower LDL cholesterol to at least 100 mg/100 ml.[48] Although a change in eating habits is the first recommendation for treatment of coronary patients with lipoprotein abnormalities, many coronary patients require drug therapy to achieve this LDL cholesterol level. In the Coronary Drug Project, a trial of 8341 men who had suffered MIs, patients receiving nicotinic acid had a significant reduction in recurrent nonfatal MIs compared with control subjects. The reduction was still apparent 15 years after the trial.[52] Blankenhorn and others[53] also studied 162 men after coronary artery bypass surgery. Treatment included a diet low in fat, saturated fat, and cholesterol and a combination of colestipol and nicotinic acid or a placebo for 2 years. Atherosclerotic progression was significantly less in patients taking drugs vs. placebo. Regression of the disease also occurred in 16.2% of patients treated with colestipol-niacin vs. 2.4% of patients treated with placebo ($p < 0.02$).[53]

The major classes of drugs for treatment of lipid abnormalities include the bile acid sequestrants, colestipol and cholestyramine, nicotinic acid, and the HMG-CoA reductase inhibitors (statins) (for example, fluvastatin, lovastatin, pravastatin, and simvastatin). Others classes of drugs include the fibric acid derivatives and probucol. Although most patients with CHD have elevation of LDL cholesterol, others may have elevations of triglyceride levels or decreases in HDL levels. A 20% to 30% reduction in LDL cholesterol can most often be achieved by a single drug therapy and diet. When needed to manage severe LDL elevations or combined lipoprotein abnormalities, the combination of two drugs at lower doses may increase the drugs' effectiveness, improve a patient's compliance to therapy, and reduce the costs and side effects of these drugs. Health care professionals, especially physicians and nurses working in rehabilitation, have an opportunity to provide education about specific medications, monitor side effects, tailor behavioral strategies to enhance compliance, and monitor ongoing problems with medications.

Cigarette smoking

Continued cigarette smoking is associated with recurrent fatal and nonfatal events in patients with CHD.[54,55] For example, Sparrow and others[56] found an 18.8% mortality rate 6 years after MI in men who quit smoking compared with a 30.4% mortality rate in those who maintained or resumed their smoking status after infarction. Stopping smoking may reduce mortality rates by as much as 50%.[57]

In cardiac patients the rates of cessation after an event such as an MI are approximately 50% when the physician and rehabilitation team are committed to smoking cessation efforts.[58] Recidivism (recurrence) rates may be quite high, however, and some studies have indicated that smokers often resume their habit immediately on hospital discharge.[59]

Interventions for smoking cessation in patients with CHD have primarily consisted of physician advice; few studies have incorporated the use of behavior-modification techniques. Nurses, however, have effectively initiated smoking-cessation counseling during hospitalization, with significant results. In one study,[10] nurses provided a relapse-prevention behavior-counseling program at the bedside accompanied by self-help materials. Follow-up counseling after hospital discharge occurred through monthly telephone calls for 6 months after the MI. At 1 year, the biochemically confirmed cessation rate was 71% in the intervention group compared with 45% in patients treated through usual care, a statistically significant difference.[10] Applying the same approach in a multiple-risk-factor intervention program beginning in the hospital more recently resulted in a similar outcome at 1 year.[42]

Because smoking may be the single most important lifestyle change to reduce subsequent morbidity and mortality rates, rehabilitation personnel should give significant attention to smoking cessation in the hospital. Multicomponent strategies incorporating behavioral techniques, strong physician advice, and the use of nicotine replacement therapy (that is, nicotinic gum or nicotine patch) appear to achieve greater long-term cessation rates.

Stress

Many patients feel that stress, often work-related, is an important factor in causing their event. Although controversy still exists over the link among stress, type A behavior, and CHD, with both positive and negative findings from major research studies,[60] excessive stress generally makes people feel bad. The type A behavior pattern has been the most extensively researched variable relevant to CHD. Characterized by excessive competitive drive and impatience, the component of type A that appears to be most strongly linked to CHD is hostility or anger.[61,62] It appears that other type A characteristics are of lesser importance.

A few intervention strategies have been successful in modifying type A behavior, including hostility, in patients with CHD. Such interventions have incorporated combined exercise and cognitive behavioral programs and stress-management courses.[63,64] Further study is needed, however, to determine the effect of behavioral strategies on the reduction of hostility in patients with established CHD and the long-term results of these interventions. Simple relaxation tapes that incorporate deep breathing and deep muscle relaxation exercises if used on a regular basis may also produce the desired effect of making people feel better.[65] For some, this technique may prove as useful as more elaborate programs.

Because excessive stress and underlying hostility often make people feel uncomfortable, it is important that rehabilitation personnel screen for these problems. Standard instruments such as the Cook-Medley Hostility Scale[66] or the Structured Type A Interview[63] can be used to detect such findings. In addition, asking patients directly by interview or questionnaire to rate how stressed or angry they feel may provide insight into the need for intervention. Patients may benefit from individual or group stress-management programs, counseling with a therapist, biofeedback, and other relaxation and communication techniques.

Alcohol

Although alcohol use is not an independent risk factor for CHD, it can cause major problems and lead to more difficulty with compliance with other lifestyle modifications if consumption rates are high. In patients suffering CHD, alcohol may produce atrial and ventricular dysrhythmias and impaired left ventricular functioning.[67] Alcohol in moderate doses may exert a positive effect on raising the HDL cholesterol subfraction[68]; however, heavy consumption is associated with adverse lipid and lipoprotein levels.[69] Moreover, heavy consumption of alcohol (more than 3 drinks/day) may increase systolic and diastolic blood pressures.[70] Because of its negative effect on blood cholesterol levels and blood pressure in addition to other potential health problems, the U.S. Departments of Agriculture and Health and Human Services recommend no more than 2 drinks/day for men or 1 drink/day for women.[51]

About 8% to 10% of adults consider themselves alcoholic, and many more may drink heavy amounts of alcohol socially. Rehabilitation personnel have the ability to adequately assess alcohol abuse by using instruments such as the CAGE questionnaire[71] or the Michigan Alcoholism Screening Test.[72] Patients who receive a firm, unequivocal message about the importance of treatment and who have the support of families are more likely to seek help. Adequate referral is appropriate to enhance psychosocial and physical recovery.

OTHER REHABILITATION ISSUES
Sexual Activity

Another issue for coronary patients after an MI or coronary artery surgery is resumption of sexual activity. Although physicians, nurses, and other rehabilitation personnel view sexual activity as an important topic of discussion, the subject continues to be neglected, leaving patients with many fears and anxieties. A study conducted in the 1980s indicates that even though patients may not be sexually active, education about this topic is of importance to them.[73]

The physiologic demands of sexual intercourse in coronary patients are relatively modest, with the average heart rate during sexual intercourse being approximately 117 beats/min.[74] If patients have undergone predischarge treadmill testing after MIs and achieved similar heart rates without significant abnormalities, they should be cleared for resumption of sexual activity at this time. If patients suffer angina pectoris, resumption may be delayed a few weeks, and appropriate medications, such as long-acting nitrates, may be prescribed to be taken before intercourse. Prophylactic nitroglycerin may also be indicated for patients who experience angina during sexual intercourse.

In counseling, patients should be told about the physiologic effects of sexual activity on the heart, provided with specific information about timing and resumption, made aware of warning signs and symptoms that may occur during sexual activity, and appropriately referred for sexual problems, which may be long-standing. The spouse or partner who may have many different concerns and issues should also be present for the educational session.

Sexual problems are common after an MI or coronary artery surgery. The frequency of sexual intercourse, for example, may decrease by 24% to 75% in middle-aged men after MIs.[75] The most commonly cited reasons for dysfunction are symptoms of fatigue and angina, psychologic fears that the MI has damaged the heart or fear of another MI, and medications such as β-blocking agents and diuretics that cause sexual impairment.[76] Although cardiac rehabilitation programs improve functional capacity, it is unclear whether exercise has a positive impact on sexual functioning, including interest and desire. It is known, however, that failure by health care professionals to discuss this topic may lead to sexual dysfunction.[77]

Because patients may be reluctant to initiate discussion about this subject, it is important that rehabilitation team members take an adequate sexual history, provide counseling, and refer patients to physicians, psychologists, or sexual therapists for problems such as impotence or loss of libido.

Return to Work

Although not all patients choose to go back to work after an MI or coronary artery surgery, for many patients returning to normal activities, including work, is important. In reported studies, between 49% and 93% of patients return to work after MI.[78,79] Factors that influence the success and timing of return to work include physical, psychosocial, demographic, and clinical characteristics.[80,81] For example, individuals aged 55 to 65 years are less likely than younger patients to return to work after MI or coronary artery surgery.[82] Patients unemployed in the 3 months before the event are less likely to return, which may reflect the unemployed patient's poor health status.[83] A common misconception is that blue-collar workers with CHD cannot return to work because of the physical demands of their jobs.[84] However, heavy labor in this country is performed by less than 20% of workers, many of whom are younger. Thus the percentage of people with CHD who perform heavy labor is quite small.

Rehabilitation team members can play an instrumental role in influencing the success and timing of patients' return to work. Enhancing patients' perceptions about their health, physical capacity, and prognosis may influence their decision about returning to work. Moreover, working closely with physicians to promote their advice may help.

Perceived health status after MI and coronary artery surgery has actually correlated with return to work independent of actual health status.[79,85] Although patients may perceive that they have a poor prognosis, in reality most patients have a good prognosis because of the technologic advances over the past decade, including thrombolytic therapy. Patients are more likely to return to work if they are given a treadmill test early in the course of recovery to determine the prognosis, explicit advice about outcome, and counseling to alleviate misconceptions about occupational tasks. Rehabilitation personnel are in a unique position to provide this information because they are often involved in conducting treadmill testing and providing or reinforcing the counseling thereafter.

A physician's advice can strongly influence the success and timing of reemployment. In the past, the physician's perceptions about a patient's return to work was very subjective and often incorrect. In some studies, for example, physicians overestimated the patient's likelihood of a recurrent cardiac event, including death, in the 6 months after infarction. Physicians estimated the likelihood of an event to be 20%, but the actual event rate was 3.5%.[86] Patients are influenced by the advice of their physician. If the physician's views are pessimistic or if patients do not receive explicit information, they rarely resume activities quickly. Encouraging physicians to provide explicit information and to use prognostic criteria to help make decisions is important to the patient's recovery. In a randomized clinical trial, patients whose physicians provided a treadmill test and explicit instructions about results, prognosis, and timing of return to work and who received reinforcement of these instructions from rehabilitation staff members returned to work at a median of 51 days compared with 75 days in patients receiving usual care.[86] Shortening the time of return in this case provided a substantial cost saving to the patient and employer.

SUMMARY

The goals of rehabilitation are to improve the quality of life for the patient with CHD by eliminating physical or psychologic barriers that may impede recovery. Rehabilitation has advanced over the past 2 to 3 decades as new information has been acquired about the safety of early ambulation, exercise testing, and exercise training in this population. Modern concepts of cardiac rehabilitation now emphasize risk stratification to individualize patient management, early progressive exercise programs, and education and counseling regarding the psychologic and vocational aspects of recovery. In addition, new behavioral strategies provide support for the modification of coronary risk factors in these patients. The future of rehabilitation lies in developing new methods for the expansion of services to all patients, for it is only when *all* patients are provided with ways to enhance their quality of life that the goals of this field will have been met.

REFERENCES

1. Roberts WC, Muja M: The frequency and significance of coronary arterial thrombi and other observations in fatal myocardial infarction, *Am J Med* 52:425, 1972.
2. Markis JE and others: Myocardial salvage after intracoronary thrombolysis with streptokinase in acute myocardial infarction, *N Engl J Med* 305:777, 1981.
3. DeBusk RF and others: Identification and treatment of low-risk patients after acute myocardial infarction and coronary-artery bypass graft surgery, *N Engl J Med* 314(4):161, 1986.
4. Ades PA, Grunvald MH: Cardiopulmonary exercise testing before and after conditioning in older coronary patients, *Am Heart J* 120(3):585, 1990.
5. Hermanson B and others: Beneficial six-year outcome of smoking cessation in older men and women with coronary artery disease: results from the CASS registry, *N Engl J Med* 319:1365, 1988.
6. Haskell WL and others: Effects of intensive multiple risk factor reduction on coronary atherosclerosis and clinical cardiac events in men

and women with coronary artery disease: The Stanford Coronary Risk Intervention Project (SCRIP), *Circulation* 89:975, 1994.
7. American Association of Cardiopulmonary Rehabilitation: *Standards and guidelines for cardiac rehabilitation,* Champaign, Ill, 1994, Human Kinetics.
8. Conventino V and others: Cardiovascular responses to exercise in middle-aged men after 10 days of bed rest, *Circulation* 65:134, 1982.
9. Miller RR and others: Prevention of lower extremity venous thrombosis by early mobilization, *Ann Intern Med* 84:700, 1976.
10. Taylor CB and others: Smoking cessation after acute myocardial infarction: effects of nurse-managed intervention, *Ann Intern Med* 113:118, 1990.
11. Hentinen M: Need for instruction and support of wives of patients with myocardial infarction, *J Adv Nurs* 8:519, 1983.
12. Bramwell L: Wives' experiences in the support role after husband's first myocardial infarction, *Heart Lung* 15:578, 1986.
13. Kübler-Ross E: *On death and dying,* New York, 1969, Macmillan.
14. The Multicenter Post-Infarction Group: Risk stratification and survival after myocardial infarction, *N Engl J Med* 309:738, 1983.
15. DeBusk RF and others: Stepwise-risk stratification soon after myocardial infarction, *Am J Cardiol* 52:1161, 1983.
16. Ewart CK and others: The effects of early post infarction exercise testing on self perception and subsequent physical activity, *Am J Cardiol* 51:1076, 1983.
17. DeBusk RF: Specialized testing after recent myocardial infarction, *Ann Intern Med* 110:470, 1989.
18. Schlant RC: Guidelines for exercise testing: a report of the American College of Cardiology/American Heart Association Subcommittee of Exercise Testing, *J Am Coll Cardiol* 8:725, 1986.
19. Haskell WL, DeBusk RF: Cardiovascular responses to repeated treadmill exercise testing soon after myocardial infarction, *Circulation* 60:1247, 1979.
20. DeBusk RF and others: Medically directed at-home rehabilitation soon after clinically uncomplicated myocardial infarction: a new model for patient care, *Am J Cardiol* 57:446, 1986.
21. Miller NH and others: Home versus group training for increasing functional capacity after myocardial infarction, *Circulation* 70:645, 1984.
22. National High Blood Pressure Education Program, National Heart, Lung and Blood Institute: Working Group Report on Primary Prevention of Hypertension, *Arch Intern Med* 153:186, 1993.
23. Bjorntorp P: Exercise in the treatment of obesity, *Clin Endocrinol Metab* 5:431, 1976.
24. Pederson O and others: Increased insulin receptors after exercise in patients with insulin-dependent diabetes mellitus, *N Engl J Med* 302:886, 1980.
25. Goldberg L and others: The effects of exercise training on plasma lipids and lipoprotein levels, *Med Clin North Am* 69:41, 1985.
26. Stern JJ and others: Life adjustment post myocardial infarction: determining predictive variables, *Arch Intern Med* 137:1680, 1977.
27. Taylor CB and others: The effects of exercise training programs on psychosocial improvement in uncomplicated postmyocardial infarction patients, *J Psychosom Res* 30:581, 1986.
28. O'Connor GT and others: An overview of randomized trials of rehabilitation with exercise after myocardial infarction, *Circulation* 80:234, 1989.
29. Oldridge NB and others: Cardiac rehabilitation after myocardial infarction: combined experience of randomized clinical trials, *JAMA* 260:945, 1988.
30. Wilke NA and others: Transfer effect of upper extremity training to weight carrying in men with ischemic heart disease, *J Cardiopulmonary Rehabil* 11:365, 1991.
31. Sparling PB and others: Strength training in a cardiac rehabilitation program: a six month followup, *Arch Phys Med Rehabil* 71:148, 1990.

32. Stewart KJ and others: Three year participation in circuit weight training improves muscular strength and self-efficacy in cardiac patients, *J Cardiopulmonary Rehabil* 8:292, 1988.

33. American College of Sports Medicine: *Guidelines for graded exercise testing and exercise prescription*, Philadelphia, 1980, Lea & Febiger.

34. Pollock ML and others: *Exercise prescription for rehabilitation of the cardiac patient*. In Pollock ML, Schmidt DH, editors: *Heart disease and rehabilitation*, New York, 1979, Wiley & Sons.

35. Borg G: Physical performance and perceived exertion: Lund, Sweden, *Gleereys* 1:63, 1962.

36. Cobb LA and others: At risk for sudden death in patients with coronary heart disease, *J Am Coll Cardiol* 7:215, 1986.

37. Van Kamp SP, Peterson RA: Cardiovascular complications of outpatient cardiac rehabilitation programs, *JAMA* 256:1160, 1986.

38. Leon AS and others: Position paper of the American Association of Cardiovascular and Pulmonary Rehabilitation: Scientific evidence of the value of cardiac rehabilitation services with emphasis on patients following myocardial infarction—exercise conditioning component, *J Cardiopulmonary Rehabil* 10:79, 1990.

39. American College of Physicians: Position paper on cardiac rehabilitation services, *Ann Intern Med* 109:671, 1988.

40. Parmley WW: President's page: American College of Cardiology position report on cardiac rehabilitation, *J Am Coll Cardiol* 7:451, 1986.

41. Stevens R, Hansen P: Comparison of supervised and unsupervised exercise training after coronary bypass surgery, *Am J Cardiol* 53:1525, 1983.

42. DeBusk RF and others: A case management system for coronary risk factor modification after acute myocardial infarction, *Ann Intern Med* 120:721, 1994.

43. Watts GF and others: Effects on coronary artery disease of lipid lowering diet, or diet plus cholestyramine in the St Thomas' Atherosclerosis Regression Study (STARS), *Lancet* 339:563, 1992.

44. Pitt B and others: Pravastatin limitations of atherosclerosis in the coronary arteries (PLAC 1): beneficial effects of pravastatin on cardiovascular events, *J Am Coll Cardiol* 23:131A, 1994.

45. Conner WE, Conner SL: *The dietary treatment of hypercholesterolemia*. In Havel RJ, editor: *The Medical Clinics of North America*, Philadelphia, 1982, Saunders.

46. Jensen MD: The roles of diet and exercise in the management of patients with insulin dependent diabetes, *Mayo Clin Proc* 61:813, 1986.

47. Superko RH: The role of diet, exercise, and medication in blood lipid management of cardiac patients, *Phys Sports Med* 16:65, 1988.

48. National Cholesterol Education Program: Report of the National Cholesterol Education Program—second report of the Expert Panel on Detection, Evaluation, and Treatment of High Blood Cholesterol in Adults, *JAMA* 269:3015, 1993.

49. Bray GA: Pathophysiology of obesity, *Am J Clin Nutr* 55:4885, 1992.

50. Gordon DJ and others: Dietary determinants of plasma cholesterol change in the recruitment phase of the Lipid Research Clinics Primary Prevention Trial, *Arteriosclerosis* 2:537, 1982.

51. Second Report of the Expert Panel on Detection, Evaluation, and Treatment of High Blood Cholesterol in Adults; National Cholesterol Education Program, National Institutes of Health; National Heart, Lung, and Blood Institute, II-22, 1993.

52. Canner PL and others: Fifteen year mortality in Coronary Drug Project patients: long-term benefit with niacin, *J Am Coll Cardiol* 8:1245, 1986.

53. Blankenhorn DH and others: Beneficial effects of combined colestipol-niacin therapy on coronary atherosclerosis and coronary venous bypass grafts, *JAMA* 257:3233, 1987.

54. Aberg A and others: Cessation of smoking after myocardial infarction: effects on mortality after 20 years, *Br Heart J* 49:416, 1983.

55. Rosenberg L and others: The risk of myocardial infarction after quitting smoking in men under 55 years of age, *N Engl J Med* 313:1511, 1985.

56. Sparrow D and others: The influence of cigarette smoking on prognosis after a first myocardial infarction, *J Chronic Dis* 31:425, 1978.

57. Mulcahy R: Influence of cigarette smoking on morbidity and mortality after myocardial infarction, *Br Heart J* 49:410, 1983.

58. Schwartz JL: *Review and evaluation of smoking cessation methods: the United States and Canada, 1978-1985, Division of Cancer Prevention and Control, National Cancer Institute*, NIH Publication No 87-2940, 1987.

59. Baile WF and others: Rapid resumption of cigarette smoking following myocardial infarction: inverse relation to MI severity, *Addict Behav* 7:373, 1982.

60. Matthews KA, Haynes SG: Type A behavior pattern and coronary disease risk: update and critical evaluation, *Am J Epidemiol* 123:923, 1986.

61. Matthews KA and others: Competitive drive, pattern A and coronary heart disease: a further analysis of some data from the Western Collaborative Group Study, *J Chronic Dis* 30:489, 1977.

62. Hecker MHL and others: Coronary-prone behaviors in the Western Collaborative Group Study, *Psychosomatic Med* 2:153, 1988.

63. Friedman M and others: Alteration of type A behavior and its effects on cardiac recurrences in post myocardial infarction patients: summary results of the Recurrent Coronary Prevention Project, *Am Heart J* 112:653, 1986.

64. Schaeffer MA and others: Effects of occupational based behavioral counseling and exercise interventions on type A components and cardiovascular reactivity, *J Cardiopulmonary Rehabil* 10:371, 1988.

65. Benson H: *Beyond the relaxation response*, New York, 1985, Berkley.

66. Cook WW, Medley DM: Proposed hostility and pharisaic virtue scales for the M.M.P.I., *J Appl Psychol* 38:414, 1954.

67. Davidson DM: Cardiovascular effects of alcohol, *West J Med* 151:430, 1989.

68. Haskell WL and others: The effect of cessation and resumption of moderate alcohol intake on serum high-density-lipoprotein subfractions: a controlled study, *N Engl J Med* 310:805, 1984.

69. Leiber CS: To drink or not to drink? *N Engl J Med* 310:846, 1984.

70. Klatsky AL and others: Alcohol consumption and blood pressure: Kaiser-Permanente multiphasic health examination data, *N Engl J Med* 296:1194, 1977.

71. Ewing JA: Detecting alcoholism: the CAGE questionnaire, *JAMA* 252:1905, 1984.

72. Selzer ML: The Michigan Alcoholism Screening Test: the quest for a new diagnostic instrument, *Am J Psychiatr* 127:1653, 1971.

73. Baggs JG, Karch AM: Sexual counseling of women with coronary heart disease, *Heart Lung* 16:154, 1987.

74. Hellerstein HK, Friedman EH: Sexual activity and the post-coronary patient, *J Cardiac Rehabil* 3:43, 1972.

75. Mann S and others: The effects of myocardial infarction on sexual activity, *J Cardiac Rehabil* 1:187, 1981.

76. Kolman PB: Sexual dysfunction in the postmyocardial infarction patient, *J Cardiac Rehabil* 4:334, 1984.

77. Papadopoulos C and others: Myocardial infarction and sexual activity of the female patient, *Arch Intern Med* 143:1528, 1983.

78. Cay EL and others: Return to work after a heart attack, *J Psychosom Res* 17:231, 1973.

79. Garrity TF: Vocational adjustment after first myocardial infarction: comparative assessment of several variables suggested in the literature, *Soc Sci Med* 7:705, 1973.

80. Smith GR, O'Rourke DF: Return to work after myocardial infarction, *JAMA* 259:1673, 1988.

81. Nagle R and others: Factors influencing return to work after myocardial infarction, *Lancet* 2:454, 1971.

82. Shapiro S and others: Return to work after first myocardial infarction, *Arch Environ Health* 24:17, 1972.

83. Hammermeister KE and others: Effect of surgical versus medical therapy on return to work in patients with coronary artery disease, *Am J Cardiol* 44:105, 1979.

84. Weinblatt E and others: Return to work and work status following first myocardial infarction, *Am J Public Health* 2:169, 1966.

85. Gundle NJ and others: Psychosocial outcome after coronary artery surgery: a randomized clinical trial, *Am J Psychiatr* 137:1591, 1980.

86. Dennis CA and others: Early return to work after uncomplicated myocardial infarction: results of a randomized trial, *JAMA* 260:214, 1988.

14

Cardiovascular Drugs

Ruth Stanley

The drugs available to treat cardiovascular disease continue to increase in number and complexity. As more is learned about the physiology and pathophysiology of cardiovascular disorders, new strategies for drug therapy are developed. At present, however, few drugs are exact, precise, and specific in their action. Therefore much of drug therapy remains an art in which guidelines must be specifically tailored to meet individual needs. This chapter presents selected pharmacologic aspects of drugs used to treat cardiovascular disorders. Although some overlap is evident, the agents are grouped in general classifications according to their pharmacologic action.

CLINICAL PHARMACOKINETICS[1]

A drug exerts its pharmacologic effects when it reaches a critical concentration at a specific site of action. Factors that determine drug concentration include the processes of drug absorption, distribution, metabolism, and elimination. *Pharmacokinetics,* the quantitative study of these processes, provides a rational basis to determine the method of administration, dose strength, and dose interval.

Elimination half-life ($t_{1/2}$) is an important concept and refers to the amount of time required for the serum concentration of a given drug to decline by 50%. Elimination half-life can be altered by various disease states (for example, heart failure, renal failure, liver insufficiency) as well as concomitant drug therapy. With repeated dosing of a given drug, serum blood levels rise until equilibrium is established between the dose administered and the amount eliminated (Fig. 14-1). It normally takes five half-lives to reach steady state. Steady state can be achieved more rapidly in drugs with a long half-life if loading doses are used. Because loading doses allow a desired concentration to be achieved quickly, these large doses are preferred in acute situations in which a quick onset is necessary (for example, procainamide in ventricular tachycardia). A maintenance dose is the amount of drug administered at a given time interval to maintain a steady-state serum level.

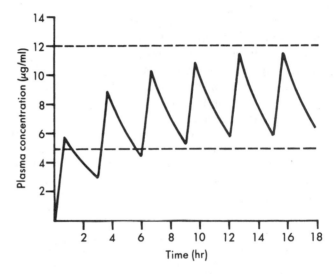

Fig. 14-1 Plasma concentration of a hypothetic drug administered at dosage intervals equal to an elimination half-life of 3 hours. Five half-lives are required to reach a steady-state level. A hypothetic range of effective plasma concentrations is illustrated by hash lines.

These concepts are important when administering antidysrhythmics or digoxin and when monitoring cardiac patients. These drugs have a therapeutic range of serum levels that produce the desired clinical effects. Concentrations above this range are likely to produce toxicity, whereas those below it are ineffective. In Fig. 14-1, the dotted lines enclose the therapeutic range of 5 to 12 mcg/ml. The trough level is 5 mcg/ml, or the lowest effective serum concentration, and the peak level is 12 mcg/ml.

Plasma drug concentrations are often used to guide therapy, but this method must be interpreted and used according to individual clinical situations. Plasma drug concentrations are especially useful in identifying toxic concentrations and determining an apparent drug failure caused by unexpectedly low plasma levels. However, for a given patient, drug toxicity may occur at a drug concentration usually considered to be therapeutic, and a subtherapeutic effect may occur at a drug concentration considered toxic. In addition, measurement of plasma drug concentration does not consider the contribution of metabolites or changes in protein binding that may contribute to the overall drug effect. Therefore tests to determine plasma drug concentrations must be approached as any other laboratory test; that is, the entire clinical picture of the patient must be considered.

A number of common variables modify therapy by affecting the relationship between drug dose and drug effects. These variables include age, weight, gender, nature of heart disease, route of drug administration, patient tolerance, physiologic milieu (for example, acid-base balance, electrolyte levels, hypoxia), and concurrent medication use. Antihypertensive, antianginal, diuretic, and vasodilating agents cannot be administered based on serum blood levels. As a result, these agents are monitored by objective measures (for example, hypotensive response, duration of action, and reduction in anginal attacks) and subjective measures (for example, side effects and quality of life). Thus the pharmacodynamic profile (effect of the drug in the body) is more important than the pharmacokinetic properties (half-life) for many classes of cardiovascular drugs. Appropriate use of these agents requires an accurate assessment of the drug's effect and the hemodynamic response to that effect.

CLINICAL PHARMACOLOGY[2,3]

The parasympathetic and sympathetic divisions of the autonomic nervous system control and regulate the cardiovascular system. The major neurotransmitter of the parasympathetic system is *acetylcholine*. The vagus nerve provides dense innervation to the heart, where cholinergic tone dominates sympathetic tone when the body is at rest. Stimulation of the parasympathetic system results in a decrease in heart rate and cardiac conduction. No parasympathetic innervation to the vasculature exists, although the vessels contain receptors and respond to locally released factors.

The major end-organ neurotransmitter of the sympathetic system is *norepinephrine*. Adrenergic receptors are classified into the two major subgroups of α receptors and β receptors. This classification is based on the differences in the physiologic actions and relative potency of the various catecholamines (for example, norepinephrine, epinephrine, isoproterenol). For the cardiovascular system, stimulation of α receptors located in the heart and smooth muscle of arterioles results in increased myocardial contractility and arteriolar vasoconstriction. β Receptors are located in the heart, arterioles (primarily skeletal muscle arterioles), and lungs. In the heart, stimulation of β receptors increases heart rate, contractility, and conduction velocity. β-Receptor stimulation of the arterioles and lungs results in dilatation.

Subclassification of α-Adrenergic Receptors

The α-adrenergic receptors have also been subclassified in α_1 and α_2 receptors, but the subclassification is not analogous to that of β receptors.

As depicted in Fig. 14-2, the adrenergic neural terminal is composed of the presynaptic sympathetic neuron, synaptic cleft, and postsynaptic effector cell. α Receptors located in the effector cell are termed *postsynaptic* or α_1 *receptors,* whereas receptors located on the nerve terminal are called *presynaptic* or α_2 *receptors.*

Stimulation of the α_1 (postsynaptic) receptors mimics the effects of norepinephrine on the effector cell, whereas inhibition of the α_1 receptor antagonizes these effects. On the other hand, the α_2 receptor serves an autoregulatory function. Stimulation of the α_2 (presynaptic) receptor inhibits the release of norepinephrine from the nerve terminal, thus diminishing norepinephrine's effects on the effector cell. Inhibition of the α_2 receptor stimulates the release of norepinephrine.

Stimulation of central α_2 adrenoreceptors in the ventrolateral medulla results in a reduction of sympathetic outflow to the periphery and is manifested clinically as a decrease in arterial blood pressure with concomitant bradycardia. In addition, central α_2 adrenoreceptor stimulation may enhance parasympathetic tone.

Finally, α receptors are present in small amounts in the coronary vasculature. The exact role of these receptors in the regulation of coronary blood flow is unclear. Stimulation of these receptors produces coronary artery vasoconstriction, thus reducing coronary blood flow. There is some evidence indicating that certain pathologic conditions (for example, coronary artery disease, angina, coronary artery spasm) may be complicated by α-mediated vasoconstriction, but there is no conclusive documentation that treatment patterns should be altered.

Subclassification of β-Adrenergic Receptors

The response of β-adrenergic stimulation or inhibition may be further subclassified into β_1 and β_2 action. This division is not complete because the activity of drugs on β_1 and β_2 receptors overlaps. However, differences in the relative potency of drugs to stimulate (agonist activity) or inhibit (antagonist activity) either β-receptor subtype allows more selective use of drugs.

The postsynaptic β_1 receptors are found primarily in the heart, and stimulation results in increased force and rate of contraction. In addition, atrioventricular (AV) nodal conduction time and refractoriness are decreased, which produces accelerated conduction of impulses through the myocardium. β_1 Receptors can be stimulated by isoproterenol, epinephrine, or norepinephrine.

Postsynaptic β_2 receptors predominate in the blood vessels and lungs. Stimulation by isoproterenol or epinephrine results in dilated arterioles and bronchioles. Presynaptic β_2 receptors mediate the positive feedback mechanism and enhance sympathetic activity at the neuronal synapse. These

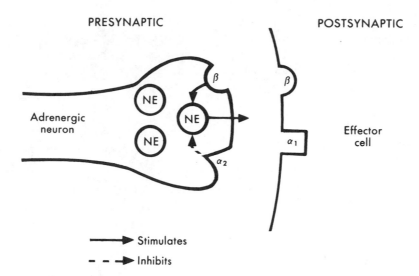

PRESYNAPTIC   POSTSYNAPTIC

→ Stimulates

- - → Inhibits

Fig. 14-2 Diagram of the adrenergic nerve terminal illustrating α_1-, α_2-, and β-adrenergic receptors in presynaptic and postsynaptic positions. Effector cell contains α_1- and β-adrenergic receptors, which interact with norepinephrine *(NE)* to produce end-organ effects. The presynaptic α_2- and β-adrenergic receptors interact with norepinephrine to stimulate (β receptor) or inhibit (α_2 receptor) further norepinephrine release.

presynaptic receptors are more sensitive to epinephrine than to norepinephrine; thus the role of these receptors in maintaining vascular tone is unclear.

INOTROPES[3-15]
Digitalis Glycosides

Digitalis preparations are the oldest and most widely used drugs in the treatment of heart disease. Many forms are available, but digoxin is the agent most often used.

Cardiovascular actions

Digitalis increases myocardial contractility, a positive inotropic effect. The mechanism by which digitalis increases myocardial contractility involves an increase in intracellular calcium levels. By inhibiting the sodium-potassium membrane pump, digitalis increases the intracellular pool of calcium ions available for excitation-contraction coupling. Catecholamines (epinephrine, norepinephrine) also increase myocardial contractility, but their mechanism of action is different from that of digitalis, as evidenced by the finding that the effects of digitalis on contractility are not inhibited by β-adrenergic blocking drugs.

The positive inotropic effects of digitalis are evident in normal and failing hearts; however, the net effect on myocardial oxygen consumption differs in these two conditions. Digitalis increases oxygen consumption in the normal, non-failing ventricle, whereas in the failing myocardium, its net effect is to decrease ventricular size and reduce wall tension, changes that decrease myocardial oxygen consumption. An additional factor that decreases myocardial oxygen consumption is the decrease in heart rate produced by digitalis, particularly in patients with atrial fibrillation.

Digitalis produces cardiac electrophysiologic effects by direct cellular actions and by indirect actions mediated through the parasympathetic nervous system. One major clinically important antidysrhythmic action of digitalis is prolongation of AV nodal refractoriness and conduction time. Digitalis shortens atrial and ventricular refractoriness and depresses normal automaticity in Purkinje fibers. These actions may produce abnormal forms of automaticity.

Digitalis has actions on the central and autonomic nervous systems. Through direct vascular and sympathetic neural actions, digitalis produces vasoconstriction. In patients treated with digitalis for heart failure, the increased cardiac output (CO) and reflex vasodilatation usually outweigh the direct effects of vasoconstriction.

Clinical uses

1. Digoxin is the most frequently used drug in this class of agents. Although it is effective in patients with congestive heart failure (CHF) and tachydysrhythmias, digoxin therapy has been questioned in patients with heart failure who have normal sinus rhythm. Patients more likely to have sustained improvements in cardiac function with chronic digoxin use typically exhibit the following characteristics: dilated and failing ventricles, impaired systolic function (ejection fraction of less than

TABLE 14-1 Digoxin Elimination

Creatinine Clearance	Approximate Half-Life	Approximate Time to Reach 90% Steady State
≤5 ml/min	3.2 days	13 days
6-15 ml/min	3.0 days	12 days
16-35 ml/min	2.5 days	10 days
36-60 ml/min	2.0 days	8 days
≥61 ml/min	1.6 days	6 days

TABLE 14-2 Factors That Affect Digoxin Serum Levels

Factor	Serum Level
Renal disease	Increased
Hepatic disease	Increased
Severe congestive heart failure	Increased
Malabsorption	Decreased
DRUG INTERACTIONS	
Quinidine	Increased
Verapamil	Increased
Amiodarone	Increased
Spironolactone	Increased
Antacids	Decreased
Kaolin-pectin preparations	Decreased
Bile acid–binding resins	Decreased

35%), a gallop of the third heart sound, and atrial enlargement. Patients with elevated filling pressures and preserved systolic function or with hypertrophic cardiomyopathy should receive digoxin only under careful supervision. See references 9-11 for a review of the literature on this subject.

2. As an antidysrhythmic agent, digoxin is effective in treating paroxysmal supraventricular tachycardia (PSVT) and in controlling ventricular rate in atrial fibrillation or atrial flutter.

Dosage and administration (Tables 14-1 and 14-2 and box)

1. The half-life of digoxin is approximately 36 hours in patients with normal renal function. The half-life increases as renal function declines and as patients require less frequent dosing to achieve therapeutic serum concentrations (for example, 0.125 mg every other day rather than 0.125 mg every day). Digoxin has a long half-life, and loading doses are indicated only for treatment of dysrhythmias. The acute inotropic effects of digoxin are minimal, so loading doses provide no therapeutic advantage and increase the risk for toxicity. Therapeutic serum concentrations are 0.5 to 2.0 ng/ml.

2. The loading dose is 0.25 mg intravenously slowly and then 0.25 mg intravenously every 6 hours to a total loading dose of 1.0 to 1.5 mg. Loading doses may also be given orally.

3. The maintenance dosage is 0.125 to 0.50 mg orally or intravenously daily. The dosage is adjusted at 1- to 2-week intervals to achieve the desired serum level and therapeutic response.

4. For accurate serum levels, the patient should be at steady state if no loading dose was given. The digoxin level should be determined 8 to 24 hours after administration or immediately before the next dose. Level analysis performed less than 6 to 8 hours after a dose is higher than the actual serum steady-state level and is useless in optimizing therapy.

5. The dosage of digoxin should be halved when quinidine, verapamil, or amiodarone are given concurrently.

FACTORS THAT INCREASE MYOCARDIAL SENSITIVITY TO DIGOXIN

Severe congestive heart failure	Pulmonary heart disease
Hypothyroidism	Myocardial ischemia
Hypokalemia	Myocardial infarction
Hypomagnesemia	Myocarditis
Hypercalcemia	Cardiomyopathies
	Valvular lesions

All of these drugs can double the serum level of digoxin.

6. Generic preparations of digoxin should be discouraged. Lanoxin products have established bioavailability and absorption patterns and should be used when possible. Lanoxin is available as tablets, caplets, an elixir, and an injection for parenteral use.

7. The blood pressure, heart rate, electrocardiogram (ECG), signs and symptoms of disease state, renal function, electrolyte levels, and serum blood levels are monitored.

Cautions and side effects (see box)

1. Cardiac dysrhythmias are the first sign of digoxin toxicity in more than 50% of toxic patients. If toxicity is suspected, the drug should be stopped, the serum digoxin and electrolyte levels determined, and an ECG obtained. Digoxin immune FAB (Digibind) is indicated for the treatment of potentially lethal digoxin intoxication (for example, severe ventricular dysrhythmias and

DIGOXIN SIDE EFFECTS

Cardiac (70% to 90%)*

Changes in rhythm (effects on cardiac automaticity and conduction)
   Premature ventricular contractions, coupled rhythm (bigeminy)
   Ventricular tachycardia; precursor of ventricular fibrillation; possibly, mechanism of sudden death in digitalis intoxication
   Nonparoxysmal AV junctional tachycardia with or without AV block
   Atrial tachycardia with or without block (most frequently seen in patients with associated potassium deficiency caused by concurrent use of thiazide diuretics)
   Possible dysrhythmias produced by digitalis excess
Effect on conduction system
   Prolonged PR interval
   Slow heart rates, including sinus bradycardia and first-, second- (type 1), and third-degree AV block
Cardiac failure

Neurologic (13% to 25%)*

Mental depression and personality changes
Abnormal visual sensations
   Color (especially brown, yellow, and green)
   Scotoma
   Blurred or dimmed vision
   Photophobia
Cerebral excitation manifested as headache, vertigo, increased irritability, convulsions
Peripheral neuritis
Generalized muscular weakness

Gastrointestinal (50% to 75%)*

Anorexia
Nausea
Vomiting
Diarrhea

Other

Gynecomastia
Allergic manifestations such as skin rash

*Frequency of occurrence with digitalis toxicity.

progressive bradydysrhythmias). Each vial of digoxin immune FAB binds approximately 0.6 mg of digoxin. For calculation of the total amount of digoxin in the body, the following equation is used:

$$\text{Digoxin in body (mg)} = \frac{(\text{Serum concentration})(5.6)(\text{Weight[kg]})}{1000}$$

To calculate the number of vials needed, use the following equation:

$$\text{Number of vials needed} = \frac{\text{Digoxin in body (mg)}}{0.6 \text{ (mg/vial)}}$$

Digoxin immune FAB is administered over 30 minutes through a 0.22-µm membrane filter. The drug may be given as an intravenous (IV) bolus if necessary.

2. If the dysrhythmia is not life threatening, the digoxin dose is held until normal sinus rhythm is restored. If digoxin therapy is to be continued, the clinician should consider using a lower dose or less frequent interval.
3. Electrolyte levels should be closely monitored when toxicity is suspected or documented. When digoxin serum levels are elevated, potassium levels are generally high. If a patient receives digoxen immune FAB, serum potassium levels fall, and supplemental potassium may be indicated. Patients with hypokalemia are acutely sensitive to digoxin and may exhibit toxicity with normal serum levels. Potassium replacement usually corrects the dysrhythmia with no change in the serum digoxin level.
4. Central nervous system and gastrointestinal side effects are more likely to occur in the older population. In addition, these adverse effects may occur with serum levels in the normal range. These effects can be controlled by decreasing the drug dosage or prolonging the interval between doses.
5. Digoxin-toxic patients are sensitive to electrical countershocks and may develop ventricular tachycardia or fibrillation if they receive electrical cardioversion.

Dopamine

Dopamine (Intropin), an endogenous catecholamine, is the immediate precursor in the synthesis of norepinephrine. The cardiovascular effects of dopamine result from actions mediated through dopamine-specific receptors and α- and β-adrenergic receptors.

Cardiovascular actions (Tables 14-3 and 14-4)

The predominant cardiovascular effects of dopamine depend on the dose administered. At doses less than 2 mcg/kg/min, dopamine-specific effects predominate. As the dose is increased, the β-adrenergic effects predominate. These effects include increases in myocardial contractility, CO, and renal blood flow (RBF) with little or no vasoconstriction. At doses greater than 7.5 mcg/kg/min, α-adrenergic effects dominate, leading to vasoconstriction and increased mean arterial pressure (MAP). Increases in systemic vascular resistance (SVR) at higher doses normally offsets improvements in CO, RBF, or pulmonary capillary wedge pressure (PCWP) and may worsen these parameters. As much as 50% of dopamine's hemodynamic actions may be produced by norepinephrine release. Dopamine exerts differing hemodynamic effects, depending on the baseline hemodynamic state of the heart. In patients with good left ventricular function, the dose-dependent effects are readily seen at the various titration doses. However, in patients with poor left ventricular function (for example, CHF), myocardial norepinephrine depletion and β-receptor down regulation combine to produce minimal β myocardial effects. Thus these patients generally have good dopaminergic responses, poor β-adrenergic responses, and strong α-adrenergic responses. Clinically, increased MAP and SVR

TABLE 14-3   Dose-Dependent Cardiovascular Effects of Dopamine

Dose (mcg/kg/min)	Receptor	Clinical Effect
0.5-2.0	Dopamine	Increased RBF and MBF; diuresis
2.0-7.5	Dopamine/β	Increased RBF and MBF; increased CO; possible decrease in PCWP
7.5-20.0	Dopamine/β α	Increased SVR and PVR Variable changes in CO, RBF, and PCWP
>20.0	α (primary) β (secondary)	Increased PVR and SVR Decreased CO, RBF, and MBF; increased PCWP

MBF, Mesentery blood flow; *PCWP*, pulmonary capillary wedge pressure; *SVR*, systemic vascular resistance; *PVR*, peripheral vascular resistance.

TABLE 14-4   Sympathomimetic Pharmacology

Drug	Adult Dose	Receptor Binding Strength			Dopamine	Relative Receptor Affinity (%)		Hemodynamic Actions		
		α	β	β₂		α	β	HR	CO	TPR
Epinephrine	1-4 µg/min	++++	++++	++++	0	50	50	↑↑	↑↑	↑
Norepinephrine	8-24 µg/min	++++	++	0	0	90	10	↑	0/↓	↑↑
Isoproterenol	2-20 µg/min	0	++++	++++	0	0	100	↑↑	↑↑	↓
Dopamine	0.2-2 µg/kg/min	+	0	0	++++	*	*	0	↑	0/↓
	2-10 µg/kg/min	++	+	+	++++			↑	0/↑	↑
	>10 µg/kg/min	++++	+++	++	++++			↑	0/↓	↑↑
Dobutamine	2.5-20 µg/kg/min	++	++++	++++	0	0	100	↑	↑↑	↓
Phenylephrine	0.04-0.2 mg/min	++++	0	0	0	100	0	0	↓	↑↑

*Varies with dosage and individual patients.
0, No effect; +, minimal effect; ++, significant effect; +++, strong effect; ++++, strongest effect; *HR*, heart rate; *TPR*, total peripheral resistance; ↑, increased; ↑↑, greatly increased; ↓, decreased.
From Kinney MR and others: *AACN's clinical reference for critical care nursing*, ed 3, St.Louis, 1993, Mosby.

occur at lower dosage ranges. For these reasons, dopamine is usually combined with inotropes (for example, dobutamine) or other sympathomimetic vasopressors (for example, norepinephrine) to achieve optimal hemodynamic effects when the condition appears refractory to dopamine alone. When this agent is used alone or with another agent, it is important to accurately assess baseline hemodynamics and altered hemodynamics secondary to drug therapy.

Clinical uses

1. The unique hemodynamic effects of dopamine make it an important agent in the treatment of cardiogenic, septic, or traumatic shock.

2. Low-dose (0.5 to 2.0 mcg/kg/min) dopamine alone or with other inotropic agents is used to treat chronic CHF that has been refractory to treatment with diuretics and digitalis. Such therapy is temporary and used only until more definitive long-term treatment can be formulated.

3. Doses greater than 7.5 mcg/kg/min are effective in hemodynamically significant hypotension but should be avoided in patients with CHF unless another selective inotropic agent (for example, dobutamine) is used concomitantly.

4. Dopamine is useful in treating hemodynamically significant hypotension when IV therapy is indicated.

TABLE 14-5	Inotropes	
Drug	**Dilution**	**Dose (mcg/kg/min)**
Dopamine	400 mg/250 ml IV fluid	0.5-20.0
Dobutamine	500 mg/250 ml IV fluid	2.5-20.0
Amrinone	500 mg/250 ml IV fluid	2.5-20.0
Milrinone	50 mg/250 ml IV fluid	0.375-0.750

Dosage and administration (Table 14-5)

1. Dopamine is administered intravenously and is compatible with all IV fluids. Dopamine can be concentrated for patients on volume restriction, but caution should be exercised when mixing more than 1600 mg in 250 ml of IV fluid.
2. Dopamine infusions should be given through a central line when possible. If local extravasation exists, tissue necrosis occurs. The clinician should immediately treat the area with small, local injections of phentolamine given as a total dosage of 5 to 10 mg. Phentolamine is maximally effective if used within 6 hours of the extravasation and is useless if used after 24 hours.
3. Doses should be adjusted based on hemodynamic monitoring. The CO, ECG, PCWP, MAP, SVR, blood pressure, heart rate, renal function, electrolyte levels, and signs and symptoms of the disease state are monitored.
4. Doses should be titrated upward according to the clinical situation (see Table 14-3). For titration off of dopamine, the dosage is reduced by 1 to 5 mcg/kg/min every 15 to 30 minutes. The clinician should allow time for the patient to react hemodynamically to the change in dose. As the dose is titrated to below 5 mcg/kg/min, some patients may become hypotensive. If they are hemodynamically stable, the drip is stopped with no further titration. If they are hemodynamically compromised, the rate is increased to the previous dose and titrated at lower increments of 1 to 2 mcg/kg/min.
5. Dopamine is inactivated in alkaline solutions.
6. Dopamine is compatible with aminophylline, bretylium, calcium chloride, dobutamine, heparin, lidocaine, potassium chloride, epinephrine, isoproterenol, and verapamil.
7. Monoamine oxidase inhibitors may increase the effects of dopamine, necessitating lower doses of dopamine for production of the desired hemodynamic response.
8. If vasopressor doses are used, maintainance of adequate circulating blood volume is essential. If the patient has hypovolemia, vasoconstricting doses may worsen cardiac function.
9. In patients with good left ventricular function immediately after coronary artery bypass graft, low-dose dopamine and fluids may cause less tachycardia than dobutamine alone when used to augment cardiac function.
10. Dopamine can be combined with inotropic and vasodilating agents to produce greater increases in CO and greater reductions in PCWP.
11. Although dopamine is available in a syringe, it must be diluted before use. The dose should not be administered via IV push.
12. Doses of 50 mcg/kg/min or more may be necessary in some patients. However, the blood pressure and SVR of most patients reach a plateau at a given dose, and increments in dose do not affect either. If the patient still has hypotension, administration of a more potent vasopressor such as phenylephrine or norepinephrine should be initiated.
13. Dopamine given at low doses is becoming one of the primary clinical uses of the drug. Low-dose infusions of 0.5 to 3.0 mcg/kg/min augment urine output and antagonize the vasoconstrictive action of norepinephrine and other vasoconstricting catecholamines.

Cautions and side effects

1. The most serious adverse side effect of dopamine is the genesis or exacerbation of dysrhythmias.
2. Dopamine, especially in higher doses, may increase myocardial oxygen consumption and cause further myocardial ischemia in coronary artery disease. Dopamine may precipitate angina pectoris.
3. Occasionally, low doses (for example, 0.5 to 2.0 mcg/kg/min) may produce vasodilatation and hypotension.
4. Other side effects of dopamine include nausea, vomiting, headache, restlessness, and tremor.
5. Concomitant use of other sympathomimetics increases the incidence of side effects. The smallest effective dose should always be used to reduce the risk of toxicity.

Dobutamine

Dobutamine (Dubutrex) is a synthetic catecholamine designed to achieve positive inotropic effects without the chronotropic and peripheral vasoconstricting effects caused by other sympathomimetic agents.

Cardiovascular actions

Dobutamine is a selective β_1 agent that directly stimulates β receptors to increase contractility. The hemodynamic changes seen with this agent are increased CO, decreased PCWP, and increased RBF (see Table 14-4). The magnitude of change in RBF and PCWP is directly related to the magnitude of change in CO. Dobutamine produces a greater increase in left ventricular contractility and stroke volume (SV) with less change in myocardial oxygen demands than dopamine, isoproterenol, norepinephrine, or epinephrine. In patients with poor left ventricular function, dobutamine induces a reflex reduction in SVR and produces little change in the heart rate. Dobutamine has no dose-dependent effects and is the preferred inotropic agent because of its consistent effects on CO and myocardial oxygen demand.

In comparing dopamine and dobutamine, the hemodynamic differences seen after surgery are related to left ventricular function. In normally functioning left ventricles, dobutamine is more chronotropic than dopamine when producing equivalent inotropic responses. In volume-loaded ventricles, both agents are equally effective in enhancing the inotropic response, but dobutamine does so with a greater reduction in SVR and pulmonary vascular resistance. In patients with poor left ventricular function and myocardial failure, dobutamine improves coronary blood flow and myocardial oxygen supply to a greater degree than the oxygen demand elicited by increased contractility. After surgery, dobutamine improves SV and myocardial blood flow while reducing PCWP with less chronotropy than dopamine in patients with poor myocardial contractility.

Clinical uses

1. Dobutamine is the agent of choice for emergency treatment of severe heart failure resulting from various etiologies, especially in shock states caused by direct myocardial decompensation.
2. When shock is caused by vascular collapse and marked vasodilatation, such as that in anaphylactic shock, the absence of vasoconstrictor effects argues against the use of dobutamine alone. Dobutamine should be reserved for patients with combined ventricular dysfunction and elevated filling pressures and used with appropriate vasopressors.
3. In patients with poor left ventricular function after coronary artery bypass graft, dobutamine improves SV and decreases filling pressures with less positive chronotropy than dopamine.
4. Dobutamine is the preferred inotrope in patients after cardiac transplant because its action does not depend on myocardial stores of norepinephrine.

Dosage and administration (see Table 14-5)

1. Dobutamine is administered intravenously and is compatible in all IV fluids. Dobutamine can be concentrated up to a maximum of 1250 mg in 250 ml of IV fluid for patients on volume restriction.
2. Dobutamine solutions may develop a pink discoloration that increases with time. This discoloration results from a slight oxidation of the drug, and no significant loss of drug potency occurs if diluted solutions are used within 24 hours of preparation.
3. Doses should be initiated at 2.5 to 5.0 mcg/kg/min and titrated according to desired response. Doses that increase the heart rate by more than 10% over baseline values should be used cautiously because of the

potential increase in myocardial oxygen demands. Doses up to 50 mcg/kg/min have been used, but most patients respond at doses between 2.5 and 20 mcg/kg/min.
4. Intermittent therapy may be useful in some patients with chronic CHF. Doses of 1.5 to 15 mcg/kg/min for 4 to 72 hours weekly have provided sustained clinical and hemodynamic benefit in some patients. However, this therapy should be used cautiously until patients who respond best can be clinically identified.
5. Dobutamine is compatible with atropine, dopamine, epinephrine, heparin, isoproterenol, lidocaine, norepinephrine, and procainamide.
6. Dobutamine can be titrated to 2.5 to 5 mcg/kg/min every 15 to 30 minutes. The clinician should allow time for the patient to react hemodynamically to the change in dose.
7. Dobutamine is inactivated in alkaline solutions.
8. Doses should be adjusted based on hemodynamic response. The CO, ECG, PCWP, SVR, heart rate, blood pressure, MAP, renal function, electrolyte levels, and signs and symptoms of the disease state are monitored.
9. Dobutamine can be combined with other inotropic and vasodilating agents to produce greater increases in CO and greater reductions in PCWP and SVR.
10. Most cases of extravasation produce no signs of tissue damage or necrosis. There is only one case report of dermal necrosis with extravasation.
11. Tolerance develops in some patients after 72 hours of therapy and can be overcome by increasing the dosage or altering concomitant drug therapy. When a plateau is reached at a given dosage in critically ill patients, another inotropic agent (for example, milrinone or amrinone) may be added to augment cardiac function.

Cautions and side effects

1. Dobutamine may increase heart rate, blood pressure, and the risk of dysrhythmias. Thus constant monitoring of these parameters and prompt dosage reduction is mandatory if these effects occur.
2. Occasionally, nausea, headache, angina pectoris, and dyspnea occur.
3. Dobutamine is contraindicated in idiopathic hypertrophic subaortic stenosis.

Phosphodiesterase Inhibitors

Amrinone (Inocor) and milrinone (Primacor) increase contractility by a mechanism that is distinct from the mechanisms of digitalis, dopamine, and dobutamine.

Cardiovascular actions

Amrinone and milrinone inhibit myocardial cellular phosphodiesterase and increase the availability of calcium in the myocardium. Also, these agents are vasodilators and reduce SVR by an unknown mechanism. The resulting hemodynamic effects are decreased SVR (direct effect) and

PCWP and increased CO and RBF. These effects are comparable to those of dopamine and dobutamine and are additive when amrinone or milrinone are used with these agents. Although amrinone and milrinone are potent inotropes with unique hemodynamic profiles, they remain second-line agents because of their toxicity and propensity to increase myocardial oxygen demand more than dobutamine. Investigational oral forms have been associated with increased mortality rates secondary to acute worsening of heart failure or dysrhythmias. There has been some speculation that prolonged IV use may be detrimental, but this theory has not been clinically substantiated. Amrinone and milrinone are excellent short-term inotropic agents that should be used with careful monitoring.

Clinical uses

1. Both agents are indicated for the treatment of CHF and cardiogenic shock.
2. These agents have additive inotropic effects when combined with dobutamine or dopamine.

Dosage and administration (see Table 14-5)

1. Amrinone should be administered in one-half normal saline or normal saline at dilutions of 3 mg/ml or less. Amrinone is light sensitive and should be covered after dilution.
2. Milrinone is compatible in most IV fluids at concentrations up to 50 mg in 250 ml of IV fluid.
3. The loading dose for amrinone is 0.75 mg/kg IV bolus over 5 to 30 minutes. Hemodynamic collapse secondary to vasodilatation may occur in some patients; caution should be used. This bolus may be repeated every 30 minutes based on response. The loading dose of milrinone is 50 mg/kg over 10 minutes. After an IV loading dose, peak effects are seen in several minutes. If no loading dose is administered, the peak effects of these agents may take at least 7 hours.
4. The maintenance dosage for amrinone is 5 to 20 mcg/kg/min. For milrinone it is 0.375 to 0.75 mcg/kg/min.
5. Milrinone is eliminated renally, and the maintenance dosage should be decreased proportionately to the decrease in renal function.
6. Both agents should be adjusted for the desired hemodynamic response. The CO, ECG, PCWP, SVR, heart rate, MAP, electrolyte levels, renal function, and signs and symptoms of disease state are monitored.
7. Amrinone is incompatible with furosemide.
8. Intermittent IV amrinone therapy has been attempted in patients with end-stage CHF. At present, this approach is discouraged.
9. The duration of hemodynamic effects with amrinone and milrinone is 60 to 90 minutes with bolus dosing or discontinuation of IV drip. Therefore titration of these agents is more difficult than that with dopamine or dobutamine. Both agents should be titrated slowly (for

example, 1 to 5 mcg/kg/min for amrinone and 0.025 to 0.1 mcg/kg/min for milrinone) every 60 to 90 minutes. More time may be necessary between titrations if the patient has altered renal or hepatic function or has been given these agents for more than 3 days. Doses are typically more difficult to titrate if the patient has a low CO and a high PCWP. Neither of these agents should be abruptly stopped; the patient's condition may decompensate rapidly, requiring a bolus dose of these agents to be sustained. The hemodynamic changes that occur with dose reductions should be carefully monitored and the process slowed if the desired hemodynamic response cannot be maintained. It may take 24 to 48 hours to withdraw therapy successfully in some patients.

Cautions and side effects

1. Amrinone causes a dose-dependent, asymptomatic thrombocytopenia in up to 4% of patients. The frequency increases with doses greater than 18 mg/kg/day. Platelet counts return to normal within 2 to 7 days after decreasing the dose or discontinuing therapy. In most cases a reduction in dose is sufficient. Since the reaction is not secondary to an immune response, platelet transfusions can be used in patients in whom the dose cannot be titrated. Milrinone induces thrombocytopenia in 1% of patients. The use of concomitant antiplatelet agents should be monitored closely.
2. Milrinone induces or exacerbates ventricular dysrhythmias in approximately 12% of patients. Of these dysrhythmias, 8% are asymptomatic increases in premature ventricular contractions, and 4% are increases in ventricular tachycardia. Milrinone increases AV nodal conduction and may be detrimental in some patients. The drug should be discontinued in patients who develop these side effects.
3. Other side effects common to both agents include nausea, headache, angina, hypotension, and increased liver enzyme levels.
4. When compared with the catecholamines, the relatively long half-lives of milrinone and amrinone and the subsequent delayed steady state with changes in infusion rates make these agents less useful in the critical care areas.

SYMPATHOMIMETICS[2,3,6-8,12,13] (see Table 14-4)
Epinephrine

Epinephrine (Adrenalin, others) is an important endogenous hormone that is produced and released by the adrenal gland in response to stress.

Cardiovascular actions

Epinephrine binds very strongly to α and β receptors. In the heart, epinephrine stimulates α_1 receptors to increase contractility, AV nodal and Purkinje fiber conduction, and sinoatrial (SA) nodal firing (see Table 14-4). Epinephrine may also accelerate firing of ectopic foci. As a result, epinephrine significantly increases myocardial oxygen demands. α_2-Receptor stimulation results in prolonged vasodilatation and bronchodilatation because of the drug's strong affinity for this receptor. This action is clinically important at low doses (for example, 0.005 to 0.02 mcg/kg/min), resulting in reduced vascular resistance. The diastolic blood pressure falls, but the systolic is maintained if there is an adequate circulating blood volume to maintain CO. Epinephrine also stimulates α receptors, and vasoconstriction predominates with dosages greater than 0.02 mcg/kg/min. α Stimulation results in increased SVR, peripheral vascular resistance (PVR), and MAP, all of which increase the workload of the heart.

Clinical uses

1. Epinephrine is most often used clinically during cardiac arrest, septic shock, and cardiogenic shock to stimulate cardiac pacemaker activity and increase contractility.
2. Epinephrine is often the drug of choice in the immediate treatment of anaphylaxis or reversible bronchospasm.
3. Epinephrine may also be used after coronary artery bypass grafting or in patients on intraaortic balloon pumping devices to augment CO and MAP.

Dosage and administration (Table 14-6)

1. Prediluted syringes with 1:10,000 solution for IV bolus during cardiac arrest are to be administered every 5 minutes as needed.
2. Prediluted epinephrine in 1:1000 solution for subcutaneous (SC) injection during anaphylaxis can be repeated every 5 to 10 minutes. The same dose is used for bronchospasm, but it is repeated every 20 to 30 minutes.
3. Epinephrine is compatible in most IV fluids. IV drips can be mixed by adding 1 to 4 mg to 250 ml of IV fluid. Solutions may be concentrated for patients on volume restriction, but caution should be used.

TABLE 14-6   Sympathomimetics

Drug	Dilution	Dose
Epinephrine	4 mg/250 ml IV fluid	0.05-0.5 mcg/kg/min
Norepinephrine	8 mg/250 ml IV fluid	2.0-24 mcg/min
Isoproterenol	1 mg/250 ml IV fluid	0.5-20.0 mcg/min
Phenylephrine	5 mg/250 ml IV fluid	0.04-0.06 mg/min

4. β-Adrenergic effects predominate at dosages less than 0.02 mcg/kg/min. IV dosages of 0.05 to 0.07 mcg/kg/min are recommended for α-adrenergic effects. The dose is titrated to the desired response. Dosages as high as 0.5 mcg/kg/min can be used when necessary to achieve the desired vasopressor response.
5. Epinephrine is compatible with dopamine, dobutamine, norepinephrine, and potassium.
6. If given by endotracheal administration, the drug is delivered deeply into the airway, and 1 mg is given initially.
7. Epinephrine is unstable in alkaline solutions.
8. The clinician should avoid using epinephrine if it is discolored or has precipitated in the IV fluid.
9. Epinephrine is useful with other agents but should be discontinued as soon as possible to avoid excessive metabolic demands on the heart.
10. The CO, MAP, SVR, ECG, blood pressure, heart rate, PCWP, and electrolyte levels are monitored.

Cautions and side effects

1. Newer advanced cardiac life-support guidelines by the American Heart Association promote the use of high-dose epinephrine (0.1 mg/kg IV push every 3 to 5 minutes) for patients whose conditions are unresponsive to intermediate dosages (2.0 to 5.0 mg IV push every 3 to 5 minutes) or escalating dosages (1.0 to 5.0 mg IV push 3 minutes apart).
2. Epinephrine may exacerbate ventricular dysrhythmias.
3. Some drug reactions may be disturbing to the patient; these include fear, anxiety, and tension.
4. Epinephrine may precipitate myocardial ischemia because of the inability of coronary blood flow to meet increased myocardial oxygen requirements.
5. Epinephrine may produce headache, tremor, and weakness.
6. RBF, glomerular filtration rate, and sodium excretion are usually reduced after the administration of epinephrine.
7. Epinephrine drips may reduce serum potassium levels by as much as 0.8 mEq/L. ECG changes are usually apparent as well, placing the critically ill patient at risk for serious dysrhythmias.
8. Epinephrine should be administered through a central venous line when possible because of the potential for ulceration with infiltration. When infiltration occurs, the site should be treated with local injections of phentolamine (5 to 10 mg total dosage). The best results are achieved when phentolamine is used within 6 hours of the extravasation, but it may be given up to 24 hours with some benefit.

Norepinephrine

Norepinephrine (Levophed, others) is the biosynthetic precursor to epinephrine and a neurotransmitter in the sympathetic nervous system.

Cardiovascular actions

Norepinephrine stimulates primarily α but also β receptors (see Table 14-4). Very low doses produce mainly β_1-adrenergic effects, resulting in increased contractility, chronotropy, and cardiac conduction. Norepinephrine often exerts a predominant α-adrenergic stimulating effect, resulting in increased PVR and MAP. CO usually remains unchanged or decreased because of the increased PVR and vagally mediated reflex reduction in heart rate. Coronary blood flow increases, whereas RBF and cerebral, visceral, and skeletal blood flow diminish.

Clinical uses

1. Norepinephrine is used to treat hypotension, septic shock, and cardiogenic shock. It increases MAP and SVR in septic shock, often without compromising CO.
2. Norepinephrine may be especially useful when hypotensive states are accompanied by low SVR and normal or slightly elevated CO, despite adequate volume resuscitation.

Dosage and administration (see Table 14-6)

1. Norepinephrine is compatible in most IV fluids. From 4 to 8 mg may be added to 250 ml of IV fluid. More concentrated solutions can be used, but they may lose their potency more rapidly.
2. The drug should not be used if a precipitate forms in the bottle or the solution has a brown discoloration.
3. The usual maintenance dose is 2 to 24 mcg/min. The rate is adjusted according to the patient's hemodynamic response and using the lowest effective dose.
4. The CO, MAP, heart rate, PCWP, SVR, renal function, signs of vasoconstriction, and electrolyte levels are monitored.
5. Norepinephrine is administered through a central line when possible. Extravasation with tissue necrosis can occur rapidly in a peripheral line. If this occurs, 5 to 10 mg of phentolamine is injected into the area as soon as possible. Phentolamine is most effective if used within the first 6 hours and is useless after 24 hours.
6. Typically norepinephrine is added to therapy after dopamine and should be discontinued as soon as possible. The dose is titrated according to the patient's hemodynamic response, and 15 to 30 minutes should be allowed between adjustments in the dose.
7. Norepinephrine is compatible with heparin, magnesium, dopamine, dobutamine, potassium, calcium, epinephrine, isoproterenol, and verapamil.
8. An adequate blood volume should be maintained when this agent is used. Hypovolemia may increase the cardiac workload and lead to ischemia.
9. Norepinephrine may be added to gastric lavage solutions in the treatment of acute gastrointestinal bleeding. The dose is 16 mg in 200 ml of iced saline.
10. In nonseptic conditions, norepinephrine is a potent renal vasoconstrictor. Low-dose dopamine (0.5 to 3.0 mcg/kg/min) antagonizes the renal vasoconstrictive effects of norepinephrine, and the clinical combination of norepinephrine and dopamine may be advantageous in patients with renal compromise.

Cautions and side effects

1. Anxiety, respiratory difficulty, and transient headaches may result.
2. Overdose may cause severe hypertension with headache, photophobia, angina, heavy sweating, and vomiting.
3. Cardiac dysrhythmias may be produced or exacerbated.
4. Reflex bradycardia may occur in some patients, but typically the heart rate is increased.
5. Norepinephrine has additive sympathomimetic side effects when used with other catecholamines.

Isoproterenol

Isoproterenol (Isuprel, others) is a synthetic, direct-acting, nonspecific β-adrenergic agonist.

Cardiovascular actions

Isoproterenol causes almost exclusive β-adrenergic receptor stimulation and acts on β_2 (smooth muscle and bronchiole) and β_1 (heart) receptors (see Table 14-4). Isoproterenol relaxes the smooth muscle of bronchi, skeletal muscle vasculature, and alimentary tract. In the heart, it increases heart rate, conductivity, and contractility. Isoproterenol lowers PVR and decreases diastolic arterial pressures. The net hemodynamic effect is to elevate CO and systolic pressure and to decrease MAP and diastolic arterial pressure. Myocardial oxygen consumption rises significantly with isoproterenol administration, and its use is discouraged with the availability of more selective inotropic agents.

Clinical uses

1. Isoproterenol is most often used to enhance pacemaker activity and improve AV conduction during episodes of sinus bradycardia or AV block.
2. In certain cardiogenic shock states, isoproterenol may be used to increase CO and decrease peripheral vasoconstriction. Isoproterenol is not indicated in the treatment of cardiogenic shock caused by acute myocardial infarction.
3. In bronchospastic lung disease, isoproterenol may be used by inhalation to produce bronchodilatation.

Dosage and administration (see Table 14-6)

1. Isoproterenol is compatible in most IV fluids. From 1 to 4 mg can be diluted in 250 ml of IV fluid. Exposure to air, light, or increased temperature may cause a pink discoloration, and the solution should be discarded.

Caution should be used with concentrations greater than 10 mg in 250 ml of IV fluid.

2. Hemodynamic effects are typically seen with doses ranging from 0.5 to 20 mcg/min. However, doses exceeding 30 mcg/min have been used in advanced shock. The lowest possible dose should be used to achieve the therapeutic response.

3. The drug should be titrated every 15 to 30 minutes according to hemodynamic response, which allows time for patient response to the change in dose.

4. Isoproterenol is compatible with dopamine, dobutamine, calcium, heparin, potassium, epinephrine, norepinephrine, and verapamil.

5. The ECG, CO, heart rate, blood pressure, and electrolyte levels are monitored.

Cautions and side effects

1. Isoproterenol increases myocardial oxygen consumption and may precipitate myocardial ischemia.

2. Cardiac dysrhythmias, including sinus tachycardia, premature ventricular complexes, ventricular tachycardia, or ventricular fibrillation, are common with the use of isoproterenol.

3. In hypovolemia the vasodilating effects of isoproterenol may produce hypotension.

4. Headache, flushing of the skin, angina, nausea, tremor, dizziness, weakness, and sweating may result.

5. Patients with symptomatic coronary artery disease, hypertrophic cardiomyopathy, and cardiac dysrhythmias are particularly susceptible to the adverse cardiac effects from isoproterenol.

Phenylephrine

Phenylephrine (Neo-Synephrine) is a synthetic agent that stimulates predominantly α receptors.

Cardiovascular actions

Phenylephrine increases total PVR and blood pressure by directly stimulating α receptors (see Table 14-4). Blood flow to vital organs, skin, and skeletal muscle is usually reduced. With prolonged use, circulating blood volume may decrease, which leads to increased myocardial demand. The predominant effect of phenylephrine on the heart is bradycardia, which results from a reflex increase in vagal tone secondary to the change in arterial pressure. The bradycardia can be blocked by atropine.

Clinical uses

1. Phenylephrine is typically used to treat PSVT. The hypertensive response increases vagal tone and may terminate the dysrhythmia.

2. Hypotension caused by peripheral vasodilatation, such as that seen with ganglionic blocking agents or spinal anesthesia, may be reversed by phenylephrine.

3. Phenylephrine is also useful in treating hypotension caused by left ventricular outflow obstruction in hypertrophic cardiomyopathy.

4. Phenylephrine is not indicated for the treatment of the usual forms of cardiogenic shock.

Dosage and administration (see Table 14-6)

1. Phenylephrine is compatible in most IV fluids. From 5 to 20 mg may be diluted in 250 ml of IV fluid for continuous infusion. Solutions should not be used if they are brown or contain a precipitate.

2. For continuous IV infusion in severe hypotension or shock, the maintenance dose is 0.04 to 0.06 mg/min. Larger doses may be necessary to stabilize the patient's condition (for example, 0.1 to 0.2 mg/min). The rate is adjusted to the lowest possible effective dose for the desired hemodynamic response.

3. For supraventricular tachycardia a bolus dose of 0.5 to 1 mg IV push followed by 1 to 2 mg (if no response occurs in 60 to 90 seconds) is sufficient to terminate the dysrhythmia.

4. Phenylephrine is compatible with lidocaine and potassium.

5. The ECG, blood pressure, heart rate, CO, SVR, MAP, PCWP, urine output, peripheral vasoconstriction, renal function, and electrolyte levels are monitored.

6. The dose is titrated every 15 minutes, and the drug is discontinued as soon as possible to prevent hypovolemia and hypoperfusion to the extremities.

7. Phenylephrine has an additive effect when used with other vasopressors.

Cautions and side effects

1. Excessive dosage may produce headache, excessive hypertension, severe bradycardia, and vomiting.

2. Phenylephrine may also cause restlessness, anxiety, tremor, and nervousness. These effects are additive to those of the other sympathomimetics.

3. Phenylephrine should not be administered to patients with hypertension for the treatment of PSVT.

α-ADRENERGIC BLOCKERS[2,12]

α-Adrenergic blocking agents directly and selectively block the stimulation of α-adrenergic receptors.

Cardiovascular actions

The effects of these agents are most prominent in the peripheral vascular beds, where vasoconstrictor responses are inhibited and vasodilatation results. α-Adrenergic blocking agents may accelerate the heart rate by reflex effects from peripheral vasodilatation or by direct effects to increase norepinephrine release from cardiac α_2-receptor inhibition. The α-adrenergic blocking agents discussed here are phenoxybenzamine (Dibenzyline) and phentolamine (Regitine). Prazosin, doxazosin, and terazosin are oral α-adrenergic blockers and are discussed in the section on vasodilators. Phenoxybenzamine inhibits α_1 receptors, and phentolamine inhibits α_1 and α_2 receptors.

Phenoxybenzamine has a slow onset of action (several hours), and the cumulative effects of daily administration appear in 7 days. Once α-adrenergic blockade is accomplished, it is complete and present for 3 to 4 days after discontinuation of the agent. Phenoxybenzamine reverses the pressor effect of epinephrine and competitively blocks the vasoconstrictor effects of norepinephrine. Unlike phenoxybenzamine, phentolamine has a rapid onset of action and a short duration of action. Phentolamine incompletely blocks α_1 and α_2 receptors and is more effective in blocking the effects of circulating norepinephrine or epinephrine than in antagonizing responses at the adrenergic nerve ending. Blood pressure response depends on the drug's vasodilating effect and its weak β-agonist effect.

Clinical uses

1. α-Adrenergic blocking agents are indicated to inhibit the excessive α-adrenergic stimulation that occurs from an endogenous source, such as that which occurs during treatment of pheochromocytoma, or from an exogenous source, such as that which occurs when catecholamines are administered to treat shock.
2. α-Adrenergic blockers also have been used as direct vasodilators to reverse the peripheral vasoconstriction that accompanies low CO states, systemic hypertension, and peripheral vascular insufficiency.
3. Phentolamine is used to prevent dermal necrosis and sloughing after extravasation of norepinephrine, phenylephrine, or dopamine.

Dosage and administration

1. Phenoxybenzamine is available in oral form and is primarily used for the treatment of pheochromocytoma. The usual initial dosage, 10 mg twice a day, is increased every other day until an adequate response is achieved. The normal maintenance dosage is usually 20 to 40 mg 2 or 3 times a day, but some patients may require higher doses.
2. Phentolamine is available as an injectable powder for solution only. Phentolamine is primarily used in the diagnosis of pheochromocytoma or for prevention of dermal necrosis. The usual dose for pheochromocytoma is 5 mg intravenously or intramuscularly. A continuous IV drip can be given at a rate of 0.1 to 2.0 mg/min, but an IV bolus dose of 5 to 10 mg is recommended by the manufacturer for the treatment of adrenergic hypertensive crisis. The dose for dermal necrosis is 5 to 10 mg injected directly into the extravasated area. Phentolamine can be reconstituted using normal saline.

3. The use of phentolamine for essential hypertension is not recommended because most conditions become refractory to the drug's antihypertensive effect.
4. Phentolamine is contraindicated in patients with myocardial infarction.
5. The ECG, blood pressure, heart rate, and side effects are monitored.

Cautions and side effects

1. As with all vasodilators, the blood pressure may fall precipitously. Maintenance of adequate volume status minimizes part of this problem.
2. Other side effects of α-adrenergic blockers include acceleration of heart rate, miosis (constriction of the pupil), nasal stuffiness, inhibition of ejaculation, sedation, nausea, and vomiting.
3. Phentolamine and phenoxybenzamine may cause abdominal pain and exacerbate peptic ulcer disease.
4. Most of the side effects are dose related and may be controlled by decreasing the dose. Many effects seen with phenoxybenzamine decrease as therapy is continued.

CENTRAL α AGONISTS[3, 12, 14, 16-19]

These agents stimulate central α_2 receptors in the vasomotor center of the medulla oblongata.

Cardiovascular actions

α-Receptor stimulation centrally inhibits norepinephrine release in the brain and peripheral sympathetic system. This inhibition results in decreased sympathetic activity, increased vagal stimulation, and decreased release of norepinephrine, epinephrine, and renin. When combined with β blockers, these agents further lower heart rate by enhancing vagal activity. Central α agonists produce a fall in the resting blood pressure, with reflex control of capacitance vessels remaining intact, which maintains CO during exercise. RBF is maintained with these agents because of a fall in renal vascular resistance. Methyldopa is slightly different from the other agents because it is a prodrug and must be metabolized to the active form. One of the metabolites acts as a false neurotransmitter that is stored and released by the nerve terminals. Because the body stores this metabolite, the onset of methyldopa activity is delayed, and the duration is prolonged.

Clinical uses

1. These agents are used to treat chronic hypertension.
2. Clonidine can be used for hypertensive urgencies.
3. Methyldopa can be used in toxemia.

Dosage and administration (Table 14-7)

1. Initial doses for these agents should be low and the dose slowly titrated to the desired response. Suggested initial starting dosages are as follows: clonidine, 0.1 mg

TABLE 14-7   Central α_2 Agonists

Agent	Trade Name	Dose	Dosage Schedule*	Form	Onset (min)	Peak (hr)	Duration (hr)
Clonidine	Catapres	0.2-1.2 mg/day	bid, tid	Oral	30-60	2-4	6-24
Guanabenz	Wytensin	4-32 mg/day	bid	Oral	60	2-4	6-12
Guanfacine	Tenex	1-3 mg/day	qd	Oral	60-120	3-4	24
Methyldopa	Aldomet	1-3 g/day	bid, tid	Oral, IV	120-180	3-6	8-24

*_bid_, Twice a day; _tid_, three times a day; _qd_, every day.

twice a day; guanabenz, 4 mg twice a day; guanfacine, 1 mg every day; methyldopa, 500 mg twice a day.

2. The dosage of clonidine needed for hypertensive urgency is initially 0.2 mg orally followed by 0.1 mg orally every hour (up to 0.8 mg) until the desired response is achieved. The onset of action and peak effect of this agent are gradual; thus the observed initial hypotensive effects reflect the first dose rather than the most recent dose. Further hourly doses are held until the total effect of the cumulative doses can be assessed. Most patients require a total of 0.4 mg or less for adequate hypertensive response. Patients experiencing abrupt withdrawal of clonidine may require more drug and adjunct therapy to control their blood pressures.

3. When given intravenously for toxemia, the usual dosage of methyldopa is 250 to 500 mg every 6 hours to a maximum of 1 g every 6 hours.

4. When given in high doses, these agents may increase blood pressure by stimulating peripheral α receptors. Therefore these agents should not be given in doses higher than recommended.

5. These agents should never be used with one another.

6. The blood pressure, heart rate, electrolyte levels, and side effects are monitored.

7. Clonidine transdermal patches are useful in noncompliant patients. Patches are changed once a week, and most patients respond to patches that deliver 0.1 to 0.2 mg/day.

8. Clonidine may also be used in alcohol, nicotine, and opiate withdrawal syndromes. Doses should be titrated to control symptoms without inducing hypotension.

9. These agents should be tapered slowly when discontinued. The tapering schedule depends on the dose and duration of therapy. Higher doses given over longer periods require more gradual tapering (for example, reduction of a clonidine dose by 0.2 mg at weekly intervals). Most patients can be easily tapered off the drug in 2 weeks with no adverse effects.

10. These agents are excellent antihypertensive drugs because they do not affect most risk factors for coronary artery disease. They have no effect on electrolyte or lipid levels and maintain exercise capacity and RBF in most patients.

11. Central α agonists are more efficacious in older patients, black patients, and obese patients.

Cautions and side effects

1. All these agents may produce rebound hypertension and should not be abruptly discontinued. Patients who are also taking β blockers are especially susceptible to severe hypertension if they stop taking the central α agonist. Rebound hypertension occurs more often with clonidine than with guanabenz, guanfacine, and methyldopa, and it rarely occurs with clonidine doses of less than 0.3 mg/day. Patients who have rebound hypertension should have the drug reinstituted immediately. If necessary, IV labetalol or nitroprusside can be used with the oral agent if the patient has recent-onset end-organ damage. β Blockers alone are not recommended because they may exaggerate the hypertensive response by providing unopposed adrenergic vasoconstriction from the increased norepinephrine release. In most patients, the dose can be easily controlled, and patients can be switched to oral therapy within 24 hours.

2. Clonidine patches produce very little rebound hypertension. The patches have a gradual onset that peaks in 2 to 3 days. If a patient is to be changed from oral therapy to a patch, oral therapy should be continued and tapered gradually over 2 to 3 days. This schedule prevents dramatic fluctuations in blood pressure.

3. Other major side effects associated with these agents are sedation, dry mouth, impotence, constipation, dizziness, hypotension, nasal congestion, and headache. These effects are primarily dose related and can be controlled by decreasing the dose.

4. Allergic contact dermatitis occurs more frequently with the transdermal patches, and rotation of sites may help in some patients. If dermatitis continues, the patch should be discontinued and oral clonidine gradually initiated.

5. A positive Coombs test may occur in 25% of patients taking methyldopa, but fewer than 1% develop hemolytic anemia.
6. Hepatic disease has also been associated with methyldopa use. This agent should be used with caution in any patient who has a history of hepatic disease.
7. Fluid and sodium retention usually occurs with long-term therapy, especially with higher doses.

GANGLIONIC AGENTS[2, 12, 14, 16-18]

Ganglionic agents act directly on the adrenergic ganglionic neurons.

Cardiovascular actions

There are three agents in this class: guanethidine (Ismelin), guanadrel (Hylorel), and reserpine. Guanethidine and guanadrel deplete norepinephrine from presynaptic storage granules, resulting in a reduction in PVR. These two agents also inhibit action potential–induced release of norepinephrine. Reserpine gradually depletes norepinephrine from postganglionic neurons and is considered a weak agent when used alone.

Clinical uses

1. Guanethidine and guanadrel are used in the treatment of hypertension. They are considered last-line agents because of their toxicity.
2. Low doses of reserpine combined with diuretics are beneficial in treating older patients with hypertension.

Dosage and administration

1. Guanethidine should be initiated at 10 mg/day and gradually increased in 10- to 25-mg increments at 5- to 7-day intervals. Guanadrel should be initiated at 5 mg twice a day and gradually increased to 20 to 75 mg twice a day. Reserpine should be initiated at 0.1 mg every day and increased as necessary to a dose no greater than 0.25 mg every day.
2. The dose should be titrated to the lowest possible effective dose to prevent side effects.
3. These agents are additive with other antihypertensive agents. They should be used cautiously with other agents that affect the adrenergic nervous system.
4. The blood pressure, heart rate, and side effects should be monitored.

Cautions and side effects

1. Guanethidine and guanadrel frequently cause orthostatic hypotension, which produces symptoms of dizziness, weakness, lassitude, or syncope. This is particularly hazardous in older patients.
2. Fluid retention and edema occur with guanethidine and guanadrel, which may exacerbate CHF in some patients.
3. Reserpine causes dose-related mental depression in approximately 10% of patients taking 0.25 mg/day.

Patients taking dosages greater than 0.25 mg/day experience significantly more depression and psychologic difficulties. Reserpine is contraindicated in any patient who has a history of mental depression or suicidal tendencies.
4. All these agents may cause diarrhea, abdominal pain, exacerbation of peptic ulcer disease, and epigastric distress. These adverse effects occur more often with reserpine.
5. Other adverse effects that may occur with these agents include impotence, bradycardia, and nasal congestion.
6. Drugs used in surgical anesthesia may produce profound hypotension, leading to cardiovascular collapse, when given with ganglionic blockers.

β BLOCKERS[16-21] (Table 14-8)

β-Adrenergic blocking agents act by competitive inhibition of adrenergic neuronal or hormonal action at the β receptor.

Cardiovascular actions

As a result of specific receptor interaction in the heart, β-adrenergic blocking agents inhibit increases in heart rate, AV nodal conduction, and myocardial contractility that result from β-receptor stimulation. In addition, β-adrenergic blocking agents inhibit bronchodilatation, peripheral vasodilatation, and renin release induced by adrenergic stimulation. Although these are the most clinically significant effects, β-adrenergic blocking agents act in all organs to inhibit the effects of β-receptor stimulation.

Propranolol was the first β-adrenergic antagonist to achieve widespread clinical use. Multiple agents are now available, all having the primary effect of blocking β receptors. The differences in clinical pharmacologic effects of these agents may be categorized according to their relative selectivity for β_1 receptors, intrinsic agonist activity, relative lipid solubility, and membrane-stabilizing effects. Each agent also has a unique pharmacokinetic profile and potency that determine its dosage strength and administration schedule. These properties of the available β-adrenergic blocking agents are listed in Table 14-8.

The term *cardioselectivity* is used to describe a β blocker that has predominant effects on β_1 receptors and therefore has its major effects on the heart. The most common clinical advantage of cardioselectivity is that there is less inhibition of bronchodilatation and vasodilatation, effects mediated primarily by β_2 receptors. Therefore cardioselective agents may lower the potential for bronchospasm in patients with chronic lung disease. A theoretic disadvantage of cardioselective agents is that catecholamine-induced potassium release from skeletal muscle and excretion is not blocked; hypokalemia may be more frequent. The clinical significance of this effect has not been firmly established. Selectivity for β_1- or β_2-receptor inhibition is relative, and

TABLE 14-8   β Blockers

Agent	Trade Name	Adult Oral Dosage	Adult IV Dosage	Cardio-selectivity	Intrinsic Sympathomimetic Activity	Hydrophilic Effect
Propranolol	Inderal	40-160 mg bid-qid	0.1-0.15 mg/kg given in 1.0-mg increments q5min	−	−	−
Metoprolol	Lopressor	50-100 mg bid	5 mg q5min for 3 doses	+	−	−
Atenolol	Tenormin	50-100 mg qd	5 mg q5min for 2 doses	+	−	+
Nadolol	Corgard	40-160 mg qd		−	−	+
Timolol	Blocadren	10-20 mg bid		−	−	−
Pindolol	Visken	5-30 mg bid		−	+	−
Acebutolol	Sectral	200-600 mg bid		+	+	+
Betaxolol	Kerlone	10-40 mg qd		+	−	+
Esmolol	Brevibloc		500 mcg/kg/min for 1 min and then 50 mcg/kg/min titrated up by 50 mcg/kg/min q5min; maximum dose: 300 mcg/kg/min	+	−	−
Labetalol*	Normodyne, Trandate	100-400 mg bid	IV push: 20 mg and then 40-80 mg q10-15 min; maintenance infusion: 1-2 mg/min	−	+	−
Oxprenolol	Trasicor	80-240 mg bid or tid		−	+	−
Penbutolol	Levatol	10-20 mg qd		−	+	−
Carteolol*	Cartrol	2.5-10 mg qd		−	+	+
Celiprolol*	Selecor	400 mg qd		+	+	+
Bisoprolol	Zebeta	5-10 mg qd		+	−	−

*Vasodilatory beta blockers.

bid, Twice a day; *qid*, four times a day; *q*, every; *qd*, every day; +, present; −, absent; *tid*, three times a day.

higher doses of cardioselective agents also produce inhibition at β_2-receptor sites. In addition, there is neither complete segregation nor different β-receptor subtypes in each organ; for example, 15% to 20% of cardiac β receptors are composed of β_2 receptors.

When a drug occupies a receptor site, thereby blocking that receptor site to its usual agonist, the drug itself may possess weak agonist activity or intrinsic sympathomimetic activity. One example of the clinical effects of intrinsic agonist activity is that these agents inhibit an exercise-induced increase in heart rate with a minimal effect on resting heart rate when compared with other β-adrenergic antagonists that do not possess this activity. This property may confer a slight advantage to these agents in some clinical situations, such as the treatment of hypertension. However, intrinsic agonist activity appears to preclude the use of these agents for the treatment of angina pectoris or prophylaxis after myocardial infarction.

β-Adrenergic blocking agents may be classified as primarily lipid soluble (*lipophilic*) or water soluble (*hydrophilic*). The potential importance of this property derives from the suggestion that hydrophilic compounds are less able than lipophilic compounds to cross the blood-brain barrier and thus have fewer side effects on the central nervous system. Finally, membrane-stabilizing effects are direct effects on membrane action potentials similar to those produced by quinidine or other local anesthetics. These effects probably play a minor role in the antidysrhythmic potential of β-adrenergic blocking agents. For example, in the case of propranolol, these effects are present only at very high drug concentrations.

Clinical uses

1. The goal in the treatment of angina pectoris is to decrease myocardial oxygen demands. This goal is accomplished primarily by lowering the heart rate but also by

decreasing myocardial contractility. Clinical effects appear additive to those of calcium channel blockers and nitrates. The usual goal is to lower the resting heart rate to 50 to 60 beats/min and to blunt the heart-rate response to exercise.

2. With dysrhythmias, the usual indications are to control the ventricular response to atrial flutter or fibrillation and to terminate and prevent recurrences of PSVT. β Blockers are useful in treating selected ventricular dysrhythmias, such as those induced by exercise, adrenergic excess, or digitalis toxicity.

3. After myocardial infarction, some β-adrenergic blockers reduce the mortality rate for 3 years. Agents specifically indicated for this use are timolol (Blocadren), metoprolol (Lopressor), propranolol (Inderal), and atenolol (Tenormin). IV β blockers are also useful in the early stages of acute myocardial infarction to accompany the administration of thrombolytic agents. Metoprolol and atenolol given intravenously are specifically indicated for this purpose.

4. Additional uses include the treatment of hypertrophic cardiomyopathy, cardiovascular manifestations of hyperthyroidism, and anxiety states.

Dosage and administration (see Table 14-8)

1. Metoprolol and atenolol are the primary IV agents used in early acute myocardial infarction. Metoprolol can be given as a 5-mg IV bolus every 5 minutes for a total dosage of 15 mg. Atenolol is given as a 5-mg IV bolus and repeated once for a total dosage of 10 mg. β Blockers are most efficacious in patients who have transmural anterior myocardial infarctions and who have clinical tachycardia and hypertension. These agents provide excellent adjunct therapy to thrombolytic agents and aspirin in these patients. β Blockers should be used cautiously in patients with hypotension or cardiogenic shock.

2. Oral therapy should be instituted after IV loading in patients with acute myocardial infarction. Metoprolol may be given as 50 mg orally every 6 hours for 48 hours and then 100 mg twice a day. Atenolol may be given as 50 mg orally twice a day for 48 hours, followed by 100 mg orally every day. Maintenance doses should maintain the resting heart rate in the range of 50 to 60 beats/min.

3. Therapy should be initiated with low doses and slowly titrated for the desired response. The blood pressure, heart rate, ECG, electrolyte levels, and side effects are monitored.

4. Nadolol, bisoprolol, careolol, and atenolol doses should be reduced by half in patients with creatinine clearances less than 40 ml/min. If the clearance is less than 20 ml/min, the dose may be given every other day.

5. Abrupt cessation of therapy must be avoided. Rebound hypertension or anginal pain may occur, and these agents should be gradually tapered over 2 weeks when discontinued.

6. β Blockers may be useful in some patients with CHF, but their role has yet to be determined. At present, these agents are not recommended for such patients.

Cautions and side effects

1. Because these agents decrease myocardial contractility, they may exacerbate or induce CHF in some patients. β Blockers have additive negative inotropic effects with other agents that depress contractility. Nonselective agents may worsen afterload abnormalities by increasing PVR. Therapy should be discontinued in patients who develop signs and symptoms of heart failure.

2. Because these agents depress SA and AV nodal conduction, bradydysrhythmias may occur. Symptomatic bradycardia and AV block are typically seen in patients if β blockers are administered with other drugs that depress SA or AV nodal conduction. Many patients respond to lower doses of β blocker, and therapy should be discontinued if they do not.

3. Nonselective β antagonists or high doses of cardioselective antagonists exacerbate or induce bronchospasm in some patients. Patients with histories of pulmonary disease should be monitored closely while receiving β blockers. Selective agents with intrinsic agonist activity are generally better tolerated by these patients. If bronchospasm occurs, isoproterenol should be given by inhalation therapy.

4. Peripheral vascular disease may be worsened by the use of these agents. Many patients complain of cold extremities, pain, tingling, or burning sensations in the extremities. Doses should be reduced, or agents with intrinsic agonist activity or cardioselectivity may be used as alternatives. The drug should be discontinued if these effects continue despite lower dosages.

5. β Blockers mask the hypoglycemic symptoms mediated by the adrenergic system. These agents also delay the recovery time from hypoglycemia. These effects are more prominent with the use of nonspecific agents but can be seen with all agents. Agents with intrinsic agonist activity or cardioselectivity should be used in patients with diabetes if β blockers must be used.

6. Dizziness, weakness, fatigue, nightmares, vivid dreams, insomnia, and general lassitude may be experienced by patients receiving these agents. The dose should be reduced if possible or a hydrophilic agent used when possible.

7. Other possible side effects are diarrhea, nausea, rash, and impotence.

8. β Blockers adversely affect the blood lipid profile by increasing serum low-density lipoprotein (LDL) levels and reducing serum high-density lipoprotein (HDL) levels. Agents that are cardioselective or possess intrinsic agonist activity have the least effect on serum lipid profiles and should be used in patients who are at risk for hyperlipidemia.

9. β Blockers typically reduce exercise tolerance in patients.
10. β Blockers are additive with other hypotensive agents and should be used cautiously with other agents that affect the adrenergic system.
11. Patients often complain of excessive fatigue when β-blocker therapy is initiated. It may take days to weeks for their bodies to adjust to the change.
12. Abrupt cessation of therapy may exacerbate angina, myocardial infarction, or dysrhythmias in patients with ischemic heart disease. These patients should be monitored closely. It is unclear whether slowly reducing the dose of a β blocker before discontinuation would prevent this effect. Patients who have received larger doses for longer periods appear to be at greater risk for such reactions. Doses can be gradually tapered over 1 to 2 weeks.

VASODILATORS[2,12,16-18, 22, 23]
Nitrates

This category includes nitroglycerin, isosorbide mononitrate, and isosorbide dinitrate. Nitrates relax smooth muscle, especially in vascular beds.

Cardiovascular actions

Nitrates are primarily venodilators but may also produce arteriolar dilatation at higher doses. Their major hemodynamic effect is to lower left and right ventricular filling pressures (preload), which improves exercise tolerance, pulmonary congestion, and dyspnea. CO may be increased in a failing ventricle if preload is elevated before administration of these agents. Nitrates are also potent coronary vasodilators and increase blood flow through normal, collateral, or occluded coronary arteries.

Nitrate therapy can be complicated by the development of tolerance to these agents, especially with the use of nitroglycerin, isosorbide dinitrate, or transdermal products. In the smooth muscle, nitrates are converted to nitrites, which produce vasodilatation. The successful metabolism of nitrates depends on the balance of two factors: the availability of sulfhydryl groups for the conversion and the amount of drug delivered to the vascular smooth muscle. Tolerance develops when the drug cannot be adequately metabolized because of a depletion of sulfhydryl groups. In patients with good CO, tolerance may develop rapidly because sustained amounts of drug are present in the smooth muscle. In contrast, patients with heart failure may not develop tolerance because less drug is available for metabolism, thus preventing sulfhydryl group depletion. In patients who develop tolerance to the cardiovascular actions, drug-free intervals of 8 to 16 hours allow time for the body to replenish the sulfhydryl groups.

Clinical uses

1. Nitroglycerin is the preferred drug in the treatment of acute episodes of angina pectoris because of the rapid onset of its action and its ability to decrease myocardial oxygen demands and dilate coronary vessels.
2. Nitrates are effective in the treatment of stable, unstable, and variant angina. They have additive effects to reduce anginal pain when used with calcium channel blockers or β blockers.
3. Nitrates are beneficial in the treatment of acute myocardial infarction. Nitrates improve blood flow to ischemic areas during periods of prolonged ischemia.
4. Nitrates are effective for reducing preload, thus improving pulmonary congestion in patients with CHF. They have additive effects when combined with other vasodilators.

Dosage and administration (Table 14-9)

1. Patients may complain of specific side effects at times when the drug is at its peak concentration. Shorter or longer dosing intervals may be required based on the duration of the pharmacologic effect in the individual.
2. Doses greater than those listed may be necessary and are effective in some patients with angina and heart failure.
3. Sublingual tablets should cause a burning sensation when placed under the tongue and usually produce a headache. Nitroglycerin sublingual doses or spray should be repeated every 5 minutes for 15 minutes in patients suffering from an acute anginal attack. If the pain persists, the patient should seek medical attention.
4. Nitroglycerin should be diluted in glass containers for IV administration. Unpredictable amounts of the drug may be lost in polyvinyl chloride plastic containers. Nitroglycerin injection is compatible in most IV fluids. Some injectable solutions contain large percentages of alcohol, and the solutions should never be concentrated more than 150 mg in 250 ml of IV fluids. If a precipitate or separation of the solution is noted, it should be discarded and a more dilute solution used.
5. Transdermal patches have been associated with unacceptable tolerance in a large percentage of patients. Their use should be monitored closely in patients with unstable angina.
6. If tolerance with oral dosing develops, the doses should be separated with a greater dosing interval. A twice-daily dosing schedule at 0800 and 1400 has been successfully used in many patients. This dosing scheme maintains an excellent vasodilator response with little or no tolerance in patients with angina. The sustained-release preparations are ideal for this type of dosing.
7. Doses should be gradually increased to maximize response and reduce side effects. The IV dose starts at 5 to 10 mcg/min and is titrated 5 mcg/min every 3 to 5 minutes to control chest pain and maintain systolic blood pressure at 90 mm Hg or greater.
8. Nitroglycerin tablets should be kept in the original glass container and closed tightly after each use.

TABLE 14-9   Nitrates

Agent	Onset (min)	Peak (hr)	Duration (hr)	Dose
ISOSORBIDE DINITRATE				
Sublingual	5-20	0.5-1.0	1-3	2.5-10 mg prn
Oral tablet	15-45	1-2	4-6	10-100 mg q3-6h
Sustained release	30-180	1-2	6-12	20-80 mg q6-12h
NITROGLYCERIN				
Sublingual	2-5		0.25-0.5	0.2-0.6 mg prn
Buccal	1-2	0.5	4-6	1.0-3.0 mg q4-6h
Spray	2-5		0.25-0.5	1 or 2 sprays prn
Topical paste	30-60	2-3	3-6	0.5-3.0 inches q3-6h
Transdermal patch	30-60	2-3	12-24	2.5-15 mg qd
Oral tablet	20-45	1-2	3-6	6.5-19.5 mg q4-6h
IV	<1		0.25-0.5	10-300 mcg/min
Sustained release	20-45	1-2	8-12	2.6-9.0 mg q8-12h
ISOSORBIDE MONONITRATE				
Oral tablet	30-60	1-4	8-24	20-60 mg daily

prn, As necessary; *q*, every.

Tablets should be stored in a cool, dark place and the cotton removed from the bottle. Bottles should be replaced when the tablets no longer burn under the tongue or 6 months after opening.

9. The blood pressure, heart rate, PCWP, CO, and side effects are monitored.

10. Isosorbide mononitrate, the active metabolite of isosorbide dinitrate, is associated with less tolerance than the dinitrate product. The simple dosing schedule of two doses given 7 hours apart (for example, 0700 and 1400) make this agent more appropriate for some patients.

Cautions and side effects

1. Nitrate therapy may cause postural hypotension, syncope, dizziness, headache, flushing, tachycardia, and nausea. The effects are dose related and can be alleviated by reducing the dose of nitrate. With continued therapy most patients become tolerant to these effects within 2 weeks of stable therapy. Acetaminophen can be used for headache relief.

2. Abrupt withdrawal of nitrate therapy may precipitate angina or pulmonary congestion in some patients.

3. Skin reactions requiring discontinuation of therapy have occurred in 40% of patients using transdermal patches.

4. Methemoglobinemia occurs rarely with the use of high-dose nitrates.

5. Nitroglycerin ointment and patches are rotated to reduce local rash and irritation. Coarsely haired regions are avoided, and occlusive dressings (for example, plastic wrap over ointment) are used when possible to increase the absorption of the paste.

Nitroprusside Sodium

Nitroprusside sodium (Nipride) is a vasodilating agent that acts directly on vascular smooth muscle independent of autonomic innervation.

Cardiovascular actions

Nitroprusside sodium has a balanced effect: dilating arterioles and venules equivalently, thus decreasing preload and afterload. In the failing heart, afterload reduction increases the CO with little or no decrease in MAP. Heart rate tends to remain unchanged or is slightly increased. Decreased preload resulting from venodilatation decreases PCWP. Beneficial hemodynamic effects are observed when the filling pressure and SVR are elevated before therapy and when CO is depressed, such as that which occurs in the failing myocardium. When heart function is normal or when left ventricular filling pressure is normal or low, nitroprusside sodium produces hypotension and tachycardia with little change in CO.

Clinical uses

1. Nitroprusside sodium is a potent, rapid-acting IV antihypertensive agent used to control hypertensive emergencies.
2. Nitroprusside sodium is used in patients with severe left ventricular failure who have adequate blood pressures (systolic blood pressure of at least 90 mm Hg) and elevated PCWPs. The drug is an excellent adjunct to inotropic agents when the blood pressure can be maintained. The combination of dopamine and nitroprusside sodium produces similar hemodynamic responses to that of dobutamine or amrinone alone.

Dosage and administration

1. Nitroprusside sodium is available only in parenteral form. It can be diluted in most IV fluids and concentrated for patients on volume restriction. The infusion bottle should be protected from light by an opaque wrapping.
2. The maintenance infusion rate is 0.5 to 10 mcg/kg/min. The rate should be adjusted to the patient's hemodynamic response and carefully controlled through the use of an infusion pump. Infusion rates should be kept at about 4 mcg/kg/min to avoid cyanide toxicity in patients receiving the drug for several days. Patients with normal renal function seldom develop thiocyanate toxicity with prolonged use (for example, 14 days) if the total dosage is less than 70 mg/kg. Thiocyanate levels of at least 10 mcg/ml are considered toxic.
3. Rapid infusions may cause nausea, itching, diaphoresis, restlessness, palpitations, and headache.
4. Because of the agent's short duration of action (3 to 5 minutes), titration is very easy. Adjustments in dosing can be made every 5 to 10 minutes when necessary.
5. The blood pressure, heart rate, thiocyanate levels, electrolyte levels, and side effects are monitored.

Cautions and side effects

1. Reflex tachycardia, hypotension, abdominal pain, nausea, restlessness, headache and dose-related side effects can be controlled by reducing the infusion rate.
2. Thiocyanate accumulates with long-term therapy (for example, longer than 14 days) or earlier in patients with renal dysfunction. Toxicity is initially manifested as fatigue, anorexia, nausea, headache, mental confusion, or muscle spasms. Severe toxicity leads to tachypnea, altered consciousness, convulsion, metabolic acidosis, or coma. Fatalities have been reported.
3. Nitroprusside sodium is contraindicated in patients with hypertension secondary to coarctation of the aorta or arteriovenous shunts.

Direct Arteriolar Vasodilators (Table 14-10)

These agents directly relax vascular smooth muscle more in arterioles than in veins. These agents include hydralazine, minoxidil, and diazoxide.

Cardiovascular actions

These agents are potent vasodilators that directly relax arteriolar smooth muscle, resulting in a reduction of PVR. The subsequent decrease in blood pressure produces a reflex sympathetic activation, which is manifested as an increase in heart rate, CO, and renin secretion with a redistribution of RBF. Because these changes may attenuate the antihypertensive response, these agents should be administered with a diuretic and sympatholytic agent if used for long-term therapy. They are not recommended for initial therapy or monotherapy of hypertension or heart failure.

Clinical uses

1. These agents are indicated for the treatment of hypertension that has not responded to previous therapy using diuretics, β blockers, angiotensin-converting enzyme (ACE) inhibitors, and/or calcium channel blockers.
2. These agents are indicated for cautious use in patients with low-output heart failure. Hydralazine is the primary agent in this class used for this indication because it produces less sodium and water retention when compared with the other agents.
3. These agents may be used in the treatment of hypertensive emergencies. Diazoxide is given intravenously only for this indication.
4. Hydralazine is indicated for the treatment of toxemia. Patients should be carefully monitored because many of the side effects of hydralazine resemble the clinical symptoms of eclampsia.

Dosage and administration (see Table 14-10)

1. The blood pressure, heart rate, fluid retention, electrolyte levels, and side effects are monitored.
2. Doses should be low initially and slowly titrated upward to achieve the desired response. These agents have additive effects with other hypotensive agents.
3. Minoxidil is a useful adjunct agent for controlling severe hypertension, such as in dissecting aortic aneurysms. It can be used with nitroprusside sodium and a β blocker to achieve maximum reduction in blood pressure.
4. Minoxidil is also an excellent adjunct agent in renal failure with uncontrolled hypertension. It is usually more effective than the other agents in this class.
5. Hydralazine and nitrates used together for heart failure may reduce morbidity and mortality rates for these patients. This combination therapy is an effective alternative for patients who cannot tolerate ACE inhibitors.

TABLE 14-10   Direct Arteriolar Vasodilators

Agent	Trade Name	Route	Onset (min)	Peak (hr)	Duration (hr)	Dose
Hydralazine	Apresoline	Oral,	60	2-4	6-12	25-100 mg qid
		IM,	20-40	1-2	3-8	5-10 mg q6h
		IV	10-20	0.5-1.0	3-8	5-10 mg q6h
Minoxidil	Loniten	Oral	30	4-8	12-48	5-20 mg bid
Diazoxide	Hyperstat	IV	1-2	0.03	4-24	50-150 mg q5min or infusion at 7.5-30 mg/min up to 5 mg/kg

IM, Intramuscularly; *qid,* four times a day; *q,* every; *bid,* twice a day.

6. Hydralazine given intravenously can be used in the treatment of toxemia.

Cautions and side effects

1. Hypotension may occur with these agents and may be manifested clinically by syncope, dizziness, or palpitations. Many patients experience these effects at the time of the drug's peak concentration. These adverse effects can be eliminated by reducing the dose, separating antihypertensive agents, or giving the drug with food. If the patient continues to have hypotension, the drug should be discontinued.
2. Reflex tachycardia and angina typically occur with these agents and may lead to myocardial ischemia. These agents must be used cautiously in patients with histories of coronary artery disease.
3. Sodium and water retention occur frequently and often result in weight gain. Concomitant use of diuretics is necessary to alleviate this side effect.
4. Hydralazine has produced a syndrome resembling systemic lupus erythematosus or rheumatoid arthritis in about 7% of patients. Clinical manifestations include fever, arthralgia, splenomegaly, lymphadenopathy, asthenia, malaise, pleuritic chest pain, edema, and a positive antinuclear antibody (ANA) reaction. Occasionally a rash appears. Hydralazine should be discontinued if these symptoms are noted. This reaction occurs more frequently in women and in patients who are on high-dose regimens (more than 200 mg/day).
5. Minoxidil may cause hair growth in some patients. A topical minoxidil product is available for male pattern baldness.

Doxazosin, Prazosin, and Terazosin

Doxazosin (Cardura), prazosin (Minipress), and terazosin (Hytrin) are orally effective α-adrenergic blocking agents.

Cardiovascular actions

Doxazosin, prazosin, and terazosin selectively block α_1-adrenergic receptors to reduce PVR. The net effect is the dilatation of arterioles and venules equally, which is similar to the effect of nitroprusside sodium. The cardiac acceleration after vasodilatation with hydralazine or after nonselective α-receptor blockade with phentolamine occurs less frequently with these agents. As a result of decreased SVR, CO increases and blood pressure falls in patients with hypertension and heart failure. The improvement in CO may not be maintained with chronic therapy secondary to the development of tolerance to these agent's effects.

Clinical uses

1. Doxazosin, prazosin and terazosin are used as oral vasodilators in the treatment of hypertension. Tolerance to the hypotensive effects usually does not develop.
2. These agents may be used for low-output states, but tolerance usually develops rapidly with chronic dosing. Thus these agents are not recommended for initial therapy.
3. Terazosin is approved for use in patients with benign prostatic hypertrophy.

Dosage and administration (Table 14-11)

1. These agents should be initiated with lower doses and slowly titrated to achieve the desired effect: prazosin, 1 mg orally twice a day (range, 6 to 15 mg/day); terazosin, 1 mg orally at bedtime (range, 1 to 5 mg/day); and doxazosin, 1 mg orally at bedtime (range 1 to 16 mg/day).
2. The first does should be given at bedtime to avoid first-dose syncope. Each increment in dose may precipitate syncopal episodes, and patients should be closely monitored.
3. These agents are available for oral use only.

TABLE 14-11   Peripheral α₁-Adrenergic Blockers

Agent	Trade Name	Onset (min)	Peak (hr)	Duration (hr)	Dose	Dose Schedule
Doxazosin	Cardura	90	2-3	24	2-16 mg/day	qd
Prazosin	Minipress	90	1-3	10	6-15 mg/day	bid-tid
Terazosin	Hytrin	90	1-2	12-24	2-20 mg/day	qd-bid

qd, Once daily; *bid,* twice daily; *tid,* three times daily.

4. Blood pressure, heart rate, and side effects should be monitored.
5. The full antihypertensive effect of these agents may not be achieved for 2 to 4 weeks.
6. These agents are additive with other hypotensive agents and synergistic with calcium channel blockers. The combination of these agents is especially beneficial in black, older, and obese patients with hypertension who have renal insufficiency.

Cautions and side effects

1. First-dose syncope usually occurs 30 to 90 minutes after the initial dose. The patient should be informed of this effect and should avoid rising suddenly. Patients who have hypovolemia are more likely to have syncope with these agents. Patients should avoid driving or hazardous tasks for 12 to 24 hours after the first dose.
2. Other adverse reactions include dizziness, headache, drowsiness, nausea, lethargy, fluid retention, urinary incontinence, and palpitations.
3. Most side effects are dose related and can be relieved by reducing the dose.

DIURETICS[12,14-19,23] (Table 14-12)

Diuretic agents increase the elimination of salt and water by the kidney.

Cardiovascular actions

Diuretics are classified into several different types of agents and differ primarily in their mechanism of action and potency. All agents reduce sodium and water reabsorption, which leads to a decreased circulating blood volume and left ventricular filling pressure (preload). Blood pressure is initially reduced by the change in plasma volume and CO, but long-term treatment with diuretics results in reduced PVR, which occurs after the plasma volume has normalized. Potassium-sparing diuretics and acetazolamide are weak agents and are often ineffective when used alone. Thiazides are moderately effective but are useless when the creatinine clearance is less than 30 ml/min. Although it is a thiazide derivative, metolazone is

effective in renal impairment and useful in combination therapy. The loop diuretics are the most potent diuretic agents and eliminate more free water than the others. Loop diuretics can be given alone or with other diuretics in any patient population.

Clinical uses

1. Diuretics are used in the chronic treatment of hypertension. These agents are especially effective in older, black, and obese patients with hypertension and can be used alone or with other antihypertensive agents.
2. Diuretics are indicated for the chronic and acute treatment of heart failure. Although they are effective in reducing the symptoms of failure, diuretics have no direct effect on the failing myocardium.
3. Diuretics are also indicated for edema and chronic renal insufficiency.

Dosage and administration

1. Thiazide diuretics are often advocated as the preferred agents for the initial diuretic treatment of hypertension, edema, or mild heart failure. Some commonly used agents are listed in Table 14-12. Thiazides appear to have a more potent hypotensive effect initially because of the greater loss of sodium compared with free water with diuresis. Thiazides are synergistic with ACE inhibitors and β blockers.
2. Loop diuretics are preferred over thiazides as initial therapy in patients with renal insufficiency or symptoms of pulmonary congestion. For acute pulmonary edema, a bolus dose of furosemide (0.5 to 1 mg/kg) can be given initially and then doubled in 2 hours if an inadequate response is obtained.
3. Dosages should be low initially and slowly adjusted according to response. Dosages of hydrochlorothiazide greater than 100 mg/day (or 1000 mg/day for chlorothiazide) are ineffective for further increasing diuresis. If the condition is unresponsive, a loop diuretic should be initiated and the thiazide stopped. Once patients appear refractory to loop diuretics, combination therapy (metolazone and a loop di-

TABLE 14-12   Commonly Used Diuretics

Agent	Trade Name	Route	Onset (min)	Peak (hr)	Duration (hr)	Dose (mg/day)
Thiazides						
Chlorothiazide	Diuril	Oral	60-120	3-6	6-12	500-1000
		IV	15	0.5	2	250-1000
Hydrochlorothiazide	Hydrodiuril	Oral	60-120	3-6	6-12	12.5-100
Metolazone	Zaroxolyn	Oral	60-120	3-6	12-24	5-20
Loop Diuretics						
Ethacrynic acid	Edecrin sodium	IV	30	2	6-12	50-400
Bumetanide	Bumex	Oral	30-60	1-2	4-6	1-10
		IV	5-10	0.5-1.0	2-3	1-10
Furosemide	Lasix	Oral	30-60	1-2	6-8	40-1500
		IV	5-10	0.5-1.0	2	40-1500
Torsemide	Demadex	Oral	30-60	1-2	6-12	5-80
		IV	5-10	0.5-1.0	6	5-80
Potassium Sparing Diuretics						
Amiloride	Midamor	Oral	120	10	24	5-10
Spironolactone	Aldactone	Oral	Gradual	72	48-72	25-200
Triamterene	Dyrenium	Oral	120-240	6	9-24	100-300
Acetazolamide	Diamox	Oral	60	2-4	8	250-500

uretic) should be used. Chlorothiazide is the only thiazide available parenterally and may be used as an alternative to metolazone.

4. Patients with poor renal function respond better to larger daily doses than to smaller, twice-daily doses.

5. Fluid removal is more difficult in patients with low albumin levels because of decreased colloid osmotic pressures. Patients should have fluids removed slowly to prevent volume depletion. A good general rule is 1 kg/day weight loss in most patients and 0.5 kg/day in patients with ascites.

6. Patients unresponsive to furosemide may be switched to bumetanide, which is 40 times more potent than furosemide (for example, 1 mg of bumetanide equals 40 mg of furosemide). However, the ratio could be as high as 1 mg of bumetanide to 120 mg of furosemide in patients with renal insufficiency. Thus some patients respond because of the higher dose. All the same, many patients respond well to alternating loop diuretics and seem to maintain a better diuresis than with chronic use of one agent for an extended time.

7. Patients receiving IV diuretics should be switched to oral therapy as soon as possible. Many patients with long-term heart failure require extremely large oral doses because of renal insufficiency and poor oral absorption. Diuretic doses may be altered significantly by the concurrent use of potent vasodilators.

8. The blood pressure, heart rate, urine output, PCWP, renal function, electrolyte levels, and side effects are monitored.

9. Torsemide has a longer duration of action than furosemide and is not associated with rebound antidiuresis. However, torsemide provides no clinical advantage over furosemide or bumetanide in the majority of patients requiring loop diuretic therapy.

10. The use of loop diuretic drips is becoming more predominant in critical care units. When the condition does not respond adequately to diuretics (for example, in hypoalbuminemia, hyponatremia, and renal insufficiency), the patient may require excessive doses. Often labeled "resistant" to diuresis, these patients are excellent candidates for continuous IV drips when intermittent therapy fails. Furosemide has been used more commonly, and the dosage range for drips is 0.05 to 0.15 mg/kg/hr. Dosages as high as 1.0 mg/kg/hr have been used in some patients with no untoward effects. The dosage range for bumetanide has not been established, but currently used dosages range between 0.25 and 1.0 mg/hr.

Cautions and side effects

1. Hypokalemia is the most common and serious adverse effect of these agents (except for the potassium-sparing agents). The use of these agents typically reduces

the serum potassium level by 0.5 to 1 mEq/L, depending on the preexisting level and body stores. Levels should be carefully monitored and potassium replaced accordingly (see section on potassium).

2. The most common adverse effect of potassium-sparing diuretics is hyperkalemia. These agents should be avoided in patients with renal insufficiency. Stopping the diuretic should return the potassium level to normal.

3. Other adverse effects of these agents include hyponatremia, hypomagnesemia, abnormalities in uric acid and calcium levels, fatigue, hypovolemia, and metabolic alkalosis. Most of these effects are dose related and can be minimized by reducing the diuretic dose.

4. Loop diuretics may cause ototoxicity if given parenterally in high doses over short periods. The risk is greatest with ethacrynic acid and least with bumetanide. Doses should be administered no faster than 40 mg/min for furosemide, 1.0 mg/min for bumetanide, 20 mg/min for torsemide, and 2.5 mg/min for ethacrynic acid.

5. Thiazide diuretics may produce glucose intolerance in patients with borderline diabetes or in older patients. The serum glucose concentration should be carefully monitored in patients receiving high doses of these agents.

6. Thiazide diuretics increase serum LDL cholesterol and triglyceride levels and reduce HDL cholesterol levels. These effects may be deleterious in patients with existing coronary artery disease. A notable exception to this is indapamide, which has minimum effects on serum lipid levels.

7. Patients receiving diuretics may experience reductions in their exercise capacity. As the plasma volume normalizes with continued therapy, this effect should lessen.

8. Patients who develop hypokalemia with these agents typically have low magnesium levels. If the magnesium levels are low, oral or parenteral magnesium therapy is necessary before potassium supplementation, or the potassium levels remain low despite replacement therapy (see section on magnesium).

9. Because acetazolamide is a carbonic anhydrase inhibitor, it may cause metabolic acidosis and can be used to treat diuresis-induced alkalosis.

10. Loop diuretic drips that are continued without appropriate monitoring place patients at risk for severe volume depletion and hypokalemia. The volume status and renal function of all patients receiving continuous drips should be carefully monitored, and some institutions have placed 24-hour automatic stop times to prevent inadvertent volume depletion.

ACE INHIBITORS[4, 5, 8, 16-18, 24-28] (Table 14-13)

The ACE inhibitors are potent, orally active agents that block the conversion of angiotensin I to angiotensin II.

Cardiovascular actions

The agents in this class are equally effective at equipotent doses. All competitively inhibit ACE, thereby blocking the formation of angiotensin II, a potent endogenous vasopressor. Angiotensin II also stimulates the sympathetic nervous system and the release of aldosterone, a hormone that retains sodium and eliminates potassium. By lowering angiotensin production, these agents produce acute and sustained reductions in preload and afterload. These agents reduce MAP, right atrial pressure, and left ventricular end-diastolic volume and pressure; they increase CO and SV.

TABLE 14-13   ACE Inhibitors

Agent	Trade Name	Onset (hr)	Peak (hr)	Duration (hr)	Dosage (mg)
Captopril	Capoten	0.5	1-1.5	8-24	6.25-100 q8-12 hr
Enalapril	Vasotec	3-4	4-8	12-24	2.5-40 q12-24 hr
Lisinopril	Zestril, Prinivil	3-4	6-8	24	2.5-40 q24 hr
Benazepril	Lotensin	1	1-4	24	10-40 q24 hr
Fosinopril	Monopril	1	1	12-24	10-40 q12-24 hr
Quinapril	Accupril	0.5-1	1-2	24	5-20 q12-24 hr
Ramipril	Altace	1-2	2-4	12-24	1.25-20 q12-24 hr
Perindopril	Aceon	1	—	24	4-16 q24 hr

q, Every.

The reduction in aldosterone results in mild diuresis and less volume expansion with continued use.

Clinical uses

1. These agents are indicated for the treatment of hypertension. They are synergistic with thiazide diuretics and additive with other hypotensive agents. They are indicated as first-line therapy. ACE inhibitors are particularly efficacious in young, white men with hypertension and in diabetic patients with or without diabetic nephropathy.
2. These agents are indicated for the treatment of CHF. They are the only form of therapy that significantly reduces the morbidity and the mortality rates associated with CHF. ACE inhibitors can be used for initial therapy instead of diuretics or digitalis. The hemodynamic effects of these agents are additive to those of other vasodilating or inotropic agents. Early initiation of therapy in patients with asymptomatic left ventricular hypertrophy may delay the progression of the failing myocardium.
3. Captopril is used after myocardial infarction to improve physical performance in patients with evidence of left ventricular dysfunction.
4. Captopril is used to slow the progression of diabetic nephropathy in diabetic hypertension.

Dosage and administration (see Table 14-13)

1. Dosages should be low initially and slowly titrated upward to the desired response. Patients with CHF may be especially sensitive to these agents and require smaller doses at extended intervals (for example, captopril, 6.25 mg every 12 hours). The hypotensive effects of these agents should be carefully monitored in this population, especially during the peak effect.
2. The dose in patients with renal insufficiency should be titrated carefully to avoid worsening of renal function secondary to hypotension. Diabetic nephropathy and hypertension are typically seen together, and ACE inhibitors are beneficial in reducing proteinuria, blood pressure, and mortality in patients with diabetes. Interestingly, recent studies have shown that ACE inhibitors lower urinary protein excretion in normotensive patients with diabetes and that this reduction is independent of a decrease in systemic blood pressure.
3. Patients with CHF receiving these agents may need the diuretic dose adjusted when ACE inhibitors are initiated. If these agents are given while the patient has hypovolemia, they may worsen cardiac and renal function. Patients on severe salt-restriction diets should be monitored closely and the restrictions eased if necessary. The manufacturer suggests holding diuretic therapy for 1 week, if possible, before initiating ACE inhibitor therapy in patients whose conditions are stable.

4. The blood pressure, heart rate, renal function, CO, PCWP, electrolyte levels, and side effects are monitored.
5. These agents do not adversely affect the serum lipid profile.
6. These agents maintain exercise tolerance in patients with hypertension and improve quality of life.
7. ACE inhibitors and β blockers should not be used concurrently for additive hypotensive effects. These agents are rarely additive and produce more adverse effects when used concomitantly.
8. Captopril has a favorable effect on the dysfunctioning myocardium after myocardial infarction by reducing the ischemic burden, increasing the work capacity, preventing dilatation of the left ventricle, and improving systolic function.

Cautions and side effects

1. Higher doses of these agents produce significantly more adverse effects. Patients with preexisting renal dysfunction are at higher risk to develop adverse effects than other patients.
2. Proteinuria, azotemia, and renal insufficiency rarely occur in patients with normal renal function who receive standard doses. The onset of these conditions is usually after the third month of chronic therapy but may occur more rapidly if the patient is receiving diuretics or becomes hypotensive.
3. Some patients may develop a persistent nonproductive cough while receiving these agents. If a cough occurs, patients may be switched from one agent to another. Fosinopril appears to cause less of an incidence of cough than the other ACE inhibitors and can be successfully used when other agents have produced this side effect.
4. Other adverse effects that may occur include dizziness, eosinophilia, neutropenia, angioedema, rash, nausea, metallic taste, and headache. These agents should be stopped if the patient develops angioedema or neutropenia. The other adverse effects are usually self-limiting and disappear with continued therapy.
5. Hypotension occurs if the patient has sodium depletion, hypovolemia, or hyperreninemia or is overdosed. A reduction in dose and fluid replacement restores blood pressure in most patients.
6. Hyperkalemia may develop in some patients, especially those with renal insufficiency. Potassium supplements and potassium-sparing diuretics should be used cautiously.

CALCIUM CHANNEL BLOCKERS[16-18, 21, 29, 30] (Tables 14-14 and 14-15)

Calcium channel blockers inhibit the transmembrane influx of extracellular calcium ions across the membranes of myocardial and smooth muscle cells.

TABLE 14-14   Calcium Channel Blockers

Agent	Trade Name	Route	Onset (min)	Peak (hr)	Duration (hr)	Dosage (mg)	Cardiovascular Actions					
							Vasodilation					
							Peripheral Effects	Coronary Effects	Cerebral Effects	Contractility	Heart Rate	AV Nodal Conduction
Diltiazem	Cardizem	Oral	30-90	0.5-1	6-10	30-120 q6-8 hr	+	+++	+	0, ↓	0, ↓	↓
		SR	Gradual	6-11	12-24	120-480 q12-24 hr						
		IV	2-5	0.25	1-2	0.25-0.35 mg/kg initially as bolus followed by 5-15 mg/hr infusion up to 24 hours						
Verapamil	Isoptin, Calan, Verelan	Oral	30	0.5-1	6-8	40-120 q6-8 hr	++	+	+	↓↓	0, ↓	↓↓
		SR	Gradual	5-7	12-24	120-480 q12-24h						
		IV	1-5	0.25-0.5	2-4	5-10 mg IV bolus followed by 5- mg/hr infusion						
Nifedipine	Procardia, Adalat	Oral	30-90	0.5-2	4-8	10-30 q6-8 hr	+++	++	++	↓, reflex ↑	0, reflex ↑	0
		SR	Gradual	—	24	30-90 q24 hr						
		SL	10-30	0.5-1	3-4	10-20 prn						
Nicardipine	Cardene	Oral	20-30	0.5-2	6-8	20-40 q8 hr	+++	++	+	↓, reflex ↑	0, reflex ↑	0
		IV	1-5	15	4-6	5 mg/hr ↑ by 2.5 mg/hr q5 min up to 15 mg/hr; reduce to 3 mg/hr maintenance						
Nitrendipine	Baypress	Oral	30-90	1-2	8-24	10-40 q12-24 hr	+++	++	++	↓, reflex ↑	0, reflex ↑	0
Nimodipine	Nimotop	Oral	—	0.5-1	4-6	60 q4h for 21 days	+	+	+++	0	0	0

q, Every; *SR*, sustained release; *SL*, sublingual; *prn*, as necessary.
↑, Increase; *0*, no change; ↓, decrease; +, mild; ++, moderate; +++, potent.

TABLE 14-15   Second-Generation Calcium Antagonists*

Drug	Trade Name	Adult Oral Dosage	Negative Inotropic Effects	Systemic Vasodilation	Vasodilatory Side Effects	Adverse Effects	Comments
Amlodipine	Norvasc	2.5-1.0 mg qd	0	++	+	Peripheral edema; dizziness; flushing; tachycardia and headache less than with other DHPs	Long-acting once-daily therapy
Felodipine	Plendil	5-10 mg qd	+	++	++	Peripheral edema; headache; dizziness; flushing; fatigue	Higher doses poorly tolerated; twice-daily therapy usually necessary
Isradipine	DynaCirc	2.5-10 mg bid	0	++	++	Ankle edema; fatigue; facial flushing; arthralgias; headache	Doses for angina are 2.5-7.5 mg tid; increased ADR with higher doses
Nisoldipine	Baymycard	10 mg qd or bid	0	++	++	Ankle edema; flushing; headache; dizziness	May be better tolerated

*All are dihydropyridine (DHP) derivatives with more selectivity for vascular smooth muscle.
qd, Every day; *bid,* twice daily; *tid,* three times daily; *ADR,* adverse drug reactions.
0, no effect; +, minimal effect; ++, maximal effect.
From Kinney MR and others: *AACN's clinical reference for critical care nursing,* ed 3, St Louis, 1993, Mosby.

Cardiovascular actions

Each of the calcium antagonist agents exerts its pharmacologic action by slightly different actions on the calcium channel, which results in variable hemodynamic effects (see Table 14-14). Nifedipine, nicardipine and nitrendipine are primarily peripheral vasodilators with less of an effect on coronary or cerebral blood flow. These three agents have no direct electrophysiologic properties and alter cardiac conduction only as a reflex action to afterload reduction. Diltiazem moderately decreases AV nodal conduction and is a potent coronary vasodilator. Diltiazem has minimal effects on peripheral vascular tone and tends to produce vasodilatation primarily when vasoconstriction is present. Verapamil has the most potent effects on heart rate and conduction and vasodilates coronary and peripheral smooth muscle. Nimodipine is primarily a cerebral vasodilator with no effect on peripheral, coronary, or conducting tissues; it is indicated only for the treatment of subarachnoid hemorrhage. All these agents except nimodipine have negative inotropic effects on the myocardium; verapamil possesses the greatest and diltiazem the least.

Second-generation DHPs (see Table 14-15) are more vasoselective for vascular smooth muscle and coronary vasculature. These properties may improve efficacy and reduce reflex-mediated adverse effects. These agents have significantly less negative inotropic effects than first-generation agents.

Clinical uses

1. All these agents except nimodipine are approved for the treatment of hypertension. All agents are equally efficacious, and the choice of agent should be based on adverse effects and hemodynamic profiles of the various agents. Calcium channel blockers are useful as initial therapy and particularly beneficial in older, black, and obese patients with hypertension. These agents are additive with other antihypertensive agents and synergistic with doxazosin, prazosin, and terazosin.
2. All these agents except nimodipine are useful in the treatment of stable, unstable, and vasospastic angina. Calcium channel blockers are the preferred agents for vasospastic angina. These agents have additive effects when combined with nitrates or β blockers.

3. Diltiazem is beneficial in reducing morbidity and mortality in patients with non-Q-wave infarctions. The usefulness of calcium channel blockers in transmural infarctions is unclear, and their use may be harmful in some patients.

4. Nimodipine is indicated for the prevention of cerebral vasospasm after subarachnoid hemorrhage. Therapy should be initiated within 96 hours of the cerebrovascular accident and continued for 21 days.

5. Verapamil and diltiazem are indicated for the treatment of supraventricular dysrhythmias. They can be used with digoxin to control ventricular rate in patients with atrial flutter and atrial fibrillation.

6. Verapamil is effective in treating hypertrophic cardiomyopathy.

7. Nicardipine is the first and only IV DHP available for the control of postoperative hypertension and hypertensive crisis.

Dosage and administration (see Tables 14-14 and 14-15)

1. Therapy is initiated with low doses, and the dose is titrated according to response. For rapid, effective control, the patient's condition should be stabilized by intermittent oral dosing before the clinician switches to sustained-release preparations.

2. Older patients may be sensitive to the effects of these agents and should be carefully monitored at the initiation of therapy.

3. These agents may worsen heart failure and should be carefully monitored in patients with histories of left ventricular dysfunction.

4. These agents do not adversely affect the serum lipid profile and improve quality of life.

5. These agents improve exercise tolerance in most patients.

6. The blood pressure, heart rate, ECG, electrolyte levels, and side effects are monitored.

7. Verapamil can be given intravenously for supraventricular dysrhythmias. The dosage is 5 to 10 mg as an IV bolus over 2 to 3 minutes, repeated every 30 minutes as needed. If necessary, verapamil can be given by constant infusion at a rate of 1 to 10 mg/hr. The infusion rate should be carefully adjusted to the lowest possible dosage that controls the dysrhythmia.

8. When mixed for continuous IV infusion, verapamil should not be concentrated more than 1 mg/ml. Verapamil is compatible for mixing in most IV fluids.

9. Verapamil is compatible with aminophylline, bretylium, calcium, digoxin, lidocaine, procainamide, atropine, dopamine, dobutamine, epinephrine, heparin, isoproterenol, nitroglycerin, norepinephrine, potassium, propranolol, and quinidine.

10. Diltiazem can be given intravenously for supraventricular tachycardia. A loading dose of 0.25 to 0.35 mg/kg should be given and followed by a continuous infusion of 10 to 15 mg/hr. Diltiazem infusions are recommended for 24 hours or less. The patient should be switched to oral therapy as soon as possible, and the following are considered equivalent dosages for drip rates: infusion, 5 mg/hr, 180 mg/day orally; infusion, 7 mg/hr, 240 mg/day orally; and infusion, 11 mg/hr, 360 mg/day orally. Doses greater than 15 mg/hr are not recommended. Diltiazem can be diluted as 250 mg in 250 ml of IV fluid for a final concentration of 1 mg/ml.

11. For rapid control of blood pressure, nicardipine given intravenously can be initiated at 5 mg/hr and increased by 2.5 mg/hr every 5 to 15 minutes up to a maximum dose of 15 mg/hr. Once the blood pressure is controlled, the rate should be reduced to 3 mg/hr and titrated by 1.0 to 2.5 mg/hr to maintain the blood pressure in the desired range. Oral therapy should be instituted as soon as possible. The peripheral infusion site must be changed every 12 hours to prevent phlebitis. Nicardipine can be diluted as 25 mg of nicardipine in 240 ml of IV fluid for a final concentration of 0.1 mg/ml.

Cautions and side effects

1. Verapamil is associated with the largest incidence of side effects but is usually well tolerated in most patients. Fewer than 6% of patients require discontinuation of the drug because of side effects. Constipation occurs in fewer than 9% of patients. Major hemodynamic and severe conduction abnormalities occur in fewer than 2% of patients, but the concomitant use of β blockers increases this incidence. Hypotension may occur with parenteral use, and IV administration of calcium before verapamil prevents hypotension without blocking the drug's dysrhythmic effect.

2. Nifedipine, nicardipine, and nitrendipine have major side effects related to their vasodilatory properties. Dizziness, flushing, headache, syncope, and lightheadedness may occur in up to 25% of patients and are generally dose related. A reduction in dose alleviates these symptoms. Peripheral edema occurs less frequently than with other vasodilators.

3. Most of these agents worsen heart failure; the exception is amlodipine.

4. Rash occurs in about 1% of patients receiving diltiazem. Bradydysrhythmias rarely occur with the use of this agent alone but are more frequent when it is combined with another agent that slows myocardial conduction.

5. Nifedipine, nicardipine, and nitrendipine may paradoxically worsen angina pain secondary to a reflex increase in sympathetic tone. Verapamil occasionally worsens angina pain if the patient develops hypotension or bradycardia and has poor left ventricular function.

6. Verapamil increases digoxin levels almost twofold in some patients. Digoxin levels should be carefully monitored with initiation of verapamil therapy, and the digoxin dose should be halved if the patient is not receiving quinidine concomitantly.

7. Other side effects common to these agents include nausea, headache, dizziness, and rash.

8. Diltiazem and nicardipine increase serum cyclosporine levels, necessitating careful monitoring of these patients to prevent cyclosporine toxicity.

9. Second-generation DHPs are associated with fewer side effects than nifedipine, nitrendipine, or nicardipine.

10. Amlodipine may be more beneficial in heart failure or left ventricular dysfunction than the other calcium channel blockers. Amlodipine appears to provide superior afterload reduction with none of the negative inotropic effects commonly seen with the other calcium channel blockers.

THROMBOLYTIC AGENTS[12,31-33] (Table 14-16)

Thrombolytic agents act directly to lyse formed thrombi.

Cardiovascular actions

All thrombolytic agents stimulate the conversion of plasminogen to plasmin by various mechanisms. Plasmin degrades fibrin, fibrinogen, and other procoagulant proteins, causing the breakdown of fresh thrombi. Streptokinase, urokinase, and anisoylated plasminogen streptokinase activator complex (APSAC) bind directly to circulating plasminogen, prompting the conversion to plasmin. Tissue plasminogen activator (TPA) binds specifically to fibrin in the thrombus and converts entrapped plasminogen to plasmin, initiating local thrombolysis. Thus TPA is more clot specific than the other agents. Although these agents are distinctly different when compared regarding clot specificity, reperfusion, and potency, confusion exists over the importance of these characteristics. No one agent has proved to be superior to any other agent in reducing morbidity and mortality rates if used within 6 hours of the onset of chest pain in acute myocardial infarction. It appears that the concomitant use of adjunct therapy such as anticoagulants, antiplatelets, β blockers, or ACE inhibitors is more important than the choice of thrombolytic used. All these agents produce bleeding to the same extent and must be used with adjunct heparin and/or aspirin therapy to prevent reocclusion.

Clinical uses

1. These agents are used in acute myocardial infarction to lyse obstructive thrombi in coronary arteries. These agents appear to be most efficacious in transmural anterior myocardial infarctions. Data suggest that these agents lower the incidence of mortality by 20% to 25%. This effect is additive with that of β blockers, antiplatelet agents, and heparin. These agents should be initiated within the first 6 hours of the onset of chest pain.

2. Streptokinase and urokinase are indicated for the treatment of deep vein thrombosis (DVT) and pulmonary embolism. The effectiveness of these agents is diminished in patients with thromboses of more than 5 days.

3. Urokinase can be used to clear occluded catheters. The dose is 5000 IU injected with a tuberculin syringe into the catheter; the clinician should aspirate the fluid after 20 to 30 minutes and repeat if necessary.

Dosage and administration (see Table 14-16)

1. Heparin should be initiated immediately after the completion of TPA infusions (see section on heparin for dosing). Heparin should be initiated 3 to 6 hours after completion of streptokinase infusions to minimize bleeding. The activated partial thromboplastin time (APTT) should be kept at 2 times the control value.

2. Aspirin therapy should be initiated within 24 hours of admission. The addition of aspirin, 81 mg (reduced strength) or 325 mg (regular strength), does not significantly increase the risk of bleeding with concurrent thrombolytic therapy. Aspirin significantly reduces the incidence of reocclusion.

3. β Blockers should be initiated within 6 hours of the onset of chest pain for maximal benefit (see section on β blockers).

4. Contraindications to thrombolytic therapy include active internal bleeding, intracranial neoplasm, severe hypertension (systolic blood pressure greater than 180 mm Hg or diastolic blood pressure greater than 110 mm Hg), recent (within 2 months) cerebrovascular event, recent (within 10 days) surgery, organ biopsy, trauma, prolonged cardiopulmonary resuscitation, or hemostatic defects.

5. Known allergy or recent exposure (within 6 months) to streptokinase or APSAC precludes the use of either agent.

6. Relative contraindications include recent (within 10 days) abdominal procedure, gastrointestinal hemorrhage, or bacterial endocarditis.

7. Older patients have a greater mortality rate associated with acute myocardial infarction, and the use of these agents may provide greater benefits in this population. However, the use of thrombolytics in the older adult is limited by the higher risk for bleeding side effects. Older patients are at greater risk for hemorrhage, and thrombolytic agents should be cautiously used in patients 75 years or older.

8. During dilution of these agents, the vials should not be shaken. These compounds are protein substances and foam when shaken. The vials should be gently rolled between the hands.

9. The blood pressure, heart rate, ECG, chest pain, APTT, electrolyte levels, and bleeding are monitored.

TABLE 14-16   Thrombolytic Agents

Agent	Trade Name	Dose (after MI)	Dose (DVT/PTE)	Reocclusion (%)	Reperfusion (%)	Clot Specificity	Bleeding Complications	Expense
Streptokinase	Streptase, Kabikinase	1.5 million IU over 1 hr	250,000 IU over 30 min and then 100,000 IU/hr for 24-72 hr	20	65	+	++++	+
Alteplase (TPA)	Activase	60 mg over 1 hr (6-10 mg in first 1-2 min) and then 20 mg/hr for 2 hr for total dose of 100 mg	—	20	70	+++	++++	++++
Urokinase	Abbokinase	—	4400 IU/kg IV load over 10 min and then 4400 IU/kg/hr for 12 hr	<10	66	++	++++	+++
Anistreplase (APSAC)	Eminase	30 units intravenously over 3-5 min	—	<10	68	++	++++	++

MI, Myocardial infarction; *DVT/PTE,* deep vein thrombosis/pulmonary thromboembolism; *IU,* International Units; *TPA,* tissue plasminogen activator; *APSAC,* anisolated plasminogen streptokinase activator complex.
+, Weakly positive; ++, positive; +++, strongly positive; ++++, very strongly positive.

Cautions and side effects

1. Hemorrhage is a major complication in 3% to 10% of patients receiving thrombolytic agents, and none of these agents has any clear advantage over the other. Cryoprecipitate, fresh frozen plasma, packed red blood cells, and platelets may be necessary, and the patient's blood should be typed and cross-matched on admission. Packed red cells are useful in patients with hematocrits less than 25%, but cryoprecipitate is the best blood product for correction of the lytic state after thrombolytic therapy. A total of 10 units of cryoprecipitate raises the fibrinogen level about 0.7 g/L and the factor VIII level about 30%. The fibrinogen levels are maintained at greater than 1.0 g/L. Occasionally, antifibrinolytic therapy may be necessary, but it should not be routinely used.

2. Intracranial hemorrhage occurs in 0.5% to 1.5% of patients.

3. Most bleeding is minor and consists of oozing around the catheter or venipuncture sites. Pressure should be applied to these areas, and manipulation of arterial lines should be avoided.

4. Allergic reactions may occur with APSAC or streptokinase. Patients can receive diphenhydramine (Benadryl) or steroids before thrombolytic administration to prevent this reaction.

5. Transient hypotension may occur with these agents and can be corrected by volume replacement. Hypotension associated with streptokinase infusions may be related to the infusion rate, which should be reduced if the blood pressure drops significantly.

HEPARIN [2, 12, 31-35] (Tables 14-17 and 14-18)

Anticoagulants inhibit the action or formation of one or more of the clotting factors and are used to prevent and treat a variety of thromboembolic disorders. Heparin is one of the agents in this class.

Cardiovascular actions

Heparin is a naturally occurring substance, but its physiologic role has not been completely elucidated. In pharmacologic doses, heparin predominantly affects blood coagulation and blood lipid levels. It inhibits thrombin and fibrin formation by activating antithrombin III and produces prolongation of clotting time, prothrombin time (PT), and APTT. Heparin also inhibits the platelet aggregation induced by thrombin. Heparin clears plasma lipids by activating lipoprotein lipase, but the clinical significance of this action is not fully understood.

Standard preparations of heparin are extracts of porcine mucosa or bovine lung and are heterogenous with molecular weights ranging from 5000 to over 30,000. The introduction of low-molecular-weight heparins (LMWHs), derivatives of standard heparin that have a molecular weight of closer to 5000, has changed the prophylaxis and treatment of DVT. LMWHs have a preferential inhibitory effect on factor Xa rather than thrombin. Standard heparin products have an factor Xa–to–thrombin ratio of 1:1, whereas LMWH ratios vary from 4:1 to 2:1. LMWHs are safe and potentially more effective than standard heparin products for the prophylaxis and treatment of DVT. LMWHs do not require APTT measurements and can be given once or twice a day.

Clinical uses

1. Heparin is indicated for the treatment of thrombophlebitis, pulmonary embolism, DVT, catheter maintenance, and acute myocardial infarction with or without thrombolytics. LMWH is indicated for the prophylaxis and treatment of only DVT.

2. Heparin should be administered after initial thrombolysis to maintain patency in acute myocardial infarctions. Heparin should be initiated after streptokinase or urokinase therapy in patients with DVT or pulmonary embolism.

TABLE 14-17	Heparin Rate Chart*	
Weight (kg)	Drip Rate (units/hr) Calculated for 15 units/kg/hr	Drip Rate (ml/hr) (40 units/ml drip)
50-52	760	19
53-54	800	20
55-57	840	21
58-60	880	22
61-62	920	23
63-65	960	24
66-68	1000	25
69-70	1040	26
71-73	1080	27
74-76	1120	28
77-78	1160	29
79-81	1200	30
82-84	1240	31
85-86	1280	32
87-89	1320	33
90-92	1360	34
93-94	1400	35
95-97	1440	36
98-100	1480	37
>100	1520	38

*Based on weight for standard heparin drips 20,000 units/500 ml (40 units/ml).

TABLE 14-18   Heparin Titration Schedule to Maintain APTT in Therapeutic Range

PTT (sec)	Patient Control Ratio (using 26 sec as control)	Atrial Fibrillation (40 units/ml drip)	DVT/PTE/AMI/CVA (40 units/ml drip)	Angioplasty/Prosthetic Valve/Stent Placement (40 units/ml drip)
<30	<1.2	2500-unit bolus, increase 200 units/hr (5 ml/hr)	2500-unit bolus, increase 200 units/hr (5 ml/hr)	5000-unit bolus, increase 200 units/hr (5 ml/hr)
31-34	1.2-1.3	Increase 160 units/hr (4 ml/hr)	Increase 160 units/hr (4 ml/hr)	2500-unit bolus, increase 200 units/hr (5 ml/hr)
35-39	1.3-1.5	Increase 80 units/hr (2 ml/hr)	Increase 80 units/hr (2 ml/hr)	Increase 200 units/hr (5 ml/hr)
40-52	1.5-2.0	No change	No change	Increase 120 units/hr (3 ml/hr)
53-65	2.0-2.5	Decrease 120 units/hr (3 ml/hr)	No change	No change
66-78	2.5-3.0	Decrease 200 units/hr (5 ml/hr)	Decrease 120 units/hr (3 ml/hr)	Decrease 120 units/hr (3 ml/hr)
79-91	3.0-3.5	Hold drip 1 hr, decrease 200 units/hr (5 ml/hr)	Decrease 200 units/hr (5 ml/hr)	Decrease 200 units/hr (5 ml/hr)
>91	>3.5	Hold drip 1 hr, decrease 200 units/hr (5 ml/hr)	Hold drip 1 hr, decrease 200 units/hr (5 ml/hr)	Hold drip 1 hr, decrease 200 units/hr (5 ml/hr)

DVT/PTE/AMI/CVA, Deep vein thrombosis/pulmonary thromboembolism/acute myocardial infarction/cerebrovascular accident.

3. Heparin may be beneficial in reducing chest pain in unstable angina, but its use is controversial.
4. The use of heparin after angioplasty is controversial. Reocclusion may occur less frequently in patients who receive 24 to 72 hours of therapy after this procedure. The APTT should be kept at 2 to 2.5 times the control value.
5. Heparin is used subcutaneously to prevent DVT in patients who are temporarily on bedrest.

Dosage and administration (see Tables 14-17 and 14-18)

1. Heparin is administered intravenously or subcutaneously. Oral administration is ineffective, and intramuscular (IM) administration is usually not recommended because it may produce local hemorrhage. LMWH is administered only by SC injection.
2. Anticoagulant doses of heparin are determined by clotting time or APTT, both of which are maintained at 1.5 to 2.5 times the control value. Continuous infusions of heparin are associated with fewer hemorrhagic side effects than intermittent injections because a more stable anticoagulant effect is maintained.
3. Patients should be given a loading dose before initiation of a continuous heparin infusion. Patients with total body weights of less than 100 kg can be given 5000 units via IV bolus, whereas patients with total

body weights of greater than 100 kg can be given 7500 units via IV bolus. The infusion rate should be initiated at 15 units/kg/hr, with a maximal initial rate of 1520 units/hr (see Table 14-17 for a weight chart to convert the rate for a standard drip for 20,000 units in 500 ml of IV fluid). Table 14-18 lists appropriate dosage adjustments for the various disease states in which heparin infusions are used.
4. The first APTT should be performed 6 hours after the initiation of the continuous heparin infusion and every 6 hours until the APTT is stabilized in the desired range. After it is stabilized, the APTT should be monitored once or twice a day or 6 hours after any change in the heparin infusion rate.
5. The conditions of patients with coronary stents are more difficult to control secondary to adjunct therapy with aspirin, warfarin, dextran, and dipyridamole. Patients should receive the same loading dose and initial rate as listed. It is recommended that the APTT be monitored every 6 hours for the first 48 hours and then return to the twice- or once-daily measurements.
6. LMWH, 30 mg subcutaneously twice a day, can be given for the prevention of DVT. It should not be administered by IM or IV injection. For the treatment of DVT, 1 mg/kg every 12 hours has been used investigationally in clinical trials. The APTT is useless in

monitoring the anticoagulant effects of LMWH. There is no routine laboratory method for measuring the anticoagulant effects of LMWH.

7. Heparin can be administered intermittently via the IV or SC route (5000 to 10,000 units every 4 to 6 hours). SC sites should be rotated.

8. For prevention of thrombosis, the heparin dose is 5000 units subcutaneously every 12 hours.

9. The heparin clearance rate is proportional to the dose administered because larger doses have a longer half-life. The anticoagulant effects of a single IV dose of heparin last an average of 3 to 4 hours.

10. Heparin is the preferred anticoagulant in pregnant or lactating women because it does not cross the placenta or appear in maternal milk. LMWH is not recommended and should not be used.

11. The APTT, bleeding, hematocrit, platelet count, and infusion rate for heparin are monitored. In patients receiving LMWH, bleeding, hematocrit, and platelet counts are monitored.

12. Heparin is compatible in most IV fluids, and a standard dilution is 20,000 units in 500 ml of IV fluid.

13. Heparin is compatible with calcium, dopamine, dobutamine, isoproterenol, lidocaine, methylprednisolone, norepinephrine, potassium, and epinephrine.

Cautions and side effects

1. Hemorrhage is the predominant side effect, and LMWH and heparin are contraindicated in active bleeding or hemorrhagic tendencies. The occurrence of hemorrhage during any type of heparin therapy should initiate a search for a pathologic bleeding site.

2. The anticoagulant effects of heparin are reversible by the administration of protamine sulfate. Doses of 1.0 to 1.5 mg of protamine sulfate antagonizes approximately 100 units of heparin, but the dose requirements fall quickly as time increases after the last dose. In most cases, discontinuation of heparin is sufficient therapy to correct anticoagulant effects. However, the anticoagulant and hemorrhagic effects of LMWH are not as easily reversible with protamine. Protamine does not bind to the low-molecular-weight components, and it is unclear whether any or only partial neutralization occurs with protamine sulfate usage in patients receiving LMWH.

3. Minor bleeding and bruising are normal complications that should not preclude the use of any heparin compound.

4. Thrombocytopenia occurs in 5% to 15% of patients receiving heparin and is seen more often with bovine-derived heparin. Thrombocytopenia usually develops within 1 to 20 days (average, 5 to 9), and heparin should be discontinued if the platelet count falls below 100,000/mm³. When LMWH was initially developed, it was theorized that thrombocytopenia would not be a complication of therapy, making LMWH use safe in patients with heparin-induced thrombocytopenia. Unfortunately, this has not been investigated thoroughly with properly designed trials, and there is evidence that LMWH may cross-react with plasma from patients with recent heparin-induced thrombocytopenia. In addition, the administration of LMWH has been associated with the development of thrombocytopenia in previously unexposed patients. Thus the risk of thrombocytopenia with LMWH or standard heparin products should be carefully assessed and monitored in all patients receiving these agents.

5. Long-term heparin therapy has been associated with alopecia, osteoporosis, neuropathy, and priapism.

WARFARIN [2,12,36,37] (Tables 14-19 through 14-21 and box)

Anticoagulants inhibit the action or formation of one or more of the clotting factors and are used to prevent and treat a variety of thromboembolic disorders. Warfarin is one of the agents in this class.

Cardiovascular actions

Warfarin interferes with the hepatic synthesis of vitamin K–dependent clotting factors, resulting in the reduction of clotting factors II, VII, IX, and X. The anticoagulant effects depend on the half-lives of the clotting factors, (50, 6, 24, 36 hours, respectively); the reduction in the rate of syn-

---

TABLE 14-19   Initial Determination of a Conservative Warfarin Maintenance Dose From Load*

PT Ratio†	Suggested Starting Dose for Maintenance Therapy
1.2	10 mg
1.3	7.5 mg
1.4	7.5 mg
1.5	7.5 mg
1.6	5.0 mg
1.7	5.0 mg
1.8	5.0 mg
1.9	5.0 mg
2.0	5.0 mg
2.1	2.5 mg
2.2	2.5 mg
2.3	2.5 mg
2.4	2.5 mg

*The patient should receive 7.5 to 10 mg orally for 3 consecutive nights. The initial maintenance dose is estimated from the PT on the morning of the fourth day of therapy (morning after the third loading dose). This dose is an estimate of the maintenance dose, and PT/International Normalized Ratio (INR) should be followed closely until the patient has reached steady state on any dose (1 week for most regimens, 2 weeks for alternating regimens).
†Morning after third loading dose of 7.5 to 10 mg.

TABLE 14-20 Initial Determination of Warfarin Maintenance Dose from Load for More Rapid Achievement of Therapeutic PT/INR*

PT Ratio†	Suggested Starting Dose for Maintenance Therapy	Suggested Follow-up for Drawing First PT INR After Discharge
1.2	10 mg	3 days
1.3	10/7.5 mg	1 week
1.4	7.5/7.5/10 mg	1 week
1.5	7.5 mg	3 days
1.6	7.5/7.5/5 mg	1 week
1.7	5/7.5 mg	1 week
1.8	5/5/7.5 mg	1 week
1.9	5 mg	3 days
2.0	5/5/2.5 mg	1 week
2.1	5/2.5 mg	1 week
2.2	2.5/2.5/5 mg	1 week
2.3	2.5 mg	3 days
2.4	2.5/1.25 mg	1 week

*The patient must receive 10 mg orally for 3 consecutive nights. The initial maintenance dose is estimated from the PT on the morning of the fourth day of therapy (morning after the third dose of 10 mg orally at bedtime). This dose is an estimate of the maintenance dose, and the PT/INR should be followed closely until the patient has reached steady state on the dose as indicated above.
†Morning after the third dose of 10 mg.
INR, International Normalized Ratio.

thesis of the clotting factors determines the clinical response. The initial prolongation of the PT is usually secondary to factor VII reduction (short half-life or 6 hours), but the steady state anticoagulant effects are not seen for 3 to 7 days as the other factors are depleted. Thus warfarin drug effects are very individualized, and it is difficult to standardize dosing practices.

Warfarin has gained new popularity in the last 5 years with the emergence of data showing that low therapeutic dosages are effective in the prevention and treatment of a variety of cardiovascular disorders that precipitate emboli. Warfarin reduces morbidity and mortality in patients with atrial fibrillation, myocardial infarction, and cardiomyopathy.

Clinical uses

1. Warfarin is indicated in the prophylaxis and treatment of DVT, PTE, and atrial fibrillation with embolism.
2. Warfarin is indicated as an adjunct agent in the prophylaxis of systemic emboli after myocardial infarction or coronary artery bypass grafting.
3. Warfarin is used in the treatment of cardiomyopathy and severe coronary artery disease, for the prevention of restenosis after coronary stent placement or angio-

plasty, and for the prevention of embolic stroke in patients with previous histories of embolic stroke.
4. Warfarin is used to prevent recurrent transient ischemic attacks in patients unable to tolerate aspirin therapy or whose conditions have not responded to it.
5. Warfarin is also used in the treatment of patients with prosthetic cardiac valve replacement to prevent the formation of emboli.

Dosage and administration (see Tables 14-19 to 14-21 and box)

1. Because the pharmacokinetic and pharmacodynamic effects of warfarin are so complex, studies have shown that experienced professionals are more likely than computer programs to accurately adjust dosing. There are *no* algorithms that accurately predict dosing in all patients, and most algorithms in use (computer or graph) are inaccurate in more than 35% of patients. There is no simple way to dose warfarin. It is important to avoid dramatic swings in the PT/International Normalized Ratio (INR) because these fluctuations jeopardize patient care outcomes.
2. For administration of warfarin to a patient, the rate of rise is the best indicator of maintenance dose. Most patients can be given 7.5 to 10 mg for 2 to 3 consecutive days, with maintenance therapy initiated on the third or fourth day. See Tables 14-19 and 14-20 for two suggested algorithms for initiation of therapy based on a loading dose. Older adults (over 65 years) and women are generally more sensitive to warfarin's anticoagulant effects, so the smaller dose of 5.0 or 7.5 mg is recommended. In addition, patients who have received therapeutic doses of dipyridamole, aspirin, or dextran within 24 hours may exhibit a greater-than-normal rise in the PT/INR with conventional loading doses; thus smaller initial dosages with close, consistent follow-up may be necessary because the PT/INR may drop in 1 to 2 weeks. Many patients who receive warfarin initially may also receive heparin for 3 to 6 days until a "therapeutic" PT/INR is achieved. It should be noted that the PT/INR may be falsely elevated with concurrent therapy and may decline significantly when heparin is discontinued. When heparin is discontinued, a PT/INR performed 6 hours or later is more accurate.
3. The INR measurement may be inaccurate for the first 4 to 6 weeks of therapy, especially in the older adult and when heparin has been used; therefore most clinicians find it helpful to follow the PT initially and use the INR after therapy is stabilized 1 to 2 months later. The box shows the relationship of PT to INR.
4. Considering that it may take 1 to 2 weeks to reach steady state at any given dose, warfarin therapy is often not stabilized before discharge. Realistically, it is rarely necessary to keep a patient hospitalized to adjust war-

TABLE 14-21   PT Measurement After Discharge*

PT Measurement (Desired Range: 1.3-1.5 × Control)	PT Measurement (Desired Range: 1.5-2.0 × Control)	Directions
FIRST MEASUREMENT (2-5 DAYS AFTER DISCHARGE)		
>2.2 × control	>2.5 × control	Hold for 1-2 doses. Reduce weekly dose by 5 mg/wk. Repeat PT in 3 days.
1.8-2.1 × control	2.3-2.4 × control	Hold for 1-2 doses. Reduce weekly dose by 2.5 mg/wk. Repeat PT in 1 wk.
1.6-1.7 × control	2.1-2.2 × control	Hold for 1 dose. Resume previous regimen. Repeat PT in 1 wk.
1.3-1.5 × control	1.5-2.0 × control	Do not change dose. Repeat PT in 1 wk.
<1.3 × control	<1.5 × control	Give extra dose for 1-2 nights. Increase dose by 2.5 mg/wk. Repeat PT in 1 wk.
Normal PT	Normal PT	Reload with 7.5 to 10 mg at bedtime for 3 nights. Increase dose by 5 mg/wk. Repeat PT in 1 wk.
SECOND MEASUREMENT (3-7 DAYS AFTER INITIAL LEVEL)		
>2.2 × control	>2.5 × control	Hold for 2-3 doses. Reduce weekly dose by 5 mg/wk. Repeat PT in less than 1 wk.
1.8-2.1 × control	2.3-2.4 × control	Hold for 2 doses. Reduce weekly dose by 2.5 mg/wk. Repeat PT in 1 wk.
1.6-1.7 × control	2.1-2.2 × control	Hold for 1 dose. Resume previous regimen. Repeat PT in 1 wk.
1.3-1.5 × control	1.5-2.0 × control	Do not change dose. Repeat PT in 2 wk.
<1.3 × control	<1.5 × control	Give extra dose for 1-2 nights. Increase dose by 2.5 mg/wk. Repeat PT in 1 wk.
Normal PT	Normal PT	Give load 10 mg for 3 nights. Increase dose by 5 mg/wk. Repeat PT in 1 wk.

*All levels should be evaluated for exogenous and endogenous factors that may alter the PT before any change in therapy is initiated.

Continued.

farin therapy, and with appropriate follow-up, most conditions can be stabilized within 1 to 3 weeks in an outpatient setting. The initial maintenance dose is not that critical because it is only an estimate; it is important to start someone on a standard dose and institute appropriate follow-up for dosage adjustments. The first PT/INR should be performed 2 to 5 days after discharge.

5. The keys to warfarin maintenance therapy are to follow trends, expect and allow fluctuations in laboratory results without making dosage changes, and use small incremental dosage changes. Warfarin requirements

TABLE 14-21   PT Measurement After Discharge—cont'd

PT Measurement (Desired Range: 1.3-1.5 × Control)	PT Measurement (Desired Range: 1.5-2.0 × Control)	Directions
THIRD MEASUREMENT (7-21 DAYS AFTER INITIAL LEVEL)		
>2.2 × control	>2.5 × control	Hold for 2-3 doses. Reduce weekly dose by 5 mg/wk. Repeat PT in 1 wk.
1.8-2.1 × control	2.3-2.4 × control	Hold for 2 doses. Reduce weekly dose by 2.5 mg/wk. Repeat PT in 1-2 wk.
1.6-1.7 × control	2.1-2.2 × control	Hold for 1 dose. Resume previous regimen until 2 consecutive measurements are elevated and then reduce dose by 2.5 mg/wk. Repeat PT in 1-3 wk.
1.3-1.5 × control	1.5-2.0 × control	Do not change dose. Repeat PT in 3 wk.
<1.3 × control	<1.5 × control	Determine compliance. Reload with 10 to 15 mg for 3 nights. Increase dose by 5 mg/wk. Repeat PT in 1 wk.
Normal PT	Normal PT	Give 15 mg for 3 nights. Increase dose by 10 mg/wk. Repeat PT in 1 wk.
MAINTENANCE DOSAGE ADJUSTMENTS		
>2.2 × control	>2.5 × control	Hold for 2-3 doses. Assess bleeding. Assess drug therapy interactions. Reduce weekly dose by 5 mg/wk. Repeat PT in less than 1 wk.
1.8-2.1 × control	2.3-2.4 × control	Hold for 2 doses. Assess bleeding. Assess drug therapy interactions. Reduce weekly dose by 2.5 mg/wk. Repeat PT in 1-3 wk.
1.6-1.7 × control	2.1-2.2 × control	Hold for 1 dose. Assess bleeding. Assess drug therapy interactions. Resume previous regimen. Repeat PT in 2-4 wk. If elevated a second time, reduce dose by 1.25-2.5 mg/wk.
1.3-1.5 × control	1.5-2.0 × control	Do not change dose. Repeat PT in 3-6 wk.
<1.3 × control	<1.5 × control	Give extra dose for 1-2 nights. Resume previous regimen. Repeat PT in 2-4 wk. If low a second time, increase dose by 1.25-2.5 mg/wk.
Normal PT	Normal PT	Assess compliance. Assess drug therapy interactions. Give load 10 mg for 3 nights. Increase dose by 5 mg/wk if compliant. Repeat PT in 1 wk.

RELATIONSHIP OF PT TO INR

$$\text{PT ratio} = \frac{\text{Patient's PT}}{\text{Laboratory control PT}}$$

$$\text{INR} = (\text{PT ratio})$$

frequently change with long-term therapy, but these changes may be seasonal or temporary (for example, with influenza or a cold, after a vaccine or antibiotic therapy, and with an exacerbation of CHF). Anticipated fluctuations secondary to short-term drug therapy, colds or influenza, or exacerbation of CHF should be conservatively managed by holding doses when necessary and then reinstituting the previous regimen if it was "therapeutic" before the anticipated changes.

6. If a change is necessary, a good rule of thumb is that it should be no greater than 10% of the total weekly dosage, or 5 mg/wk in most patients. Often, dosage changes of 2.5 mg/wk provide the most accurate adjustment in drug therapy. To achieve small dosage reductions, alternating dosage schedules must be implemented. Table 14-21 lists suggested guidelines for initial PT measurements in the first month and for maintenance therapy.

7. It is important to avoid drug-free days and uneven alternating schedules. For example, 5 mg every other day is *not* the same as 2.5 mg every day. With this regimen, the PT/INR is difficult to follow because it is virtually impossible to reach steady state. An analogous situation is administering aminoglycosides, randomly missing a daily dose, and analyzing daily serum blood levels. Examples of appropriate alternating schedules follow: 5 mg/2.5 mg; 5 mg/5 mg/2.5 mg; 5 mg/5 mg/5 mg/2.5 mg; and 5 mg/day except 2.5 mg on Sunday.

8. To increase compliance, warfarin dosing calendars are necessary adjuncts to therapy when alternating schedules are used, and patients should be encouraged to bring them to their clinic visit.

9. New patients should be followed weekly (or every 2 weeks if on alternating schedules) until the PT/INR is in the desired range. Weekly PT/INR checks are continued until the patient's condition is stabilized for 2 consecutive weeks; then the time interval is increased to 2 or 3 weeks. Once it is therapeutic, this interval can be increased to 4 to 6 weeks for well-stabilized conditions. If the PT/INR is outside the desired range, the warfarin dosage should be re-evaluated (not necessarily changed) and the interval between laboratory measurements modified if necessary. Again, the clinician should keep in mind that it is common for patients to have fluctuations of 1 to 3 seconds in their PTs at any given time and that cor-

rection may require only adding or deleting a dose for a day before resuming the previous regimen.

10. Dosage changes are usually necessary only when the PT/INR is extremely high or low, repeatedly outside the therapeutic range, or altered by concomitant long-term drug therapy. It is more difficult to establish a patient's warfarin requirements when the dosage is constantly altered and steady state is never achieved.

11. Another reminder is that patients on alternating schedules (for example 5 mg/2.5 mg, 5 mg/5 mg/2.5 mg, and 5 mg/5 mg/5 mg/2.5 mg) may require 2 to 3 weeks to reach steady state and that checking the PT/INR before this time may not reflect the final effect of such a dosage regimen.

12. Patients are often good judges of their own response to therapy based on how they "feel" when taking the drug. It is necessary and helpful to chart a patient's response to any given dose and maintain that flow sheet in the chart. This type of flow sheet aids in determining future dosage adjustments, identifying seasonal changes, and documenting responses to any given dosage. Many of the bleeding complications with warfarin are secondary to poor compliance, and flow sheets assist in recognizing noncompliant patients.

Cautions and side effects (see boxes)

1. Bleeding occurs in up to 30% of patients receiving warfarin, with the incidence of fatal or life-threatening bleeding ranging from 2% to 8%. Bleeding often occurs in the gastrointestinal tract, soft tissues, and urinary tract. Risk factors for increased bleeding include age (over 65), female gender, high-intensity therapy, a history of stroke or gastrointestinal bleeding, a serious comorbid disease, the first month of therapy, and atrial fibrillation. Bleeding may be reduced by using less

ANTICOAGULATION SCALE FOR ASSESSMENT OF BLEEDING AND BRUISING

1. No signs of symptoms of bleeding or bruising
2. Acceptable minor bleeding or bruising:

Gum bleeding	Oozing from puncture sites
Mild hemoptysis	Pink or streaked nasal discharge
Bleeding from hemorrhoids	Increased menstrual bleeding
Petechiae	Ecchymosis
Easy bruising	Subconjunctival hemorrhage
Larger bruises	Minor hematoma

3. Unacceptable major bleeding or bruising:

Gross hematuria	Hematemesis
Gross hemoptysis	Black or tarry stools
Occult rectal bleeding	Excessive menstrual bleeding
Hemarthrosis	Cerebral bleeding
Major hematoma	Retroperitoneal bleeding
Adrenal hemorrhage	Occult nose bleeding

MAJOR DRUG INTERACTIONS WITH WARFARIN

Increased Effect

Amiodarone
Cephalosporins given intravenously
Erythromycin
Metronidazole (Flagyl)
Lovastatin
Fluconazole
Trimethoprim and sulfamethoxazole (Bactrim)
Salicylates (ASA)
NSAIDs
Cimetidine
Vitamin E (large quantities)
Androgens

Decreased Effect

Barbiturates
Carbamazepine
Cholestyramine
Griseofulvin
Rifampin
Vitamin K (in foods or drug products)
Aminoglutethimide

ASA, Acetylsalicylic acid; *NSAIDs*, nonsteroidal antiinflammatory drugs.

intense therapy when applicable and by making incremental adjustments in therapy.

2. See the box for a suggested outcome scale for monitoring bleeding complications. Unacceptable or serious major bleeding or bruising warrants close attention to dosing adjustments and the source of the bleeding. To follow insidious gastrointestinal blood loss, measurement of complete blood counts or hemocult tests can be done at 6- to 9-month intervals.

3. There are several important drug interactions with warfarin (see box). Concomitant use of warfarin with any of these medications should be cautiously monitored.

4. Warfarin is contraindicated in pregnancy.

5. The most serious side effect other than bleeding is "purple toe syndrome," which is characterized by the release of plaque emboli that occlude peripheral circulation. Although this syndrome is rare, patients who develop it do so in the first 2 weeks of therapy. Warfarin should be discontinued if this side effect occurs. Patients with known protein C deficiency are at increased risk for developing this complication and should be carefully monitored when warfarin therapy is indicated.

6. Erratic intake of vitamin K–containing food and drug products may alter the anticoagulant effects of warfarin. Patients should be instructed to maintain a consistent intake of these foods or products while receiving warfarin.

ANTIPLATELET AGENTS[38-40]

The demonstrated and the hypothesized effects of platelets suggest that these blood elements play an important role in several cardiovascular disorders, including the genesis of atherosclerotic plaque, coronary artery thrombosis, coronary spasm, and arterial thromboembolism. Therefore drugs that interfere with platelet function are potentially valuable therapeutic agents.

Cardiovascular actions

Antiplatelet drugs prolong platelet survival and interfere with the metabolism of prostaglandins and thromboxane, agents that affect the ability of platelets to aggregate and initiate thrombosis. Effects on the prostaglandins contained in vascular endothelium may also influence the net result of antiplatelet drugs. The major antiplatelet agents in use are aspirin and dipyridamole. Aspirin is an irreversible inhibitor of cyclooxygenase, and dipyridamole increases cyclic adenosine monophosphate. Both decrease the aggregation of platelets, but neither affect platelet adhesion. Dipyridamole is a weak agent and is ineffective when used alone in most patients. Aspirin is the most effective oral antiplatelet agent in use.

Clinical uses

1. Aspirin can be used alone or with dipyridamole for the treatment of acute myocardial infarction, coronary bypass grafting, and cardiac valvular replacement.

2. Aspirin reduces the mortality rate associated with acute myocardial infarction by 20%.

3. Aspirin reduces the incidence of myocardial infarction and mortality by approximately 50% in patients with existing unstable angina.

4. Aspirin has not been shown to be effective in the primary prevention of coronary artery disease. The results of several studies indicate that the risk of infarction may be decreased but that the risk of hemorrhagic stroke may be increased.

Dosage and administration

1. Dipyridamole is ineffective alone and should be given with aspirin in dosages of 25 to 75 mg 3 times/day.

2. Reduced-strength doses of aspirin (81 mg) may be used if patients have difficulty tolerating the 325-mg strength. Enteric forms of multiple strengths of aspirin are available for patients who have difficulty tolerating the gastrointestinal side effects of aspirin products. Enteric-coated products are recommended in patients who require aspirin therapy but have a history of peptic ulcer disease or gastroesophageal reflux disease.

3. Some controversy has surrounded the ideal dose of aspirin. Small doses (for example, 81 mg) effectively inhibit cyclooxygenase without significantly affecting prostaglandins. However, low doses have been clinically

ineffective in some patients. Doses greater than 1000 mg may increase the incidence of side effects, with no greater antiplatelet effects than with 325 mg. The current recommended doses for any indication vary between 325 mg every day and 325 mg 3 times a day. Most clinical trials have used one of these two dosing schemes, and the recommendations are based on these clinical trials.

Cautions and side effects

1. Aspirin produces gastrointestinal disturbances in some patients. These side effects can be minimized by giving the drug with food or antacid or by using an enteric-coated preparation. Occult gastrointestinal bleeding or mucosal lesions are rare with the doses recommended for antiplatelet therapy.
2. Other dose-related side effects of aspirin are tinnitus, hearing loss, hepatotoxicity, renal insufficiency, rash, hematologic abnormalities, and anemia. These effects are rarely seen at the doses used for antiplatelet therapy.
3. Aspirin sensitivity occurs in less than 1% of the general population but in about 20% of patients with chronic urticaria and 4% of patients with chronic asthma. Mild to moderate bronchospasm may occur 15 to 30 minutes after ingestion of aspirin. Patients with known sensitivity should avoid aspirin use.
4. Adverse effects with dipyridamole are transient and dose related and resolve with continued therapy. These effects include headache, dizziness, nausea, peripheral dilatation, flushing, weakness, rash, pruritus, and aggravation of angina.

ANTIDYSRHYTHMICS [2, 12-14, 19, 41, 42]

An increasing number of antidysrhythmic drugs have become available for general clinical use. Specific electrophysiologic and pharmacologic features of these agents are presented in Tables 14-22 and 14-23. This discussion focuses on selected clinical aspects of the use of these agents.

Disopyramide

Disopyramide (Norpace) is a class IA antidysrhythmic similar to procainamide and quinidine.

Cardiovascular actions

See Table 14-22 for specific electrophysiologic effects. Disopyramide increases SVR and exerts a negative inotropic effect on the myocardium. The combination of these effects may lead to significant left ventricular failure in some patients. Also, disopyramide has systemic and myocardial anticholinergic properties that modify its electrophysiologic profile. For example, these anticholinergic effects may produce acceleration of the sinus rate or enhancement of AV nodal conduction.

TABLE 14-22   Electrophysiologic Effects of Antidysrhythmic Agents*

Agent	Sinus Rate	PR Interval	QRS Complex	QT Interval
Disopyramide	0, ↑	0, ↑	↑	↑
Procainamide	0	0, ↑	↑	↑
Quinidine	0, ↑	0, ↑	↑	↑
Lidocaine	0	0	0	0
Mexiletine	0	0	0	0
Tocainide	0	0	0	0, ↓
Phenytoin	0	0	0	0, ↓
Flecainide	0	↑	↑	↑
Propafenone	0	↑	↑	0
Propranolol	↓	0, ↑	0	0, ↓
Amiodarone	↓	↑	0, ↑	↑
Bretylium	0, ↑	0	0	0
Verapamil	0, ↓	0, ↑	0	0
Diltiazem	0, ↓	0, ↑	0	0
Sotalol	↓	0, ↑	0	0, ↓

*See Table 14-23 for names and classes of dysrhythmic agents.
↑, Increase; ↓, decrease; 0, no change.

Clinical uses

1. Disopyramide is used in the treatment of ventricular and supraventricular dysrhythmias. It is effective in 50% to 60% of patients.
2. The role of disopyramide in antidysrhythmic therapy remains to be defined. Many physicians believe that this agent should be reserved for use when the other class IA or IB agents fail.

Dosage and administration (see Table 14-23)

1. The dosage of disopyramide should be adjusted in patients with creatinine clearances less than 40 ml/min. The following is a guideline for initial therapy in patients with renal impairment:

Creatinine clearance	Dose
30 to 40 ml/min	100 mg every 8 hours
15 to 30 ml/min	100 mg every 12 hours
Less than 15 ml/min	100 mg every 24 hours

The extended-release capsules are not recommended for patients with creatinine clearances less than 40 ml/min.
2. Trough levels should be ascertained when indicated. Steady-state levels are achieved 48 hours after initiation of therapy in patients with normal renal function.
3. Patients may be given an oral loading dose of 300 mg followed by 150 mg every 6 hours. This dosing scheme

TABLE 14-23   Antidysrhythmic Agents

Agent	Trade Name	Class	Administration and Dosage	Plasma Elimination Half-Life (hr)	Plasma Concentration (mcg/ml)
Disopyramide	Norpace	IA	Oral: 100-300 mg q6hr	4-8	3-8
			SR: 150-300 mg q12hr	8-12	
Procainamide	Procan, Pronestyl	IA	IV load: 10-15 mg/kg at 20-50 mg/min	—	4-8
			Infusion: 1-4 mg/min	3-4	
			Oral: 250-1000 mg q3-4hr	3-4	
			SR: 500-2000 mg q6hr	6-8	
Quinidine	Quinaglute, Duraquin	IA	IV load: 5-8 mg/kg at 0.3 mg/kg/min	—	2-5
			Oral: 200-600 mg q6-8hr	6-11	
			SR: 324-648 mg q6-12hr	6-12	
Lidocaine	Xylocaine	IB	IV load: 1-2 mg/kg	—	1.5-6
			Infusion: 1-4 mg/min		
Mexiletine	Mexitil	IB	Oral: 150-400 mg q8hr	12	0.5-2
Tocainide	Tonocard	IB	Oral: 400-800 mg q8hr	12	4-10
Phenytoin	Dilantin	IB	IV load: 10-15 mg/kg at 20-50 mg/min		10-20
			Oral: 100-200 mg q8hr		
Flecainide	Tambocor	IC	Oral: 50-200 mg q12hr	16-20	—
Propafenone	Rythmol	IC	Oral: 150-300 mg q8hr	3-6	—
Propranolol	Inderal	II	IV load: 0.1-0.15 mg/kg in 1-mg increments q3-5min		—
			Oral: 40-120 mg q6hr	4	
Amiodarone	Cordarone	III	Oral load: 800-1600 mg/day for 7-10 days		1.5-3.5
			Oral: 200-600 mg/day		
Bretylium	Bretylol	III	IV load: 5-10 mg/kg		—
			Infusion: 1-4 mg/min	8-10	
Verapamil	Isoptin, Calan	IV	IV load: 5-10 mg		—
			Infusion: 1-10 mg/hr	3-8	
			Oral: 40-120 mg q6-8hr	3-8	
Diltiazem	Cardizem, Dilacor	IV	IV load: 0.25-0.35 mg/kg initially as a bolus followed by 5-15 mg/hr infusion up to 24 hours		—
			Oral: 30-120 q6-8hr	4-6	
			SR: 120-480 q12-24hr		
Sotalol	Betapace	II	80-160 mg bid	12	

q, Every; *SR,* sustained release; *bid,* twice daily.

is not recommended because of the higher incidence of adverse effects.
4. The dose is adjusted to the ECG and the patient's response.
5. The ECG, blood pressure, heart rate, and side effects are monitored.

Cautions and side effects

1. The most common adverse effects of disopyramide are anticholinergic and may require reductions in the dose or cessation of therapy. Dry mouth is usually transient and decreases with continued administration. Other anticholinergic effects include constipation; dry nose, eyes,

and throat; and blurred vision. The most serious effect is urinary retention, and patients with benign prostatic hypertrophy are at particular risk.

2. Heart failure may be precipitated in some patients and is characterized by weight gain, shortness of breath, orthopnea, and edema. Heart failure develops in approximately 15% of patients with no histories and in 80% of patients with histories of left ventricular dysfunction. The drug should be stopped if symptoms develop.

3. As with other antidysrhythmics agents, disopyramide is dysrhythmogenic and may precipitate AV block or ventricular dysrhythmias. The drug should be discontinued if the dysrhythmias worsen or new dysrhythmias appear.

4. Other side effects include hypoglycemia, headache, general fatigue, and rash.

Procainamide

Procainamide (Procan, Pronestyl) is a class IA antidysrhythmic similar to quinidine and disopyramide.

Cardiovascular actions

See Table 14-22 for specific electrophysiologic effects. Procainamide is a ganglionic blocker and may decrease systemic blood pressure, especially with parenteral administration. Procainamide may have a direct negative inotropic effect, but contractility is not depressed at therapeutic serum concentrations. The anticholinergic properties of procainamide are much weaker than those seen with disopyramide or quinidine.

Clinical uses

1. Procainamide is indicated for the treatment of atrial and ventricular dysrhythmias. The drug is efficacious in 60% to 80% of patients.

2. Procainamide is a primary agent in the treatment of atrial and ventricular dysrhythmias. Combination therapy with agents outside of class IA may be more efficacious and less toxic for complex ventricular dysrhythmias.

3. The toxicity of this agent may limit its long-term use in some patients.

Dosage and administration (see Table 14-23)

1. Procainamide may be given orally, intravenously, or intramuscularly. IM doses must be given every 4 hours to maintain therapeutic serum concentrations.

2. The dose of procainamide should be adjusted in patients with renal dysfunction. The following guidelines can be used when initiating therapy:

Creatinine clearance	Dosage
20-50 ml/min	500 mg every 6 hours orally or 1 to 2 mg/min intravenously
Less than 20 ml/min	250 to 500 mg every 6 hours orally or 0.5 to 1 mg/min intravenously

3. Procainamide has an active metabolic, *N*-acetylprocainamide (NAPA) that is eliminated renally. NAPA may accumulate in patients with renal insufficiency, and serum levels should be monitored (normal range, 10 to 20 mcg/ml). NAPA has class III antidysrhythmic properties.

4. Oral regular-release capsules should be used to initiate therapy. Sustained-release products can be given when switching from IV, IM, or chronic oral therapy. The sustained-release dose is one fourth of the total dose given every 6 hours.

5. Blood levels can be checked 10 to 24 hours after the initiation of parenteral or oral therapy with regular-release capsules. The clinician should wait 24 to 48 hours for steady-state levels in patients receiving the sustained-release products. Trough levels should also be checked.

6. When using an IV drip, the clinician should avoid doubling or tripling the rate if possible. A bolus of 2 mg/kg for each 1 mcg/ml increase in the serum level desired should be reinfused, and the infusion rate is increased accordingly. With bolus dosing, the clinician should not exceed a rate of 50 mg/min to avoid hypotension. Continuous infusions may also be adjusted according to weight (for example, 0.02 to 0.08 mg/kg/min).

7. IM therapy may be painful, and absorption is variable.

8. The dose is adjusted according to the ECG and the patient's response.

9. The ECG, heart rate, blood pressure, serum levels, and side effects are monitored.

10. Procainamide is stable in most IV fluids; standard concentration is 2 g in 500 ml of IV fluid.

11. Procainamide is compatible with atropine, dopamine, dobutamine, heparin, lidocaine, potassium, and verapamil.

Cautions and side effects

1. Approximately 50% of patients develop a positive ANA reaction within 2 to 18 months of starting therapy. Patients with a positive ANA may develop a lupuslike syndrome characterized by polyarthralgia, arthritis, pleural effusions, dyspnea, fever, chills, myalgia, skin lesions, headache, fatigue, and nausea. Therapy should be discontinued if symptoms develop. If symptoms are severe or persistent, administration of corticosteroids may be beneficial.

2. Patients receiving more than 4 g/day may complain of nausea, vomiting, and anorexia. Procainamide can be given with food, snacks, or antacids. Sustained-release preparations may reduce these effects, especially in patients receiving more than 2 g/day. It should be noted that the wax matrix for the sustained-release preparations often appears in feces.

3. Procainamide may be prodysrhythmic in 10% of patients. Torsades de pointes occurs more often in patients with hypokalemia. If new dysrhythmias appear or dysrhythmias worsen, procainamide should be discontinued. The risk for prodysrhythmic effects is increased with larger doses.
4. Other adverse effects include agranulocytosis, thrombocytopenia, neutropenia, rash, urticaria, headache, and dizziness.

Quinidine

Quinidine (Quinaglute, Dura-Tabs) is a class IA antidysrhythmic similar to disopyramide and procainamide.

Cardiovascular actions

See Table 14-22 for specific electrophysiologic effects. Quinidine is a ganglionic blocker, and decreases in blood pressure occur more often with high plasma concentrations and IV administration. Quinidine has myocardial anticholinergic properties similar to disopyramide but few systemic effects. At therapeutic serum levels, quinidine does not depress myocardial contractility despite its direct negative inotropic effect.

Clinical uses

1. Quinidine is used in the treatment of atrial and ventricular dysrhythmias. It is effective in 60% to 70% of patients.
2. Quinidine may be combined with agents from other classes for more effective, less toxic treatment of complex dysrhythmias.

Dosage and administration (see Table 14-23)

1. IM administration should be avoided because of erratic absorption and precipitation of the drug at the injection site.
2. Three different salts of quinidine are marketed. The sulfate salts contain 83% quinidine base, whereas the gluconate and polygluconate salts contain 60% to 65% quinidine base. When switching from one preparation to another, it is important to ensure that the patient receives the same amount of quinidine base regardless of the salt form.
3. Patients can receive oral loads of quinidine if necessary, but this is discouraged because of the high incidence of adverse effects.
4. Maintenance dosage can be achieved by intermittent IV doses given every 6 hours. Each dose should be given over 60 minutes or at a rate no faster than 15 mg/min.
5. Quinidine has two active metabolites that accumulate with renal dysfunction. Direct assays measure quinidine and metabolites, whereas extractable assays measure only quinidine. The metabolites may exhibit activity with accumulation, but this is more prominent in renal failure rather than mild renal insufficiency. Extractable levels should be monitored in most patients.
6. Steady-state levels are achieved 24 hours or more after therapy is started. Trough levels should be checked.
7. The dose should be adjusted according to the ECG, the patient's response, and serum levels.
8. The blood pressure, heart rate, ECG, serum levels, and side effects are monitored.
9. Quinidine increases digoxin levels almost twofold when these drugs are given concurrently. The digoxin dose should be halved, with the initiation of quinidine and serum digoxin levels checked after 3 days.

Cautions and side effects

1. Adverse gastrointestinal effects occur in 50% ot 85% of patients receiving quinidine salts and may necessitate cessation of therapy. The most common effects are nausea, diarrhea, anorexia, abdominal pain and cramps, colic, bitter taste, and vomiting. These effects are generally not dose related and result primarily from local irritation. Quinidine can be given with food or antacids, and loperamide may be necessary for temporary control of diarrhea. Changing from the sulfate to the gluconate salt may be beneficial in a limited number of patients. If tolerance to these effects is not evident in 1 to 2 weeks, the drug may need to be discontinued.
2. Cinchonism, an idiosyncratic reaction, may occur in patients after the initiation of therapy. Clinical manifestations are tinnitus, headache, vertigo, fever, lightheadedness, tremor, and altered vision. The dose should be reduced or the drug stopped if symptoms continue.
3. Quinidine may cause one-to-one conduction in patients with atrial fibrillation or flutter; this effect is secondary to the drug's anticholinergic properties. Tachycardia can be prevented by prior digitalization.
4. Quinidine is prodysrhythmic in approximately 10% of patients. Torsades de pointes may appear in patients with hypokalemia. Therapy should be discontinued in patients who develop new dysrhythmias or whose dysrhythmias worsen.
5. Leukopenia and thrombocytopenia may develop within 3 months of therapy. The drug should be stopped; blood counts return to normal in 1 to 2 weeks.
6. Other adverse effects include fever, hepatotoxicity, rashes, and hemolytic anemia.

Lidocaine

Lidocaine (Xylocaine) is a class IB antidysrhythmic similar to mexiletine and tocainide.

Cardiovascular actions

See Table 14-22 for specific electrophysiologic effects. Lidocaine has no effect on autonomic tone or cardiac contractility. It is a central nervous system depressant.

Clinical uses

1. Lidocaine is indicated for the treatment of ventricular dysrhythmias. It is effective in 70% to 80% of patients.
2. Lidocaine is used prophylactically in acute myocardial infarction to prevent ventricular dysrhythmias.
3. Lidocaine may be beneficial with other antidysrhythmics of another class for treating acute refractory ventricular dysrhythmias.

Dosage and administration (see Table 14-23)

1. Lidocaine is available for parenteral use only.
2. IM injections can be used if necessary, and absorption is more rapid from the deltoid muscles. Repeated and frequent dosing is necessary with IM therapy.
3. The clearance of lidocaine decreases with continued therapy. Serum levels and signs of toxicity should be closely monitored, especially in patients with poor renal function.
4. Steady-state levels are achieved 6 hours after changes in the dose or the initiation of therapy.
5. Lidocaine is stable in most IV fluids; a standard dilution is 2 g in 500 ml of IV fluid. Drips can be concentrated for patients on volume restriction.
6. Lidocaine is compatible with aminophylline, bretylium, calcium, digoxin, dopamine, dobutamine, heparin, potassium, procainamide, and verapamil.
7. The ECG, heart rate, blood pressure, serum levels, and side effects are monitored.

Cautions and side effects

1. Serious adverse effects requiring discontinuation are uncommon. Most are dose related and can be eliminated by reducing the dose.
2. Major central nervous system side effects include headache, drowsiness, dizziness, disorientation, confusion, lightheadedness, nervousness, and tremors. Muscle twitching and seizures may occur with toxicity.
3. Lidocaine is prodysrhythmic in some patients and should be discontinued if dysrhythmias worsen.
4. Hypersensitivity reactions may occur rarely.

Mexiletine

Mexiletine (Mexitil) is a class IB antidysrhythmic similar to lidocaine and tocainide.

Cardiovascular actions

See Table 14-22 for specific electrophysiologic effects. Mexiletine has no autonomic or negative inotropic effects. Mexiletine is a central nervous system depressant.

Clinical uses

1. Mexiletine is indicated for the treatment of ventricular dysrhythmias. The efficacy of this agent alone is only about 50%. With other antidysrhythmics or another class, mexiletine may be efficacious in 80% to 90% of patients.

Dosage and administration (see Table 14-23)

1. The clearance of mexiletine is reduced in renal failure, and the dose should be halved or the interval extended.
2. Oral loads are not recommended because of intolerable side effects in most patients.
3. Steady-state levels are achieved 24 to 48 hours after the initiation of therapy or a change in therapy. Trough levels should be checked. Serum levels are poorly correlated to therapeutic effect and are more useful for determining toxicity rather than therapeutic benefit.
4. Doses greater than 1200 mg/day are associated with a higher incidence of toxicity.
5. The ECG, heart rate, blood pressure, and side effects are monitored.
6. The dose is adjusted according to the patient's response, side effects, and ECG.

Cautions and side effects

1. Central nervous system side effects occur in up to 40% of patients receiving mexiletine. Neurologic toxicities include fine hand tremor, dizziness, lightheadedness, nervousness, paresthesias, confusion, blurred vision, and memory loss. Most of these effects are dose related, and the dose should be reduced to minimize symptoms. If seizures occur, the drug is discontinued.
2. Gastrointestinal side effects are common and include nausea, vomiting, abdominal pain, diarrhea, and anorexia. These effects may be related more to the amount of the dose (for example, 150 mg vs. 200 mg) than to the total dose. Doses should be given with meals, antacids, or snacks. Smaller doses or shorter intervals may be necessary.
3. Mexiletine may worsen cardiac dysrhythmias or induce new dysrhythmias. The drug should be discontinued if this occurs.
4. Other rare effects include rash, hair loss, impotence, and arthralgia.

Tocainide

Tocainide (Tonocard) is a class IB antidysrhythmic similar to lidocaine and mexiletine.

Cardiovascular actions

See Table 14-22 for specific electrophysiologic effects. Tocainide slightly increases SVR and has a small negative inotropic effect. However, the administration of tocainide has not been associated with clinical evidence of worsening heart failure. The significance of these effects remains to be determined.

Clinical uses

1. Tocainide is indicated for the treatment of ventricular dysrhythmias. It is 60% to 70% efficacious alone or with other antidysrhythmics of another class.
2. The precise role of tocainide in antidysrhythmic therapy remains to be established. It may be most beneficial in patients responsive to lidocaine and unresponsive to class IA agents alone.

Dosage and administration (see Table 14-23)

1. Loading may occur using the oral route, but this is usually not necessary and causes more toxicity.
2. Steady-state levels are achieved after 3 days of therapy, and trough levels should be checked.
3. Dosages should be halved or the dosing interval increased for patients with renal failure.
4. The dose should be adjusted according to the ECG, the patient's response, and side effects.
5. The ECG, blood pressure, heart rate, serum levels, and side effects are monitored.
6. If tablets are halved, the exposed portion may cause tingling or numbness in the mouth. This is not serious and can be diminished by taking the tablet after swishing antacids in the mouth.
7. Adverse effects increase with dosages greater than 1200 mg/day.

Cautions and side effects

1. From 30% to 50% of patients experience central nervous system toxicity, which includes tremors, dizziness, paresthesias, lightheadedness, slurred speech, and lethargy. These effects are usually dose related, and the dose should be reduced to minimize symptoms.
2. Seizures, psychosis, and hallucinations have occurred and necessitate discontinuation of the drug.
3. From 2% to 25% of patients experience gastrointestinal effects, the most frequent being nausea, anorexia, vomiting, and diarrhea. The drug should be given with food or antacids or the dose reduced if possible.
4. Dysrhythmias may occur in up to 10% of patients, and the drug should be stopped if this occurs.
5. Other adverse effects include bone marrow depression, pulmonary disease, and rash.

Flecainide

Flecainide (Tambocor) is a class IC antidysrhythmic.

Cardiovascular effects

See Table 14-22 for specific electrophysiologic effects. Flecainide has a moderate negative inotropic effect, which is more pronounced in patients with coronary heart disease or left ventricular failure. Flecainide has no autonomic effects.

Clinical uses

1. Flecainide is effective in the treatment of supraventricular and ventricular dysrhythmias in 80% to 90% of patients.
2. Flecainide may adversely affect morbidity and mortality rates in patients with asymptomatic ventricular dysrhythmias after myocardial infarction.
3. Flecainide is a potent agent and should be used cautiously with other antidysrhythmics.

Dosage and administration (see Table 14-23)

1. The clearance of flecainide is decreased in patients with renal failure, and the dose should be decreased accordingly.
2. Doses greater than 400 mg/day are associated with significantly greater toxicity than lower doses. Dosages should be increased every 3 to 5 days; more rapid titration may result in serious toxicity.
3. Steady-state levels are achieved in 3 to 5 days; trough levels should be checked.
4. Flecainide may increase digoxin and propranolol levels.
5. The ECG, blood pressure, heart rate, and side effects are monitored.
6. The dose should be increased according to the patient's response, the ECG, and side effects.

Cautions and side effects

1. From 10% to 30% of patients experience dizziness and visual difficulties. Other common central nervous system effects include headache, fatigue, tremor, paresthesias, spots before the eyes, and blurred vision. These effects are usually dose related and can be minimized by reducing the dose.
2. Flecainide is prodysrhythmic in 10% to 15% of patients, and the drug should be discontinued if these effects occur.
3. The drug's negative inotropic effects may exacerbate heart failure in patients with serum levels greater than 1.0 ng/ml, ejection fractions less than 35%, and complex ventricular dysrhythmias. Patients should be monitored closely and the drug discontinued if the condition becomes symptomatic.
4. Gastrointestinal toxicity, including anorexia, vomiting, nausea, and diarrhea, may occur in up to 10% of patients. These effects can be minimized by giving the drug with food or antacids.
5. Other less frequent side effects include rash, impotence, and blood dyscrasias.

Propafenone

Propafenone (Rythmol) is a unique class IC agent that also has calcium channel and β-blocking activity.

Cardiovascular actions

See Table 14-22 for specific electrophysiologic effects. Propafenone has β-sympatholytic activity about one-fortieth the potency of propranolol. At very high doses, propafenone also blocks calcium channels. Propafenone has moderate negative inotropic effects.

Clinical uses

1. Propafenone is indicated for the treatment of life-threatening ventricular dysrhythmias.
2. The use of propafenone is not indicated in patients with less severe ventricular dysrhythmias.

Dosage and administration (see Table 14-23)

1. The therapeutic effect is poorly correlated to serum concentrations.
2. After initiation of therapy at 150 mg every 8 hours, the dose is increased at 3- to 4-day intervals. The safety and efficacy of doses greater than 900 mg/day have not been established.
3. Propafenone has a saturable first-pass absorption, and its bioavailability may increase with larger doses.
4. The drug increases serum digoxin concentrations.
5. Propafenone may increase the anticoagulant effect of warfarin.
6. The ECG, heart rate, blood pressure, and side effects are monitored.

Cautions and side effects

1. Some 20% of patients require discontinuation secondary to side effects.
2. The most common side effects are dizziness, headache, altered taste, nausea, and constipation. Most are dose related, and reductions in dose alleviate symptoms.
3. About 10% of patients experience prodysrhythmic effects and should be discontinued from propafenone therapy.
4. Propafenone may exacerbate heart failure in patients with preexisting left ventricular dysfunction. Patients should be monitored for signs and symptoms of failure and the drug stopped if they occur.
5. Other adverse effects include paresthesias, vivid dreams, elevated liver enzyme levels, blood dyscrasias, and alopecia.

Sotalol

Sotalol (Betapace) exhibits both class II and class III antidysrhythmic properties.

Cardiovascular actions

See Table 14-22 for specific electrophysiologic effects. The β-blocker activity is not cardioselective and is maximal at doses between 320 and 640 mg/day. The class III elec-trophysiologic effects are seen at dosages of at least 160 mg/day. Sotalol is a potent negative inotropic agent.

Clinical uses

1. Sotalol is indicated for the treatment of documented ventricular dysrhythmias that are considered life threatening if left untreated.

Dosage and administration (see Table 14-23)

1. The dose of sotalol should be adjusted in older adults and in patients with compromised renal function using the following chart:

Creatinine clearance	Dosing interval
>60 ml/min	12 hr
30-60 ml/min	24 hr
10-30 ml/min	36-48 hr
<10 ml/min	Individualize

2. Serum blood levels are not useful when assessing the efficacy of therapy.
3. The dose should be slowly titrated every 3 days as needed for therapeutic effect. The recommended initial dosage is 80 mg twice a day. Most patients respond to total dosages of 160 to 320 mg/day given in divided doses. Some patients have required dosages as high as 640 mg/day.

Cautions and side effects

1. Caution should be used when combining sotalol with class IC antidysrhythmics, calcium channel blockers, digoxin, or any drug that prolongs the QT interval.
2. The prodysrhythmic effect of sotalol increases with increased dosages. The incidence of torsades de pointes increases from 1.6% to 5.8% as the dose increases from 320 to 640 mg/day.
3. Many side effects are dose related, and a reduction in the dose minimizes these effects. Common side effects are dyspnea, rhythm disturbances, fatigue, dizziness, asthenia, headache, lightheadedness, sleep disorders, nausea, vomiting, diarrhea, shortness of breath, and extremity pain.
4. Prodysrhythmic events must be anticipated with initiation of therapy and every upward titration of dose. Most events occur within 7 days of dosage changes.
5. Other side effects common to β blockers can be seen with sotalol (see section on β blockers).

Amiodarone

Amiodarone (Cordarone) is a class III antidysrhythmic.

Cardiovascular actions

See Table 14-22 for specific electrophysiologic actions. Amiodarone has sodium channel blocking and β-sympatholytic activity but no parasympathomimetic activity. The reduction in blood pressure and coronary resistance is more pronounced with IV therapy. Amiodarone does not appear to produce substantial changes in left ventricular function even though it is a mild negative inotropic agent.

Clinical uses

1. Amiodarone is indicated for the treatment of supraventricular and ventricular dysrhythmias. It is more than 90% effective in most patients.
2. Amiodarone may be used cautiously with other antidysrhythmics.

Dosage and administration (see Table 14-23)

1. Amiodarone distributes extensively into tissue and concentrates in fat, liver, muscle, spleen, and kidney tissue.
2. The half-life of the drug is approximately 40 to 80 days with chronic dosing. Amiodarone can be measured in the serum for up to 50 days after the cessation of therapy.
3. Serum blood levels are poorly correlated to therapeutic effect.
4. Patients should receive a loading dose over 7 to 10 days, followed by daily maintenance therapy. The goals are to use the lowest possible dose to terminate the dysrhythmia and prevent adverse effects. The dose should be adjusted according to the patient's response, the ECG, and toxicity.
5. Amiodarone increases digoxin levels, and the digoxin dose should be halved with concomitant therapy.
6. Amiodarone increases the anticoagulant effect of warfarin; the dose of warfarin should be reduced with concomitant therapy.
7. The ECG, blood pressure, heart rate, and toxicity are monitored.

Cautions and side effects

1. Amiodarone causes side effects in 100% of patients receiving the drug. Most effects occur at doses greater than 400 mg/day and with prolonged therapy; 25% of patients require cessation of therapy.
2. Corneal microdeposits occur in 50% to 100% of patients with chronic therapy. Vision is normally not affected, and the deposits disappear if the drug is discontinued. Methylcellulose eyedrops may be used for the discomfort.
3. Photosensitivity occurs in 1% to 50% of patients, and patients should avoid direct sunlight.
4. Dysrhythmias may be exacerbated by this agent in 10% of patients. The drug should be stopped if this occurs.
5. Up to 15% of patients develop pulmonary problems consisting of interstitial infiltrates, dyspnea, cough, and fibrosis. The drug should be stopped immediately, and steroids can be used if necessary.

6. About 25% of patients develop hypothyroidism or hyperthyroidism. The patient should be treated appropriately for the condition while amiodarone administration is continued.
7. Gastrointestinal disturbances, including nausea, vomiting, constipation, and anorexia, occur in up to 30% of patients. The drug can be given with food or antacids and at more frequent intervals during the day to minimize these effects.
8. Central nervous system disturbances may include sleep disorders, tremors, headache, and peripheral neuropathy. Reductions in dose usually minimize these effects.
9. Abnormal liver function tests occur in up to 20% of patients receiving chronic therapy. These alterations are usually benign but should be followed.

Bretylium

Bretylium (Bretylol) is a class III antidysrhythmic.

Cardiovascular actions

See Table 14-22 for specific electrophysiologic effects. Bretylium causes initial catecholamine depletion. In addition, there is a rise in blood pressure, heart rate, and contractility, which is followed by hypotension and decreased myocardial conduction.

Clinical uses

1. Bretylium is most efficacious for ventricular fibrillation.
2. Bretylium may be used for ventricular tachycardia but is usually less effective than other antidysrhythmic agents.

Dosage and administration (see Table 14-23)

1. A rapid IV push of the loading dose should be avoided because it may induce nausea and vomiting if the patient is alert.
2. The drug should be used cautiously if hypotension is present.
3. Bretylium is stable in most IV fluids and can be concentrated for patients on fluid restriction.
4. Bretylium is compatible with potassium, quinidine, verapamil, dopamine, and dobutamine.
5. The ECG, blood pressure, heart rate, and side effects are monitored.

Cautions and side effects

1. Hypotension is the most frequent adverse reaction and often occurs within the first hour of therapy. Hypotension may continue despite the cessation of therapy, and the patient should be monitored.
2. Other side effects include vertigo, lightheadedness, nausea, and diarrhea.

ANTILIPEMIC AGENTS[2,12,14,43]
Bile Acid–Binding Resins

Cholestyramine and colestipol are anion exchange resins with similar mechanisms of action.

Cardiovascular actions

See Table 14-24 for specific antilipemic effects. These agents bind bile acids in the intestines to form insoluble complexes, which are excreted in the feces. The loss of bile acids leads to increased production of bile acids in the liver and increased LDL receptors, which increases LDL uptake. These agents reduce LDL serum concentrations by 15% to 30%. They have no direct cardiac effects.

Clinical uses

1. Bile acid–binding resins are indicated primarily for the management of type IIa hyperlipidemia.
2. These agents are additive with other antilipemic agents and can be used with other agents when necessary.
3. Bile acid–binding resins may increase triglyceride levels and should not be used alone in patients with combined hyperlipidemia and hypertriglyceridemia.

Dosage and administration (see Table 14-24)

1. Cholestyramine and colestipol should not be taken in the dry powder form. The bulk powder should be mixed with moisturized pulpy fruit (for example, applesauce, crushed pineapple) or a minimum of 120 ml of fluid.
2. These agents are also available in flavored powders for reconstitution and chew bars.
3. These agents may alter the absorption of fat-soluble vitamins and folic acid.
4. Oral medications should be taken at least 1 hour before or 4 to 6 hours after these agents when possible. These agents are usually given in two to four divided doses before meals or at bedtime. Concomitant doses of medication should be avoided when possible.
5. The lipid-lowering effects of these agents are dose related. It is important to start with lower doses and titrate at monthly intervals.
6. Combination therapy with niacin or lovastatin may produce up to a 60% reduction in baseline LDL levels.
7. Serum LDL, HDL, and triglyceride levels and side effects are monitored.

Cautions and side effects

1. The most common adverse effects involve the gastrointestinal tract, especially with the use of high doses or in patients older than 60 years of age.
2. Constipation occurs in approximately 20% of patients receiving cholestyramine and colestipol. Constipation may become severe, especially in older adults, and lead to impaction. These agents should be given with bran cereal, stool softeners, or other soluble dietary fibers in patients who develop symptoms.
3. Other less common adverse gastrointestinal effects include abdominal pain and distention, gas, bloating, nausea, diarrhea, anorexia, exacerbation of hemorrhoids, indigestion, and heartburn. Many of these effects disappear with continued therapy.
4. These agents may alter fat absorption in doses larger than 24 g/day of cholestyramine and 30 g/day of colestipol. Serum electrolyte levels may also be affected at these doses.
5. Other adverse effects include rash, sour taste, and elevation of liver function enzymes.

TABLE 14-24	Antilipemic Agents					
Agent	**Trade Name**	**LDL**	**HDL**	**Triglycerides**	**Daily Dose**	**Time Necessary for Maximal Effect (Weeks)**
Cholestyramine	Questran	↓	0, ↑	0, ↑	12-24 g	2-4
Colestipol	Colestid	↓	0, ↑	0, ↑	15-30 g	2-4
Niacin (nicotinic acid)	Various	↓	↑	↓	1.5-6 g	3-5
Gemfibrozil	Lopid	↓	↑	↓	600-1200 mg	3-4
Clofibrate	Atromide-S	↓	0, ↑	↓	1-2 g	3-4
Probucol	Lorelco	↓	↓	0	500-1000 mg	4-12
Lovastatin	Mevacor	↓	0, ↑	0, ↓	20-80 mg	2-4
Pravastatin	Pravachol	↓	0, ↑	0, ↓	10-40 mg	2-4
Simvastatin	Zocor	↓	0, ↑	0, ↓	5-40 mg	2-4
Fluvastatin	Lescol	↓	0, ↑	0, ↓	20-40 mg	2-4

↓, Decrease; ↑, increase; 0, no change.

Niacin

Niacin (Nicotinic Acid) is an effective antilipemic agent in doses greater than 1 g/day.

Cardiovascular actions

See Table 14-24 for specific antilipemic effects. The exact antilipemic mechanism of niacin is unknown but is thought to be related to increased activity of lipoprotein lipase, decreased esterification of triglycerides, or inhibition of lipolysis in adipose tissue. Niacin reduces triglycerides by 20% to 80%, reduces LDL levels by 15% to 30%, and increases HDL levels. These effects are dose related.

Clinical uses

1. Niacin is used alone or in combination with other antilipemic drugs for the treatment of types IIa, IIb, III, and V hyperlipoproteinemia. It is the drug of choice for types IIb, III, IV, and V.
2. Niacin has additive effects when given with other antilipemic agents.

Dosage and administration (see Table 14-24)

1. Niacin is administered orally, preferably with meals.
2. The initial dose should be 500 mg 3 times a day, with 325 mg of aspirin given 30 minutes before each dose. Doses should be gradually increased at monthly intervals. Most patients experience transient side effects with the initiation of therapy; tolerance normally develops within 1 to 2 weeks.
3. Serum LDL, HDL, and triglyceride levels and side effects are monitored.
4. Slow-release products are usually not effective in reducing the initial adverse effects of this agent, and they may be hepatotoxic.
5. The dose of niacin should be maximized before combination therapy is used.

Cautions and side effects

1. Most side effects of niacin are dose related and are minimized with reductions in dose.
2. The most common side effects are cutaneous flushing, pruritus, burning or tingling, and dyspepsia. These effects usually occur within 30 minutes of ingestion and are present for 30 to 60 minutes. These effects are minimized by giving 325 mg of aspirin 30 minutes before each dose. Single doses greater than 500 mg are necessary to develop tolerance within 1 to 2 weeks. As the dose is titrated upward, the reaction may recur, and the patient should be treated prophylactically with aspirin.
3. Gastrointestinal effects may include nausea, vomiting, diarrhea, dyspepsia, peptic ulceration, and abdominal discomfort. These effects can be reduced by giving the drug with food or antacids.
4. Other side effects of niacin include cholestasis, hepatotoxicity, hyperglycemia, elevations in hepatic enzyme levels, hyperpigmentation, hyperuricemia, and hypotension.

Fibric Acid Derivatives

Gemfibrozil and clofibrate have similar mechanisms of action.

Cardiovascular effects

See Table 14-24 for specific antilipemic effects. These agents increase the activity of lipoprotein lipase, which increases the rate of catabolism of very-low-density lipoprotein (VLDL) and intermediate-density lipoprotein (IDL) to LDL. These drugs may also increase the rate of removal of these lipoproteins from plasma. Gemfibrozil and clofibrate produce a 5% to 15% reduction in LDL.

Clinical uses

1. Gemfibrozil and clofibrate are alternatives to niacin therapy in types III, IV, and V hyperlipidemia.
2. Gemfibrozil may also be used in types IIb and V hyperlipidemia for combination therapy.
3. These agents are used primarily for hyperlipidemias associated with hypertriglyceridemia.
4. These agents are effective with other antilipemic agents.

Dosage and administration (see Table 14-24)

1. Gemfibrozil has a lower incidence of adverse effects and may be preferred over clofibrate in most patients.
2. These agents are available only orally and can be given daily in two equal doses.
3. Doses should be low initially and given before the morning and evening meals. Doses should be titrated at monthly intervals.
4. Serum LDL, HDL, and triglyceride levels and side effects are monitored.

Cautions and side effects

1. Clofibrate may increase twofold the incidence of cholelithiasis and cholecystitis in patients receiving long-term therapy. Thromboembolism, cardiac dysrhythmias, and intermittent claudication may also occur. Because of an increased incidence of morbidity and overall mortality rate in clinical trials, clofibrate is not the drug of choice for any type of hyperlipidemia. This agent should be used as an alternative agent or in combination therapy only.
2. Other adverse effects associated with clofibrate include nausea, diarrhea, weight gain, skin rash, alopecia, weakness, impotence, influenza-like syndrome, increased hepatic enzyme levels, and decreased libido.
3. Clofibrate displaces highly protein-bound drugs and may precipitate toxicity when used with warfarin, phenytoin, or tolbutamide.
4. Adverse gastrointestinal effects are often seen with gemfibrozil use and include abdominal pain, nausea, diarrhea, flatulence, and epigastric pain.

5. Other adverse effects of gemfibrozil include headache, blurred vision, dizziness, eosinophilia, cholelithiasis, rash, musculoskeletal pain, mild anemia, hyperglycemia, and leukopenia.
6. As with clofibrate, gemfibrozil may potentiate the anticoagulant effects of warfarin.
7. Both these agents may have additive toxicity when given with lovastatin; this effect is manifested as musculoskeletal weakness or rhabdomyolysis.

Probucol

Probucol (Lorelco) is structurally unrelated to any of the other antilipemic agents.

Cardiovascular actions

See Table 14-24 for specific antilipemic actions. Probucol combines with LDL cholesterol in the plasma, producing a particle that is more rapidly removed than normal LDL. Probucol may increase the activity of the reverse transport system, thereby reducing HDL concentrations in the plasma. This agent has no effect on triglyceride levels.

Clinical uses

1. Probucol is used as an alternative agent in the treatment of type IIa hyperlipidemia.
2. The drug may be useful in some patients with type III hyperlipidemia but is generally less effective than fibric acid derivatives.
3. Probucol is useful with other antilipemics. The manufacturer recommends that probucol not be given with clofibrate or gemfibrozil because of increased toxicity and lack of additional benefits.

Dosage and administration (see Table 14-24)

1. Probucol is administered orally and should be given in two equal doses with the morning and evening meals.
2. Increases in dose should be at 3-month intervals to allow maximal effects from a single dose to occur.
3. Serum LDL, HDL, and triglyceride levels and side effects should be monitored.

Cautions and side effects

1. Probucol has a low incidence of side effects, and most are mild and transient.
2. About 10% of patients experience gastrointestinal side effects, including diarrhea, flatulence, nausea, abdominal pain, indigestion, and vomiting. These effects seldom require discontinuation of therapy.
3. Probucol may prolong the QT interval on the ECG, and serious dysrhythmias have been reported. ECGs should be obtained before and periodically during therapy.
4. Probucol decreases HDL serum concentrations. The significance of this effect is unclear.
5. Other adverse effects include eosinophilia, paresthesias, and rash.

3-Hydroxy-3-Methylglutaryl Coenzyme A Reductase Inhibitors

This class of agents (3-hydroxy-3-methylglutaryl coenzyme A [HMG-CoA] reductase inhibitors) differs in structure and pharmacologic activity from the other antilipemic agents. The agents in this class are lovastatin (Mevacor), pravastatin (Pravachol), simvastatin (Zocor), and fluvastatin (Lescol).

Cardiovascular actions

See Table 14-24 for specific antilipemic actions. These agents competitively inhibit the HMG-CoA reductase, thereby decreasing the endogenous synthesis of cholesterol. These agents may also increase hepatic LDL receptors, resulting in a greater uptake of LDL from the plasma. These drugs produce a dose-related 25% to 45% reduction in LDL levels.

Clinical uses

1. These drugs can be used as monotherapy in type IIa or IIb hyperlipidemia.
2. These agents are effective with niacin and bile acid–binding resins. Caution should be used when combining any of these drugs with clofibrate or gemfibrozil because of the increased risk for musculoskeletal toxicity.

Dosage and administration (see Table 14-24)

1. These agents are available for oral use only and should be administered once or twice a day. Daily doses should be given at bedtime for best results.
2. The dose should be low initially and titrated at monthly intervals.
3. All of these agents should be used cautiously with immunosuppressants because of the increased risk of myopathy.
4. Serum LDL, HDL, and triglyceride levels and side effects should be monitored.

Cautions and side effects

1. The most frequent adverse effects of all these agents are gastrointestinal and include flatulence, abdominal pain, diarrhea, and dyspepsia. Simvastatin appears to have a lower incidence of gastrointestinal side effects when compared with lovastatin, pravastatin, and fluvastatin.
2. Mild elevations in liver enzyme function tests may occur within 6 weeks of therapy and usually do not necessitate cessation of therapy. Increases of more than 3 times the upper limit of normal values indicate toxicity, and the drug should be stopped. Liver function tests should be monitored periodically during therapy.
3. Creatinine kinase elevations are seen in approximately 11% of patients, but myalgia and muscle cramps have been reported in only 1% to 3% of patients. Patients should be advised to report muscle weakness, pain, or

tenderness. The drug should be promptly discontinued if these symptoms are present.

4. Eye opacities have appeared in some patients, but no clinically important loss of visual acuity has occurred during drug therapy. Ophthalmic examinations should be performed periodically in patients receiving this drug.

5. Other adverse effects include blurred vision, headache, dizziness, insomnia, malaise, and rash.

6. The long-term side effects of these agents appear to be minimal.

MISCELLANEOUS AGENTS[2,3,12,13,44]
Atropine

Atropine is a parasympatholytic agent.

Cardiovascular actions

Atropine blocks activity in portions of the parasympathetic nervous system by inhibiting the action of acetylcholine. In the heart, atropine principally increases the rate of automatic discharge of the SA node and shortens the refractory period and conduction time of the AV node. A lesser effect, particularly in the atria, may be to increase contractility.

Clinical uses

1. Atropine is indicated to block unwanted effects of vagal tone such as symptomatic sinus bradycardia, sinus bradycardia associated with increased ventricular ectopy during acute myocardial infarction, or AV block caused by increased vagal tone.

2. Atropine may be used in cardiac arrest to antagonize the parasympathetic drive.

Dosage and administration

1. Atropine is administered intravenously, usually in an initial dose of 0.5 to 1.0 mg by rapid injection. Additional increments of 0.5 mg are administered until the desired effects are obtained, unwanted side effects are controlled, or a total dosage of 2.0 to 2.5 mg is reached.

2. Smaller doses or slower administration of atropine may evoke a vagomimetic effect that produces sinus node slowing and AV conduction delay.

3. Atropine administered through an endotracheal tube is slowly absorbed, and drug concentrations in the serum and at the site of action are low. Thus larger doses, usually twice the IV dose, are required to achieve therapeutic responses.

4. The cardiovascular effects of atropine given intravenously are short lived, and chronic therapy is not indicated. Pacemaker placement should be considered in anyone who requires long-term control of bradydysrhythmias.

5. The ECG, blood pressure, heart rate, and side effects are monitored.

Cautions and side effects

1. Many of the side effects of atropine are dose related and may produce systemic effects for several hours after administration.

2. Usual side effects are urinary retention, dryness of skin and mucous membranes, bronchial secretions, pupillary dilatation, acute glaucoma, tachycardia, blurred vision, and mydriasis.

3. Atropine-induced sinus node acceleration during acute myocardial infarction may precipitate further ischemia, which may lead to ventricular dysrhythmias and ventricular fibrillation after atropine administration.

4. Doses greater than 5 mg may produce speech disturbances, swallowing difficulties, ataxia, confusion, delirium, or hallucinations.

Edrophonium

Edrophonium (Tensilon) is a parasympathomimetic agent.

Cardiovascular actions

Edrophonium is a cholinergic drug that acts by inhibiting the action of acetylcholinesterase, the enzyme that degrades acetylcholine. Cardiac effects of edrophonium are similar to those produced by enhanced vagal tone. Edrophonium decreases the sinus nodal discharge rate, increases the refractoriness and conduction time of the AV node, and decreases myocardial contractility.

Clinical uses

1. Edrophonium is used primarily to terminate episodes of PSVT when other vagal maneuvers such as carotid sinus massage or the Valsalva maneuver are ineffective.

2. Edrophonium may also be used to treat sinus tachycardia secondary to sympathomimetic use.

Dosage and administration

1. Edrophonium is administered as a 5- or 10-mg IV bolus. A test dose of 1 to 2 mg may be given initially.

2. The effects of edrophonium begin within 30 to 60 seconds after administration and may last as long as 10 minutes.

3. A continuous infusion of 0.25 to 2.0 mg/min may be used if prolonged effects are desired.

4. Atropine antagonizes the effects of edrophonium.

5. The ECG, blood pressure, heart rate, respiratory rate, and side effects are monitored.

Cautions and side effects

1. Enhanced vagal tone may aggravate preexisting conditions of intestinal obstruction, bronchial asthma, or urinary obstruction; edrophonium should be avoided in these circumstances.

2. Side effects are mainly secondary to vagal overactivity and may include nausea, perspiration, salivation, bronchial spasm, slow pulse, and hypotension.
3. To counteract potential life-threatening complications, atropine should be immediately available when edrophonium is used.

Sodium Bicarbonate

Sodium bicarbonate is a major extracellular buffer that provides the physiologic control of acid-base balance. Bicarbonate metabolism is regulated primarily by the kidney, and the bicarbonate system is one of many acid-base systems.

Clinical use

1. Sodium bicarbonate is used to correct metabolic acidosis.

Dosage and administration

1. Sodium bicarbonate is administered at 1 mEq/kg every 10 minutes during cardiopulmonary resuscitation until circulation is restored. When possible, administration should be guided by repeated measurements of arterial blood pH.
2. Sodium bicarbonate should be administered through a separate IV line because it may inactivate many agents, particularly the catecholamines.
3. Sodium bicarbonate precipitates calcium, and the line should be thoroughly flushed if these agents are given through the same IV line during an emergency.

Cautions and side effects

1. Treating acidosis with bicarbonate does not alter the underlying defect that caused the acidosis, such as cardiogenic shock or ventricular fibrillation.
2. Overdoses of bicarbonate produce a metabolic alkalosis.
3. The large sodium load administered with sodium bicarbonate may worsen preexisting CHF.

Potassium

Potassium is a major intracellular cation found principally in muscle, including cardiac tissue. The greatest amount of total body potassium is located within the cells, and intracellular concentration is approximately 30 times the extracellular concentration. Despite this, the extracellular or serum potassium concentration usually correlates well with the total body potassium level in stable, steady-state conditions. Renal function provides the major regulation of body potassium. Certain metabolic diseases, kidney diseases, diarrhea, vomiting, diuretic therapy, or infusions of potassium-free fluids that increase extracellular fluid volume may reduce serum potassium levels. Elevated serum levels are caused by acidosis, renal failure, massive tissue necrosis, major catabolic states, and the inadvertent administration of potassium.

Cardiovascular actions

Potassium plays a major role in the maintenance of normal cellular excitability and conduction. Hypokalemia prolongs the recovery of excitability; this is manifested as a prolonged QT interval on the ECG and slows the AV and intraventricular conduction times. Premature ventricular complexes and disorders of AV conduction may occur. Hyperkalemia increases the rate of repolarization (shortened QT interval on the ECG) and at progressively higher levels first increases and then decreases excitability and conduction velocity. Therefore potassium administration may initially facilitate conduction but later may produce AV conduction delay and slow intraventricular conduction.

Clinical use

1. Potassium supplements are used in the prevention or treatment of potassium depletion.

Dosage and administration

1. Since potassium loss in the urine parallels sodium loss to some degree, the restriction of dietary sodium helps mitigate potassium loss.
2. Potassium chloride, which also replenishes chloride ions lost during diuresis and during sodium chloride restriction, is the preferred salt for oral administration.
3. Potassium can be replaced by oral or parenteral administration. The dose should be adjusted to the patient's needs. A serum potassium concentration of 3 mEq/L implies a total body deficit of approximately 300 mEq. Each subsequent 1 mEq/L decrease in serum concentration indicates an additional deficit of 200 to 400 mEq.
4. Changes in extracellular pH produce a reciprocal effect on plasma potassium concentrations. A change in pH of 0.1 unit can be accompanied by a change in the opposite direction of 0.6 mEq/L of serum potassium.
5. IV administration of potassium should be no more concentrated than 60 mEq/L and infused at a rate no greater than 20 mEq/hour. Concentrated solutions should be given through central lines only and carefully monitored.
6. For serum potassium concentrations greater than 2.5 mEq/L, a maximum dose of 200 mEq/day should not be exceeded. For serum potassium concentrations less than 2.5 mEq/L, a maximum dose of 400 mEq/day should not be exceeded.
7. The usual adult oral dosage for replacement is 40 to 100 mEq/day. Doses larger than 40 mEq should be separated if given in oral tablet form because the matrices of these tablets may form a complex that causes esophageal ulceration.

8. Oral potassium solutions should be diluted before administration. Orange, apple, and tomato juice and carbonated drinks help mask the salty taste.

9. Peak elevation of serum potassium levels occurs 1 hour after administration (2 hours for sustained-release products), and the effect on the serum potassium level is seen primarily in the first 3 hours.

10. Potassium supplements are also found in some salt substitutes and in bananas and citrus fruit.

11. Many forms and preparations of oral potassium are available. Care should be taken that the proper amount of potassium is administered if different products are used.

12. IV infusions of potassium may cause pain or burning at the infusion site. The solution should be further diluted, and the patient should be carefully monitored for signs of phlebitis or local tissue necrosis. If there is any suspicion of extravasation or infiltration, the IV access site should be moved and treated promptly.

13. Renal function, serum potassium levels, ECG, and side effects are monitored.

14. Second-degree AV block is generally a contraindication to potassium use. However, in the case of digitalis-induced atrial tachycardia with AV block, potassium administration may slow the atrial rate and restore sinus rhythm without worsening the AV block.

15. Potassium is contraindicated in patients who have severe renal impairment, untreated Addison disease, acute dehydration, heat cramps, acidosis, and preexisting hyperkalemia from any cause.

16. Patients with concurrent hypomagnesemia should receive magnesium replacement as well. Serum potassium levels are not corrected if the patient has a magnesium deficiency.

Cautions and side effects

1. Rapid potassium infusion produces sinus bradycardia, depression of intrinsic pacemakers, and slowing of AV conduction to the point of block.

2. Adverse symptoms reported with potassium therapy are nausea, vomiting, diarrhea, and abdominal discomfort.

3. Hyperkalemia may occur after administration of potassium, especially with impaired renal function. Hyperkalemia may manifest as weakness, paresthesias, decreased blood pressure, and ECG changes. Cardiac dysrhythmias ranging from heart block to cardiac arrest caused by ventricular fibrillation or ventricular asystole may occur.

4. ECG manifestations of hyperkalemia include a peaked, narrowed T wave and shortened QT interval. As toxicity increases, the QRS complex widens, the PR interval lengthens, and the P wave may diminish in size or disappear.

Magnesium (Tables 14-25 and 14-26)

Magnesium is the second most common intracellular cation and is essential for the activity of multiple metabolic pathways and enzyme systems. The total body content of magnesium is 2000 mg, with less than 1% being found in the serum. Therefore serum magnesium levels may not accurately reflect intracellular stores. The total serum magnesium concentration ranges from 1.7 to 2.4 mg/100 ml (1.4 to 2.0 mEq/L) in adults. Normal dietary intake is 25 to 30 mg/day.

Hypomagnesemia can be caused by excessive gastrointestinal losses, reduced oral intake, drug-induced losses, renal losses, and many disease states. Signs and symptoms of magnesium deficiency are rare when total serum magnesium levels are above 1.5 mg/100 ml. Levels below 1.0 mg/100 ml are most commonly associated with complaints of muscular spasms, paresthesias, and weakness.

Cardiovascular actions

Cardiovascular manifestations of hypomagnesemia may include heart failure, coronary artery spasms, dysrhythmias, and hypotension. Severe magnesium depletion can result in central nervous system effects ranging from coma, disorientation, apathy, and depression to seizures. Finally, hypomagnesemia may cause hypokalemia and intracellular potassium depletion.

Clinical uses

1. Magnesium is used in the prevention and treatment of hypomagnesemia.

2. Magnesium is indicated in the treatment of toxemia.

3. Magnesium is indicated in the treatment of hypokalemia when magnesium depletion is suspected.

4. Magnesium is considered the drug of choice in the treatment of torsades de pointes.

Dosage and administration (see Tables 14-25 and 14-26)

1. The recommended daily maintenance dosage for adults is 0.4 mEq/kg/day orally or 0.1 to 0.2 mEq/kg/day parenterally.

2. See Tables 14-27 and 14-28 for dosing recommendations and magnesium content of various products.

Cautions and side effects

1. Serum levels of 4 to 10 mEq/L are associated with muscle weakness, loss of deep tendon reflexes, and hypotension.

2. Serum levels of greater than 15 mEq/L are associated with respiratory paralysis, widening of the QRS complex, dysrhythmias, and complete heart block.

3. IM injections are commonly painful, so the IV or oral routes are recommended when appropriate.

4. Magnesium should be given no faster than 2 g/min intravenously.

TABLE 14-25   Therapy of Magnesium Deficiency

Degree of Deficiency	Day	Suggested Dosage*
Asymptomatic magnesium deficiency		Magnesium sulfate, 3 g (24 mEq magnesium) orally every 6 hr OR Milk of Magnesia, 10 ml (27 mEq magnesium) orally every 6 hr
Symptomatic deficiency without life-threatening condition	1	Intramuscular route (50% magnesium sulfate): 2.0 g (16 mEq) every 4 hr for 6 doses OR Intravenous route (10% magnesium sulfate): 6.0 g (48 mEq) in any IV solution over 4 hr and then an additional 4 g (32 mEq) infused intravenously over remainder of day
	2-5	Intramuscular route: 1.0 g (8 mEq) every 4-6 hr OR Intravenous route: 5.0 g infused intravenously every 24 hr
Symptomatic, life-threatening condition	1	2.0-4.0 g (16-32 mEq) intravenously over 2-4 min followed by 10 g over remainder of 24 hr
	2-5	5.0 g infused intravenously every 24 hr

*Assumes normal renal function.

TABLE 14-26   Magnesium Content of Various Drugs

Product	Magnesium Content	
	mg	mEq*
ORAL		
Milk of Magnesia, 10 ml	324	27
Gelusil Suspension, 5 ml	82	6.8
Gelusil M Suspension, 5 ml	82	6.8
Gelusil II, 5 ml	164	13.7
Maalox Suspension, 5 ml	82	6.8
Maalox Plus, 5 ml	82	6.3
Maalox TC Suspension, 5 ml	124	10.3
Mylanta, 5 ml	82	6.8
Mylanta II, 5 ml	164	13.7
Chelated Magnesium Tablets 500 mg	100	8.3
Magnesium Complexed Tablets	133	11.1
Magnesium citrate solution, 5 ml	46.2-56.5	3.9-4.7
PARENTERAL		
Magnesium sulfate injection		
10%, 10 ml (1 g)	97.56	8.1
50%, 2 ml (1 g)	97.56	8.1

*1 mEq magnesium ion weighs 12 mg.

Adenosine

Adenosine (Adenocard) is an endogenous purine nucleoside.

Cardiovascular actions

Adenosine vasodilates coronary arteries, reduces atrial contractility, depresses SA and AV nodal activity, and inhibits the stimulating effect of catecholamines on the myocardium.

Clinical uses

1. Adenosine is indicated for the conversion of PSVT to normal sinus rhythm, including PSVT associated with accessory bypass tracts. It is more than 90% effective for termination of tachycardias that involve the AV node as part of the reentry circuit.
2. The ultimate place in therapy for this agent remains to be determined. It is used for PSVT when verapamil is contraindicated or ineffective.

Dosage and administration

1. Adenosine is available for IV use only.
2. Adenosine is usually administered as a 6-mg rapid IV bolus given over 1 to 2 seconds. If the first dose does not result in conversion to normal sinus rhythm within 1 to 2 minutes, 12 mg should be given as a rapid IV bolus. An additional 12 mg may be administered if necessary.
3. Caution should be used in patients with asthma, since bronchoconstriction has been reported after inhaled adenosine.
4. The ECG, blood pressure, heart rate, and side effects should be monitored.

Cautions and side effects

1. Frequently reported side effects are facial flushing (18%), dyspnea (12%), retrosternal chest pressure (7%), and dysrhythmias preceding conversion to normal sinus rhythm.
2. Most side effects are transient, lasting less than 1 minute, and are reported by patients as being minor.
3. The conditions of patients receiving theophylline may be refractory to adenosine.
4. Patients receiving dipyridamole may be acutely sensitive to the effects of adenosine, necessitating lower initial doses.

REFERENCES

1. Winter ME: *Basic clinical pharmacokinetics,* Spokane, Wash, 1985, Applied Therapeutics.
2. Gilman AG, Goodman LS: *The pharmacological basis of therapeutics,* ed 8, New York, 1990, Pergamon.
3. Chernow B, editor: *The pharmacologic approach to the critically ill patient,* ed 3, Baltimore, 1994, Williams & Wilkins.
4. Katz AM: Changing strategies in the management of heart failure, *J Am Coll Cardiol* 13(3):513, 1989.
5. Parmley WM: Pathophysiology and current therapy of congestive heart failure, *J Am Coll Cardiol* 13(4):771, 1989.
6. Feldman AM, Bristow MR: The beta-adrenergic pathway in the failing human heart: implications for inotropic therapy, *Cardiology* 77(suppl 1):1, 1990.
7. Katz AM: Cardiomyopathy of overload: a major determinant of prognosis in congestive heart failure, *New Engl J Med* 322(2):100, 1990.
8. Ventura HO and others: Current issues in advanced heart failure, *Med Clin North Am* 76(5):1057, 1992.
9. Kelly RA: Cardiac glycosides and congestive heart failure, *Am J Cardiol* 65:10E, 1990.
10. Gheorghiade M, Zarowitz BJ: Review of randomized trials of digoxin therapy in patients with chronic heart failure, *Am J Cardiol* 69:48G, 1992.
11. Packer M and others: Withdrawal of digoxin from patients with chronic heart failure treated with angiotensin-converting enzyme inhibitors, *New Engl J Med* 329(1):1, 1993.
12. American Society of Hospital Pharmacists: *American hospital formulary service,* Bethesda, Md, 1994, The Society.
13. Trissel LA: *Handbook on injectable drugs,* Bethesda, Md, 1990, American Society of Hospital Pharmacists.
14. Knoben JE, Anderson PO, editors: *Handbook of clinical drug data,* ed 6, Hamilton, Ill, 1988, Drug Intelligence Publications.
15. Stanley R: Drug therapy of heart failure, *J Cardiovasc Nurs* 4(3):17, 1990.
16. Eselin JA, Carter BL: Hypertension and left ventricular hypertrophy: is drug therapy beneficial? *Pharmacotherapy* 14(1):60, 1994.
17. Houston MC: New insights and new approaches for the treatment of essential hypertension: selection of therapy based on coronary heart disease risk factor analysis, hemodynamic profiles, quality of life, and subsets of hypertension, *Am Heart J* 117(4):911, 1989.
18. Houston MC: New insights and approaches to reduce end-organ damage in the treatment of hypertension: subsets of hypertension approach, *Am Heart J* 123(5):1337, 1992.
19. Morganroth J and others: *Cardiovascular drug therapy,* St Louis, 1986, Mosby.
20. Frishman WH: Beta-adrenergic blockers, *Med Clin North Am* 72(1):37, 1988.
21. Strauss WE, Parisi AF: Combined use of calcium channel and beta-adrenergic blockers for the treatment of chronic stable angina, *Ann Intern Med* 109:570, 1988.
22. Elkayam U: Tolerance to organic nitrate: evidence, mechanisms, clinical relevance, and strategies for prevention, *Ann Intern Med* 114(8):667, 1991.
23. Cohn J: *Drug treatment of heart failure,* New York, 1983, Advanced Therapeutics Communications.
24. Kostis JB: Angiotensin converting enzyme inhibitors. I. Pharmacology, *Am Heart J* 166(6):1580, 1988.
25. Kostis JB: Angiotensin converting enzyme inhibitors. II. Clinical use, *Am Heart J* 166(6):1591, 1988.
26. Lewis EJ and others: The effect of angiotensin-converting enzyme inhibition on diabetic nephropathy, *New Engl J Med* 329(20):1456, 1993.
27. Hollenberg NK, Raij L: Angiotensin-converting enzyme inhibition and renal protection, *Arch Intern Med* 153:2426, 1993.
28. Sogaard P and others: Effects of captopril on ischemia and dysfunction of the left ventricle after myocardial infarction, *Circulation* 87(4):1093, 1993.
29. Gibson RS: Current status of calcium channel blocking drugs after Q-wave and non Q-wave myocardial infarction, *Circulation* 80(suppl IV):107, 1989.
30. Weiner DA: Calcium channel blockers, *Med Clin North Am* 72(1):83, 1988.
31. Bang NU and others: After coronary thrombolysis and reperfusion, what next? *J Am Coll Cardiol* 14(4):837, 1989.

32. Sane DC and others: Bleeding during thrombolytic therapy for acute myocardial infarction: mechanisms and management, *Ann Intern Med* 111:1010, 1989.

33. Kim CB, Braunwald E: Potential benefits of late reperfusion of infarcted myocardium, *Circulation* 88(5pt1):2426, 1993.

34. Hirsh J, Levine MN: Low molecular weight heparin, *Blood* 79(1):1, 1992.

35. Simonneau G and others: Subcutaneous low-molecular weight heparin compared with continuous intravenous unfractionated heparin in the treatment of proximal deep vein thrombosis, *Arch Intern Med* 153:1541, 1993.

36. Hirsh J and others: Oral anticoagulants: mechanism of action, clinical effectiveness, and optimal therapeutic range, *Chest* 102(4):312S, 1992.

37. Levine MN and others: Hemorrhagic complications of anticoagulant treatment, *Chest* 102(4):352S, 1992.

38. Stein B and others: Platelet inhibitor agents in cardiovascular disease: an update, *J Am Coll Cardiol* 14(4):813, 1989.

39. Hennekens CH and others: The benefits of aspirin in acute myocardial infarction, *Arch Intern Med* 154:37, 1994.

40. Willard JE and others: The use of aspirin in ischemic heart disease, *New Engl J Med* 327(3):175, 1992.

41. Wellens HJ, Bragadin P: Treatment of cardiac arrhythmias: when, how, and where? *J Am Coll Cardiol* 14(6):1417, 1989.

42. Epstein AE and others: Mortality following ventricular arrhythmia suppression by encainide, flecainide, and moricizine after myocardial infarction (CAST trial), *JAMA* 270(20):2451, 1993.

43. Lipid Research Clinics Investigators: The lipid research clinics coronary primary prevention trial: results of 6 years post-trial follow-up, *Arch Intern Med* 152:1399, 1992.

44. Arsenian MA: Magnesium and cardiovascular disease, *Prog Cardiovasc Dis* 35(4):271, 1993.

CHAPTER 15

Home Care of Patients with Cardiac Disease

Doris F. Glick

PERSPECTIVES ON HOME CARE

Home care, the fastest growing sector of the health care system, provides a major portion of acute health care in the United States. In recent years, one third of the hospital beds in America have been effectively replaced by home care providers. The length of stay at the hospital has been reduced by 35% to 50%, and in most hospitals, patient census has fallen to about 65%.[1] Patients with cardiac disease have always been cared for to some extent at home; however, as a consequence of ongoing trends in the health care system, more care is provided for very seriously ill patients in their homes.

Cardiac care is customarily envisioned as technologically sophisticated, and home care has been transformed to incorporate the latest advances in science and technology and advanced practice clinicians. Remarkable advances in technology have enabled earlier hospital discharge after cardiac events or surgery, ambulatory care for patients awaiting transplant, and long-term home care for patients with congestive failure or those receiving prolonged anticoagulation therapy. Miniaturization of equipment, home electrocardiographic (ECG) monitors, ambulatory infusion devices, and life-sustaining pharmaceutic agents have made it possible for seriously ill patients to be cared for at home.[2] An increasing number of agencies and a diversity of providers deliver home-based services designed to address the needs of these cardiac patients and their families.

Development of Home Care

Since the beginning of recorded history, societies have recognized certain people who provided care for the sick at home. The earliest known visiting nurse was Phoebe, whose visits to the ill in their homes was recorded in the Bible in Paul's letters to the Romans (Romans 16:1-2). In the modern era, William Rathbone established the first visiting nurse association in Liverpool, England, in 1859. Rathbone consulted his friend, Florence Nightingale, whose recommendations continue to form the conceptual basis of home health services. Nightingale emphasized the importance of family-focused care, need for patient teaching, and concern for environmental conditions. She believed that nurses practicing in the home required advanced education in addition to the skills acquired in the hospital.

In the United States, visiting nurse associations were first established in 1856 in Boston and Philadelphia. These formed the foundation of modern community health nursing practice. In 1893, Lillian Wald and Mary Brewster established the Henry Street Settlement House in New York City to care for the sick poor at home.

From that time until the early 1960s, high-quality, low-cost home care services were provided by two types of agencies. Visiting nurse associations were private or voluntary nonprofit agencies that provided care for the sick at home. Public health agencies were supported by public funds and regulated through legislation at the local, state, and federal levels. Public health agencies focused primarily on control of communicable diseases and on health promotion and disease prevention. What home care they provided for the sick tended to focus on teaching the family or other care providers to care for their sick member rather than on the direct provision of care. Throughout this time, home care remained a small segment of the total health care system.[3,4]

In the 1960s, establishment of the Medicare and Medicaid systems provided some reimbursement for community health agencies to provide illness care, and the demands for home care began to increase. A profound impact on the delivery of home care occurred in the 1980s. The federal government in 1984 introduced the change from cost reimbursement to prospective payment for financing hospital services. This innovation initiated the trend of discharging patients from hospitals much earlier in their course of recovery.[5] Moreover, patients with many severe or acute illnesses or elective surgery were no longer admitted to a hospital. As a result, by the latter part of the 1980s, there was a significant increase in the severity of illness among patients being cared for at home, and this trend continues today. Frequently these patients are older, have multiple medical diagnoses, and require complex care. Home care services thus have become increasingly focused on severe illness and high-tech care.

Parallel to these trends, physicians have moved away from house calls. Physicians have tended to function more and more in hospitals since the physician shortage created by World War II made home visits an inefficient means to use scarce resources. Gradually, technologic advances required practice to take place in the hospital rather than in the home. Today economic incentives encourage physicians to practice in acute care institutions, and there is no formal reimbursement for physician participation in home care.[6]

Because of the changes that have occurred in health care reimbursement in recent years and with more older and sicker patients being cared for in their own homes, there has been a notable increase in the number of home health care agencies. Proprietary agencies have been established along with the nonprofit visiting nurse associations and public health departments to provide home care services. One year after Medicare was enacted in 1966, 1753 home health care agencies were certified by Medicare. By 1974, there were 2237, a 48% increase,[7] and by 1989, according to the National Association for Home Care, that number had reached 10,850.[8] This is a growth of 500% in 15 years. By 1992, on any given day in the United States, 1,237,100 patients received home care.[9]

The cost of home care accounts for an escalating proportion of the total health care budget in the United States. In 1991, expenditures for home health care reached $12 billion, 29% above that for 1990,[10] and by 1993, home health care was a $15 billion industry.[11] According to the Health Care Financing Administration (HCFA) that oversees Medicare, expenditures for home care will continue to increase. Although the annual growth in total health care expenditures is projected to be 8.5%, estimates indicate that expenditures for home care will grow at a rate of 12.1% per year.[12] Thus home health is the most rapidly growing segment of the health care system.

Scope of Home Health Services

Home care is an array of services brought to people in their own homes to restore health or manage illness. The focus is on family-centered care, patient teaching, home environment, multidisciplinary health care, and return to an optimal level of health. Because most patients are chronically ill and older, Medicare provides reimbursement to home health care agencies for 75% to 80% of all home care services. The remainder of the agencies are reimbursed by Medicaid, private insurance companies, and in some cases, by the patients themselves. Medicare reimburses the following services[13]:

1. Parttime or intermittent nursing care provided by or under the supervision of a registered professional nurse
2. Physical, occupational, or speech therapy
3. Management and evaluation of the patient care plan
4. Medical social services under the direction of a physician
5. Parttime or intermittent services of a home health aide, as permitted by the regulations
6. Medical supplies (other than drugs and biologic agents such as serum and vaccinations) and the use of medical equipment
7. Medical services provided by an intern or resident enrolled in a teaching program in hospitals affiliated or under contract with a home health agency
8. Outpatient services that cannot be readily provided in the patient's home

Medicare does not pay for home services performed by immediate relatives or by members of the household. It does not cover 24-hour nursing care, drugs and biologic agents, home-delivered meals, homemaker services, or blood transfusions. Moreover, Medicare does not pay for custodial care (care not requiring professional skills), drugs and devices not approved by the Food and Drug Administration (FDA), and services or devices that are experimental.[14]

Costs and Benefits of Home Care

More comprehensive third-party payment has led to health care delivery at home, and the HCFA has estimated that one third of all patients admitted to a hospital could be adequately cared for by home care. The cost of home care, even high-tech care, is usually less expensive than hospital care. According to estimates by the National Association for Home Care, the daily cost in 1987 for rather intensive treatment at home was $25 to $100 per day vs. $300 to $500 for similar care in a hospital. The monthly cost for skilled nursing care at home was $750 versus $2000 in a hospital.[12] Since then, the average expense for a home care visit has increased (Table 15-1).

Public sources financed 75% of all expenditures for home care in 1990, up from 50% in 1970.[13] Payment sources for home care follow: Medicare, 44.7%; Medicaid 27.1%; self-pay, 12.7%; private health insurance, 7.6%; and nonpatient revenue sources, 7.5%.[15]

Many ill people would rather be treated in their own homes than in a hospital. There is an ongoing trend for people to assume more responsibility for their own well-being and to be more sophisticated regarding self-care. The increasing ability of the health care system to deliver complex technical care in the home has contributed to the growing public acceptance of this mode of care. Families usually appreciate having their loved one at home with them, and patients who are cared for at home can enjoy a more normal lifestyle. They can see family and friends,

TABLE 15-1	Average Expense for a Home Care Visit*	
Expense	1987	1993
Average	49	66
Nurse	62	84
Therapist	57	77
Aide	34	46
Homemaker	33	34
Other professional	56	75

*In dollars.

From Starr B: Refurbishing home care, *Business Health* 12(1):40, 1994.

sleep in their own beds, and be surrounded by things that are meaningful, such as pets, the telephone, music, the television, books, a garden, and other personal possessions. They can manage their own schedules, be free from the regimented and impersonal environment of the hospital, and perhaps most important, have the gratification of being in control of their own lives.[16]

A survey was commissioned by Olsten Health Care of Westbury, New York, to examine attitudes and opinions among Americans who had experienced home care. Findings indicated that 92% think that providers of home care are knowledgeable and capable, 90% think that home care enables patients to recuperate more quickly from illnesses, and 98% think that the home provides a more comfortable environment for terminally ill patients.[17]

Despite these benefits, home care is frequently long term and can represent a considerable emotional, social, and financial burden on the patient and family. The costs to family and friends who provide care at home are usually underestimated.[18] Among people over age 65, about 30% live alone,[19] and as many as a third of all patients receiving home health services live alone. Older women constitute the majority of such patients.[20] Being ill at home alone can be a frightening experience for these patients who are likely to feel isolated, lonely, and worried about being able to reach help in an emergency. Many electronic communication devices are available to assist frail older or ill individuals in summoning help.

At least another third of all home health patients are cared for at home by spouses. This care-giving spouse is likely to be older and female and may be feeble and in poor health. Caring for the ill spouse is an emotional and physical stressor, and the patient's illness imposes stressful alterations of established roles within the marriage. The remainder of home health patients are cared for by other family members, such as children, siblings, parents, or significant others. The ability to cope varies from couple to couple or family to family and depends on the availability of family and social support systems, on the quality of home services provided, and on the availability of services that can provide family members with temporary respite from the burden of providing continuous care. One study of spouses and families who manage family members with terminal illnesses found that 33% of the relatives were at risk of failing health status because of age or illness.[21]

Thus home care is frequently long term and can represent a considerable financial and emotional burden to the patient and family. Although advances in medicine and refinements of high-tech interventions contribute greatly to the potential for extended survival, the costs to the family may be a significant source of stress and a drain on their coping ability.

CONTINUITY OF CARE

Continuity of care is the connection and coordination of all health care services used by a patient. Well-planned continuity of care prevents duplication and fragmentation of services and ensures that each patient receives the most appropriate care. It assists patients to achieve their maximal health potential with the least discomfort and stress. Planned coordination of care reduces health care costs by ensuring cost-efficient use of services.[22] Effective continuity of care requires collaboration and cooperation among all the agencies and disciplines involved in a patient's care.

Case Management

Case management is a concept that enables continuity of care. The basic purpose of case management is to "integrate, coordinate and advocate for individuals, families and groups requiring extensive services."[23] Its fundamental focus is coordination of care.

Case management has been described as a clinical system that "focuses on the achievement of patient outcomes within effective and appropriate time frames and resources. Case management focuses on the entire episode of illness, crossing all settings in which the patient receives care."[24]

Case management is a role that provides a patient with one practitioner responsible for the active coordination of care in a manner that maximizes the contributions of several disciplines and services. It is a technology that produces tools and techniques to organize the timing and sequencing of care. It is a process that views the multiple needs of the patient from an episode-focused perspective across a continuum of care, providers, and settings. It is also a service that enables patients to make informed decisions and to optimally use existing health care resources in the most cost-effective manner. The goal of case management is to move the patient and family toward optimal outcomes of care.[23]

A case-management plan is a complete protocol for interventions appropriate for an episode of a specific illness.

It shows the relationships among patient problems, medical and nursing processes, clinical work, timing and length of stay, and costs of care. A critical path is an abbreviated form of the case management plan that depicts, on one page, the "key incidents that must occur in a predictable and timely order to achieve an appropriate length of stay."[25] Critical paths provide physicians and nurses with tools to monitor the plan and flow of care.[25]

Discharge Planning: Collaboration Among Agencies

A specific component of the case-management process, discharge planning facilitates the transition of patients from an acute care setting to home by coordinating the patient's need for continuing services, equipment, and supplies; family and social support; and education. This process should begin when a patient is admitted to an acute care institution. The American Nurses' Association defines discharge planning as[26]

> that part of the continuity of care process which is designed to prepare the patient or client for the next phase of care and to assist in making any necessary arrangements for that phase of care, care by family members or care by an organized health care provider.

The American Hospital Association describes discharge planning as "an interdisciplinary hospital-wide process that should be available to aid patients and their families in developing a feasible post-hospital plan of care."[27] Standards have been established by the Joint Commission of Accreditation of Healthcare Organizations (JCAHO) that address patients' rights to continuity of care. JCAHO site visits seek to confirm that discharge planning takes place and that its effectiveness is evaluated by the institution.[28]

Discharge planning consists of assessment of individual needs, of patient teaching, and when ongoing care is required, of the home environment; identification of a caregiver; and identification of appropriate community resources. Assessment for discharge should focus on health care needs, expected severity of illness at discharge, age, living arrangements, and anticipated need for instruction. Some patients, such as those over age 65, those who live alone, those likely to have a decrease in level of functioning after discharge, or those who require complex care, can be identified as high-risk patients. When it is determined that a patient or family cannot provide self-care without assistance, referrals to home care and other appropriate community agencies should be made. Early identification of the anticipated length of stay in the hospital establishes a framework within which coordination of resources, education, and referrals must take place.[29]

The purpose of patient education is to teach self-care. Factors associated with the ability of the patient to provide adequate self-care include the medical diagnosis, nursing diagnosis, functional limitations, knowledge levels and intellectual capabilities, and anxiety levels.

When a patient is incapable of self-care, a caregiver must be identified if possible. Although identification of a caregiver who is competent, able, and willing is frequently critical to the patient's well-being, locating such a person may be difficult. Caregivers may be family members. Many people live alone or live with a spouse who also has health problems or functional limitations. Others may live with caregivers who work outside the home or have other responsibilities and demands on their time. Some caregivers may be poorly taught or simply unable to learn to carry out the necessary care effectively. Although situations occur in which patients at home are neglected, improperly cared for, or even abused, in most cases caregivers in the home provide effective, dedicated, and competent care. Indeed, home caregivers are a generally unrecognized but vital link in today's health care system.

Assessment of the home environment is an important component of discharge planning. Even today, some people live without indoor plumbing, and many homes have inadequate heat. The lack of a cooling system or the presence of stairs can present special problems for the cardiac patient. Factors such as space, safety, and level of repair, all affect the adequacy of care at home, especially when special equipment is required.[29]

Hospital discharge planners must keep up-to-date regarding the availability of agencies that provide home health services for patients in their service area and should maintain close links with community agencies. Effective interagency collaboration helps ease the transition for patients and families from one site of care to the next. The discharge planners' knowledge of available community services, supplies, equipment, and other resources is crucial in determining the extent to which the patient's needs are met after leaving the hospital.

Home Health Care Team: Collaboration Among Disciplines

Interdisciplinary collaboration is a necessity in the provision of home health services. No single discipline can effectively respond to all of the needs for home care, and Medicare-certified agencies are required to document interdisciplinary services. Interdisciplinary collaboration requires a comprehensive approach in which health care professionals relate effectively and cooperatively with each other. It implies effective communication, shared problem solving, and joint decision making by an integrated team.[30]

Each patient has an individualized care plan. Effective collaboration ensures that the patient's needs are met in the most appropriate manner, without overlap among disciplines. Successful interdisciplinary collaboration requires that all members of the health care team be competent practitioners in their respective disciplines. The roles and responsibilities of the disciplines involved in home health care are established by Medicare regulations, state licensing boards, and professional organizations. These disciplines and their respective responsibilities follow.[7]

Physician

Each patient who receives home health services must be under the care of a physician. Although a nurse may make an assessment visit without physician approval, every plan of care must be "certified" by a physician *before* care is provided for Medicare to reimburse for services. If care is to continue, the plan of care must be recertified by the physician in collaboration with home care professionals at least every 60 days.

Nurse

The nurse receives the referral information, usually from a physician or hospital discharge planner and makes an initial evaluation visit. At this visit the nurse interviews the patient and caregiver to determine the types and amount of services needed. Assessment includes a psychosocial and medical history, a physical examination of the patient, and an assessment of the adequacy of the environment. Medications are reviewed. The agency services are explained and the availability of insurance and/or Medicare eligibility is evaluated. Treatments may be provided, if needed. Based on this initial evaluation visit, the plan of care is established.

From the first interview, the emphasis of home health nursing is on maximizing self-care abilities. This focus is a hallmark of home nursing and represents one of the fundamental differences between home nursing and hospital nursing. While the patient is in the hospital, the nurse provides care; in the home the nurse teaches self-care to the patient and the family or another care provider. In fact, the home health nurse may be the patient's only contact with the health care system.

Subsequent nursing visits provide skilled nursing care services, teach patient care, supervise home health aides, coordinate other services, and update the plan of care as needed. The nurse serves as case manager, monitors the status of the patient, and ensures that adequate care is provided. As patient problems increase in complexity and demands for sophisticated technologic skills and services escalate, home health nurses have many issues to address. These nurses must maintain a holistic approach that includes the emotional needs and social well-being of the patient and family.

Physical therapist

When it is needed, maintenance, preventive, and restorative treatment is provided by physical therapists who have baccalaureate degrees and are licensed in the state in which they practice. Treatment may include muscle strengthening, restoration of mobility, control of spasticity, gait training, or active-passive resistive exercises. Included in the job of the physical therapist is teaching the treatment regimen to the patient and family, collaborating with other health care professionals, and participating in patient care conferences.

Occupational therapist

Services for patients who need assistance in achieving their optimal level of functioning in activities of daily living are provided in the home by occupational therapists. These practitioners are educated at the baccalaureate level and are registered by the National Occupational Therapy Association. Occupational therapists assist patients in restoring the muscle strength and mobility required for functional skills, with special focus on the upper extremities. They teach self-care activities, remove barriers, and provide adaptive equipment when needed. Occupational therapists collaborate with other team members and participate in patient care conferences.

Speech pathologist

Patients with communication problems related to speech, language, or hearing may receive home services by a speech pathologist who holds a master's degree and is certified by the American Speech and Hearing Association. Services include evaluating speech and language abilities and teaching the patient and family how to develop optimal levels of communication. Speech pathologists may also address eating or swallowing problems.

Social worker

Assistance with social, emotional, and environmental factors that relate to the health and well-being of the patient and family may be provided by a social worker. In home health care, the social worker usually holds a master's degree in social work. Social workers assist people in identifying and using appropriate community resources. They may assist with applications for aid, be involved in crisis intervention, assist in obtaining needed equipment and supplies, and provide guidance in addressing financial problems.

Home health aide

Patients who need assistance with personal hygiene may receive the services of a home health aide. Supervised by the nurse, the home health aide must have experience as an aide and have special training in providing home care. Services include assistance with personal hygiene and walking, meal preparation, and light housekeeping chores. The home health aide implements the plan of care and reports to the supervising nurse.

Homemaker

Although similar to the home health aide, the homemaker focuses on housekeeping chores. Services include home maintenance, shopping, cooking, and companionship.

Community Resources

In addition to the customary home health services described, other services are sometimes available to assist the ill or infirm at home. The availability of these services varies from community to community. The services may have long waiting lists, so they may not be available to all patients who could benefit from them.

The family caring for an ill member at home may be helped by special home care courses and materials prepared by the American Red Cross. Materials for patient education that address health promotion and approaches to caring for patients with cardiac diagnoses are available through the American Heart Association.

Homemaker or chore services may be available through community agencies such as senior citizens, the American Red Cross, or the Long Term Care Project. These services may also be provided by private groups or churches. Such groups may also provide transportation. Meals on Wheels is available in many communities to provide home-delivered meals to older adults or infirm people. Some grocery stores and pharmacies provide home delivery.

Medical equipment and supplies for home use are available through private vendors. Under certain conditions, Medicare pays for some equipment used in the home. For example, for Medicare to cover the cost of a hospital bed for home use, the patient must spend at least 50% of the time in bed. Similar restrictions apply to other equipment and supplies. Many home health agencies and equipment vendors maintain a loan closet to provide supplies and equipment to patients who need but cannot afford them. Sometimes supplies are donated by private individuals or organizations.[29]

A program called the *Vial of Life Program* is available in some communities. Emergency information and medical history are recorded on a medical information form that is tucked into a plastic vial and stored on the right side of the top shelf of the refrigerator. A decal attached to the outside of the door of the refrigerator alerts an ambulance crew that the information is inside. Such a system is particularly useful for older adults and for people who live alone.

Emergency electronic systems are available in many communities. An electronic device that can be activated in an emergency is either worn or placed in a strategic location in the home, such as beside the bed or in the bathroom. Activation of the system alerts an operator to call for emergency services and may also alert the patient's family or physician.[31]

In all cases, families should be instructed to post emergency numbers near their telephone. Patients should be provided with a card that describes their diagnoses, treatments, and when relevant, the most effective means of controlling the dysrhythmias. Patients who are not homebound should be encouraged to carry this card and wear a medic alert bracelet.

An innovation in the provision of health services is the establishment of adult day-care centers. These centers provide care for adults who are not capable of caring for themselves alone at home during the day but who are able to leave home. This service offers respite for overburdened caregivers and those who must go to work or to other responsibilities during the day. Services are usually available on an hourly, daily, or weekly basis, and include nursing supervision, meals, planned activities, socialization, and assistance with bathing and other activities of daily living.

ASSESSMENT FOR HOME CARE

Assessment for home care consists of collecting data about the patient and family as bases for planning the treatment regimen to meet the patient's needs in the home. The assessment includes information about the family's ability to provide necessary care, observations about the adequacy of the home environment, and the availability of support systems and community resources.

Family

Cardiac illness of a family member is a major life stressor on the entire family, and families vary greatly in their ability to cope. Household routines and lifestyles are usually disrupted, and roles of the members as they relate to each other are likely to be altered. Although it is the cardiac patient who initially enters the health care system, it is the family that ultimately provides the context for recovery or long-term care. The family or lack thereof profoundly affects the individual's response to illness and may determine whether home care is a viable option. Patients who live alone require special support and services to manage their self-care. These patients are at greater risk for rehospitalization or admission to long-term care facilities than patients with caretaker families.

The concept of family is broadly defined in the health care literature. *Family* generally implies a social system of two or more people who coexist and who share mutual affection and mutual responsibility.[32] This definition includes traditional nuclear families, single-parent and step families, and any other couple or group who share a valued relationship characterized by commitment, mutual decision making, and shared resources. According to U.S. Bureau of Labor statistics, the traditional family configuration of a father who is employed and a woman who stays home as wife and mother constitutes only about 13% of the households in the United States. Of the remaining households, 16% are married couples who have children and who both work, 16% are single-parent families, 23% are married couples living alone, 23% are single-person households, 6% are households with extended families, and all others compose the remainder.[33]

The patient and family may not realize the full impact of the illness while the patient is in the hospital. The major adjustments must occur when the patient returns home.

Frequently the patient and family must deal with issues for which they are not prepared. The degree of adjustments to lifestyle is determined by the severity of the illness and the associated degree of disability, the amount of care that must be provided by others, the kind of equipment and environmental alterations required, and the availability and use of appropriate health care services. *Home care* frequently implies that those in the home must cope with a crisis that has no closure. The ability of family members to provide care is directly related to their levels of anxiety and methods of coping with stress. The cultural, racial, ethnic, and religious identities of family members contribute to their health beliefs and to their style of coping with illness. The level of education affects comprehension about the disease process and determines the level at which health teaching must be provided. Families are usually able to provide effective basic health care if properly instructed by health care professionals.[34] Because families vary in their patterns of coping, assessment of the ability to cope is a first step in the provision of home care.

Families must deal with several tasks to cope with the long-term illness of a member.[32,35] First, they must learn to prevent or manage a crisis. This is especially relevant for families of patients with cardiac disease who are at risk for life-threatening dysrhythmias or cardiac arrest.

Second is the task of regimen management. The difficulty inherent in this task depends on the degree of modification of the usual daily routine required by the patient's illness and the extent to which this modification affects family members. The more assistance the patient requires in providing self-care, the greater the demands for other family members to modify their daily routines.

The third task is symptom control. Success is contingent on the judgment of the patient and family in dealing with symptoms as they occur. Adequate teaching is necessary to allay fears and to provide information about palliative measures.

The fourth task is to deal with temporal and role disruption. Patients suddenly spending more time at home, deprived of former activities, must find new ways to occupy time. Moreover, the illness may bring major changes in the roles of family members in relationship to each other. Roles of economic provider, housekeeper, or decision maker within the household may be profoundly altered by the illness and may require adjustment by all family members.

Fifth, families must cope with the trajectory of the illness. For example, some cardiac patients may recover, others remain at a diminished level of health, some slowly decline, and a few experience sudden death.

The sixth family task is to overcome social isolation. Impaired functioning, diminished energy, altered body image, and time-consuming therapeutic regimens may interfere with social relationships. In many cases, the caregiver becomes isolated at home with the patient and has no respite.

The final task is that of finding adequate financial resources to pay for necessary treatment and daily care and to compensate for possible loss of income. Cardiac illness of a family member can last many years and may severely drain the economic resources of the family.

Home care differs from hospital care in that in the institution the roles and the realm of control of each health care provider are well defined. The hospital is their "territory," and the patient is the "guest" outsider. Health care providers control the terms and the timing of the situation. When the home is the health care setting, it is the "territory" of the household members. They are in control and have their designated roles, and the home health care provider is the "guest" outsider. The patient and other members of the household control the circumstances and the timing of the care provided.

Assessment of the family should include a description of the family, including household members and members of the patient's support system who may be involved in providing care or support. The roles of each member, especially in nontraditional families, and the tasks they assume in caring for the patient should be clarified. Family dynamics should be observed and decision makers and caretakers identified. As typical family size decreases and more women are employed outside of the home, fewer caregivers are available at home.[36] The caregiver and other family members involved in the patient's day-to-day care should be assessed to determine their ability to provide the needed care.[6]

Assessment should also address environmental issues and access to care. For example, the availability of a telephone and an automobile determines the degree to which the patient and family can communicate with and use the health care system. Even today, not all households have access to these conveniences.

The ability of the family to provide care depends on their level of understanding of cardiovascular disease and of the patient's therapeutic regimen. They should understand the importance of preventing complications and know what therapeutic measures contribute to that end. They should be able to provide the patient with the necessary diet, medications, and activity and should be able to carry out necessary interventions, such as accurate monitoring of pulse, blood pressure, and if necessary, status of an artificial pacemaker. In some cases, it may be necessary for a caregiver to learn complex technical skills.

Household members who are willing and capable should be encouraged to learn techniques of basic life support (BLS). Classes are frequently available through community agencies or the local affiliate of the American Heart Association or American Red Cross. When necessary, special instructions should be provided for resuscitating a patient with a tracheostomy or laryngectomy. The home health nurse should assess and document the BLS skills of family members and make referrals for annual refresher courses and opportunities to practice. The patient's risk for cardiac or respiratory arrest should routinely be monitored.[37]

Patient

The need for home care results from an acute exacerbation or complication of a chronic disease.[38] In the majority of cases, the patient was hospitalized before admission for home care. Being discharged from the hospital is an experience that may be regarded with ambivalence by most patients. On one hand, patients are relieved to have survived a life-threatening cardiac crisis. On the other hand, leaving the security of the hospital may generate fear and apprehension. Patients who have a major cardiac event such as a myocardial infarction may fear a recurrence. They may wonder whether recovery at home is possible, whether family members will manage to provide the necessary care, and whether professional help will be available if it is needed. The history of the sudden onset of heart disease for many patients compounds these fears.

Mental status, especially that of older patients, should be evaluated at each visit. Once survival from a cardiac event is ensured, many patients become depressed. Uncertainty, worry, and a sense of loss can result in depression when the patient returns home. Symptoms may include insomnia, cognitive changes, diminished libido, restlessness, and possibly recurring thoughts of death. The problems usually diminish or disappear within 3 months as strength and feelings of well-being return.[39] Psychologic symptoms of physiologic imbalances also occur. Side effects of medications may cause such symptoms. For example, even at nontoxic levels, digitalis may be associated with delirium in older adults.[40]

Assessment of the cardiac patient at home emphasizes factors that relate to controlling the disease process and modifying cardiovascular risks. The history should focus on issues germane to management of the cardiac patient at home (see box).

Physical assessment of the cardiac patient at home should include measurement of blood pressure in both arms as the patient sits and stands. Readings should be taken twice, at least 10 minutes apart. Heart sounds should be evaluated for rate, rhythm, quality, and extra sounds, and the radial pulse is evaluated for pulse deficit. Breath sounds should be evaluated for rate, quality, and the possibility of rales. Skin color and peripheral pulses should be assessed. Abnormal signs such as peripheral edema or neck vein distention should be evaluated. Weight should be measured and, if relevant, intake and output records reviewed. The evaluation should include symptoms of cardiac insufficiency, such as dyspnea, orthopnea, chest pain, nausea, dizziness, decreased appetite, or excessive fatigue.[41]

Blood testing may be indicated for homebound patients for many reasons. Patients with congestive failure who are taking diuretics may require periodic electrolyte, blood urea nitrogen, and creatinine measurements. Pa-

---

ASSESSMENT CRITERIA OF THE CARDIAC PATIENT AT HOME

History of symptoms, specifically:
  Chest pain: onset, precipitating factors, duration, location and radiation, means of relief, and any associated symptoms
  Weakness, faintness, headaches, dizziness
  Cyanosis
  Dyspnea, orthopnea
  Palpitations
  Edema
  Changes in visual fields
History of heart disease, hypertension, or diabetes
Family history, especially of cardiovascular diseases and risks
Relationships with family and close friends, support system
Occupation, work environment, and relationships
Leisure and recreational activities
Exercise type and amount
Diet history, especially fats, salts, and total calories
Knowledge level about current health problems
Ability to carry out self-care
Ability to utilize available resources
Psychosocial reaction to disease status and ability to cope

From Caliandro G: *Adults with coronary artery disease.* In Caliandro G, Judkins BL, editors: *Primary nursing practices,* Glenview, Ill, 1988, Scott Foresman.

---

tients on digitalis or other cardiopulmonary medications may need monitoring of serum levels. Periodic prothrombin times will be indicated for patients on anticoagulation medication.[42]

In general, all patients with cardiac disease are at risk for congestive heart failure. Homebound patients should be monitored for the following cardinal signs of congestive heart failure.[43]

1. Fatigue and anorexia are among the earliest signs of cardiac decompensation.
2. Palpitations can be a source of great anxiety for the patient, and, if dysrhythmias are frequent, they can compromise cardiac output.
3. Dyspnea, hyperpnea, or both result from pulmonary congestion and increase the work of breathing.
4. Paroxysmal nocturnal dyspnea is caused by changes in fluid dynamics and reduced cardiac output resulting from being in the prone position. This sudden occurrence may be accompanied by confusion related to cerebral hypoxia. The condition may prevent the patient from getting enough rest and is associated with serious potential for injury, especially among older adults.
5. Orthopnea and dyspnea on exertion may occur.
6. Generalized or pitting edema of the extremities occurs frequently, as does jugular venous distention and a third heart sound.

Patients at risk for congestive failure should be advised to call the nurse or physician if their shoes become too tight, usual tasks or activities of daily living become difficult, extra sleep is needed, and urination at night becomes more frequent.[43]

Nursing diagnoses derived from the assessment data reflect the physiologic status of the patient and the psychosocial condition of the patient and family. Physiologic and psychosocial nursing diagnoses likely to occur among cardiac patients and the etiology and defining characteristics for each are presented in Tables 15-2 and 15-3.[44]

PLAN OF CARE

The plan of care is based on the assessment data and the patient's medical and nursing diagnoses. The care plan is a problem-solving model that incorporates the patient's needs for care, the prescribed medical regimen, and the patient's and family's perceptions of the illness.

Documentation of the Treatment Plan

The home health plan of treatment must be developed and thoroughly documented to meet guidelines for Medicare reimbursement and to meet state and federal regulatory requirements for agency certification and recertification. Each patient's plan of care is developed by the nurse and must be recertified by the physician every 60 days. In addition, for the agency to be reimbursed for services provided, the patient must be certified to be confined to home and in need of intermittent professional skilled care.[46]

The plan of care must include the following components.[45]

1. *Diagnosis:* The diagnosis indicates the principal medical diagnosis most closely related to the current plan of treatment. The diagnosis, expressed in the appropriate ICD-9-CM Code, may relate to the most recent hospitalization of the patient but must relate to home care services provided. In the case of multiple diagnoses, the one representing the greatest need for home care services should be used.
2. *Medications:* The list of medications includes the dose, frequency, and route for each drug. New prescriptions and changes in prescriptions must be indicated.
3. *Surgical procedures:* The nurse lists the procedures related to the care provided, with the date of the surgery.
4. *Other pertinent diagnoses:* Only diagnoses that relate to the patient's plan of treatment are listed in order of seriousness. Medicare uses these diagnoses to justify payment or denial of payment for services rendered.
5. *Functional limitations:* Medicare reimburses for services only if a patient is homebound.
6. *Mental status:* The nurse describes the patient's ability to function within the home.
7. *Nutritional requirements:* TPN may be listed here or in the section on medications.
8. *Prognosis:* Medicare continues to reimburse only if the patient's condition is improving.
9. *Prescriptions:* The list of prescriptions indicates the disciplines and treatments prescribed and includes the frequency of services to be provided.

Adherence to the treatment regimen is a crucial issue for patients being cared for at home. Patients are more likely to comply in a hospital under the supervision and direction of professional care providers than in their own homes, where it is easier to slip back into former habits and routines. Some of the reasons identified for nonadherence to prescribed treatment follow[47]:

1. The patient is intimidated by the magnitude of the treatment program.
2. The patient feels better and thinks that there is no need for the treatment.
3. The patient thinks that treatment will not help.
4. The patient cannot afford the cost of the treatment.
5. The patient does not trust or respect the health care providers.
6. The patient is forgetful, a common occurrence among older adults.

Diet

Special dietary needs of the patient at home affect the entire family. Because many of the risk factors for cardiac disease are familial, the entire family may benefit from a diet conducive to heart health. Family members are likely to share past dietary patterns that have put the patient at risk and may share unhealthy lifestyles that also include obesity, insufficient exercise, smoking behavior, and genetic predispositions. The crisis of having an ill member may motivate other members of the family to want to modify their own risk factors by changing behaviors and diet.

Decisions must be made about whether the whole family will share the patient's dietary restrictions, perhaps adding seasonings on an individual basis, or whether special food will be prepared for the patient. In general, the degree of restriction required by the patient (for example, amount of sodium permitted) determines the impact on the rest of the household. The nurse should identify, as the target for diet teaching, the household member who does the grocery shopping and the person who cooks the meals.

In addition to the specific dietary restrictions prescribed for an individual, a dietary plan for all cardiac patients should consider the following factors[41]:

1. A diet that is high in fiber (such as vegetables, fruit, whole grains, and bran) promotes bowel elimination and prevents the tendency to use the Valsalva maneuver and the discomfort of constipation. Such foods also aid in weight control, if this is a problem.

TABLE 15-2   Potential Nursing Diagnoses of the Patient With a Chronic Cardiac Condition: Physiologic

Nursing Diagnoses	Etiologies	Defining Characteristics
Activity intolerance	Decreased cardiac reserve	Verbal report of fatigue or weakness; abnormal HR, BP, or ECG response to activity; exertional discomfort or dyspnea
Decreased cardiac output	Alteration in heart rate or rhythm, preload, afterload, or contractility	HR, BP, or ECG changes; dysrhythmias; fatigue; color changes of skin or mucous membranes; oliguria; diminished peripheral pulses; cold, clammy skin; rales; dyspnea; restlessness
Fluid volume deficit	Fluid restriction; diuretics	Increased serum sodium levels; increased HR; increased Hgb and Hct; decreased pulse pressure; dry skin; thirst
Fluid volume excess, relative or actual	Compromised regulatory mechanisms secondary to decreased cardiac output; excessive fluid and/or sodium intake	Edema; weight gain; intake level greater than output level; third heart sound; shortness of breath; rales; jugular venous distention; decreased Hgb and Hct; changes in electrolyte levels and BP
Impaired gas exchange	Alveolar-capillary membrane changes secondary to pulmonary vascular congestion	Confusion; restlessness; anxiety; altered arterial blood gas levels; HR changes
Potential for infection	Altered primary defenses secondary to surgical incisions and invasive catheters and lines	Changes in white blood count and differential; erythema, edema, pain, purulence at site; fever
Potential for injury	Risk of pericarditis and/or myocardial rupture after myocardial infarction; side effects of medications; generalized weakness of chronic illness secondary to decreased cardiac reserve	Changes in vital signs; difficulty ambulating; change in mental status; history of injury or accident; evidence of injury
Altered nutrition, less than body requirements	Decreased appetite; early satiety secondary to physical presence of implanted device	Weight loss; pale conjunctival and mucous membranes; poor muscle tone; reported decreased food intake
Altered nutrition, more than body requirements	Decreased metabolic needs secondary to sedentary and debilitated lifestyle; maladaptive coping	Weight gain; increased triceps skinfold; observed dysfunctional eating patterns
Pain (chronic or acute)	Myocardial ischemia	Verbal complaints of pain; moans, crying, restlessness, grimace; rigid muscle tone; diaphoresis; HR, BP, or respiratory rate changes; pupillary dilatation
Self-care deficit	Physical limitations secondary to decreased cardiac reserve	Inability to perform bathing, dressing and grooming, feeding, or toileting
Sexual dysfunction	Actual or perceived activity intolerance secondary to decreased cardiac reserve; fear of recurrence of dysrhythmias, pain, or cardioversion or defibrillation during coitus; side effects of medications	Reported difficulties, limitations, or changes in sexual behaviors or activities
Impaired skin integrity	Surgical incision and invasive catheters and lines; prolonged bedrest	Disruption of skin surface; destruction of skin layers; invasion of body structures
Altered tissue perfusion	Decreased cardiac output, interruption of arterial blood flow secondary to coronary artery disease, cerebral vascular disease, or peripheral vascular disease; embolus	Diminished pulses; cold skin; decreased function of affected organ

HR, Heart rate; *BP*, blood pressure; *Hgb*, hemoglobin (count); *Hct*, hematocrit.

TABLE 15-3   Potential Nursing Diagnoses of the Patient With a Chronic Cardiac Condition: Psychosocial

Nursing Diagnoses	Etiologies	Defining Characteristics
Impaired judgment	Disability requiring change in lifestyle; inadequate support systems; impaired cognition; assault to self-esteem; incomplete grieving	Verbalization of nonacceptance of health status change; inability to problem solve or set goals; lack of movement toward independence
Anxiety	Threat of death; threat of chronic, life-altering condition; necessity of high-tech treatments and their side-effects; financial concerns	Verbalization of increased tension, fear, uncertainty, concerns; decreased verbalization; inability to concentrate and understand or retain information; poor eye contact; trembling; facial tension; perspiration; voice quivering; extraneous movement; pupil dilatation; restless, hostile, or withdrawn appearance
Body image disturbance	Change in body function; physical scarring; presence of pacemaker, implantable cardioverter defibrillator, ventricular assist device; limitations of debilitated condition	Verbalization of change in lifestyle; negative feelings about body; focus on past appearance or function
Ineffective individual and/or family coping	Situational crisis; personal vulnerability; lack of knowledge of personal and community resources; inadequate or incorrect information or understanding; preoccupation with managing emotional conflicts; prolonged illness that exhausts supportive capacity	Verbalization of inability to cope or ask for help; inability to meet role expectations; inability to meet basic needs; inability to problem solve; destructive behavior toward self or others; inappropriate use of defense mechanisms; overprotectiveness of significant other or caregiver
Ineffective denial	Fear	Delay of seeking or refusal of health care to the detriment of health; lack of perception of personal relevance of symptoms or danger; refusal to discuss condition; minimization of severity of condition and its consequences; disregard recommendations and treatments
Diversional activity deficit	Prolonged limiting condition; chronic fatigue; lack of supportive resources	Statements related to boredom; inability to participate in past or usual hobbies and activities
Altered family processes	Situation transition secondary to chronic illness	Family inability to meet physical, emotional, spiritual needs of members; inability to express and accept feelings; inability to demonstrate respect for individual members' autonomy; lack of appropriate family decision-making process; inability to accept or receive help; failure of family to accomplish current or past developmental task; failure to adapt to change or deal with experiences constructively
Fear	Realization of mortality and vulnerability for chronic, debilitating condition	Apprehension; verbalization of fatalism; extreme emotion; verbalization of need to contact people and "put affairs in order"
Grieving	Anticipated or actual loss of person, function, status, and livelihood	Expression of distress at potential loss; guilt, anger, sorrow; change in eating habits, sleep patterns, and activity level; altered communication; interference with life functioning; developmental regression
Altered growth and development	Effects of physical disability and resultant dependence; inadequate caretaking; indifference; environmental and stimulation deficiencies	Delay or difficulty in performing motor, social or expressive skills typical of age; inability to perform self-control activities; flat affect; listlessness

TABLE 15-3   Potential Nursing Diagnoses of the Patient With a Chronic Cardiac Condition: Psychosocial—cont'd

Nursing Diagnoses	Etiologies	Defining Characteristics
Altered health maintenance	Lack of or change in communication skills; lack of ability to make deliberate and thoughtful judgments; perceptual or cognitive impairments; ineffective coping; dysfunctional distress; lack of material resources; self-neglect of caregiver	Demonstrated lack of knowledge regarding basic health practices; lack of adaptive behaviors for change in health status or environment; reported or observed lack of equipment and financial and other resources
Impaired home maintenance management	Impaired cognitive or emotional functioning; lack of knowledge; inadequate support systems; insufficient finances	Verbalization or observation of lack of necessary equipment or aids; evidence of hazards in the home; insufficient provision or handling of food, wastes, clothes, and linen; inappropriate household temperature
Hopelessness	Failing or deteriorating physical condition; long-term stress; abandonment; prolonged wait for treatment (transplantation)	Passivity; decreased verbalization; decreased affect; lack of initiative; decreased response to stimuli; decreased appetite; increased sleep; lack of involvement in care
Knowledge deficit	Lack of exposure to information; information misinterpretation; cognitive limitation; lack of interest in learning; inappropriate level or amount of information; lack of reinforcement	Verbalization of knowledge deficit; inaccurate follow-through of instruction; inaccurate performance of test
Noncompliance	Misunderstanding of instructions or importance of treatment and regimen; physical or financial inability to follow through with treatment and regimen; frustration, denial	Verbalization or observation of deviation from regimen; evidence (complication) of lack of treatment and regimen; lack of knowledge of regimen; lack of available personal and community resources
Powerlessness	Need for therapeutic regimen; physical deterioration despite compliance; lack of control over availability of treatment (organs); physical dependency; overprotectiveness of significant other or caregiver	Verbal expressions of lack of control over outcome or self-care; apathy; nonparticipation in care or decision making; expressions of dissatisfaction or frustration, resentment, anger, and guilt
Altered role performance	Debilitating physical limitations on work, parental, and sexual relationships; overprotectiveness of significant other or caregiver	Self-verbalization of dissatisfaction with role performance
Situational low self-esteem	Chronic illness	Self-negating verbalizations; expressions of shame, guilt, and uselessness
Sleep pattern disturbance	Paroxysmal nocturnal dyspnea; therapeutic regimen; stress	Verbal complaints of not feeling rested, inability to sleep; dark circles under eyes; yawning
Social isolation	Limited physical mobility; therapeutic isolation; environmental barriers; absence of available significant others or peers; communication barriers; altered thought processes	Absence of supportive family and friends; sad, dull affect; lack of communication; withdrawal; expression of feelings of solitude or rejection
Spiritual distress	Loss of faith in God or belief system; isolation from religious ties	Expression of concern with meaning of life and death and belief systems; anger toward God; questions about meaning of suffering and own existence; inability to participate in own religious practices

2. Most cardiac patients benefit from restriction of high-sodium food to avoid fluid retention. Patients need to learn to avoid "hidden" salt, such as that in processed foods, pickled foods, salty snacks, and foods containing monosodium glutamate.
3. Patients who are taking potassium-depleting diuretics may benefit from foods high in potassium, such as bananas, tomatoes, raisins, and potatoes.
4. Limitation of caffeine intake from coffee, tea, colas, and chocolate helps avoid unnecessary sympathetic nervous system stimulation.
5. Avoidance of cholesterol and saturated fats found in eggs, meats, cheese, and whole milk products may limit the progression of atherosclerosis. Total fat should be limited to less than 30% to 40% of total caloric intake.
6. Restriction of sugar, alcohol, and total calories aids in weight control, if this is necessary.

Patients on sodium-restricted diets may choose to use salt substitutes. Commercially available salt substitutes usually contain potassium salts. These products may safely enhance the palatability of food for most patients, and those who are taking diuretics may benefit from the supplemental potassium. However, patients already taking potassium substitutes, those on potassium-sparing diuretics, and those who may have a moderate degree of renal failure should use these products with caution. In these circumstances, serum potassium levels might be monitored or nonpotassium salt substitutes used instead.[42]

Patients are more likely to comply with long-term dietary restrictions if prior eating preferences and cultural and religious aspects of diet are incorporated into the diet plan. A diet consisting of modifications of familiar foods is more palatable than a diet based on new and different foods. In addition, the family's economic constraints, as well as the availability of foods, must be considered in the diet plan. It is futile to recommend fresh fruits or seafood, for example, if they are unaffordable or unavailable.

Medications

Patients with cardiac problems must frequently adhere to complex regimens for medication administration at home. The extent and accuracy of following the prescribed medication schedule is related to several factors in the home situation. Nonadherence may occur because a patient or caregiver does not understand how or when the drugs are to be taken. They may not understand why the drugs are important. They may not be able to remember to take them, or they may be confused. Patients may resist taking a medication because they experience side effects that are difficult to discuss with the physician or nurse (such as decreased libido associated with antihypertensives). Some patients may not adhere because they cannot manage the cost of the drugs, and some patients, especially older adults, may have difficulty opening containers.

The home medication regimen begins with a nursing evaluation of the potential of the patient or caregiver to administer the necessary medications. Special consideration should be given to cognitive ability, motivation, dexterity, financial resources, and ability to obtain refills. The patient should be evaluated for the effects of the medications, possible side effects, and potential for misuse of over-the-counter drugs. Patients taking antihypertensives, for example, should be warned against using over-the-counter antihistamines without first consulting the physician.

Teaching addresses individual needs. The nurse should emphasize the importance of taking the prescribed drugs and should instruct the patient about the correct dose, route, and time. The patient should be taught the action of the drug and the possible side effects. Audiovisual aids are helpful, and most patients benefit from written materials aimed at the individual's level of understanding.

Patients who must take frequent doses of medications usually benefit from dispenser boxes that can be labeled and prefilled on a weekly basis. These can be purchased at a pharmacy or may be made from egg cartons that are cut and pasted to accommodate the dosage schedule required (for example, two or four times a day). Others may prefer a calendar or tally sheet that can be checked off. Such assistance is frequently appreciated even by fully cognizant patients or caregivers who must deal with a repetitious daily routine and many other demands on their attention.[41]

Patients taking digitalis should be taught to monitor their own pulses and to identify changes in rate or rhythm. They should be advised to withhold the digitalis and notify the physician if the rate drops below 60 beats/min, if a regular pulse becomes irregular, or if an irregular pulse changes. Patients should be aware of the signs and symptoms of digitalis toxicity: anorexia, nausea, vomiting, diarrhea, or visual changes. Patients taking diuretics are at increased risk of digitalis toxicity because of potassium depletion.

Some patients who have been hospitalized with a cardiovascular diagnosis are discharged on anticoagulant therapy. Home care includes assessing for signs of overdose such as severe bruising, bleeding gums, nosebleeds, blood in the urine, tarry stools, headaches, or visual or motor changes; patients on this therapy should be taught these warning signs. Patients should be advised to use electric razors rather than sharp blades, to use soft toothbrushes, and to avoid cuts or trauma. Aspirin should not be used by these patients.[48]

Pain Management

Pain experienced by the cardiac patient at home is likely to be the pain of angina related to myocardial ischemia or the postoperative pain of a sternal incision. In some instances, it may be necessary to differentiate between these two types of pain. Patients often describe the pain of angina as aching, squeezing, burning, tightness, or choking; it frequently radiates to the shoulder, arm, neck or jaw. Ischemic pain may be accomplished by nausea, epigastric burning, diaphoresis, fatigue, anxiety, or palpitations. On the other hand, incisional pain is likely to occur only with deep breaths. A history that describes the pain, its usual patterns, precipitating factors, and methods of relief may be useful to the nurse in evaluating the type of pain and planning the appropriate intervention.

The pain of angina is relieved by measures that enhance myocardial oxygenation, either by improving delivery of oxygen to the myocardium or by decreasing its demand for oxygen. This can be accomplished by having the patient rest in a head-up position, either sitting or in a semi-Fowler position. Lying prone increases venous return and consequently myocardial wall tension and consumption of oxygen. If rest alone does not relieve the pain, sublingual nitroglycerin may be administered at 5-minute intervals up to 3 times. Nitroglycerin causes vasodilatation, which decreases venous return and subsequent coronary workload and increases myocardial oxygen supply as a result of dilatation of the coronary vessels. The patient should contact immediately the physician or an ambulance if three doses of nitroglycerin do not relieve the pain. Patients should be warned that nitroglycerin may cause headaches and that they should remain seated when taking it to avoid syncope and falls. This is especially critical for patients who live alone or who have osteoporosis.

The patient or caregiver should understand that nitroglycerin has a short shelf life and needs to be replaced about every 3 months. It should be kept in a dark bottle and refrigerated to prevent rapid deterioration. The patient may carry a few day's supply, and household members should know where the tablets are stored.

Other coronary vasodilators may be prescribed for some patients. For example, long-acting nitrates in the form of patches or slow-release capsules may be used to promote more consistent coronary artery vasodilatation. The patient should know how to use these properly. A β-adrenergic blocker that decreases myocardial oxygen consumption (for example, propranolol) may be prescribed to decrease the frequency of anginal attacks.[48]

Prevention of angina pain, especially that of stable angina, may be possible if precipitating factors can be identified. The possible influence of diet (especially caffeine), smoking, emotional stress, exercise, temperature changes, blood pressure levels, and diabetic control should be evaluated. Interventions may then be devised to assist the patient in avoiding the precipitating factor or learning to handle the situation more effectively. These may entail lifestyle changes that may be acceptable to the patient and appropriate to the situation. Measures that may help include increasing aerobic capacity by regular moderate exercise, learning to better cope with stress, stopping cigarette smoking, eating smaller meals more frequently, reducing weight, avoiding temperature extremes, and learning to pace daily activities.

When pain is due to incisional discomfort resulting from cardiac surgery, the patient may have rapid, shallow respirations in an attempt to ease the discomfort. Ineffective breathing patterns may result. These patients should use the analgesics prescribed to prevent severe discomfort. The analgesics may be taken ahead of time to better enable the patient to do deep-breathing exercises. This is a problem of limited duration that will be resolved when the chest heals.[49]

Activity and Rest

Patients must be homebound for home care to be reimbursed by third-party payers, and therefore they are likely to have limited activity tolerance. Prior hospitalization and immobility from prolonged bedrest may result in decreased physical work capacity as evidenced by hyperventilation and decreased cardiac reserve. Other possible effects of immobility are diminished vasomotor reflex, increased potential for thromboembolism, nitrogen and protein loss, and loss of skeletal muscle mass. The activity level of a homebound cardiac patient may be further curtailed by signs and symptoms of overexertion, such as shortness of breath or chest pain, by anxiety and misunderstanding, or by another complicating diagnosis such as diabetes, arthritis, or chronic pulmonary disease.

In general, a patient should be encouraged to get as much exercise as can be tolerated. Physical activity assists in overcoming the deconditioning effects of immobility, increases aerobic capacity, contributes to the relief of anxiety and depression, and helps improve self-esteem and body image.[49]

Initial assessment of activity tolerance focuses on the ability to perform normal activities of daily living without distress. Other activities such as climbing stairs or talking on the telephone contribute to daily well-being. Blood pressure and pulse may be monitored before and after exercise to determine tolerance levels. A decrease in blood pressure by more than 20 mm Hg, increase of pulse rate by more than 20% of the resting rate or a rate above 120 beats/min, and the development of chest pain are indications that the activity level should be decreased.

In general, activity levels should be increased gradually, according to the individual's diagnosis and potential for cardiac rehabilitation. If the patient is not participating in a cardiac rehabilitation program, the plan of treatment should include specific guidelines for home care in regard to pulse limits, specific activities, and precautions.

The patient should plan for periods of rest and relaxation between activities. For severely ill and debilitated patients, this may necessitate pacing activities of daily living. Patients should know how to assess their own level of fatigue. Isotonic exercises, such as lifting, and activities that involve holding the arms over the head for a long time, such as curling hair, should be avoided. Quiet leisure activities such as watching TV, listening to music, working at a computer, or reading should be encouraged. As tolerance for activity increases, gradually increasing distances while walking may be advisable. Patients should be cautioned to avoid extremes of temperatures, such as walking outside in very hot or cold weather.[41,49]

Sexual Activity

Men and women with cardiac disease are prone to sexual dysfunction. Problems such as decreased libido, impotence, or orgasmic dysfunction may be caused by medications, organic problems, anxiety, depression, or poor self-esteem. These problems may be exacerbated for patients who have had cardiac crises such as myocardial infarctions or bypass surgery because of lack of knowledge and because of the reluctance of health care professionals to deal with this issue.

Cardiac patients may have a variety of fears: death during sexual intercourse, inadequate sexual performance, another infarction caused by sexual activity, and diminished sexual ability caused by illness and aging. They may fear that medical advice prohibits sexual activity. These fears may become heightened when information about sexuality is omitted from extensive patient teaching protocols. Yet few patients are sufficiently comfortable to approach the physician or nurse with these concerns.

Some drugs frequently prescribed for cardiac patients have side effects that interfere with sexual functioning. The likelihood of such problems varies among individuals and depends on factors such as dosage of the drug, possible interactions with other drugs or foods, the weight of the patient, rates of absorption and excretion, and compliance with the medication regimen. The most common drugs causing sexual problems are the antihypertensives. The thiazide diuretics, spironolactone, methyldopa, guanethidine, and furosemide have been associated with impotence, diminished libido, impaired arousal, and retarded ejaculation.[49] Although most of the available information on sexual side-effects of drugs comes from studies of men, similar problems have been reported in women.

Previous sexual patterns should be taken into consideration when advising cardiac patients about return to sexual activity. This requires an ongoing professional relationship with the patient, good rapport and trust, and a nonjudgmental attitude. It should be noted that although sexual response may be slower with advancing age, there is no physiologic cause for sexual activity to stop because of age.

The sexual partner is likely to have many of the same fears as the cardiac patient, and the partner may try to avoid sexual activities to protect the patient. It may help therefore to include the patient's partner when providing information about return to sexual functioning.

Coitus with the usual partner is physiologically equivalent to activities such as a brisk walk or climbing a flight of stairs. It has been equated to 5 metabolic equivalents (METs) of work on an exercise stress test. Advice to patients should be based on consultation with the physician. Generally, patients who can sustain heart rates of 110 to 120 beats/min with no shortness of breath or anginal pain may resume sexual activity. This is most likely to include patients who have had myocardial infarctions or cardiac surgery whose recoveries are not complicated by cardiac failure or dysrhythmias.

Patients should be advised to resume sexual activity gradually and only after activities such as walking moderate distances or climbing stairs can be done comfortably. Sexual activity causes the least amount of stress when it occurs in familiar surroundings with the usual partner. Gradual foreplay helps the heart prepare for coitus. The patient should assume comfortable positions during sexual activity and avoid positions that cause isometric muscle contractions. Activity should be slowed or stopped if chest pain or shortness of breath occurs. Sexual activity should be avoided soon after eating because food intake diverts blood flow to the gastrointestinal organs. Likewise, alcohol, which decreases cardiac output, should be avoided. The cardiac patient and sexual partner should be encouraged to communicate their feelings about sex openly and frankly with each other. Such candid sharing helps to avoid misunderstandings and false impressions that frequently occur under these circumstances.[49]

Psychosocial Considerations

Some families have a tendency to overprotect their ill member. Although all family members are prone to this behavior, it is frequently seen in wives of cardiac patients. These families become overindulgent in providing care, making decisions without involving the patient, and become overly cautious in their efforts to limit the patient's behavior. Acting out of fear and anxiety, such families become overbearing and are a hindrance to the patient's sense of self-control. Some patients may rebel against this treatment, behave recklessly, and take unnecessary chances to regain a sense of control over their lives. Others may become more dependent than their condition warrants and succumb to a sense of hopelessness.

Loss of personal control and a sense of powerlessness result from the disabling effects of the aging process and chronic illness. The perception of control over life is critical to self-management of a chronic illness. Control enhances the ability to recover from illness or to maintain well-being and prevent deterioration. Control is the belief that individuals can influence the events in their lives and can manipulate some parts of their environment. Perceived control may enhance the patient's ability to cope with illness and its possible complications. Families should be helped to understand that the patient's sense of control may be augmented by planning personal daily activities, rather than having others plan the day. Daily scheduling, however, may have to revolve around the treatment regimen and can become problematic when the patient depends on a caregiver to perform these activities.[50]

Knowledge and understanding contribute to a sense of control. Patient teaching that provides information about the illness and its symptoms and management can modify the sense of loss of control associated with anxiety about the unknown. Likewise, the provision of anticipatory guidance can help the patient and caregiver prepare for unfamiliar situations.

Patients should always be consulted about decisions that relate to their care. Caregivers should be assisted to understand that the patient's ability to cope is directly related to participation in decisions and a resulting sense of control over daily life.

HOME CARE FOR PATIENTS WITH TECHNICALLY COMPLEX NEEDS

In no other area are the changes in health care more obvious than in the complex and sophisticated field of medical technology that has been introduced into home health care. Recent advances in cardiac treatment have put special demands on home health nurses to develop advanced practice expertise to manage complex and high-tech interventions in the home and to educate patients and caregivers to handle complicated therapeutic regimens.

Pacemakers

A permanent artificial pacemaker may be inserted for patients who have permanent dysfunction of the cardiac conduction system that cannot be controlled by drugs. This heart block may be secondary to myocardial infarction, surgery, or trauma. Patients with rhythm disturbances such as severe bradycardia, sick sinus syndrome, or attacks of Stokes-Adams disease may also be candidates for pacemaker insertion to maintain normal rate and adequate cardiac output.

Pacemaker insertion is a surgical procedure that takes place in a hospital or 1-day surgery center. Although patient education begins at that time, anxiety, problems in communication, or hearing deficits may limit patient understanding about pacemaker function and care. Education is thus a major priority for home care after pacemaker insertion, and it begins with assessment of patient and family levels of anxiety and understanding.

The patient probably returns home from the hospital without a dressing on the suture line. The area should be checked by the home health nurse for redness, drainage, or pain, which indicate infection of the incision or the subcutaneous pocket. The patient should be assessed for symptoms that occurred before insertion of the pacemaker (for example, chest pain, dyspnea, dizziness, and edematous ankles).

The patient should be aware that electrical stimulation from the pacemaker may result in cardiac, skeletal, or diaphragmatic contraction. For example, pectoral or rectus abdominis muscle groups may be stimulated. This can be corrected by lowering the pacing threshold while maintaining cardiac capture. Diaphragmatic stimulation resulting in phrenic nerve contraction and hiccoughs may occur if the heart wall is thin. This problem usually resolves over time as fibrous tissue forms over the electrode tip. Diaphragmatic stimulation can also result from myocardial perforation or from cardiac tamponade—a life-threatening situation resulting in failure to capture.[51]

Although some patients go home the day of surgery with little or no restriction of activity, others may have bedrest prescribed for a period after pacemaker insertion to avoid electrode dislodgement. After that time, fibrosis begins to secure the electrode to the endocardium. Incision discomfort, if present, is mild, and acetaminophen is likely to provide sufficient relief. Vigorous motion, especially of the arms, should be avoided for 6 weeks to prevent displacement of the electrode. After 6 weeks, all normal activity, including sexual activity, may be resumed. The patient may swim and engage in sports, but activities that could cause chest trauma (for example, contact sports) should be avoided.

The patient and caregiver must know how to take a resting pulse for 1 full minute each day and to record it if asked to do so. Ideally this should be done seated on the side of the bed before arising each morning. They should know the normal rate of the pacemaker and understand that the pulse may exceed that rate; any pulse rate below that rate may indicate a failing generator and should be reported. It should be noted that pacemakers with a rate hysteresis feature do go below the normal rate. A physician may request that a magnet be placed over the generator while taking a pulse. This puts the pacemaker in a fixed-rate mode so that the pulse rate indicates the pacemaker function. This technique carries a slight risk of triggering ventricular dysrhythmias and should never be done by the patient alone. Battery depletion may be evident if there is a decrease in the basic pacing rate, and a lead fracture may be indicated if there are intermittent periods of pacing alternating with periods of failure to pace. Battery depletion and lead fracture require surgical intervention to be corrected.[51]

Patients who live long distances from the physician or clinic or who have difficulty traveling may have their pacemakers checked via telephone using a special telephone transmitter. The transmitter has wrist electrodes that convert heart impulses to electronic signals that can be transmitted via the telephone. When the pacemaker clinic calls the patient at a prearranged time, the patient puts on the wrist electrodes and turns on the transmitter; the clinic is able to print out a record of the patient's ECG. Many clinics have 24-hour service so that patients can call at any time if they have problems or concerns about the status of their pacemaker function.

Patients with permanent pacemakers should be taught to avoid exposure to electromagnetic fields that could interfere with pacemaker function. For example, malfunctioning engines, power tools and equipment, dental equipment, and inadequately shielded microwave ovens can affect pacemaker function. Some radio frequencies, especially 3.5 and 28.5 megahertz (MHz) used by ham or citizens band radio operators, can cause problems. Generally, well-maintained household appliances are safe. Work and specialized settings should be evaluated on an individualized basis because the degree of risk varies with the type of signal generated by the electric device and the type of artificial pacemaker used. Patients should know that if a device causes symptoms such as fainting or dizziness, they should immediately move away from the source. They should also understand that electronic metal detectors, such as those used in airports and libraries, may be triggered by a pacemaker, but pacemaker function will not be affected.[37] However, handheld metal detectors such as "frisk wands" do contain magnets and should be avoided if possible.

Clinical environments or health care therapies with potential electromagnetic interference with pacemaker functioning include diathermy, electrocautery, diagnostic ultrasound, defibrillation, radiation therapy, positron emission tomography, nuclear magnetic resonance, magnetic resonance imaging, transcutaneous electrical nerve stimulation, acupuncture, lithotripsy, and ultrasonic scalers used in dental offices.[51] Patients must be taught to notify health care providers of their permanent pacemakers before undergoing such therapies so that precautionary measures may be taken.

Home ECG

Home ECG monitoring devices can provide critical information about changes in rhythm or the cardiovascular status of the patient at home. Devices such as wrist ECG monitors have been successfully used to monitor the status of ambulatory patients. Lightweight, 12-lead ECG machines may be used in the home to provide additional information.[2] Small, computerized devices that can be carried by a patient and used to register cardiac episodes have been tested. The average delay in starting a recording, however, makes these devices of limited use for short cardiac episodes. The practical use of these devices may be limited to verifying functional cardiac disorders or in cooperative patients having dysrhythmic episodes that occur infrequently and last at least 1 minute.[52] Researchers continue to search for solutions for physiologic monitoring in daily life settings. Attempted solutions include automatic ECG monitoring using electrodes installed inside the wall of a bathtub or a toilet set.[53]

A Holter monitor may be worn at home for 12 to 24 hours to record an ambulatory ECG while the patient engages in normal daily activities. Such recording is helpful in detecting and documenting intermittent dysrhythmias or those that occur only during certain daily activities.

The home health nurse should explain to the patient and family the reasons for the procedure, answer questions, and help reduce anxiety about the equipment. The patient, or if necessary the caregiver, should keep a log of all activities and events that occur while the monitor is in place and any symptoms or sensations that arise. The patient should be encouraged to perform normal daily activities, except for showering. The recorder should be protected from water and should not be dropped. Electrodes that come loose should be reapplied and taped in place. It is important to confirm that the patient understands where to go to have the monitor removed at the designated time.[37]

Supplemental Oxygen

Patients with chronic hypoxemia may require administration of oxygen at home. Typically these patients suffer from inadequate cardiac output, chronic obstructive pulmonary disease, or both. Many home health patients suffer from a combination of cardiac and respiratory problems. Oxygen is available for use in cylinders, oxygen concentrators, and liquid oxygen systems. Home oxygen use requires a physician's prescription.

Oxygen cylinders are the most common mode of home oxygen use. These stationary tanks weigh about 150 pounds and are 5 feet high. A gauge indicates the amount of oxygen remaining in the tank. Such a cylinder, used at a flow rate of 2 L/min, lasts about 50 hours.

Oxygen concentrators, available in floor or tabletop models, concentrate oxygen that is removed from the room air. This is the most expensive mode of delivery unless the patient requires large amounts of oxygen. The rental and use of this system equals the cost of about 8 to 10 cylinders per month. If an oxygen concentrator is used, an oxygen cylinder should be kept at hand in case of a power failure.

Mobile patients may have a liquid oxygen system. Large, stationary units weighing about 70 pounds store oxygen under pressure as a liquid. Smaller, portable canisters can be refilled from these home units. The portable unit lasts up to 16 hours and may be carried with the patient away from home.

Oxygen is usually administered via nasal cannula rather than a mask because it does not have to be removed for the patient to eat or drink. Generally hypoxemia resulting from cardiac insufficiency is relieved by oxygen at 1 to 2 L/min by nasal cannula. A cannula delivers oxygen at a concentration of approximately 24% to 44%. A humidifier should always be attached to the tank to moisturize the dry oxygen gas.

Because of the costs resulting from wasteful inefficiency of continuous flow of conventional oxygen delivery, several oxygen-conserving devices have been developed. The transtracheal oxygen catheter, for example, can provide an average of 55% reduction of oxygen flow. This device requires a minor surgical procedure to create a minitracheostomy site for the insertion of a small-bore oxygen catheter. This provides a larger anatomic reservoir and thereby reduces dead space and expiratory loss of oxygen. In addition, it eliminates nasal irritation caused by a nasal cannula and is less conspicuous.[54] Patients and family must be able to care for the minitracheostomy site and the catheter and assess for possible complications of mucous plugging, subcutaneous emphysema, cellulitus, catheter malplacement, and hemoptysis.

Other oxygen-conserving devices such as the reservoir nasal cannula and pendant reservoir cannula work by storing oxygen during expiration and delivering a bolus during early inspiration. While reducing oxygen flow 35% to 75%, these devices may reduce patient adherence because of their bulky mustache appearance. A more popular oxygen-conserving device is the demand valve, which is noninvasive and relatively inconspicuous. This device can reduce oxygen flow by 55% to 88% by restricting delivery to inspiration.[54] Initial costs for oxygen-conserving devices are greater than for traditional delivery systems and may not be reimbursed; however, the long-term savings may justify their use.

Assessment of the patient requiring home oxygen should include a cardiovascular and respiratory history, with attention to smoking and environmental irritants. Arterial blood gas levels should be evaluated before oxygen therapy is begun. It is important that the family and patient understand that the oxygen should be used only as directed and that the use of more may be harmful.

Periodic assessment by the home health nurse should include respiratory status; the nurse should look for signs of dyspnea and tachycardia and indications of hypoxia such as dizziness, restlessness, or confusion. The nasal mucosa should be checked for irritation from the nasal prongs. Signs of oxygen toxicity may be similar to those of hypoxia. Ongoing monitoring of blood gas levels is indicated to evaluate the course of the disease, to assess any change of clinical status that may be related to the cardiopulmonary system, and to facilitate changes in the oxygen prescription. If oxygen saturation is monitored by pulse oximetry, concurrent values must be documented and reconciled with the results of the baseline blood analysis before reliance on the pulse oximeter analysis.[55]

Safety teaching must be a high priority for home care when oxygen is in use. The oxygen should be stored and used at least 10 feet away from open flames, such as gas stoves, heaters, or wood burners. No one should smoke within 10 feet of the equipment. Electric equipment used near the oxygen system should be grounded with a three-pronged plug. Electric appliances such as razors and hair dryers should not be used near the oxygen. Clothing or night clothes made of nylon and wool blankets should not be used to avoid sparks from static electricity. Aerosols should not be used in the area.

Home care for a patient using oxygen is likely to require some financial counseling for the patient and family. It must be determined if and how much of the cost of the oxygen and equipment will be paid by a third-party payer such as Medicare. The cost of the different types of equipment should be compared, and the options of renting or purchasing the equipment should be considered. In addition, the home must have adequate storage space. Oxygen cylinders require storage away from heat, sunlight, and flammable materials. Liquid oxygen should be stored in a well-ventilated area because small amounts are likely to escape.

Family members must be taught to use and maintain the equipment and to safely store the oxygen. In addition, they must know how and when to reorder oxygen cylinders.[37]

Intravenous Therapy

Significant improvements in biomedical, nursing, and pharmacologic care have greatly increased survival rates after a cardiac event; however, survivors frequently depend on some form of long-term pharmacologic or technologic therapy. The chronically ill cardiac patient is likely to need many medications. Oral diuretics, vasodilators, and glycosides are the traditional treatments of choice for the home patient with congestive heart failure. Despite use of these therapies, patients are prone to develop symptoms that require hospital admission for intravenous administration of diuretics, inotropes, angiotensin-converting enzyme (ACE) inhibitors, and vasodilators. Until recently, the accepted standard of care for patients receiving intravenous inotropic or vasoactive therapy has been admission into a critical care unit for close cardiac monitoring.[56] The cycle of exacerbation, hospitalization, treatment, stabilization, and discharge is often repetitive and short in duration.

Efforts to contain rising costs for in-hospital acute care and improvements in infusion devices and intravenous catheter technology have resulted in a significant expansion in the types and number of infusion therapies delivered by home care providers.[57] Advances in these services have made possible home delivery of total parenteral nutrition, antibiotic and antiinfective therapy, chemotherapy, intravenous and intraspinal pain medication administration, and blood product administration.[57,58]

Improvements in home infusion services for patients with chronic cardiac conditions have led to the home use of such high-tech drugs as dopamine,[59] dobutamine,[59-62,64,65] nitroglycerin,[59,63] and amrinone.[56,59] The use of these therapies has allowed chronically ill individuals who are severely compromised to return to their homes, families, and lives. Although many of these individuals return to the comforts of home for an optimal death experience, others return home to await heart transplantation. Still others may need these therapies only intermittently during periods of exacerbation. Regardless of the prognosis, high-tech home care delivers cost-effective quality care while improving the quality of life for individuals and families.[64]

Although it is not a widespread practice, the home use of intravenous inotropic and vasoactive medications is becoming more prevalent and is an attractive, cost-effective alternative for selected patients with chronic cardiac conditions. Safety is the primary concern for the use of such therapy at home.[58] Treatment should be implemented within a structured home health care program that has established standards and protocols for discharge planning from acute care to home care, client admission criteria, delivery of care, and client and caregiver education.

Intravenous inotropic and vasoactive therapy is initiated in the acute care setting, where the patient's condition is monitored for the effect of the therapy and is stabilized. If weaning from the drug is impossible and the patient's condition is otherwise stable, home care arrangements may be made for long-term pharmacologic support. Collaborative efforts of the home health care service with the cardiovascular advanced practice nurse, the primary nurse, the social worker, and the cardiologist are necessary to facilitate the extensive discharge planning for this special need.[56] Issues that must be addressed before delivery of home intravenous therapy include patient selection, intravenous therapy needs, service options for provision of needed therapy, type of infusion device, type and site of venous access for delivery of therapy, identification of the caregiver and caregiver limitations, access to health care for emergency backup, storage of medications and solutions, psychosocial needs, and education.[58]

Inotropic therapy in the home using dopamine, dobutamine, and amrinone enhances cardiac contractility and output in an effort to prevent exacerbation of symptoms that would necessitate hospital admission. The goal of inotropic therapy at home is to use the smallest dose possible to relieve symptoms. The dosages are individualized based on body surface area and titrated to achieve the desired effect (relief of symptoms) within limits. Patients are weighed daily and dosages recalculated if there is a 5-pound weight gain or loss. Dopamine therapy in home care is typically restricted to doses producing dopaminergic and β-receptor stimulation (2 to 5 mcg/kg/min) that cause renal vasodilatation and increased cardiac contractility. Dopamine doses that produce α-receptor stimulation (10 mcg/kg/min or more) and cause peripheral vasoconstriction are avoided. Dobutamine and amrinone, although not dose specific in their effects, are maintained at the lowest possible dose.

The home health care nurse evaluates hemodynamic stability noninvasively through assessment of blood pressure, pulse pressure, heart sounds, jugular venous distention, breath sounds, peripheral edema, skin color, level of consciousness, and toleration of activities of daily living. Changes in cardiac function are reported to the collaborating cardiologist for appropriate alterations of the medication regimen. Weekly blood tests determine blood urea nitrogen, creatinine, and electrolyte levels.[62]

Nitrate therapy used for the treatment of angina on an outpatient basis is typically achieved through sublingual tablets, buccal spray, or topical patches. Occasionally, such attempts to relieve symptoms are unsuccessful and necessitate intravenous administration of nitroglycerin in the hospital. Patients with refractory unstable angina are therefore frequently seen in the emergency room. Such patients as well as patients suffering from nocturnal angina may benefit from intermittent intravenous home infusion of nitroglycerin.[59,63] Since tolerance and dependence on nitrate therapy may occur, an intermittent approach to therapy is recommended so that nitrate-free periods can take place. Often such home infusions are administered only at night. Although it is well tolerated by most patients, intravenous nitroglycerin may cause reversible yet significant hypotension as well as bradycardia, postural syncope, and headache. Accordingly, proper administration of nitroglycerin must include dosage control and monitoring of blood pressure and heart rate. Dosages are individualized and based on blood pressure tolerance and relief and prevention of symptoms. Because plastic fluid bags and tubing absorb nitroglycerin, glass bottles and polyvinyl chloride tubing is required.

Home inotropic therapy is accomplished through an implanted ventral venous access port, a tunneled central venous line (Hickman catheter), or a peripherally inserted central catheter placed before discharge from the acute care setting.[57] Hickman catheters offer the advantages of not needing to be changed and having a low potential for infection. In addition, a double-lumen Hickman catheter allows a second port for drawing blood specimens and administering additional medications.[61] Nitroglycerin therapy does not require central venous access and thus may be provided through peripheral sites. Inotropic and vasoactive intravenous therapies require the use of an infusion pump to regulate flow. Some patients require continuous therapy, whereas others do not because their symptoms may be successfully managed by alternating a specified time on the therapy with a specified time off the therapy (for example, 2 hours on, 3 hours off).[62] For such scheduled regimens, the home infusion pumps are preprogrammed with the dosage and an infusion schedule.[57] Programmable, portable infusion pumps make home infusion therapy manageable and convenient for the patient and family, but the high cost of infusion pumps and supplies are a major barrier for many potential home care recipients.[64]

The level of treatment that can be delivered at home depends on the patient's ability and motivation, the accessibility of family support and their capability of involvement, and the availability of the professional home health team (mutually determined by collaborative team and patient and family agreement). The education of the professional home health nurse must include the knowledge and skill required for the safe, competent, and effective delivery of such high-tech infusion therapy. Equally important is the education of the patient and caregivers. When adequate support systems are in place, the patient and caregiver can usually become independent in the overall administration of the therapeutic regimen.[57]

Education of the patient and caregiver should begin before discharge from the acute care setting. Effective patient education may even result in predischarge mastery of tasks such as pump programming and troubleshooting, assembly of tubing, and mixing of medications and solutions. Frequently, however, patients are discharged with little knowledge of the technical aspects of the therapy and must rely heavily on the professional home health nurse until necessary knowledge is acquired and the responsibilities can be assumed by the patient or caregiver. Regardless of where and when learning takes place, the patient and caregiver must know the rationale for the therapy, the desired effects and side effects and assessment thereof, programming and troubleshooting of the infusion pump, assembly of the infusion tubing, dosages of medications, mixing of the infusion, adjustment of infusion rate relative to weight change, and care and management of the venous access site. Needed skills can be taught and evaluated through demonstration and return demonstration of these skills.

Once the patient and caregivers assume patient care responsibilities, the home health nurse may decrease the length and number of home visits. However, the nurse is available at any time to assist the patient and caregiver, who must be knowledgeable in the plans for follow-up care and emergency support arrangements.

The most common problem associated with home inotropic therapy is infection of the venous access site, which is treated with antibiotics administered orally.[62] Since inotrope therapy is administered only through a central venous port, the risk of infiltration associated with short, peripherally placed catheters is negligible. Examples of patient- and family-reported problems that may occur include pump problems, patient or caregiver lack of knowledge, nonavailability of supplies, caregiver anxiety, and problems with reimbursement.[58]

Because increasing numbers of patients are discharged from the acute care setting with intravenous therapy, arrangements for home therapy with inotropic and vasoactive medications must be made on an individual basis and under close scrutiny.[58] Safety is the primary concern for such high-tech care, and a structured program must be implemented to ensure comprehensive care to meet the special needs of these patients.

Implantable Cardioverter Defibrillators

Implantable cardioverter defibrillators (ICDs) are surgically placed pulse generators capable of recognizing and treating life-threatening ventricular dysrhythmias by countershocking the heart. Patients with ICDs have special needs on returning into the community. The patient with an ICD has extensive education before discharge; however, reinforcement and additional education are needed once the patient is at home. Initial education includes detection and prevention of infection of the operative site. Ongoing education addresses actions to take when the device discharges, follow-up and emergency care, activity guidelines, and avoidance of magnets and electromagnetic interference.

Patients may be instructed to notify the cardiologist or electrophysiologist each time their hearts are cardioverted/defibrillated. Frequent shocks over a short period may necessitate a visit to their physician or hospitalization. Frequent inappropriate shocks may indicate a need to reprogram the ICD. Frequent appropriate shocks may indicate the need to change or add antidysrhythmic medications or treat an underlying chemical or metabolic disorder.[66] Patients and families are instructed to seek emergency medical care any time that symptoms are unrelieved by cardioversion/defibrillation. Symptoms necessitating medical attention include palpitations, tachycardia, shortness of breath, chest pain, or syncope.

Patients should carry identification cards and wear identification tags and bracelets that identify them as patients with ICDs. Patients and families are also encouraged to carry instruction sheets, including phone numbers of the cardiologist or electrophysiologist, when traveling or seeking emergency medical care. Families are informed that the device is of secondary consequence in the event that cardiopulmonary resuscitation or external cardioversion is required.

Activity guidelines for the patient with an ICD may include restriction from driving, a limitation that for some patients can cause significant stress related to loss of control and independence.[65] Resumption of activities of daily living, including sexual intercourse, should be encouraged as soon as the patient feels ready. Patients should be told that a shock during sexual intercourse is rare but possible if the heart rate exceeds the programmed cutoff rate and other programmed detection criteria are met. The subsequent shock, however, will not harm their partner. Similarly, if the patient's heart rate during normal exercise exceeds the programmed rate and other detection criteria, they may receive a shock. Therefore the patient should know the ICD cutoff rate, ways to monitor the heart rate during exercise, ways to pace exercise to target heart rate, and information needed to notify the physician if such instances of cardioversion/defibrillation occur during exercise. The ICD cutoff rate for cardioversion/defibrillation may merely need to be increased or other programmed parameters adjusted. Diagnostic tests may be needed to distinguish between sinus tachycardia during exercise and a tachydysrhythmia. The patient should be encouraged to resume all tolerated physical activities with the exception of rough physical contact sports.[66]

Magnets are used in the clinical setting to activate, deactivate, and test the ICD. A potential danger for some patients is that of environmental exposure to magnetic fields that could inadvertently deactivate the device without the patients' knowledge or cause premature depletion of the batteries.[66] Patients may need to be taught the significance of avoiding magnets and magnetic fields and be alerted to concerns regarding certain medical procedures. For example, magnetic resonance imaging is sometimes contraindicated, and with some devices electrocautery can be performed only after the ICD is deactivated. Appliances and devices that should be avoided are the same as for the permanent pacemaker.

The physiologic aspects of care for patients and their families, although significant, are dwarfed when compared with their psychosocial and emotional needs. Issues that may be of special concern include the recurrence of a sustained tachycardic event and the associated syncope, apprehension about the possibility of cardioversion and anxiety about the sensation of being shocked, worry about whether the device will work when needed, and fear of sudden death.[65,66] Other causes of anxiety include concern about clothes not fitting, fear of changes in mental functioning (primarily loss of memory), overprotectiveness of the significant other, sleep disturbances, eating problems, and a sense of loss of control.[65,67] The primary psychosocial concerns of the significant others of patients with ICDs are fear of death, preparation for death, family and role changes, overprotectiveness, and fear if the patient is driving.[65] Although most concerns diminish over time,[65,67] these patients and families need education, social support, and enhancement of effective coping strategies.

Ventricular Assist Devices

Increased technology in the area of mechanical circulatory support, coupled with the shortage of donor hearts, has created a population of patients who are being bridged to transplant with implanted ventricular assist devices (VADs). The duration of this bridge has been documented to be as long as 233 days,[68] and thus the focus of care has shifted from acute to chronic support of patients on VADs. Although most of these patients remain in the hospital until transplantation, there have been attempts to place some individuals in "out-of-hospital facilities" or "homelike but safe" outpatient settings, usually apartment-like facilities close to the hospital that provide varying degrees of medical and engineering support.[69,70] Such attempts improve patient perceptions of physical functioning, increase affect and life satisfaction, improve mood, decrease depression and anxiety, increase the patient's confidence in personal capabilities, and increase physical activities.[70] Although this living arrangement is likely to cause the patients' caregivers to feel a sense of increased burden and responsibility, both patients and caregivers have reported experiencing a deepening of the quality of their relationship.[70] Thus chronic care of the patient in an outpatient setting may improve quality of life, empower the patient and family to regain some sense of control, and dramatically limit the cost of care during the sometimes lengthy bridge to transplantation.

Education for the chronic use of VAD begins when the patient is identified as a transplant candidate, continues through the preoperative and postoperative phases of implantation of the VAD, and extends throughout the entire bridge experience. The extensive educational needs of patients and families must be met in the acute phase of care if a patient is to be discharged to an outpatient setting for chronic care. Patients and families must become competent in using the VAD console, monitoring battery time and changing of batteries, preventing stress on the driveline and kinking of the tubing, performing sterile dressing changes at the driveline exit site, implementing the physical rehabilitation protocol, monitoring vital signs, monitoring for complications, and appropriately using medications (anticoagulants, antiplatelets, and gut decontaminants, in addition to any other medications needed such as diuretics, antidysrhythmics, and antihypertensives).[69] Effective use of emergency procedures, including backup from nursing, biomedical engineering, and emergency medical personnel, must be understood.

The psychosocial and emotional concerns of these patients and families are likely to include fear of death, stress related to a chronic illness, loss of control over shortages of donor organs, fear of the unknown related to use of the VAD, fear of complications, concerns about facing a lifetime of dependency on the medical community, financial concerns, loss of role in family, loss of career, and social isolation. Although some of these concerns may be alleviated through discharge to an outpatient setting, these issues should be addressed through education, ongoing counseling and support, referral to psychologic and religious experts, and involvement in social support groups of patients awaiting cardiac transplantation and transplant recipients.

Although the number of patients returning to the community is limited and the care of these patients is well structured and controlled by the transplant center, the discharge of patients demonstrates the emergence of high-tech capabilities into home care. The potential for greater numbers of patients needing such highly technologic home care is high with continued advances in research and development, coupled with financial constraints on in-patient care. This heightened level of care places great importance on safety and requires a structured home program incorporating case management, collaborative networks, discharge planning and education, admission criteria, established standards and protocols, financial support, and research.

DYING AT HOME

In recent years, there has been a trend among dying patients to prefer to spend their final days (or months) at home. This trend parallels other changes that have occurred in the health care system. Hospitals today have become oriented toward more intensive care of the critically ill, and for many patients this high-tech environment is no longer warranted. For many chronically ill or dying patients, palliative care is the best that can be offered. These patients need comfort, communication, and competent caregivers. Often this kind of care can best be provided at home, where the patient can experience a comfortable life for as long as possible. When death is inevitable, it can occur in familiar surroundings with the support of family and friends.[4]

The trend has occurred in the context of major changes in the way that health care is funded. Dying at home, especially when the illness is long term, is a more economically feasible alternative than hospitalization.[71] The hospice movement has provided momentum to this trend, and Medicare now provides benefits for hospice care.

The hospice movement in the United States is grounded on the work of Dame Cicely Saunders, the English nurse and physician who founded St. Christopher's Hospice in London in 1968. Hospice is a concept that aims to provide palliative, symptomatic care rather than aggressive treatment. The goal is to relieve pain and keep the patient comfortable and conscious. Care might be provided in the patient's home or in a hospice; in either case, the atmosphere is relaxed and homelike.[72] Care is provided by a team of professionals and volunteers who address the needs of the patient and family for physical caring and emotional, spiritual, social, and financial assistance.

Because of the manner in which hospice care is funded, the majority of patients who participate in the program are cancer patients. To be eligible for reimbursement for hospice care, the patient must have a prognosis of death within less than 6 months. Although such a prognosis is possible for many cancer patients, the course of cardiac disease is usually less predictable. Thus although more people die of cardiac disease than any other cause, death is more likely to be sudden and unplanned, and few cardiac patients participate in a hospice program.

The unexpectedness of cardiac death frequently places a family in a sudden crisis for which they are not prepared. The family facing the potential or actual loss of a member experiences the grief process before they can reach a renewed equilibrium. Grief is the intense emotional suffering that a person feels as a result of being deprived of something that is valued. This may be the loss of a significant person, a valued object, or a part of oneself, or it may be a developmental loss. Engle[73] described three stages of grief and mourning that a family is likely to experience: shock and disbelief, awareness of the loss, and restitution.

When a loss occurs, especially if it is unanticipated, family members are likely to be stunned and disorganized. Emotions may be paralyzed, and people may feel out of contact with reality as they make necessary arrangements. Soon the loss becomes real, and each person in his or her own way feels anguish, pain, anger, and denial. People may feel varying degrees of helplessness and hopelessness. If family members blame themselves for the death of a loved one, they may feel guilty; others may direct anger at health care providers for not saving the patient. Finally, restitution begins, and families begin to accept the reality of their loss and learn new ways of coping. Ultimately family equilibrium is restored as other family members take over the roles formerly belonging to the deceased member.

When life-threatening situations provide time, family members may prepare for the loss of a member. When facing a potential loss, people experience anticipatory grief. In this circumstance, the loss may be rehearsed in fantasy many times. This process may sometimes help people deal with the loss when it occurs.[33]

Patients who realize that they are approaching their own death also experience the grief process. Kübler-Ross[74] identified five stages of grief likely to be experienced by a patient: denial and isolation, anger, bargaining, depression, and acceptance.

When death seems inevitable, it may be appropriate to provide anticipatory guidance for the patient and family. In addition, the caregiver should be given phone numbers and instructions for handling an emergency. The home care team should be aware of local regulations regarding the handling of a home death. This information can be obtained from the local police department or from the medical examiner's office.

If death occurs during a home visit, rescue procedures should be initiated, according to policy. The physician should be notified. The health care providers should stay with the family until the body has been removed, providing support, offering assistance in contacting the funeral director, and assisting and supporting the family while the body is removed.[75]

The family's religious orientation should be accepted and supported. Some religions require ritual acts associated with the death process. These rituals include special rites or anointing of the sick, or they may require special washing and handling of the body after death. These requirements should be known and the wishes of the family respected.[72]

RESEARCH NEEDS

Home care presents researchers with many challenges. Home health research generally aims to find improved ways to ensure cost-effective delivery of high-quality health care. Research needs fall into three areas: quality of care, financing, and technology.

As the health care system continues to change, more agencies are being established to meet the needs for illness care at home, and more people will depend on this mode of health care delivery. It is estimated that 4 million Americans, most of whom are older, require assistance in performing activities of daily living.[76] At the same time, there is an emphasis on the use of complex technology in the home. As this trend evolves, quality-assurance systems are needed to promote the delivery of safe, high-quality care for all patients. Such systems must focus on the delivery of safe, competent, and sophisticated care for the acutely ill patient, as well as on the delivery of appropriate and compassionate care for the chronically ill or older patient.

Studies are needed to establish the most effective treatment protocols for home care of patients with specific cardiac diagnoses and to assess the outcome potential for subgroups. Research questions address tracking patients over time to better understand the trajectory of illness; measuring need, predictors, and demand for home care; and developing tools for assessing needs and monitoring care.[77] Norms are needed as bases for decision making for older patients with advanced disease who need supportive care or who can be rehabilitated. Likewise, for younger patients, criteria are needed regarding the most appropriate type and amount of home care to maximize the potential for long-range positive outcomes. Studies that examine ways to enhance the potential for self-care are needed. Examination of patterns of referral can contribute to determination of the most effective site of care at various levels of illness.

The financing of care is a critical issue in the health care system and health care reform is evolving. Regulations governing reimbursement are restrictive, and they limit the type and amount of care that people receive. The government is faced with the quandary of how to reconcile budget constraints, lower taxes, and decrease government spending with public demands for health care and increasing health care costs.[6] The health care system is faced with the challenge of finding ways to provide the best care for the least cost. Some of these issues present ethical questions that cannot be directly answered by research. For example, what portion of the burden of the cost of care should fall on the consumer, and what portion should be borne by the government? On the other hand, research must provide information that forms the context in which these decisions are made. Studies are needed to find the most cost-effective means of providing care for patients with common diagnoses. The outcomes of care and long-range consequences must be evaluated. For example, at what point in the course of an illness can patients be discharged from a service without increasing their chances of relapse and readmission? What are the most effective referral patterns? Finally, studies are needed to determine the most effective models for interagency and interdisciplinary cooperation to ensure continuity of services without duplication.

As technologic advances enhance the ability of hospitals to manage serious illnesses, research must find ways to adapt these technologies for home use. Sophisticated technology used in the home must be cost effective and must be designed simply enough to be managed by families and nonprofessional caregivers. Studies that address how to efficiently provide equipment for home use and how to effectively train home care users are needed. Special attention should be given to providing safe, compassionate, and humane care in the home while maintaining cost-effective services and appropriate use of technologic advances.

REFERENCES

1. Vidaver VS: A position for home care, *Caring* 12(6):5, 1993.
2. Lenane J: High-tech cardiac home care, *Caring* 13(2):29, 1994.
3. Keating SB, Kelman GB: *Home health care nursing: concepts and practice,* Philadelphia, 1988, Lippincott.
4. Lancaster J: *History of community health and community health nursing.* In Stanhope M, Lancaster J, editors: *Community health nursing: process and practice for promoting health,* St Louis, 1988, Mosby.
5. Report to Congress: *Impact of the Medicare hospital prospective payment system,* Washington DC, 1986 Annual Report, Health Care Financing Administration.
6. Haddad AM: *High tech home care: a practical guide,* Rockville Md, 1987, Aspen.
7. Garvey E, Logue JH: *The community health nurse in home health and hospice care.* In Stanhope M, Lancaster J, editors: *Community health nursing: process and practice for promoting health,* St Louis, 1988, Mosby.
8. Home health care: profile, *Am Nurse* 22(2):24, 1990.
9. Home health and hospice care: United States, 1992, *MMWR* 42(42):820, 1993.
10. Anderson K: Is it still home sweet home care? *Business Health* 11(1):42, 1993.
11. Gould DA, Haslanger KD: Home care prospects in an era of health care reform, *J Ambulatory Care Manage* 16(4):9, 1993.
12. Selby TL: Home health care finds new ways of caring: skilled RNs meet patient needs as agencies flourish, *Am Nurse* 22(2):1, 1990.
13. Helbing C and others: Home health agency benefits, *Health Care Financ Rev* Medicare and Medicaid Statistical Supplement:125, 1992.
14. *The Medicare 1994 handbook,* DHHS Health Care Financing Administration, US Publication No HCFA 10050, 1994.
15. Letsch SW and others: National health expenditures, *Health Care Financ Rev* 14(2):1, 1991.
16. Malloy C: *Overview of acute care nursing in the home.* In Malloy C, Hartshorn J, editors: *Acute care nursing in the home: a holistic approach,* Philadelphia, 1989, Lippincott.
17. Currents: survey suggests home care can reduce America's skyrocketing health care costs, *Hosp Health Networks* 67(15):26, 1993.
18. Hanger HC and others: The cost of returning home, *NZ Med J* 106(964):397, 1993.
19. Cafferata GL: Marital status, living arrangements, and the use of health services by elderly persons, *J Gerontol* 42(6):613, 1987.
20. Glick DF: *An analysis of the relationship between utilization of home health services and nursing diagnosis as a measure of patient health problems,* unpublished doctoral dissertation, 1987, The Pennsylvania State University, University Park, Penn.
21. Wilkes E: Dying now, *Lancet* 1(8383):950, 1984.
22. Steffl BM, Eide I: *Discharge planning handbook,* 1981, Charles B Slack.
23. Bower KA: *Case management by nurses,* Kansas City, Mo, 1992, American Nurses Publishing.

24. Zander K: The 1990's: core values, core change, *Frontiers Health Serv Manage* 7(2):28, 1990.

25. Zander K: Nursing case management: strategic management of cost and quality outcomes, *J Nurs Admin* 18(5):23, 1988.

26. *Continuity of care and discharge planning program,* New York, 1975, American Nurses Association.

27. *Guidelines: discharge planning,* Chicago, 1984, American Hospital Association.

28. *Accreditation manual for hospitals,* Chicago, 1983, Joint Commission on the Accreditation of Hospitals.

29. Smith CD: *Discharge planning.* In Malloy C, Hartshorn J, editors: *Acute care nursing in the home: a holistic approach,* Philadelphia, 1989, Lippincott.

30. Mariano C: The case for interdisciplinary collaboration, *Nurs Outlook* 37(6):285, 1989.

31. Harris MD: *Home care.* In Caliandro G, Judkins BL, editors: *Primary nursing practice,* Glenview, Ill, 1988, Scott, Foresman.

32. Hanson SMH: *Family nursing and chronic illness.* In Wright LM, Leahey M, editors: *Families and chronic illness,* Springhouse, Penn, 1987, Springhouse.

33. Bozett FW: *Family nursing and life threatening illness.* In Leahey M, Wright LM, editors: *Families and life-threatening illness,* Springhouse, Penn, 1987, Springhouse.

34. Orem DE: *Nursing concepts of practice,* New York, 1980, McGraw-Hill.

35. Stauss AL, Glasser BG: *Chronic illness and quality of life,* St Louis, 1975, Mosby.

36. Seigel H: Nurses improve hospital efficiency through risk assessment model at admission, *Nurs Manage* 19(10):38, 1988.

37. Walsh J and others: *Manual of home health care nursing,* Philadelphia, 1987, Lippincott.

38. Folden SL: Caring for older homebound adults: a chronic illness perspective, *J Home Health Care Pract* 2(1):57, 1989.

39. Friedman JA: *Home health care,* New York, 1986, Norton.

40. Goldberg PB, Roberts J: Rational drug regimens for the elderly patient, *Med Clin North Am* 67(2):323, 1983.

41. Rovinski CA, Zastocki DK: *Home care: a technical manual for the professional nurse,* Philadelphia, 1989, Saunders.

42. Babitz LE, Kahn ML: *Cardiac disease.* In Bernstein LH and others, editors: *Primary care in the home,* Philadelphia, 1987, Lippincott.

43. McGurn W: *People with cardiac problems: nursing concepts,* Philadelphia, 1981, Lippincott.

44. Thompson K: *Potential nursing diagnoses of the chronic cardiac patient,* unpublished paper, Charlottesville, Va, 1994, University of Virginia.

45. Marrelli TM: *Handbook of home health standards and documentation guidelines for reimbursement,* St Louis, 1988, Mosby.

46. *HCFA Medicare Home Health Agency Manual,* transmittal no. 203, Washington, DC, 1987, Health Care Financing Administration.

47. Carney KL: Heart-smart home care with cardiac clinical specialists, *Caring* 13(2):32, 1994.

48. Gaul AL: *Cardiovascular disease.* In Hogstel MD, editor: *Home nursing care for the elderly,* Bowie, Md, 1985, Brady.

49. Pratt N: *Alterations in circulation.* In Malloy C, Hartshorn J, editors: *Acute care nursing in the home: a holistic approach,* Philadelphia, 1989, Lippincott.

50. Miller JF, Oertel CB: *Powerlessness in the elderly: preventing hopelessness.* In Miller JF, editor: *Coping with chronic illness,* Philadelphia, 1983, Davis.

51. Stewart JV, Sheehan AM: Permanent pacemakers: the nurse's role in patient education and follow-up care, *J Cardiovasc Nurs* 5(3):32, 1991.

52. Fechter P: Advantage of ECG self-recording by the patient, *Schweizerische Medizinische Wochenschrift* 121(41):1488, 1991.

53. Togawa T and others: Physiological monitoring techniques for home health care, *Biomed Sci Instrument* 28:105, 1992.

54. Shigeoka JW: Oxygen-conservers, home oxygen prescriptions, and the role of the respiratory care practitioner, *Respiratory Care* 36(3):178, 1991.

55. AARC clinical practice guideline: oxygen therapy in the home or extended care facility, *Respiratory Care* 37(3):918, 1992.

56. Moore J: Intravenous amrinone therapy at home for the patient with chronic congestive heart failure, *Focus Crit Care* 15(6):32, 1988.

57. Chambers M: Home infusion partners with managed care, *Caring* 12(6):54, 1993.

58. McAbee RR and others: Home intravenous therapy: issues. I. *Home Health Care Serv Q* 12(3):59, 1991.

59. Clark B (personal communication with Brenda Clark, RPh, Home IV Care, Charlottesville, Va, Feb 23, 1994).

60. Gorski LA, Schmidt TB: Home dobutamine therapy, *J Home Health Care Pract* 2(4):11, 1990.

61. Phillips P: Home dobutamine: an alternative for patients awaiting cardiac transplant, *Canadian Nurse* 88(10):13, 1992.

62. Sohl LL, Applefeld MM: A new direction for dobutamine, *Nursing* 20(10):42, 1990.

63. Noble NT, Lewinski JC: Nocturnal angina: home intravenous nitroglycerin therapy, *Cardiovasc Nurs* 25(5):25, 1989.

64. Bruera E: Ambulatory infusion devices in the continuing care of patients with advanced diseases, *J Pain Symptom Manage* 5(5):287, 1990.

65. Sneed NV, Finch N: Experiences of patients and significant others with automatic implantable cardioverter defibrillators after discharge from the hospital, *Prog Cardiovasc Nurs* 7(3):20, 1992.

66. Veseth-Rogers J: A practical approach to teaching the automatic implantable cardioverter-defibrillator patient, *J Cardiovasc Nurs* 4(2):7, 1990.

67. Dunbar S: New research to help people with ICDs cope with life, *AACN News,* August 3, 1993.

68. Abou-Awdi NL: Thermo cardiosystems left ventricular assist device as a bridge to cardiac transplant, *AACN Clin Iss Crit Care Nurs* 2(3):545, 1991.

69. Capretta CJ and others: Nursing management and rehabilitation of chronic ventricular assist device patients, *Prog Cardiovasc Nurs* 7(4):16, 1992.

70. Dew MA and others: Life quality in the era of bridging to cardiac transplantation: bridge patients in an outpatient setting, *ASAIO* 39(2):145, 1993.

71. Lemkin P: The newest treatment in home care, *Caring* 13(2):22, 1994.

72. Miller MC: *Spirituality, beliefs, values and practices.* In Malloy C, Hartshorn J editors: *Acute care nursing in the home: a holistic approach,* Philadelphia, 1989, Lippincott.

73. Engle GL: *Psychological development in health and disease,* Philadelphia, 1962, Saunders.

74. Kübler-Ross E: *On death and dying,* New York, 1969, Macmillan.

75. Stewart R: *Manual of community and home health nursing,* Boston, 1987, Little Brown.

76. *NCHSR home health research,* National Center for Health Services Research program note, Sept 1989.

77. Raphael C, Angelicola M: Research and development: the center for home care policy and research, *Caring,* 12(9):62, 1993.

Index

A

A wave, assessment of, 26
AAI pacemaker, *223*, 228, 228t
AAIR pacemaker, 224, 228t
AAT pacemaker, *223* 228, 228t, 237
Abbokinase; *see* Urokinase
Abdomen, assessment of, 38-39
Aberrant ventricular conduction, 162
Accelerated idioventricular rhythm, 96t-97t, 144-145, *145, 146, 201*
   significance of, 144-145
   treatment of, 145
   and ventricular tachycardia, *202*
Accupril; *see* Quinapril
Accuracy, diagnostic studies and, 42
ACE inhibitors; *see* Angiotensin-converting enzyme inhibitors
Acebutolol, 430t
Aceon; *see* Perindopril
Acetaminophen, 433
Acetazolamide, 437t
Acetylcholine, 7, 416
ACLS; *see* Advanced cardiac life support
Actin, 1
Activase; *see* Alteplase
Activity
   cardiac rehabilitation and, 406-408
   in health history, 18, 19
   home care and, 483-484
   pulseless electrical, *314, 322*
Acupuncture, smoking cessation and, 264
Acute inferior myocardial infarction, dysrhythmias and, *176*
Acute myocardial infarction (AMI), 287-296, *288, 320*
   complications of, 296
   persistent hypotension and, 289
   persistent pain and, 289
   PTCA in treatment of; *see* Percutaneous transluminal coronary angioplasty
   pulmonary edema and, 289
   serious dysrhythmias and, 289
   thrombotic therapy for, *290,* 290-292
   treatment of, 289-296
Acute pulmonary edema, 297, *319*
Acute rejection, cardiac transplantation and, 396, *396,* 396t
Acute renal failure (ARF), 370
Adalat; *see* Nifedipine
Adenocard; *see* Adenosine
Adenosine, 323t, 468
   cardiac transplantation and, 392
   cardiovascular actions of, 468
   cautions and side effects of, 468
   clinical uses of, 468
   dosage and administration of, 468
   stress testing with, 45
Adenosine triphosphate (ATP), 1
Adjustment to illness, 16
Admission note to coronary care unit, *278*
Adrenalin; *see* Epinephrine
α-Adrenergic blockers, 416, *417,* 426-427
   cardiovascular actions of, 426-427
   cautions and side effects of, 427
   clinical uses of, 427
   dosage and administration of, 427
β-Adrenergic blockers, 416-417, 430
   for angina, 287

β-Adrenergic blockers—cont'd.
   for dilated cardiomyopathy, 380
   for hypertrophic cardiomyopathy, 383
β-Adrenoreceptor blockers for angina, 287
Adult respiratory distress syndrome (ARDS), 368, 369-370
Advanced cardiac life support (ACLS), 311, *312*
Afterload, 9, 366-367
Age as risk factor for coronary artery disease, 258
AHA; *see* American Heart Association
Aidcheck, 330
Alarm control system in coronary care unit, 282
Albumin, decreased preload and, 366
Alcohol
   cardiac rehabilitation and, 410-411
   hypertension and, 259-260
   as risk factor for coronary artery disease, 267
Aldactone; *see* Spironolactone
ALG; *see* Antilymphocyte globulin
Alprazolam, 333
Altace; *see* Ramipril
Alteplase, 444t
Ambulatory ECG, *47,* 47-48, *48*
Ambulatory monitoring, 47-48
American Cancer Society, 268
American College of Cardiology, 408
American College of Physicians, 408
American Heart Association (AHA), 256, 268, 310, 318
American Lung Association, 268
American Red Cross, 311, 318, 475
AMI; *see* Acute myocardial infarction
Amiloride, 437t
Amiodarone, 453t, 454t, 459-460
   adult respiratory distress syndrome and, 368
   for AV nodal reentry, 112
   cardiovascular actions of, 459-460
   cautions and side effects of, 460
   clinical uses of, 460
   dosage and administration of, 460
   for premature ventricular complexes, 138
   Qtc interval and, 65
   for ventricular tachycardia, 141
Amlodipine, 441t, 443
Amplitude
   electrocardiography and, 64
   of pulse, 22
Amrinone, 299, 323t, 421t
Anacrotic notch, 22
Anatrial tachydysrhythmia, *190*
Angina, 286-287, 483
   atypical, *181, 213*
   crescendo, 286
   diagnosis of, 286-287
   exertional, 286
   preinfarction, 286
   Prinzmetal, *181, 213,* 286
   progressive, 286
   stable, 257, 286
   treatment of, 287
   unstable, 286
   variant, 258, 286
Angiography, cardiac, *55,* 55-56
Angioplasty
   percutaneous transluminal coronary; *see* Percutaneous transluminal coronary angioplasty
   unstable angina and, 287
Angiotensin II, 5

Angiotensin-converting enzyme (ACE) inhibitors, 438t, 438-439
  for acute myocardial infarction, 290
  cardiovascular actions of, 438-439
  cautions and side effects of, 439
  clinical uses of, 439
  for dilated cardiomyopathy, 380
  dosage and administration of, 439
Angle of Lewis, 27
Anistreplase, 290, 291, 444t
Annuloplasty ring, Sorin Puig Massana, *352*
Anterior descending branch of left coronary artery, 5
Antibodies, monoclonal and polyclonal, cardiac transplantation and, 393
Antibradycardia pacing, implantable cardioverter defibrillators and, 243
Antidepressants, coronary artery disease and, 333
Antidiuretic hormone, 5
Antidysrhythmic agents, 112, 453t, 453-460, 454t
  for accelerated idioventricular rhythm, 145
  electrophysiologic effects of, 453t
  Qtc interval and, 65
  for torsades de pointes, 144
Antiembolic hose, venous stasis and, 335
Antilipemic agents, 460-464, 461t, 463
Antilymphocyte gamma globulin (ATGAM), 393
Antilymphocyte globulin (ALG), 393
Antiplatelet agents, 452-453
  for acute myocardial infarction, 291
  cardiovascular actions of, 452
  cautions and side effects of, 453
  clinical uses of, 452
  dosage and administration of, 452-453
Antitachycardia pacing, implantable cardioverter defibrillators and, 243
Antithymocyte globulin (ATG), 393, 394t-395t
Anxiety, relief of, in coronary care unit, 277-279, *280*
Anxiolytics, 333
AOO; *see* Atrial asynchronous pacemaker
Aortic ejection sound, 31
Aortic regurgitation, 344t, *348*, 348-349
  diagnostic evaluation of, 348-349
  etiology of, 348
  murmurs of, 35, *35*
  pathophysiology of, 348, *348*
  signs and symptoms of, 348
  treatment of, 349, 350t
Aortic stenosis, 34, 343-347
  diagnostic evaluation of, 343-346
  etiology of, 343, 344t
  pathophysiology of, 343, *346*
  signs and symptoms of, 343
  treatment of, 346-347, *347*
Aortic valve, 2, 50-51
Aortic valve disease, 343-349
Apical heart rate and rhythm, assessment of, 29
Apical-radial deficit, 29
Appetite changes in health history, 20
APSAC, 444t
Aramine; *see* Metaraminol
ARDS; *see* Adult respiratory distress syndrome
ARF; *see* Acute renal failure
Arterial blood gases, assessment of, 38
Arterial blood pressure, assessment of, 25, *26*
Arterial line, 25-27
Arterial pressure, cardiogenic shock and, 305
Arterial pulses, assessment of, 22-25, *23*, *24*
Arteriography, coronary, 55, 56
Artery(ics), auscultation of, 25
Artifact
  AV block and, *210*
  dysrhythmias and, 171, *172*
  ventricular tachycardia and, *209*
Artificial cardiac pacemaker, 220-240
  asynchronous atrial, 222
  atrial demand, 222, *223*
  atrial synchronous ventricular, 222-223, *223*
  AV sequential, 223-224, *225*

Artificial cardiac pacemaker—cont'd.
  electrode systems for, 229-233
  failure of, to pace, 236-237
  follow-up for, 234
  fully automatic stimulation, 224, *225*, *226*
  and implantable cardioverter defibrillators, 220-255
  indications for, 220-221
  leads for, 229-233
    epicardial, 233
    temporary, 233, *234*
    transvenous, 232-233, *233*
  loss of sensing by, 237
  modalities for, 221-229
  mode selection for, 227-229, 228t
  NBG code for, 221t, 221-222
  nursing care of patients with, 250-252
  oversensing by, 237
  pacing at altered rate by, 237
  permanent, 220-221
  power sources for, 229
  programmability of, 229, 230t-232t
  rate-responsive, 224-227, *226*
  temporary, 221
  troubleshooting, 235-238, *236*, 239t-240t, *240*, *241*
  undesirable patient-pacemaker interactions and, 237-238, 239t-240t
  universal stimulation, 224, *225*, *226*
  ventricular asynchronous, 222
  ventricular demand, 222, *223*
Aspirin, 443, 452-453
  for acute myocardial infarction, 291
  for pericarditis, 296
  PTCA and, 294
ASVIP; *see* Atrial synchronous ventricular inhibited pacemaker
Asynchronous atrial pacemaker, 222
Asystole, *315*
Atenolol, 430t, 431
ATG; *see* Antithymocyte globulin
ATGAM; *see* Antilymphocyte gamma globulin
Atherosclerosis, coronary artery disease and, 256
ATP; *see* Adenosine triphosphate
Atria, rhythms originating in, 92
Atrial activity, identification of, supraventricular dysrhythmia with abnormal QRS complexes and, 164-165
Atrial asynchronous pacemaker (AOO), 222, 228t, 237
Atrial capture, retrograde, ventricular tachycardia with, *200*
Atrial complexes, premature; *see* Premature atrial complexes
Atrial demand pacemaker, 222, *223*, 228t
Atrial fibrillation, 94t-95t, *121*, *125*, 125-127, *126*, *179*, *194*
  significance of, 125-126
  third-degree AV block during, *206*
  treatment of, 126-127
Atrial flutter, 94t-95t, *121*-125, *122*, *123*, *124*, *184*, *192*, *193*, *321*
  coarse, *193*
  impure, *193*
  significance of, 122-123
  third-degree AV block during, *206*
  treatment of, 124-125
Atrial flutter-fibrillation, *190*, *193*
Atrial gallop, 32
Atrial synchronous ventricular inhibited pacemaker (ASVIP), 222, 228t
Atrial synchronous ventricular pacemaker, 222-223, *224*
Atrial tachycardia, *177*
  with AV block, *194*, *195*
  with block, 94t-95t
  significance of, 128
  treatment of, 128-129
  with and without AV block, *127*, 127-129, *128*
Atrioventricular (AV) block, 92, 148-154
  artifact and, *210*
  atrial tachycardia with, *194*, *195*
  complete, 96t-97t
    with ventricular escape rhythm, *175*
  first-degree, 96t-97t, 148, *148*, *149*
    significance of, 148
    treatment of, 148

Atrioventricular (AV) block—cont'd.
paroxysmal, *218*
second-degree, 148-150, *150, 151, 152, 183*
Mobitz type I, 149, *168*
significance of, 149
treatment of, 149
Mobitz type II, 149-150, *169*
significance of, 149
treatment of, 149-150
type I, 96t-97t, *204*
type II, 96t-97t, *205*
third-degree, 150-154, *152, 153, 205, 218*
during atrial flutter and atrial fibrillation, *206*
significance of, 154
treatment of, 154
Atrioventricular (AV) valve, 342
Atromide-S; *see* Clofibrate
Atropine, 464
for accelerated idioventricular rhythm, 145
for atrioventricular block, 154
for AV block, 279
cardiac transplantation and, 392
cardiovascular actions of, 464
cautions and side effects of, 464
clinical uses of, 464
dosage and administration of, 464
for Mobitz type I second-degree AV block, 149
for Mobitz type II second-degree AV block, 149
for sinus arrest, 102
Atropine sulfate, 323t
Augmented ECG leads, 66-67
Auriculopuncture, smoking cessation and, 264
Auscultation of arteries, 25
Auscultatory gap, 25
Auscultatory method of determining blood pressure, 25
Automated blood pressure monitors, 25
Automaticity, dysrhythmias and, 89, 91
Autonomic nervous system, 7
Autoregulation, 4
AV block; *see* Atrioventricular block
AV bundle, 6
AV dissociation, 161-162
AV junction, rhythms originating in, 92
AV junctional complexes, 129
premature, 129, *130*
AV junctional rhythm, 94t-95t, 129, *131, 132, 179, 195, 196*
significance of, 129
treatment of, 129
AV junctional tachycardia, nonparoxysmal, 129-133, *133*
AV nodal reentry, 94t-95t, *108*, 108-113, *109, 110, 111, 170*
significance of, 109
treatment of, 109-113
AV node, 6
A-V oxygen difference, heart failure and, 303
AV reciprocating tachycardia (AVRT), 113, *174*
AV sequential pacemaker, 223-224, *225*, 228t
AV valve; *see* Atrioventricular valve
AVRT; *see* AV reciprocating tachycardia
Axis deviation, electrocardiography and, 74
Azathioprine, 393, 394t-395t

B

Balloon-tipped PA catheter, flow-directed, bedside right-sided heart catheterization using, *53*, 53-55
BARI; *see* Bypass Angioplasty Revascularization Investigation
Barlow syndrome, 353
Baseline, electrocardiography and, 58
Basic cardiac life support (BCLS), 310-311, 339, 476
Batteries for pacemakers, 229, 246
Baymycard; *see* Nisoldipine
Baypress; *see* Nitrendipine
BCLS; *see* Basic cardiac life support

Bedside right-sided heart catheterization using flow-directed, balloon-tipped PA catheter, *53*, 53-55
Behavior
health-seeking, in health history, 16-20
type-A, coronary artery disease and, 266, 334
Benazepril, 438t
β Blockers, 429-432, 430t, 443
cardiovascular actions of, 429-430
cautions and side effects of, 431-432
clinical uses of, 430-431
dosage and adminstration of, 430t, 431
Betapace; *see* Sotalol
Betaxolol, 430t
Bifascicular block, 155-160
significance of, 160
treatment of, 160
Bigeminal pulse, 22
Bigeminy, 137
Bile acid sequestrants for lipid abnormalities, 409
Bile acid–binding resins, 460-461
cardiovascular actions of, 461
cautions and side effects of, 461
clinical uses of, 461
dosage and administration of, 461, 461t
Biofeedback, stress and, 334
Biopsy, endomyocardial, 56-57, *396*
Biphasic deflection, electrocardiography and, 58
Bisoprolol, 430t, 431
Bleeding, anticoagulation scale for assessment of, 451
Blocadren; *see* Timolol
Blood flow, coronary, 2-4, *3*
Blood gases, arterial, 38
Blood pressure, *4*
arterial, assessment of, 25, *26*
automated monitors of, 25
classification of, for adults, 259t
direct monitoring of, 25-26
indirect monitoring of, 25
manual indirect, 25
Blood testing, home care and, 477
Blood urea nitrogen (BUN), 40
BMI; *see* Body mass index
Body mass index (BMI), 409
Bogalusa Heart Study, 261, 268
Borg Scale, 407
Bowel habits, alterations in, in health history, 20
Bradycardia, *316*
sinus; *see* Sinus bradycardia
Bradycardia-tachycardia syndrome, 102
Bradykinin, 5
Bradypnea, 39
Breath sounds, assessment of, 37-38
Bretylium, 453t, 454t, 460
cardiovascular actions of, 460
cautions and side effects of, 460
clinical uses of, 460
dosage and administration of, 460
for premature ventricular complexes, 137
for ventricular flutter, 148
for ventricular tachycardia, 140
Bretylium tosylate, 323t
defibrillation and, 311
Bretylol; *see* Bretylium
Brevibloc; *see* Esmolol
Brevital; *see* Methohexital
Bronchial breath sounds, 37
Bronchovesicular breath sounds, 37
Bruising, anticoagulation scale for assessment of, 451
Bruit, 25
Bumetanide, 437t
Bumex; *see* Bumetanide
BUN; *see* Blood urea nitrogen

Bundle branch block, 92, 154-160, *156-157*, *158*
    left; *see* Left bundle branch block
    right; *see* Right bundle branch block
Bundle of His, rhythms originating in, 92
Bypass Angioplasty Revascularization Investigation (BARI), 359

C

C wave, assessment of, 26
CABG; *see* Coronary artery bypass grafting
CABRI; *see* Coronary Angioplasty versus Bypass Revascularization Investigation
CAD; *see* Coronary artery disease
Caffeine
    hypertension and, 259-260
    as risk factor for coronary artery disease, 267
CAGE questionnaire, 411
Calan; *see* Verapamil
Calcium antagonists
    for hypertrophic cardiomyopathy, 383
    second-generation, 441t
Calcium channel blockers, 60, 439-443, 440t, 441t
    for angina, 287
    cardiovascular actions of, 441
    cautions and side effects of, 442-443
    clinical uses of, 441-442
    dosage and administration of, 442
    PTCA and, 294
Calcium chloride 10%, 323t
Calcium disturbances, dysrhythmias and, 166, *168*
Calcium entry blockers, 60
Capillary refill, assessment of, 28
Capoten; *see* Captopril
Captopril, 438t, 439
    for dilated cardiomyopathy, 380
    for heart failure, 299
Cardene; *see* Nicardipine
Cardiac angiography, *55*, 55-56
Cardiac Arrhythmia Suppression Trial (CAST), 365
Cardiac assessment, 29-37
Cardiac catheterization, 55-56
Cardiac chamber size and functions, echocardiography and, 49
Cardiac cycle, normal, dysrhythmias and, 86, *87*, *88*
Cardiac death, sudden; *see* Sudden cardiac death
Cardiac electrophysiologic studies, 56
Cardiac function, regulation of, 7-9, *8*
Cardiac index, 3, 37
Cardiac neurosis, 331
Cardiac output (CO), 3, 363
    assessment of, 37
    control of, 8-9
    decreased, 369
    echocardiography and, 52
Cardiac rehabilitation
    activity duration in, 407
    activity frequency and, 408
    activity intensity in, 407
    after myocardial infarction, 402-414
    alcohol in, 410-411
    diet in, 409
    exercise benefits and training in, 406-408
    in-hospital, 403-406
        activity guidelines for, 403-404
        educational and psychologic needs in, 404
        risk stratification in, 404-406, *405*
        treadmill test in, 405-406
    management of coronary risk factors in, 408-411
    modification of lifestyle and, 408-411
    outpatient recovery period of, 406
    return to work in, 411-412
    serum cholesterol levels in, 409-410
    sexual activity and, 411

Cardiac rehabilitation—cont'd.
    smoking in, 410
    stress in, 410
    supervised vs. unsupervised, 408
Cardiac rhythms, classification of normal and abnormal, 92
Cardiac tamponade, 2
Cardiac transplant vascularity, cardiac transplantation and, 396-397
Cardiac transplantation, 387-401
    antithymocyte globulin and, 394t-395t
    azathioprine and, 393, 394t-395t
    cardiac transplant vasculopathy and, 396-397
    complications of, 395-397
    contraindications for, 388t
    corticosteroids and, 393, 394t-395t
    cyclophosphamide and, 393
    cyclosporine and, 393, 394t-395t
    donor selection and operative procedure for, 390-391, *391*, *392*
    historic events in, 387t
    immunosuppression and, 392-393, 394t-395t, 397
    infection and, 397
    listing for, and waiting for donor organ, 389-390
    long-term follow-up and, 397, 398t-399t
    malignancy and, 397
    methotrexate and, 393
    monoclonal antibodies and, 393
    muromonab-CD3 and, 394t-395t
    mycophenolate mofetil and, 393
    nursing management and, 390t, 398t-399t
    photophoresis and, 395
    plasmapheresis and, 395
    polyclonal antibodies and, 393
    postoperative care and long-term follow-up for, 391-397
    quality of life and, 397
    recipient selection for, 387-390, *388*
    referral and cardiac transplant evaluation for, 389, 390t
    rejection and, 395-396
    total lymphoid irradiation and, 393
Cardioacceleratory area, 8
Cardiogenic shock, 300-315, *319*
    arterial pressure and, 305
    defibrillation and cardioversion and, 311-315, *312-320*, *321*
    dysrhythmias and, 310-311
    electrophysiologic monitoring and, 315
    hemodynamic assessment in, 300-303, *301*, 305-310, *306*, *307*, *308*
    intraaortic balloon pumping and, 309-310, *310*
    PA end-diastolic pressure and, 300-303, *303*, *304*
    PA equipment and, 304-305
    PA pressure and, 300, *302*, 304-305
    patient care in, 304-305
    pulmonary capillary wedge pressure and, 300, 304-305
    treatment of, 306-309
Cardioinhibitory area, 8
Cardiomyopathy, 376-386
    classification of, 376, 377t, 385t
    dilated, 376-381, 377t, *378*, 385t
        clinical presentation of, 379
        diagnostic tests for, 379-380, *380*, *381*
        pathology of, 379, *379*
        pathophysiology of, 376-379, *378*
    hypertrophic, 49, 377t, *378*, 381-383, 385t
        clinical presentation of, 382
        diagnostic tests for, 382-383
        medical and surgical interventions for, 383
        pathophysiology of, 381-382, *382*
    hypertrophic obstructive, 381
    medical and surgical interventions for, 380-381
    restrictive, 377t, *378*, 383-384, 385t
        clinical presentation of, 383
        diagnostic tests for, 384, *384*
        medical and surgical interventions for, 384
        pathophysiology of, 383
    secondary, 377
Cardioplegia, 362

Cardiopulmonary bypass (CPB), surgical management of heart disease and, 360-362, *361*
Cardioselectivity, β blockers and, 429
Cardiovascular assessment, 10-41
    formulating nursing diagnoses in, 40, 41
    health history in; *see* Health history in cardiovascular assessment
    interview in; *see* Interview in cardiovascular assessment
    physical examination in; *see* Physical examination in cardiovascular assessment
Cardiovascular center, 8
Cardiovascular drugs, 415-469; *see also* specific drugs
    ACE inhibitors, 438t, 438-439
    α-adrenergic blockers, 426-427
    antidysrhythmics, 453t, 453-460, 454t
    antilipemic agents, 460-464
    antiplatelet agents, 452-453
    β blockers, 429-432, 430t
    calcium channel blockers, 439-443, 440t, 441t
    central α agonists, 427-429
    clinical pharmacokinetics and, *415*, 415-416
    clinical pharmacology of, 416-417
    diuretics, 436-438, 437t
    ganglionic agents, 429
    heparin, 445t, 445-447, 446t
    inotropes, 417-423
    miscellaneous, 464-468
    subclassification of α-adrenergic receptors and, 416, *417*
    subclassification of β-adrenergic receptors and, 416-417
    sympathomimetics, 423-426
    thrombolytic agents, 443-445
    vasodilators, 432-436
    warfarin, 447-452, 448t, 449t-450t
Cardiovascular subsystem, postoperative management of heart disease and, 363-368
Cardioversion, cardiogenic shock and, 311-315, *312-320*, *321*
Cardizem; *see* Diltiazem
Cardura; *see* Doxazosin
Careolol, 431
Carpentier mitral and tricuspid rings, *352*
Carteolol, 430t
Cartrol; *see* Carteolol
Case management, home care and, 472-473
CAST; *see* Cardiac Arrhythmia Suppression Trial
Catecholamines, 416, 417
CCU; *see* Coronary care unit
Cedilanid-D; *see* Deslanoside
Celiprolol, 430t
Centers for Disease Control and Prevention, 262-263, 264
Central α₂ agonists, 427-429
    cardiovascular actions of, 427
    cautions and side effects of, 428-429
    clinical uses of, 427
    dosage and administration of, 427-428, 428t
Central cyanosis, 28
Central venous pressure (CVP), 27-28
Chelated Magnesium Tablets, 467t
Cheyne-Stokes respiration, 39
Chlorothiazide, 437t
Cholestyramine, 409, 460-461, 461t
Cholinergic drugs for AV nodal reentry, 111
Chordae tendineae, 342
Cigarette smoking; *see* Smoking
Cine CT; *see* Ultrafast computed tomography
Circulation
    coronary, 5-6, *6*
    peripheral, assessment of, 22-28
    pulmonary, 5
    systemic, *4*, 4-5
Circulatory arrest, 315-322
    resuscitation and, 318-322, *322*, 323t-324t
Circulatory assist devices, 367-368
Circumflex branch of left coronary artery, 5
CK; *see* Creatine kinase
Class of 1989 Study, 269

Clinical pharmacokinetics, cardiovascular drugs and, 415-416
Clinical pharmacology, cardiovascular drugs and, 416-417
Clofibrate, 461t, 462
Clonidine, 428t
Clubbing, assessment of, 28, *29*
CO; *see* Cardiac output
Cognitive restructuring, stress and, 334
Colestid; *see* Colestipol
Colestipol, 409, 460-461, 461t
Collaterals, myocardial infarction and, 257
Color, skin, 28
Comfort in health history, 17
Communication in interview, 14
Complexes, electrocardiography and, 58, 60-66
Compromised family coping, 15-16
Computed tomography, ultrafast, 47
Congestive heart failure, 477-478
Continuity of care, home care and, 472-475
Contractility
    myocardial, 9
    postoperative management of heart disease and, 367-368
Cook-Medley Hostility Scale, 410
Coping behaviors
    of family, 15-16
    in health history, 15-16
    of patient, 15
Cor pulmonale, 298
Cordarone; *see* Amiodarone
Corgard; *see* Nadolol
Coronary Angioplasty versus Bypass Revascularization Investigation (CABRI), 359
Coronary arteriography, 55, 56
Coronary artery bypass grafting (CABG), 287, 292, 293, 359
Coronary artery disease (CAD), 256-275
    acute myocardial infarction and; *see* Acute myocardial infarction
    age and, 258
    alcohol intake and, 267
    angina pectoris and, 286-287
    caffeine intake and, 267
    cardiogenic shock and; *see* Cardiogenic shock
    care issues of, 334-339
    circulatory arrest and, 315-322, *322*, 323t-324t
    community resources and, 338-339
    complications of, 286-331
    daily care and, 335, *336*
    developmental issues and existential concerns and, 333-334
    discharge instructions and, 338-339
    emotional problems and, 333
    excessive concerns about health and, 332-333
    follow-up care and, 338
    gender and, 258
    glucose intolerance and, 265-266
    heart failure and, 296-299, 297t
    hospital phase of, 331-332, *332*
    hypercholesterolemia and, 260-262
    hypertension and, 258-260, *259*
    incidence, prevalence, morbidity, and mortality of, 256-258
    left ventricular failure and, 297-298, 298t
    medications and, 338
    national priorities concerning, 271
    natural history and prognosis for, 257-258
    nutrition and, 338
    obesity and, 267
    organic problems and, 333
    pathogenesis of, 256-257
    personality factors and, 266
    physical activity and, 338
    physical inactivity and, 264-265
    posthospital phase of, 332-334
    postoperative management of, 363-372
        admission to unit and, 363, *364*
        afterload and, 366-367
        cardiovascular subsystem and, 363-368
        circulatory assist devices and, 367-368

Coronary artery disease (CAD)—cont'd.
  postoperative management of—cont'd.
    contractility and, 367-368
    heart rate and rhythm and, 363-365
    infection and, 372, 374
    left ventricular afterload reduction and, 366-367
    neurologic subsystem and, 370-372
    nutrition and, 372-373
    pain and, 372, 373
    preload and, 365-366, 366t
    pulmonary subsystem and, 368-370
    renal subsystem and, 370
    right ventricular afterload reduction and, 366
  prehospital phase of, 331
  prevention of, 268-271
    in community, 269-271
    in home, 268
    in schools, 268-269
    on worksites, 269
  priorities during intermediate care and, 337-338
  problems continuing from earlier years and, 333
  psychologic adjustment to, 331-334
  race and, 258
  research needs in health promotion and, 271-272
  right ventricular failure and, 298-299
  risk factors for, 258-268
  sexual activity and, 338
  smoking and, 262-264, 338
  sociocultural considerations of, 334-335
  stress and, 266-267
  sudden cardiac death and; *see* Sudden cardiac death
  surgical management of, 359-375
    cardioplegia and, 362
    CPB and, 360-362, *361*
    intraoperative events and, 360-363
    myocardial revascularization and, 359-360
    preoperative considerations of, 360
    procedures of, *362,* 362-363, *363*
  transfer from CCU and, 337
  treatment considerations and, 334
  valvular; *see* Valvular heart disease
Coronary care unit (CCU), 276-341
  completion of database in, 279-281
  complications of coronary artery disease and, 286-331
  decrease in myocardial oxygen consumption in, 279
  equipment in, 281-286, *282*
    alarm control system of, 282
    central console of, 283
    digital display of, 282
    electric hazards of, 284-286, 285t
    electrodes of, 283-284
    filter of, 283
    interference with monitoring and, 284, *284*
    monitoring system in, 281-283
    oscilloscope in, 281, *282*
    rate display and alarm limits of, 282
    sweep speed of, 282
  establishment of intravenous access in, 277
  immediate monitoring of cardiac rate and rhythm in, 277
  priorities in admission to, 277-281, *278*
  relief of pain and anxiety in, 277-279, *280*
  summary flow sheet for, *336*
  supplemental oxygen administration in, 279
Coronary circulation, 5-6, *6*
Coronary clubs, coronary artery disease and, 339
Coronary Drug Project, 409
Coronary nodal complexes, 129
Coronary sinus complexes, 129
Corticosteroids
  cardiac transplantation and, 393, 394t-395t
  for dilated cardiomyopathy, 380
Cough, assessment of, 37
Counterpulsation; *see* Intraaortic balloon pumping
CPB; *see* Cardiopulmonary bypass
Creatine kinase (CK), myocardial infarction and, 288

Crescendo angina, 286
Culinary Hearts Kitchen, 271
Culture in health history, 16
Current pathways, implantable cardioverter defibrillators and, 248-249
CVP; *see* Central venous pressure
Cyanosis, assessment of, 28
Cyclophosphamide, cardiac transplantation and, 393
Cyclosporine, cardiac transplantation and, 393, 394t-395t
Cytoxan; *see* Cyclophosphamide

D

DCA; *see* Directional coronary atherectomy device
DDD pacemaker, 222, 225t, *226,* 227, 228, 228t, 229, 235, *236,* 237, 238
DDDR pacemaker, 224, *226,* 227-228, 228, 228t, 229, 235, 237, 238
DDI pacemaker, 223-224, 229
DDIR pacemaker, 228, 228t, 229
Decision time, coronary heart disease and, 331
Decision-making ability in health history, 16
Defensive coping behaviors, 15
Defibrillation, cardiogenic shock and, 311-315, *312-320, 321*
Defibrillator, implantable cardioverter; *see* Implantable cardioverter defibrillator
Deflections, electrocardiography and, 58-59, *60,* 64
Demadex; *see* Torsemide
Denial, acceptance of illness and, 16
15-Deoxyspergudin, cardiac transplantation and, 395
Depolarization, diastolic, dysrhythmias and, 89
Deslanoside for AV nodal reentry, 112
Dextran, low-molecular-weight, PTCA and, 294
Diabetes mellitus, non-insulin-dependent, 265
Diagnoses, nursing, 40, 41, 479t, 480t-481t
Diagnostic studies, 42-57, 46-47
  ambulatory ECG and, *47,* 47-48, *48*
  bedside right-sided heart catheterization using flow-directed, balloon-tipped PA catheter and, *53,* 53-55
  cardiac angiography and, *55,* 55-56
  cardiac catheterization and, 55-56
  cardiac electrophysiologic studies and, 56
  echocardiography and; *see* Echocardiography
  endomyocardial biopsy and, 56-57
  MI imaging and, 45-46
  myocardial perfusion imaging and, 45, *45*
  radionuclide angiocardiography and, 46, *46*
  radionuclide imaging and, *45,* 45-46
  serum enzyme levels in acute myocardial infarction and, 42-43, 43t
  stress testing and, 43-45, *44*
Diamox; *see* Acetazolamide
Diastolic depolarization, dysrhythmias and, 89
Diastolic murmurs, 35, *35,* 36t
Diastolic pressure, 4, 25
Diazepam, 279
Diazoxide, 434, 435t
Dibenzyline; *see* Phenoxybenzamine
Dicrotic notch, 22
Diet; *see* Nutrition
Digitalis, 482
  for accelerated idioventricular rhythm, 145
  for atrial fibrillation, 126
  for atrial flutter, 124, 125
  for atrial tachycardia, 128, 129
  for atrioventricular block, 148
  for AV nodal reentry, 112
  for dilated cardiomyopathy, 380
  for Mobitz type I second-degree AV block, 149
  for nonparoxysmal AV junctional tachycardia, 131
  for premature ventricular complexes, 137
Digitalis glycosides, 417-419
  cardiovascular actions of, 417
  cautions and side effects of, 418-419
  clinical uses of, 417-418
  dosage and administration of, 418, 418t
Digitalis toxicity, atrial tachycardia with AV block caused by, *195*

Digoxin, 417-419, 418t
  for AV nodal reentry, 112
  cardiac transplantation and, 392
Dilacor; *see* Diltiazem
Dilantin; *see* Phenytoin
Dilated cardiomyopathy; *see* Cardiomyopathy, dilated
Diltiazem, 440t, 443, 453t, 454t
  for angina, 287
  for hypertrophic cardiomyopathy, 383
Diphasic deflection, electrocardiography and, 58
Diphenhydramine, PTCA and, 294
Dipyridamole, 452
  for acute myocardial infarction, 291
  PTCA and, 294
  stress testing with, 45
Direct arteriolar vasodilators; *see* Vasodilators, direct arteriolar
Direct blood pressure monitoring, 25-26
Directional coronary atherectomy (DCA) device, 296
Disabling family coping, 15
Discharge planning, home care and, 473
Discomfort in health history, 17
Disopyramide, 453t, 453-455, 454t
  for AV nodal reentry, 112
  cardiovascular actions of, 453
  cautions and side effects of, 454-455
  clinical uses of, 453
  dosage and administration of, 453-454
  for long QT syndrome, 144
  for premature ventricular complexes, 138
  for torsades de pointes, 144
  for ventricular tachycardia, 141
Dissociation, AV, 161-162
Diuretics, 436-438, 437t
  cardiovascular actions of, 436
  cautions and side effects of, 437-438
  clinical uses of, 436
  for dilated cardiomyopathy, 380
  dosage and administration of, 436-437
  for heart failure, 299
  loop, 299, 366, 436-438, 437t
  potassium sparing, 437t
  thiazide, 299, 436-438, 437t
Diuril; *see* Chlorothiazide
Dobutamine, 323t, 420t, 421t, 421-422
  cardiovascular actions of, 421-422
  cautions and side effects of, 422
  clinical uses of, 422
  dosage and administration of, 422
  right ventricular afterload reduction and, 366
Dopamine, 323t, 419-421, 420t, 421t
  cardiovascular actions of, 419-420, 420t
  cautions and side effects of, 421
  clinical uses of, 420
  dosage and administration of, 421, 421t
  right ventricular afterload reduction and, 366
Doppler echocardiography, 49, 52-53
Doppler method of recording systolic blood pressure, 25
Doxazosin, 427, 435-436, 436t
  cardiovascular actions of, 435
  cautions and side effects of, 436
  clinical uses of, 435
  dosage and administration of, 435-436, 436t
Doxepin hydrochloride, 333
Dressler syndrome, 296
Drugs; *see* Cardiovascular drugs; Medications
Dsypnea, assessment of, 37
Dubutrex; *see* Dobutamine
Duraquin; *see* Quinidine
Dura-Tabs; *see* Quinidine
DVI pacemaker, 223-224, *225*, 228, 228t
DVIR pacemaker, 228, 228t
Dying at home, 491
DynaCirc; *see* Isradipine

Dyrenium; *see* Triamterene
Dyspnea, 39
  paroxysmal nocturnal, 297
Dysrhythmias, 86-219, 94t-97t
  accelerated idioventricular rhythm, 144-145, *145*, *146*
  acute myocardial infarction and; *see* Acute myocardial infarction
  analysis of, 91-92
  artifacts and, 171, *172*
  assessment of, 37
  atrial fibrillation; *see* Atrial fibrillation
  atrial flutter; *see* Atrial flutter
  atrial tachycardia; *see* Atrial tachycardia
  AV block; *see* Atrioventricular block
  AV dissociation, 161-162
  AV junctional rhythm; *see* AV junctional rhythm
  AV nodal reentry; *see* AV nodal reentry
  bifascicular block, 155-160
  bundle branch block; *see* Bundle branch block
  calcium disturbances and, 166, *168*
  cardiogenic shock and, 310-311
  classification of, 92
  determination of heart rate and, 86-89, *90*
  electrolyte disturbances and, 166, *167*, *168*
  electrophysiologic consequences of, 92-93
  electrophysiologic principles and, 89-91
  etiology of, 93
  invasive electrophysiologic studies and, 166-171, *168*, *169*, *170*, *171*
  left anterior hemiblock, 155, *217*
  left bundle branch block; *see* Left bundle branch block
  left posterior hemiblock, 155, *160*
  long QT syndrome, 144
  nonparoxysmal AV junctional tachycardia; *see* Nonparoxysmal AV junctional tachycardia
  normal cardiac cycle and, 86, *87*, *88*
  normal sinus rhythm, 93, *98*
  potassium disturbances and, 166, *167*, *168*
  preexcitation syndrome; *see* Preexcitation syndrome
  premature atrial complexes; *see* Premature atrial complexes
  premature AV junctional complexes, 129, *130*
  premature ventricular complexes; *see* Premature ventricular complexes
  respiratory sinus, *188*
  right bundle branch block; *see* Right bundle branch block
  sinus, 100-102, *101*, *102*
  sinus arrest, 102, *103*, *189*
  sinus bradycardia; *see* Sinus bradycardia
  sinus exit block; *see* Sinus exit block
  sinus tachycardia; *see* Sinus tachycardia
  sodium disturbances and, 166
  supraventricular, with abnormal QRS complexes, *162*, 162-166, *163*, *164*
  test section for, 171, *171-218*
  therapy of, 92-161
    general concepts of, 92
    hemodynamic consequences of, 92-93
    risks of, 93, 94t-97t
    slowing ventricular rate and, 92-93
  torsades de pointes; *see* Torsades de pointes
  ventricular escape beats; *see* Ventricular escape beats
  ventricular fibrillation; *see* Ventricular fibrillation
  ventricular flutter; *see* Ventricular flutter
  ventricular tachycardia; *see* Ventricular tachycardia
  wandering pacemaker, 104, *105*

E

Early repolarization, electrocardiography and, 64
Early systolic ejection click, 31-32
EAST; *see* Emory Angioplasty Surgery Trial
Eating patterns in health history, 19-20
ECG; *see* Electrocardiography
ECG leads; *see* Electrocardiography, leads in
Echocardiography, 48-53
  of aortic valve, 50-51
  applications of, 49-52

Echocardiography—cont'd.
  cardiac chamber size and functions and, 49
  cardiac output and, 52
  clinical applications of, 52-53
  Doppler, 49, 52-53
  intracardiac pressure and, 52-53
  intracardiac shunts and, 53
  of mitral valve, 49-50
  M-mode, 49, *50*
  motion, 49, *50*
  of normal heart, 49, *50, 51*
  pericardial disease and, 51
  of pulmonic valve, 51
  stress, 51-52
  techniques of, 49
  transesophageal, 49, 52, 351
  transthoracic, 48-49
  of tricuspid valve, 51
  two-dimensional, 49, *51*
  valvular functions and, 49-51
  valvular regurgitation and, 52
  valvular stenosis and, 52
ECMO, 367, 370
Economic history in health history, 16
Edecrin sodium; *see* Ethacrynic acid
Edema
  assessment of, 28
  pulmonary; *see* Pulmonary edema
Edrophonium, 464-465
  cardiovascular actions of, 464
  cautions and side effects of, 464-465
  clinical uses of, 464
  dosage and administration of, 464
Edrophonium chloride, 111
Educational needs, cardiac rehabilitation and, 404
EDV; *see* End-diastolic volume
EF; *see* Ejection fraction
Einthoven, Willem, 58
Einthoven's law, electrocardiography and, 66, *68*
Einthoven's triangle, electrocardiography and, 66, *67*
Ejection fraction (EF), 3, 46
Ejection murmurs, 34-35, *35*, 36t
Electric axis, electrocardiography and, 73-74
Electric events in heart, electrocardiography and, 69-70, *70, 71*
Electric hazards in coronary care unit, 284-286, 285t
Electric heart positions, electrocardiography and, 73-74
Electrocardiography (ECG), 23, 24, 58-85
  ambulatory, *47*, 47-48, *48*
  amplitude in, 64
  basic considerations of, 58-59
  causes of axis deviation and, 74
  deflections and, 58-59, *60*, 64
  determination of horizontal plane projection of mean QRS vector and, 74, *75*
  electrophysiologic principles of, 59-60
  home care and, 486
  intrinsicoid deflection in, 64, *64*
  leads in, 66-68
    for artificial cardiac pacemakers, 229-233, 232-233, *233*, 233
    augmented, 66-67
    hexaxial reference figure and, 67
    for implantable cardioverter defibrillators, 246-247, 246-248, 247-248, *248*
    posterior, 68
    precordial, 67-68, *68*
    precordial figure and, 67
    right precordial, 68
    standard limb, 66, *67*, 68
    temporary, for artificial cardiac pacemakers, 233, *234*
  left atrial enlargement and, 76-77, *77*
  left ventricular enlargement and, 74-76, *76*
  myocardial infarction and, *79*, 79-85

Electrocardiography—cont'd.
    evolution of, 82-85, *83, 84, 85*
    localization of, *81*, 81-82
    Q wave and, 79
    vector abnormalities and, 79-81, *80*
  P wave in, 60-61, *63*
  QRS complex in, 61-64, *63*
  QT interval in, 65, *65*
  right atrial enlargement and, 79, *79*
  right ventricular enlargement and, 77-79, *78*
  ST segment in, 64, *65*
  standardization of, 58, *59*
  T wave in, 64
  U wave in, 65-66
  vector approach to, 68-74, *69*
    electric heart positions and electric axis and, 73-74
    mean cardiac vector and, 70-71, *71*
    mean QRS axis and, 71-72, *73*
    sequence of electric events and, 69-70, *70, 71*
  waves and complexes in, 60-66
Electrodes
  for artificial cardiac pacemakers, 229-233
  in coronary care unit, 283-284
  esophageal pill, supraventricular dysrhythmia with abnormal QRS complexes and, 165-166
  for implantable cardioverter defibrillators, 246-248
Electrolyte disturbances, dysrhythmias and, 166, *167, 168*
Electrophysiologic consequences of therapy of dysrhythmias, 92-93
Electrophysiologic mapping techniques for ventricular tachycardia, 141, *142*
Electrophysiologic monitoring, cardiogenic shock and, 315
Electrophysiologic principles, dysrhythmias and, 89-91
Electrophysiologic studies (EPS)
  cardiac, 56
  invasive, dysrhythmias and, 166-171, *168, 169, 170, 171*
Electrophysiologic testing, sudden cardiac death and, 328-329
Elimination half-life of cardiovascular drugs, 415
Elimination in health history, 20
Eminase; *see* Anistreplase
Emory Angioplasty Surgery Trial (EAST), 359
Emotional integrity in health history, 17-18
Emotional problems, coronary artery disease and, 333
Emotion-focused physiologic strategies, stress and, 267
Enalapril, 380, 438t
End-diastolic volume (EDV), 3
Endocarditis, infective, 355
Endocardium, 1
Endomyocardial biopsy, 56-57, *396*
English language, reading, writing, and understanding in interview, 14
Epicardium, 2
Epinephrine, 5, 323t-324t, 416, 417, 420t, 423-424, 424t
  cardiovascular actions of, 423-424
  cautions and side effects of, 424
  clinical uses of, 424
  defibrillation and, 311
  dosage and administration of, 424, 424t
EPS; *see* Electrophysiologic studies
Equipment
  in coronary care unit; *see* Coronary care unit, equipment in
  for PTCA, 292, *293*
Ergonovine maleate, coronary artery spasm and, 287
Esmolol, 430t
Esophageal pill electrode, supraventricular dysrhythmia with abnormal QRS complexes and, 165-166
Essential hypertension, 258
Ethacrynic acid, 299, 437t
Excitation of heart, 6-7, *7, 8*
Exercise
  cardiac rehabilitation and, 406-408
  coronary artery disease and, 264-265, 335
  in health history, 19
  home care and, 483-484
Exercise stress testing, 44-45
Exertional angina, 286

F

Failure to pace, artificial cardiac pacemakers and, 236-237
Family
    coping behaviors of, 15-16
    in health history, 15
    home care and, 475-477
Fast channels, electrocardiography and, 60
Fast sodium channels, electrocardiography and, 60
Fatigue in health history, 19
Fatty streaks, coronary artery disease and, 256
Fear, stress and, 17
Felodipine, 441t
Fibric acid derivatives, 462-463
    cardiovascular actions of, 462
    cautions and side effects of, 462-463
    clinical uses of, 462
    dosage and administration of, 462
    for lipid abnormalities, 410
Fibrillation
    atrial; *see* Atrial fibrillation
    ventricular; *see* Ventricular fibrillation
Fibrous plaques, coronary artery disease and, 256
Financial support in health history, 16
Fine rales, 37-38
First heart sound, assessment of, 31-32, *33*
Five-City Project, 269-270
FK-506, cardiac transplantation and, 395
Flecainide, 453t, 458
    for AV nodal reentry, 112
    cardiovascular effects of, 458
    cautions and side effects of, 458
    clinical uses of, 458
    dosage and adminstration of, 458
    for premature ventricular complexes, 138
    for ventricular tachycardia, 141
Floppy valve syndrome, 353
Flow sheet for physical examination data, *21*
Flow-directed, balloon-tipped PA catheter, bedside right-sided heart
    catheterization using, *53*, 53-55
Fluvastatin, 410, 461t, 463-464
Fosinopril, 438t
Fourth heart sound, assessment of, 32-33, *33*, *34*
Framingham study, 259, 264
Friction rub
    pericardial, 35
    pleural, 38
Fully automatic stimulation pacemaker, 224, *225*, *226*
Furosemide, 437t
    decreased preload and, 366
    for heart failure, 299

G

Ganglionic agents, 429
    cardiovascular actions of, 429
    cautions and side effects of, 429
    clinical uses of, 429
    dosage and administration of, 429
Gas exchange, impaired, 371
Gelusil II, 467t
Gelusil M Suspension, 467t
Gelusil Suspension, 467t
Gemfibrozil, 461t, 462
Gender as risk factor for coronary artery disease, 258
GISSI study; *see* Gruppo Italiano per lo Studio Streptochinase nell'Infarto
    Miocardico study
Glasgow coma scale, 39
Global Utilization of Streptokinase or tPA for Occluded Coronary Arter-
    ies (GUSTO), 291
Glucose intolerance as risk factor for coronary artery disease, 265-266
Grieving, stress and, 17
Grieving process, 491
Gruppo Italiano per lo Studio Streptochinase nell'Infarto Miocardico
    (GISSI) study, 290
Guanabenz, 428t

Guanadrel, 429
Guanethidine, 429
Guanfacine, 428t
GUSTO; *see* Global Utilization of Streptokinase or tPA for Occluded
    Coronary Arteries

H

HDLs; *see* High-density lipoproteins
Health, excessive concerns about, coronary artery disease and, 332-333
Health care team, home care and, 473-474
Health history in cardiovascular assessment, 14-20
    activity and rest in, 18, 19
    comfort of patient in, 17
    coping behaviors in, 15-16
    culture in, 16
    current health problems in, 14
    current medications in, 14-15
    decision-making ability in, 16
    economic history in, 16
    elimination in, 20
    emotional integrity in, 17-18
    family history in, 15
    health-seeking behaviors in, 16-20
    judgment in, 16
    misconceptions of illness in, 15
    nutrition in, 19-20
    orientation and memory in, 15
    perceptions of knowledge of illness and expectations in, 15-16
    previous illness, hospitalizations, surgeries, and problems in, 14
    readiness to learn about illness in, 15
    risk factors in, 15
    role of patient in home in, 16
    self-care in, 18-19
    social history in, 16
    socialization of patient in, 16
    spiritual concerns in, 16
    stress in, 17
Health history data collection form, 11-13
Health problems, current, in health history, 14
Health-seeking behaviors in health history, 16-20
Healthy People 2000, 271
Heart
    anatomy of, 1-2, *2*, *3*
    assessment of, 29-37
    blood flow and, 2-4, *3*
    control of cardiac output and, 8-9
    coronary circulation and, 5-6, *6*
    electric events in, electrocardiography and, 69-70, *70*, *71*
    excitation of, 6-7, *7*, *8*
    fibrous skeleton of, *3*
    function of, regulation of, 7-9, *8*
    hypertrophied, *382*
    internal anatomy of, *3*
    intrinsic regulation of, 7
    normal, echocardiography and, 49-52, *50*, *51*
    pulmonary circulation and, 5
    regulation of cardiac function and, 7-9, *8*
    systemic circulation and, *4*, 4-5
Heart, Body, and Soul program, 271
Heart, Lung and Blood Institute, 261
Heart disease; *see* Coronary artery disease
Heart failure, 296-297, 297t
    congestive, 477-478
    left ventricular, 297-298, 298t
    right ventricular, 298-299
    treatment of, 299
Heart murmurs, 33-36, 36t
    of aortic and pulmonic regurgitation, 35, *35*
    assessment of, 29-36
    configuration of, *35*
    continuous, 35
    diastolic, 35, *35*, 36t
    ejection, 34-35, *35*, 36t
    holosystolic, 35, *35*, 36t

Heart murmurs—cont'd.
  intensity of, 33
  location of, 34
  midsystolic, 34-35, *35*
  pitch of, 34
  quality of, 33
  radiation of, 34
  regurgitant, 35, *35*
  systolic, 34, 36t
  timing of, 33
Heart rate, 9
  apical, 29
  calculation of, from electrocardiogram, *90*, 90t
  determination of, dysrhythmias and, 86-89, *89*, *90*
  monitoring of, in coronary care unit, 277
  postoperative management of heart disease and, 363-365
Heart Smart, 268
Heart sounds
  assessment of, 29-36, *32*, *33*, *34*
  first, 31-32, *33*
  fourth, 32-33, *33*, *34*
  second, 32, *33*
  third, 32, *33*
Heart valves, structure and function of, 342
Height and weight, 39
Helsinki Heart Study, 261
Hemiblock
  left anterior, 155, *217*
  left posterior, 155, *160*
Hemodynamic assessment in cardiogenic shock, 300-303, *301*, 305-310, *306*, *307*, *308*
Hemodynamic consequences of therapy of dysrhythmias, 92-93
Hemodynamic values, normal resting, 54
Heparin, 445t, 445-447, 446t
  for acute myocardial infarction, 291
  for angina, 287
  cardiovascular actions of, 445
  cautions and side effects of, 447
  clinical uses of, 445-446
  dosage and administration of, 446-447
Hexaxial reference figure, electrocardiography and, 67
High output failure, heart failure and, 296
High-density lipoproteins (HDLs), 260
Histamine, 5
History
  family, in health history, 15
  health; *see* Health history in cardiovascular assessment
HIV; *see* Human immunodeficiency virus
HMG-CoA; *see* 3-Hydroxy-3-methylglutaryl coenzyme A reductase inhibitors
Holodiastolic murmurs, 33
Holosystolic murmurs, 33, *35*, 35, 36t
Holter monitoring, 47-48, 486
Home care, 470-493
  activity and rest and, 483-484
  assessment for, 475-478
  benefits of, 471-472, 472t
  case management and, 472-473
  community resources and, 474-475
  continuity of care and, 472-475
  costs of, 471-472, 472t
  development of, 470-471
  diet and, 478-482
  discharge planning and, 473
  documentation of treatment plan in, 478
  dying patient and, 491
  family and, 475-477
  health care team in, 473-474
  home ECG and, 486
  home health aide and, 474
  homemaker and, 474
  implantable cardioverter defibrillators and, 489-490
  intravenous therapy and, 487-489
  medications and, 482

Home care—cont'd.
  nurse and, 474
  occupational therapist and, 474
  pacemakers and, 485-486
  pain management and, 482-483
  patient and, 477-478
  for patients with technically complex needs, 485-490
  perspectives on, 470-472
  physical therapist and, 474
  physician and, 474
  plan of, 478-485
  psychosocial considerations of, 484-485
  research needs for, 491-492
  scope of services for, 471
  sexual activity and, 484
  social worker and, 474
  speech pathologist and, 474
  supplemental oxygen administration and, 486-487
  ventricular assist devices and, 490
Home health aide, home care and, 474
Home maintenance management in health history, 19
Homemaker, home care and, 474
Hopelessness in health history, 18
Hospices, 491
Hospitalizations, previous, in health history, 14
Human immunodeficiency virus (HIV), 16
Humoral rejection, cardiac transplantation and, 396
Hydralazine, 434, 435t
  for angina, 287
  for aortic regurgitation, 349
  for dilated cardiomyopathy, 380
  for heart failure, 299
Hydrochlorothiazide, 437t
Hydrodiuril; *see* Hydrochlorothiazide
Hydrophilic β-adrenergic blocking agents, 430
3-Hydroxy-3-methylglutaryl coenzyme A (HMG-CoA) reductase inhibitors, 409-410, 463-464
  cardiovascular actions of, 463
  cautions and side effects of, 463-464
  clinical uses of, 463
  dosage and administration of, 463
Hylorel; *see* Guanadrel
Hyperacute rejection, cardiac transplantation and, 396
Hyperacute state, myocardial infarction and, 82
Hypercholesterolemia as risk factor for coronary artery disease, 260-262
Hypertension as risk factor for coronary artery disease, 258-260, *259*
Hypertrophic cardiomyopathy; *see* Cardiomyopathy, hypertrophic
Hypertrophic obstructive cardiomyopathy, 381
Hypertrophied heart, *382*
Hyperventilation, 39
Hypnosis, smoking cessation and, 264
Hypomagnesemia, 466
Hypotension, *319*
  acute myocardial infarction and, 289
Hytrin; *see* Terazosin

I

IABP; *see* Intraaortic balloon pumping
ICD; *see* Implantable cardioverter defibrillator
Idiopathic hypertrophic subaortic stenosis, 381
Idioventricular rhythm, accelerated; *see* Accelerated idioventricular rhythm
Illness
  acceptance and adjustment to, 16
  perception or knowledge of, in health history, 15-16
  previous, in health history, 14
Immunosuppression, cardiac transplantation and, 392-393, 397
Impaired gas exchange, 371
Implantable cardioverter defibrillator (ICD), 240-250
  with antitachycardia and antibradycardia pacing and shock capabilities, 243
  and artificial cardiac pacemakers, 220-255
  electrode systems for, 246-248
  follow-up for, 249-250
  home care and, 489-490
  indications for, 241-242

Implantable cardioverter defibrillator (ICD)—cont'd.
   leads for, 246-248
      epicardial, 247-248
      transvenous, 246-247, *248*
   modalities for, 242-243
   mode selection for, 243
   NBD code, 242t, 242-243
   next-generation, 243
   nursing care of patients with, 250-252
   with only shock capability, 243
   power sources for, 246
   programmability of, 243-246, 244t, *245, 247*
   with shock capability and antibradycardia pacing, 243
   sudden cardiac death and, *329, 329-331, 330*
   troubleshooting, 250
   waveforms and current pathways for, 248-249, *249*
Imuran; *see* Azathioprine
Inderal; *see* Propranolol
Indirect blood pressure monitoring, 25
Individual coping behaviors, 15
Indomethacin, 296
Infection
   cardiac transplantation and, 397
   postoperative management of heart disease and, 372-373, 374
Infective endocarditis, 355
Inferior infarction with lateral extension, 82
Inferolateral infarction, 82
In-hospital cardiac rehabilitation, 403-406
Inocor; *see* Amrinone
Inotropic therapy, intravenous, 488
Inotropism, 9
Institute of Medicine of the National Academy of Sciences, 271
Intensity of heart murmurs, 33
Intercalated discs, 1, *2*
Intermediate care unit, coronary care unit and, 337
Internal jugular vein, 26
Internodal pathways, 6
Interpolated premature complex, 134
Interuniversity Study on Nutrition and Health, 270
Intervals, electrocardiography and, 58, 88t
Interview in cardiovascular assessment, 10-14, *11-13*
   alternative forms of communication in, 14
   communication in, 14
   establishing nurse-patient relationship in, 10-14
   guiding, 10-14
   health history data collection form in, *11-13*
   intubation or speech impairment in, 14
   other languages in, 14
   reading, writing, and understanding English in, 14
Intraaortic balloon pumping (IABP)
   cardiogenic shock and, 309-310, *310*
   left ventricular afterload reduction and, 367
Intracardiac pressures, echocardiography and, 52-53
Intracardiac shunts, echocardiography and, 53
Intracoronary stents, PTCA and, 295
Intravenous access, establishment of, in coronary care unit, 277
Intravenous therapy, home care and, 487-489
Intrinsic regulation of heart, 7
Intrinsicoid deflection, electrocardiography and, 64, *64*
Intropin; *see* Dopamine
Intubation, interview and, 14
Invasive electrophysiologic studies, dysrhythmias and, 166-171, *168, 169, 170, 171*
ISIS-2, 290
Ismelin; *see* Guanethidine
Isoelectric deflection, electrocardiography and, 58
Isoenzymes, myocardial infarction and, 288
Isoproterenol, 324t, 416, 420t, 424t, 425-426
   for atrioventricular block, 154
   cardiovascular actions of, 425
   cautions and side effects of, 426
   clinical uses of, 425
   dosage and administration of, 425-426
   for Mobitz type II second-degree AV block, 149

Isoproterenol—cont'd.
   right ventricular afterload reduction and, 366
   for sinus arrest, 102
Isoptin; *see* Verapamil
Isordil; *see* Isosorbide dinitrate
Isorhythmic AV dissociation, 161
Isosorbide dinitrate, 287, 432, 433, 433t
Isosorbide mononitrate, 432, 433, 433t
Isradipine, 441t
Isuprel; *see* Isoproterenol

J

JCAHO; *see* Joint Commission of Accreditation of Healthcare Organizations
Joint Commission of Accreditation of Healthcare Organizations (JCAHO), 473
Judgment in health history, 16
Jugular vein, internal, 26

K

Kabikinase; *see* Streptokinase
Kerlone; *see* Betaxolol
Kubler-Ross, E.,491

L

L tubules; *see* Longitudinal tubules
Labetalol, 430t
Lactate dehydrogenase (LDH), 288
Languages in interview, 14
Lanoxin; *see* Digoxin
Lasix; *see* Furosemide
LBBB; *see* Left bundle branch block
LDH; *see* Lactate dehydrogenase
LDLs; *see* Low-density lipoproteins
Leads, ECG; *see* Electrocardiography, leads in
Left anterior hemiblock, 155, *217*
Left atrial enlargement, electrocardiography and, 76-77, *77*
Left bundle branch block (LBBB), 96t-97t, 155, *156-157, 163, 164, 187*
   functional, after atrial premature complexes, *209*
   significance of, 155
   treatment of, 155
Left coronary artery, 5
Left main coronary artery, 5
Left posterior hemiblock, 155, *160*
Left ventricular afterload reduction, 366-367
Left ventricular end-diastolic pressure (LVEDP), 54
Left ventricular enlargement, electrocardiography and, 74-76, *76*
Left-sided precordial leads, electrocardiography and, 67
Leisure activities in health history, 19
Len[gv]egre disease, 155
Lescol; *see* Fluvastatin
Lev disease, 155
Levatol; *see* Penbutolol
Levophed; *see* Norepinephrine
Lewis, angle of, 27
Liberalized cardiac unit, coronary care unit and, 337
Lidocaine, 324t, 453t, 454t, 456-457, *457*
   for accelerated idioventricular rhythm, 145
   for acute myocardial infarction, 291
   for atrial flutter, 117
   cardiovascular actions of, 456
   cautions and side effects of, 457
   clinical uses of, 457
   defibrillation and, 311
   dosage and administration of, 457
   myocardial infarction and, 289
   for nonparoxysmal AV junctional tachycardia, 131
   for premature ventricular complexes, 137
   for torsades de pointes, 144
   for ventricular flutter, 148
   for ventricular tachycardia, 140
Lidocaine reaction, tachydysrhythmia and, 316-318
Limb leads, standard ECG, 66, *67, 68*
Lipid Research Clinics Coronary Primary Prevention Trial, 260-261
Lipid theory, atherosclerosis and, 257

Lipophilic β-adrenergic blocking agents, 430
Lisinopril, 438t
Lithium batteries for pacemakers, 229, 246
Location of heart murmurs, 34
Long QT syndrome, significance and treatment of, 144
Longitudinal (L) tubules, 1
Long-term ECG recording, 47-48
Loop diuretics, 436-438, 437t
    decreased preload and, 366
    for heart failure, 299
Lopid; *see* Gemfibrozil
Lopressor; *see* Metoprolol
Lorelco; *see* Probucol
Loss of sensing, artificial cardiac pacemakers and, 237
Lotensin; *see* Benazepril
Lovastatin, 410, 461t, 463-464
Low-density lipoproteins (LDLs), 260
Low-molecular-weight dextran, PTCA and, 294
LVEDP; *see* Left ventricular end-diastolic pressure

M

Maalox Plus, 467t
Maalox Suspension, 467t
Maalox TC Suspension, 467t
Magnesia, Milk of, 467t
Magnesium, 466, 467t
    cardiovascular actions of, 466
    cautions and side effects of, 466
    clinical uses of, 466
    dosage and administration of, 466
Magnesium citrate solution, 467t
Magnesium Complexed Tablets, 467t
Magnesium sulfate, 324t, 467t
    defibrillation and, 311
    for torsades de pointes, 144
Magnetic resonance imaging (MRI), 47
Malignancy, cardiac transplantation and, 397
Mannitol, decreased preload and, 366
Manual indirect blood pressure, 25
Maximum impulse, point of, 29, *30*
Mean arterial pressure, 4, 25
Mean cardiac vector, electrocardiography and, 70-71, *71*
Medicaid, 470
Medical preparation, coronary heart disease and, 331
Medicare, 470, 478
Medications
    coronary artery disease and, 338
    current, in health history, 14-15
    home care and, 482
Medium rales, 38
Memory and orientation in health history, 15
MET; *see* Metabolic equivalent
Metabolic equivalent (MET), 279, 406
Metaraminol, 112
Methohexital, 311
Methotrexate, 393
Methoxamine hydrochloride, 112
8-Methoxypsoralen, 395
Methyldopa, 428t
Metolazone, 437t
Metoprolol, 430t, 431
Mevacor; *see* Lovastatin
Mexiletine, 453t, 454t, 457
    cardiovascular actions of, 457
    cautions and side effects of, 457
    clinical uses of, 457
    dosage and administration of, 454t, 457
    for premature ventricular complexes, 138
    for torsades de pointes, 144
Mexitil; *see* Mexiletine
MI; *see* Myocardial infarction
Michigan Alcohol Screening Instrument, 411
Midamor; *see* Amiloride
Midazolam, 311

Midprecordial leads, electrocardiography and, 67
Midsystolic clicks, 35
Midsystolic murmurs, 34-35, *35*
Milk of Magnesia, 467t
Milrinone, 299, 421t
Minipress; *see* Prazosin
Minnesota Heart Health Program, 269, 270
Minnesota Multiphasic Personality Inventory (MMPI) Hostility Scale, 266
Minoxidil, 299, 434, 435t
Mitral regurgitation, 35, 344t-345t, 351-353
    diagnostic evaluation of, 353
    etiology of, 351-352
    pathophysiology of, 352, *353*
    signs and symptoms of, 352
    treatment of, 353
Mitral rings, Carpentier, *352*
Mitral stenosis, 344t, 349-351
    assessment of, 35
    diagnostic evaluation of, 350-351
    etiology of, 349
    pathophysiology of, 349, *351*
    signs and symptoms of, 349-350
    treatment of, 351, *352*
Mitral valve, 2, 49-50, 342
Mitral valve disease, 349-354
    mitral regurgitation; *see* Mitral regurgitation
    mitral stenosis; *see* Mitral stenosis
    mitral valve prolapse; *see* Mitral valve prolapse
Mitral valve prolapse, 353-354
    diagnostic evaluation of, 354
    etiology of, 353
    pathophysiology of, 353
    signs and symptoms of, 353-354
    treatment of, 354
M-mode echocardiography, 49, *50*
MMPI; *see* Minnesota Multiphasic Personality Inventory Hostility Scale
Moist rales, 37
Monitoring system in coronary care unit, 281-283
Monoclonal antibodies, cardiac transplantation and, 393
Monoclonal hypothesis, atherosclerosis and, 257
Monomorphic ventricular tachycardia, repetitive, *180*
Monopril; *see* Fosinopril
8-MOP; *see* 8-Methoxypsoralen
Morphine sulfate, 279
Motion echocardiography, 49, *50*
Mouth, assessment of, 40
Movement, limitation of, in health history, 19
MRFIT; *see* Multiple risk-factor intervention trial
MRI; *see* Magnetic resonance imaging
MUGA; *see* Multiple gated acquisition blood pool imaging
Multifocal premature ventricular complexes, 137
Multiform premature ventricular complexes, 137
Multiple gated acquisition (MUGA) blood pool imaging, 46, 329
Multiple risk-factor intervention trial (MRFIT), 266
Murmurs; *see* Heart murmurs
Muromonab-CD3, 393, 394t-395t
Muscle strength, assessment of, 39
Mycophenolate mofetil, 393
Mylanta, 467t
Mylanta II, 467t
Myocardial contractility, 9
Myocardial infarction (MI), 45-46, 257
    acute; *see* Acute myocardial infarction
    cardiac rehabilitation after, 402-414
    drugs commonly used in, 323t-324t
    ECG in diagnosis of; *see* Electrocardiography, myocardial infarction and
Myocardial ischemia, unstable, 286
Myocardial oxygen consumption, decrease in, in coronary care unit, 279
Myocardial perfusion imaging, 45, *45*
Myocardial revascularization, 359-360
Myocardium, 1-2
Myofibrils, 1
Myosin, 1

N

Nadolol, 430t, 431
Nasopuncture, smoking cessation and, 264
National Cholesterol Education Program (NCEP), 261-262, 409
National High Blood Pressure Education Program Working Group, 271
National Survey of Worksite Health Promotion Activities, 269
NBD code, implantable cardioverter defibrillators and, 242-243
NBG code, artificial cardiac pacemaker and, 221t, 221-222, 242
NCEP; *see* National Cholesterol Education Program
Negative predictive value, diagnostic studies and, 42
Neostigmine, 125
Neo-Synephrine; *see* Phenylephrine hydrochloride
Neurologic functioning, assessment of, 39
Neurologic subsystem, postoperative management of heart disease and, 370-372
Neurosis, cardiac, 331
Niacin, 461t, 462
    cardiovascular actions of, 462
    cautions and side effects of, 462
    clinical uses of, 462
    dosage and administration of, 462
Nicardipine, 440t, 442, 443
Nicotine gum, smoking cessation and, 264
Nicotine-substitution therapy, smoking cessation and, 264
Nicotinic acid, 409, 461t
Nicotinic Acid; *see* Niacin
NIDDM; *see* Non-insulin-dependent diabetes mellitus
Nifedipine, 440t, 442
    for angina, 287
    for hypertrophic cardiomyopathy, 383
Nimodipine, 440t
Nimotop; *see* Nimodipine
Nipride; *see* Nitroprusside sodium
Nisoldipine, 441t
Nitrates, 432-433, 488
    for angina, 287
    cardiovascular actions of, 432
    cautions and side effects of, 433
    clinical uses of, 432
    for dilated cardiomyopathy, 380
    dosage and administration of, 431-433, 433t
    for heart failure, 299
    PTCA and, 294
Nitrendipine, 440t, 442
Nitroglycerin, 432-433, 433t
    for acute myocardial infarction, 290
    for angina, 287
    for cardiogenic shock, 309
    PTCA and, 294
Nitroglycerin paste, 287
Nitrol; *see* Nitroglycerin paste
Nitroprusside
    for acute myocardial infarction, 290
    for cardiogenic shock, 309
    for heart failure, 299
    left ventricular afterload reduction and, 367
Nitroprusside sodium, 433-434
    cardiovascular actions of, 433-434
    cautions and side effects of, 434
    clinical uses of, 434
    dosage and administration of, 434
Nodal complexes, 129
Non-insulin-dependent diabetes mellitus (NIDDM), 265
Nonparoxysmal AV junctional tachycardia (NPJT), 94t-95t, 129-133, *133, 162, 196, 197*
    significance of, 131
    treatment of, 131
Norepinephrine, 5, 7, 416, 417, 420t, 424t, 424-425
    cardiovascular actions of, 425
    cautions and side effects of, 425
    clinical uses of, 425
    dosage and administration of, 425
Normodyne; *see* Labetalol
Norpace; *see* Disopyramide

North Karelia Project, 270
Northeast Oklahoma City Cholesterol Education program, 271
Norvase; *see* Amlodipine
NPJT; *see* Nonparoxysmal AV junctional tachycardia
Nurse, home care and, 474
Nurse-patient relationship in interview, 10-14
Nursing diagnoses, 40, 41, 479t, 480t-481t
Nursing management
    on admission to coronary care unit, 364
    cardiac transplantation and, 390t, 398t-399t
    of patients with permanent cardiac pacemakers and ICDs, 250-252
    of valvular heart disease, 350t
Nutrition
    cardiac rehabilitation and, 409
    coronary artery disease and, 338
    in health history, 19-20
    home care and, 478-482
    postoperative management of heart disease and, 372-373

O

Obesity as risk factor for coronary artery disease, 267
Obstructive breathing, 39
Occupation
    cardiac rehabilitation and, 411-412
    in health history, 16
Occupational therapist, home care and, 474
Olsten Health Care, 472
Opiates, 279
Orientation and memory in health history, 15
Orthoclone OKT3; *see* Muromonab-CD3
Orthopnea, 37
Oscilloscope in coronary care unit, 281, *282*
Outpatient cardiac rehabilitation, 406
Oversensing, artificial cardiac pacemakers and, 237
Oxprenolol, 430t
Oxygen administration
    assessment of, 37-38, *38*
    in coronary care unit, 279
    history of, 38
    home care and, 486-487

P

P wave, electrocardiography and, 60-61, *63*
PA catheter, *301*
    flow-directed, balloon-tipped, 53, 53-55
PA end-diastolic pressure, cardiogenic shock and, 300-303, *303, 304*
PA pressure, cardiogenic shock and, 300, *302*, 304-305
Pacemaker, 29, *178*
    artificial cardiac; *see* Artificial cardiac pacemaker
    atrial asynchronous, 222
    atrial demand, 222, *223*
    atrial synchronous ventricular, 222-223, *224*
    AV sequential, 223-224, *225*
    fully automatic stimulation, 224, *225, 226*
    home care and, 485-486
    rate-responsive, 224-227, *226*
    ventricular asynchronous, 222
    ventricular demand, 222, *223*
    wandering, 104, *105*
        significance of, 104
        treatment of, 104
Pacing at altered rate, artificial cardiac pacemakers and, 237
Pain
    acute myocardial infarction and, 289
    angina, 483
    in health history, 17
    home care and, 482-483
    postoperative management of heart disease and, 372, 373
    relief of, in coronary care unit, 277-279, *280*
Palpation, blood pressure determined by, 25
Palpitations, pain and, 17
Pandiastolic murmurs, 33
Pansystolic murmurs, 33
PAP; *see* Pulmonary artery pressure

Papillary muscle rupture, 35
Parasystole, 92, 160-161, *161*
    significance of, 160
    treatment of, 161
    ventricular, *161, 207*
Parasystolic focus, 160
Paroxysmal AV block, *218*
Paroxysmal nocturnal dyspnea, 37, 297
Paroxysmal supraventricular tachycardia, 108, *186, 192*
Paroxysmal ventricular tachycardia, *173*
Patient
    assessment of; *see also* Cardiovascular assessment; Diagnostic studies;
        Nursing management
    cardiac, care of; *see* Coronary care unit
    coping behaviors of, 15
    decision-making ability of, 16
    home care and, 477-478
    marital status of, 16
    role of, 16
    selection of, for PTCA, 292-293
Pawtucket Heart Health Project, 270
PCWP; *see* Pulmonary capillary wedge pressure
PEA; *see* Pulseless electrical activity
Penbutolol, 430t
Percutaneous transluminal coronary angioplasty (PTCA), 292-296
    complications of, 295-296
    equipment for, 292, *293*
    indications for, 293
    mechanism of, 292
    precautions for, 293
    procedure for, 293-295, *294, 295*
    selection of patients for, 292-293
Perfusion defect, 45
Pericardial disease, echocardiography and, 51
Pericardial friction rub, assessment of, 35
Pericardial rub, 296
Pericarditis, 296
Pericardium, 2
Perindopril, 438t
Peripheral α_1-adrenergic blockers, 436t
Peripheral circulation, assessment of, 22-28
Peripheral cyanosis, 28
Personality factors as risk factor for coronary artery disease, 266
PES; *see* Programmed electric stimulation
PET; *see* Positron emission tomography
Pharmacokinetics, clinical, cardiovascular drugs and, 415-416
Pharmacology, clinical, cardiovascular drugs and, 416-417
Phenothiazines for long QT syndrome, 144
Phenoxybenzamine, 426-427
Phentolamine, 426-427
Phenylephrine, 420t, 424t, 426
    cardiovascular actions of, 426
    cautions and side effects of, 426
    clinical uses of, 426
    dosage and administration of, 426
Phenylephrine hydrochloride, 112
Phenytoin, 453t, 454t
    for nonparoxysmal AV junctional tachycardia, 131
    for premature ventricular complexes, 138
    for ventricular tachycardia, 141
Phosphodiesterase inhibitors, 422-423
    cardiovascular actions of, 422-423
    cautions and side effects of, 423
    clinical uses of, 423
    dosage and administration of, 423
Photophoresis
    cardiac transplantation and, 395
    ultraviolet-A radiation, 395
Physical activity, coronary artery disease and, 338
Physical examination in cardiovascular assessment, *20*, 20-40
    abdomen in, 38-39
    apical rate and rhythm in, 29
    arterial blood pressure in, 25, *26*
    arterial line in, 25-27, *27, 28*

Physical examination in cardiovascular assessment—cont'd.
    arterial pulses in, 22-25, *23, 24*
    auscultation of arteries in, 25, *26*
    breath sounds in, 37-38
    cardiac assessment in, 29-37
    cardiac index in, 37
    cardiac output in, 37
    central venous pressure in, 27-28
    cough and sputum in, 37
    dyspnea in, 37
    dysrhythmias in, 37
    edema in, 28
    flow sheet for data in, *21*
    Glasgow coma scale in, 39
    heart sounds in, 29-35, *32, 33, 34, 35,* 36t
        first, 31-32, *33*
        fourth, 32-33, *33, 34*
        second, 32, *33*
        third, 32, *33*
    height and weight in, 39
    laboratory data in, 40
    mouth and throat in, 40
    murmurs in, 33-35, *35,* 36t
    muscle strength in, 39
    neurologic functioning in, 39
    orthopnea in, 37
    oxygenation in, 37-38
    pacemaker in, 29
    peripheral circulation in, 22-28
    physical integrity in, 39-40
    physical regulation in, 40
    pleural friction rub in, 38
    point of maximum impulse in, 29, *30*
    pulmonary artery and pulmonary capillary wedge pressures in, 37
    pupils in, 39
    reflexes in, 39
    respiratory rate, rhythm, depth, and expansion in, 37
    senses in, 39
    serum enzyme levels in, 37
    skin integrity in, 40
    skin temperature and color in, 28, *29*
    summation gallop in, 33, *33*
    temperature in, 40
    tissue integrity in, 40
    urine studies in, 40
    venous pressure in, 26-27, *27, 28*
    venous pulse in, 26, *27*
    white blood cell count and differential in, 40
Physical inactivity as risk factor for coronary artery disease, 264-265
Physical integrity, assessment of, 39-40
Physical regulation, assessment of, 40
Physical therapist, home care and, 474
Physician, home care and, 474
Physiologic third heart sound, 32
Pindolol, 430t
Pitch of heart murmurs, 34
Plasmapheresis, cardiac transplantation and, 395
Plendil; *see* Felodipine
Pleural friction rub, 38
PMI; *see* Point of maximum impulse
Pneumothorax, 368
Point of maximum impulse (PMI), 29, *30*
Polyclonal antibodies, cardiac transplantation and, 393
Positive predictive value, diagnostic studies and, 42
Positron emission tomography (PET), 47
Posterior ECG leads, 68
Postsynaptic receptors, 416
Potassium, 465-466
    for atrial tachycardia, 128-129
    cardiovascular actions of, 465
    cautions and side effects of, 466
    clinical uses of, 465
    dosage and administration of, 465-466
    for ventricular tachycardia, 141
Potassium disturbances, dysrhythmias and, 166, *167, 168*

Potassium sparing diuretics, 437t
Power sources
   for artificial cardiac pacemakers, 229
   for implantable cardioverter defibrillators, 246
Powerlessness in health history, 18
Pravachol; *see* Pravastatin
Pravastatin, 410, 461t, 463-464
Prazosin, 427, 435-436, 436t
   for angina, 287
   cardiovascular actions of, 435
   cautions and side effects of, 436
   clinical uses of, 435
   for dilated cardiomyopathy, 380
   dosage and administration of, 435-436, 436t
   for heart failure, 299
Precordial ECG leads, 67-68, *68*
Precordium, point of maximum impulse and, 29
Predictive values, positive and negative, diagnostic studies and, 42
Preexcitation syndrome, *113*, 113-121, *114, 115,* 116, *116, 117, 118, 119, 120,* 121, *121, 208*
   significance of, 113-116
   treatment of, 116-121
Preinfarction angina, 286
Preload, 9, 365-366, *366*
Premature atrial complexes, 104-108, *105, 106, 107, 191*
   functional RBBB and LBBB after, *209*
   significance of, 108
   treatment of, 108
Premature AV junctional complexes, 129, *130*
   significance of, 129
   treatment of, 129
Premature ventricular complexes, 134-138, *135, 136, 175, 185*
   immediate suppression of, 137
   interpolated, *198*
   long-term suppression of, 138
   maintenance of suppression of, 137
   multiform, *198*
   significance of, 137
   treatment of, 137-138
Pressor drugs for AV nodal reentry, 111-112
Pressure gradient, PTCA and, 294
Presynaptic receptors, 416
Primacor; *see* Milrinone
Prinivil; *see* Lisinopril
Prinzmetal angina, *181, 213,* 286
Probucol, 461t, 463
   atherogenesis and, 257
   cardiovascular actions of, 463
   cautions and side effects of, 463
   clinical uses of, 463
   dosage and administration of, 463
   for lipid abnormalities, 410
Procainamide, 324t, 453t, 454t, 455-456
   for atrioventricular block, 148
   for AV nodal reentry, 112
   cardiovascular actions of, 455
   cautions and side effects of, 455-456
   clinical uses of, 455
   defibrillation and, 311
   dosage and administration of, 455
   for long QT syndrome, 144
   for premature ventricular complexes, 137
   Qtc interval and, 65
   for torsades de pointes, 144
   for ventricular flutter, 148
   for ventricular tachycardia, 140, 141
Procan; *see* Procainamide
Procardia; *see* Nifedipine
Programmability
   of artificial cardiac pacemakers, 229, 230t-232t
   of implantable cardioverter defibrillators, 243-246, 244t, *245, 247*
Programmed electric stimulation (PES), 328
Progressive angina, 286
Prolonged QT syndrome, 326

Pronestyl; *see* Procainamide
Propafenone, 453t, 454t, 458-459
   cardiovascular actions of, 459
   cautions and side effects of, 459
   clinical uses of, 459
   dosage and administration of, 459
Propranolol, 429, 430t, 453t, 454t
   for atrial fibrillation, 126
   for atrial flutter, 124
   for atrial tachycardia, 129
   for AV nodal reentry, 112
   for hypertrophic cardiomyopathy, 383
   for nonparoxysmal AV junctional tachycardia, 131
   for premature ventricular complexes, 138
   for ventricular tachycardia, 141
Prostaglandins, 5
Prostigmin; *see* Neostigmine
Protamine sulfate, 362
Psychologic adjustment to coronary artery disease, 331-334, *332*
Psychologic needs, cardiac rehabilitation and, 404
Psychosocial considerations, home care and, 484-485
PTCA; *see* Percutaneous transluminal coronary angioplasty
Public Health Service, 271
Pulmonary artery pressure (PAP), 37
Pulmonary capillary wedge pressure (PCWP), 53-54
   assessment of, 37
   cardiogenic shock and, 300, 304-305
Pulmonary circulation, 5
Pulmonary edema
   acute, 297, *319*
   acute myocardial infarction and, 289
Pulmonary membrane, 5
Pulmonary regurgitation, 345t, 357-358
   diagnostic evaluation and treatment of, 358
   etiology of, 357
   pathophysiology of, 357, *357*
   signs and symptoms of, 357
Pulmonary stenosis, 345t, 356-357
   diagnostic evaluation of, 356-357
   etiology of, 356
   pathophysiology of, 356, *356*
   signs and symptoms of, 356
   treatment of, 357
Pulmonary subsystem, postoperative management of heart disease and, 368-370
Pulmonary valve, 2
Pulmonary valve disease, 356-358
   pulmonary regurgitation; *see* Pulmonary regurgitation
   pulmonary stenosis; *see* Pulmonary stenosis
Pulmonary vascular resistance (PVR), 366
Pulmonic regurgitation, murmurs of, 35, *35*
Pulmonic stenosis, 34
Pulmonic valve, echocardiography and, 51
Pulse
   amplitude of, 22
   arterial, 22-25, *23, 24*
   bigeminal, 22
   large bounding, 22
   normal arterial, 22
   rate and rhythm of, 22
   small weak, 22
   venous, 26, *27*
Pulse pressure, 4, 25
Pulseless electrical activity (PEA), *314, 322*
Pulsus alternans, 22
Pulsus paradoxus, 22-24
Pupils, assessment of, 39
Purkinje fibers, 6
Purple toe syndrome, 452
PVR; *see* Pulmonary vascular resistance

Q

Q wave, myocardial infarction and, 79
QRS axis, mean, electrocardiography and, 71-72, *73*

QRS complex
  abnormal, supraventricular dysrhythmias with, *162*, 162-166, *163*, *164*
  electrocardiography and, 61-64, *63*
QT interval, electrocardiography and, 65, *65*
QT syndrome
  long, 144
  prolonged, 326
Quality of heart murmurs, 33
Questran; *see* Cholestyramine
Quinaglute; *see* Quinidine
Quinapril, 438t
Quinidine, 453t, 454t, 456
  for atrial fibrillation, 126
  for atrial flutter, 117, 124
  for atrioventricular block, 148
  for AV nodal reentry, 112
  cardiovascular actions of, 456
  cautions and side effects of, 456
  clinical uses of, 456
  dosage and administration of, 456
  for long QT syndrome, 144
  Qtc interval and, 65
  for torsades de pointes, 144
  for ventricular tachycardia, 141

R

Race as risk factor for coronary artery disease, 258
Radiation of heart murmurs, 34
Radionuclide imaging, 45-46
  MI imaging and, 45-46
  myocardial perfusion imaging and, 45, *45*
  radionuclide angiocardiography and, 46, *46*
Rales, 37-38
Ramipril, 438t
Randomized Interventional Treatment of Angina (RITA), 359
Rapamicin, 395
Rate-dependent aberration with functional LBBB, *187*
Rate-pressure product (RPP), 279
Rate-responsive pacemaker, 224-227, *226*
Rating of Perceived Exertion (RPE) Scale, 407
RBBB; *see* Right bundle branch block
Reciprocating tachycardia using accessory pathway, 94t-95t
Recombinant tissue-type plasminogen activator (rt-PA), 290, 291
Reentry, dysrhythmias and, 91
Reflexes, assessment of, 39
Registry of the International Society for Heart and Lung Transplantation, 387
Regitine; *see* Phentolamine
Regurgitant murmurs, 35, *35*
Rejection, cardiac transplantation and, 395-396
Renal subsystem, postoperative management of heart disease and, 370
Repolarizatin, electrocardiography and, 60, 64
Reserpine, 429
Respiration
  Cheyne-Stokes, 39
  rate, rhythm, depth, and expansion of, 37
  sighing, 39
  variations in, 39
Respiratory membrane, 5
Respiratory sinus dysrhythmia, *188*
Response to injury theory, atherosclerosis and, 256-257
Rest
  in health history, 18, 19
  home care and, 483-484
Restenosis, PTCA and, 295
Restrictive cardiomyopathy; *see* Cardiomyopathy, restrictive
Return to work, cardiac rehabilitation and, 411-412
Rewarming shock, hypotension and, 365
Rheumatic disease, 343
Rhonchi, 37
Right atrial enlargement, electrocardiography and, 79, *79*
Right atrial pacing, sinus arrest and, *189*
Right bundle branch block (RBBB), 96t-97t, 155, *158*, *163*
  functional, after atrial premature complexes, *209*

Right bundle branch block—cont'd.
  significance of, 155
  treatment of, 155, *159*
Right coronary artery, 6
Right ventricular afterload reduction, 366
Right ventricular enlargement, electrocardiography and, 77-79, *78*
Right-sided heart catheterization, bedside, using flow-directed, balloon-tipped PA catheter, *53*, 53-55
Right-sided precordial leads, electrocardiography and, 67
Risk factors in health history, 15
RITA; *see* Randomized Interventional Treatment of Angina
Roller coaster effect, hypotension and, 365
RPE Scale; *see* Rating of Perceived Exertion Scale
RPP; *see* Rate-pressure product
rt-PA; *see* Recombinant tissue-type plasminogen activator
Rythmol; *see* Propafenone

S

SA node, 6
Sandimmune; *see* Cyclosporine
Sarcoplasmic reticulum, 1
Scintigraphy, thallium-201, with dipyridamole, myocardial infarction and, 288
Second heart sound, assessment of, 32, *33*
Sectral; *see* Acebutolol
Sedatives for anxiety and stress, 279
Segments, electrocardiography and, 58
Selecor; *see* Celiprolol
Self-care in health history, 18-19
Self-esteem, emotional integrity and, 17
Self-perception in health history, 17
Semilunar valve, 342
Senses, assessment of, 39
Sensitivity, diagnostic studies and, 42
Serum cholesterol levels, cardiac rehabilitation and, 409-410
Serum enzyme levels
  in acute myocardial infarction, 42-43
  assessment of, 37
Serum glutamic-oxaloacetic transaminase (SGOT), myocardial infarction and, 288
Sexual activity
  cardiac rehabilitation and, 411
  coronary artery disease and, 338
  in health history, 16
  home care and, 484
SGOT; *see* Serum glutamic-oxaloacetic transaminase
Shock, cardiogenic; *see* Cardiogenic shock
Shock capability, implantable cardioverter defibrillators and, 243
Sick sinus syndrome, 102, *185*
Sighing respiration, 39
Simvastatin, 410, 461t, 463-464
Sinequan; *see* Doxepin hydrochloride
Sinus arrest, 102, *103*, *189*
Sinus bradycardia, 94t-95t, 99-100, *100*, *185*, *188*
  significance of, 99-100
  treatment of, 100
Sinus dysrhythmia, 100-102, *101*, *102*
  significance of, 101-102
  treatment of, 102
Sinus exit block, 102-104, *103*, *104*, *186*, *190*
  significance of, 102-104
  treatment of, 104
Sinus node, rhythms originating in, 92
Sinus rhythm, 94t-95t
  normal, 93, *98*, *174*, *211*, *212*, *214*, *215*, *216*, *217*
Sinus tachycardia, 93-99, 94t-95t, *99*, *187*
  significance of, 93
  treatment of, 93-99
Skin integrity, assessment of, 40
Skin temperature and color, assessment of, 28
Sleep in health history, 18, 19
Slow response, electrocardiography and, 60
Smoking
  cardiac rehabilitation and, 410
  coronary artery disease and, 338

Smoking—cont'd.
  hypertension and, 259-260
  as risk factor for coronary artery disease, 262-264
Social activities in health history, 19
Social history in health history, 16
Social worker, home care and, 474
Socialization in health history, 16
Sociocultural considerations, coronary artery disease and, 334-335
Sodium, hypertension and, 259
Sodium bicarbonate, 324t, 465
  cautions and side effects of, 465
  clinical uses of, 465
  dosage and administration of, 465
Sodium disturbances, dysrhythmias and, 166
Sorin Puig Massana annuloplasty ring, 352
Sotalol, 453t, 454t, 459
  cardiovascular actions of, 459
  cautions and side effects of, 459
  clinical uses of, 459
  dosage and administration of, 459
Specificity, diagnostic studies and, 42
Speech impairment, interview and, 14
Speech pathologist, home care and, 474
Spiritual concerns in health history, 16
Spironolactone, 299, 437t
Sputum, assessment of, 37
ST segment, electrocardiography and, 64, 65
Stable angina, 257, 286
Stanford Heart Disease Project, 269-270
Starling's law, 7
Statins, 410
Stenosis
  aortic; see Aortic stenosis
  idiopathic hypertrophic subaortic, 381
  mitral, 35
  mitral; see Mitral stenosis
  tricuspid; see Tricuspid stenosis
  valvular, 52
Step-down unit, coronary care unit and, 337
Sternal angle, 27
Steroids, 296
Streptase; see Streptokinase
Streptokinase, 443, 444t
  for myocardial infarction, 290
  myocardial infarction and, 402
Stress
  cardiac rehabilitation and, 410
  in health history, 17
  as risk factor for coronary artery disease, 266-267
Stress echocardiography, 51-52
Stress testing, 43-45, 44
Stroke volume, 3
Structured Type A Interview, 410
Sudden cardiac death, 322-331, 325
  diagnosis of, 326
  electrophysiologic testing and, 328-329
  ICD and, 329, 329-331, 330
  risk factors for, 326, 326
  treatment of ventricular dysrhythmias and, 326-328, 328
Sulfinpyrazone, 291
Summation gallop, assessment of, 33, 33
Superkids—Superfit, 268
Supraventricular dysrhythmia with abnormal QRS complexes, 162, 162-166, 163, 164
Supraventricular tachycardia, 123, 170, 172
  paroxysmal, 186, 192
Surgeries, previous, in health history, 14
Sweep speed in coronary care unit, 282
Sympathetic nervous system, 5
Sympathomimetics, 423-426
Systematic desensitization, stress and, 334
Systemic circulation, 4, 4-5
Systolic Hypertension in the Elderly Program, 259
Systolic murmurs, 34, 36t

Systolic pressure, 4, 25

T

T tubules; see Transverse tubules
T wave, electrocardiography and, 64
Tachycardia, 111, 129, 317
  atrial; see Atrial tachycardia
  AV reciprocating, 113
  nonparoxysmal AV junctional, 94t-95t, 129-133, 133
  paroxysmal supraventricular, 108
  reciprocating, using accessory pathway, 94t-95t
  sinus; see Sinus tachycardia
  supraventricular; see Supraventricular tachycardia
  toothbrush, 172
  ventricular; see Ventricular tachycardia
Tachydysrhythmia, anatrial, 190
Tachypnea, 39
Tambocor; see Flecainide
Technetium-99, MI imaging and, 45-46
TEE; see Transesophageal echocardiography
Telemetry unit, coronary care unit and, 337
Temperature
  assessment of, 40
  skin, 28
Tenormin; see Atenolol
Tensilon; see Edrophonium chloride
Terazosin, 427, 435-436, 436t
  cardiovascular actions of, 435
  cautions and side effects of, 436
  clinical uses of, 435
  dosage and administration of, 435-436, 436t
Thallium-201 scintigraphy with dipyridamole, myocardial infarction and, 288
Thiazide diuretics, 436-438, 437t
  for heart failure, 299
Third heart sound, assessment of, 32, 33
Thrill, 25
Throat, assessment of, 40
Thrombolytic agents, 443-445
  for acute myocardial infarction, 291
  for angina, 287
  cardiovascular actions of, 443
  cautions and side effects of, 445
  clinical uses of, 443
  dosage and administration of, 443, 444t
  myocardial infarction and, 402
Thrombotic therapy for acute myocardial infarction, 290, 290-292
Timing of heart murmurs, 33
Timolol, 430t
Tissue integrity, assessment of, 40
Tissue plasminogen activator (TPA), 291, 402, 444t
Tobacco; see Smoking
Tobacco-Free Schools project, 268
Tocainide, 453t, 454t, 457-458
  cardiovascular actions of, 457
  cautions and side effects of, 458
  clinical uses of, 458
  dosage and adminstration of, 458
  for premature ventricular complexes, 138
  for torsades de pointes, 144
  for ventricular tachycardia, 141
Tonocard; see Tocainide
Toothbrush tachycardia, 172
Torsades de pointes, 138, 143, 143-144, 328, 328
  significance of, 143
  treatment of, 143-144
Torsemide, 437t
Total lymphoid radiation, cardiac transplantation and, 393
TPA; see Tissue plasminogen activator
Tracheal breath sounds, 37
Trandate; see Labetalol
Transesophageal echocardiography (TEE), 49, 52, 351
Transfer from coronary care unit, 337
Transportation time, coronary heart disease and, 331

Transthoracic echocardiography, 48-49
Transverse (T) tubules, 1
Trasicor; *see* Oxprenolol
Treadmill test, cardiac rehabilitation and, 405-406
Triamterene, 299, 437t
Triaxial reference figure, electrocardiography and, 66
Tricuspid regurgitation, 35, 345t, 355-356
    diagnostic evaluation of, 355
    etiology of, 355, *355*
    pathophysiology of, 355
    signs and symptoms of, 355
    treatment of, 355-356
Tricuspid rings, Carpentier, *352*
Tricuspid stenosis, 35, 345t, 354-355
    diagnostic evaluation of, 354
    etiology of, 354
    pathophysiology of, 354, *354*
    signs and symptoms of, 354
    treatment of, 354-355
Tricuspid valve, 2, 342
    echocardiography and, 51
Tricuspid valve disease, 354-356
    tricuspid regurgitation; *see* Tricuspid regurgitation
    tricuspid stenosis; *see* Tricuspid stenosis
Tricyclic antidepressants, 144
Tropomyosin, 1
Troponin, 1
Two-dimensional (2D) echocardiography, 49, *51*
Type-A behavior, coronary artery disease and, 266, 334

U

U wave, electrocardiography and, 65-66
Ultrafast computed tomography (cine CT), 47
Ultraviolet-A radiation photophoresis (UVARP), 395
United Network of Organ Sharing (UNOS), 390
UNOS; *see* United Network of Organ Sharing
Unstable angina, 286
Unstable myocardial ischemia, 286
Urinary patterns, alterations in, in health history, 20
Urine, characteristics of, 40
Urokinase, 290-291, 443, 444t
U.S. Agency for Health Care Policy and Research, 287
UVARP; *see* Ultraviolet-A radiation photophoresis

V

V leads, electrocardiography and, 66
V wave, assessment of, 26
VAD; *see* Ventricular assist device
Valvular functions, echocardiography and, 49-51
Valvular heart disease, 342-358
    acquired, physiologic dynamics of, 344t-345t
    aortic, 343-349
    aortic regurgitation; *see* Aortic regurgitation
    aortic stenosis; *see* Aortic stenosis
    mitral regurgitation; *see* Mitral regurgitation
    mitral stenosis; *see* Mitral stenosis
    mitral valve disease; *see* Mitral valve disease
    mitral valve prolapse; *see* Mitral valve prolapse
    murmurs of, 343
    nursing treatment of, 350t
    pulmonary regurgitation; *see* Pulmonary regurgitation
    pulmonary valve disease; *see* Pulmonary valve disease
    structure and function of valves and, 342
    tricuspid regurgitation; *see* Tricuspid regurgitation
    tricuspid stenosis; *see* Tricuspid stenosis
    tricuspid valve disease; *see* Tricuspid valve disease
Valvular regurgitation, echocardiography and, 52
Valvular stenosis, echocardiography and, 52
Variant angina, 258, 286
Vasoactive chemicals, 5
Vasoactive therapy, 488
Vasoconstrictors, 5
Vasodilators, 5, 432-436
    for cardiogenic shock, 309

Vasodilators—cont'd.
    for dilated cardiomyopathy, 380
    direct arteriolar, 434-435, 435t
        cardiovascular actions of, 434
        cautions and side effects of, 435
        clinical uses of, 434
        dosage and administration of, 434-435, 435t
    for heart failure, 299
Vasomotor area, 8
Vasopressin, 5
Vasospasm, atherosclerosis and, 257-258
Vasotec; *see* Enalapril
Vasoxyl; *see* Methoxamine hydrochloride
VAT pacemaker, 222, 228t, 235, 237, 238
VDD pacemaker, 227, 228t, 235, 237, 238
Vector abnormalities, myocardial infarction and, 79-81, *80*
Vector approach to electrocardiography, 68-74, *69*
Venous pressure
    assessment of, 26-27, *27*, *28*
    central, 27-28
Venous pulse, assessment of, 26, *27*
Ventricles, rhythms originating in, 92
Ventricular assist device (VAD), home care and, 490
Ventricular asynchronous pacemaker (VOO), 222, 228t, 237
Ventricular complexes, premature; *see* Premature ventricular complexes
Ventricular demand pacemaker, 222, 223, 228t
Ventricular dysrhythmias, treatment of, sudden cardiac death and, 326-328, *328*
Ventricular escape beats, 133-134, *134*, *197*
    significance of, 133
    treatment of, 134
Ventricular escape rhythm, 133
    complete AV block with, *175*
Ventricular fibrillation, 96t-97t, 145-148, *147*, *177*, *178*, *203*, 313, 322, 325, *325*, *327*
    myocardial infarction and, 289
    significance of, 145-146
    treatment of, 146-148
Ventricular flutter, 96t-97t, 145-148, *147*, *177*, *204*
    significance of, 145-146
    treatment of, 146-148
Ventricular fusion beat, 134
Ventricular gallop, 32
Ventricular parasystole, *161*, *207*
Ventricular rate, slowing, therapy of dysrhythmias and, 92-93
Ventricular septal defects, 35
Ventricular tachycardia, 96t-97t, 138, 138-143, *139*, *142*, *171*, *182*, *183*, *184*, *199*, 313
    accelerated idioventricular rhythm and, *202*
    artifact and, *209*
    monomorphic, repetitive, *180*
    paroxysmal, *173*
    with retrograde atrial capture, *200*
    significance of, 140
    treatment of, 140-143, *142*
Verapamil, 440t, 442, 443, 453t, 454t
    for angina, 287
    for atrial fibrillation, 126
    for atrial flutter, 117, 124
    for atrial tachycardia, 128, 129
    for AV nodal reentry, 110
    for hypertrophic cardiomyopathy, 383
    for nonparoxysmal AV junctional tachycardia, 131
Verelan; *see* Verapamil
Versed; *see* Midazolam
Very low-density lipoproteins (VLDLs), 260
Vesicular breath sounds, 37
Vesnarinone, 380
Vial of Life Program, 475
Visiting nurse associations, 470
Visken; *see* Pindolol
VLDLs; *see* Very low-density lipoproteins
Volume replacement, 365, 366t
VOO; *see* Ventricular asynchronous pacemaker
VVI pacemaker, 223, 228t, *236*, *240*

VVIR pacemaker, 224, *226*, 228t, 229
VVT pacemaker, *223*, 228t, 237

W

Wandering pacemaker; *see* Pacemaker, wandering
Warfarin, 447-452, 448t, 449t-450t
    cardiovascular actions of, 447-448
    cautions and side effects of, 451-452
    clinical uses of, 448
    dosage and administration of, 447t, 448t, 448-451, 449t-450t
    major drug interactions with, 452
Waveforms, implantable cardioverter defibrillators and, 248-249, *249*
Waves, electrocardiography and, 58, 60-66
WBC count; *see* White blood cell count
Weight and height, 39
Wenckebach sinus exit block, 102
White blood cell (WBC) count, assessment of, 40

Wilson, Frank N., 58
Wolff-Parkinson-White (WPW) syndrome, 113
WPW pathway, reciprocating tachycardia using, 94t-95t

X

X wave, assessment of, 26
Xanax; *see* Alprazolam
Xylocaine; *see* Lidocaine

Y

Y wave, assessment of, 26

Z

Zaroxolyn; *see* Metolazone
Zebeta; *see* Bisoprolol
Zestril; *see* Lisinopril
Zocor; *see* Simvastatin